PRACTICE MANAGEMENT
for the
DENTAL TEAM

SEVENTH
EDITION

PRACTICE MANAGEMENT
for the
DENTAL TEAM

SEVENTH
EDITION

Betty Ladley Finkbeiner, CDA Emeritus, BS, MS
Emeritus Faculty
Washtenaw Community College
Ann Arbor, Michigan

Charles Allan Finkbeiner, BS, MS
Emeritus Faculty
Washtenaw Community College
Ann Arbor, Michigan

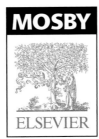

MOSBY

ELSEVIER

3251 Riverport Lane
St. Louis, Missouri 63043

PRACTICE MANAGEMENT FOR THE DENTAL TEAM   ISBN: 978-0-323-06536-8
Copyright © 2011 by Mosby, Inc., an affiliate of Elsevier Inc.

Previous editions copyrighted 2006, 2001, 1996, 1991, 1985, 1977.

ISBN: 978-0-323-06536-8

Vice President and Publisher: Linda Duncan
Executive Editor: John Dolan
Managing Editor: Kristin Hebberd
Publishing Services Manager: Julie Eddie
Project Manager: Marquita Parker
Design Direction: Charlie Seibel

Printed in China

Last digit is the print number: 9 8 7 6 5 4 3 2 1

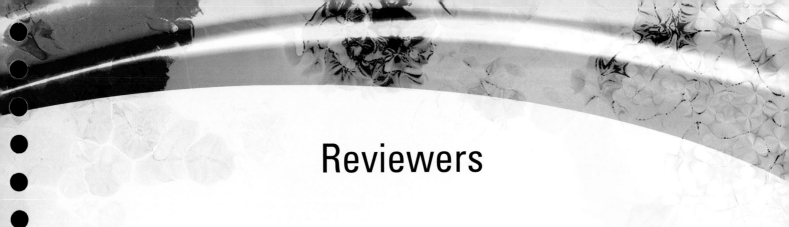

Reviewers

Carol Ann Chapman, CDA, RDH, MS
Dental Clinical Associate
Dental Hygiene Clinic
Edison State College
Fort Myers, Florida

Sharron J. Cook, CDA
Instructor, Dental Assisting
School of Health Sciences
Columbus Technical College
Columbus, Georgia

Heidi Gottfried-Arvold, BA, CDA
Program Director/Chairperson
Dental Assistant Program
Gateway Technical College
Kenosha Campus
Kenosha, Wisconsin

This edition is dedicated to

Charlotte Hanson

As our friend, mentor, and professional colleague, Charlotte has been quick to help us through many editorial crises. Although best known as a speech teacher by academic appointment, to us she has been our personal "Webster's Collegiate Dictionary, Thesaurus and objective critic."
A truer friend, one could not find.

BLF
CAF

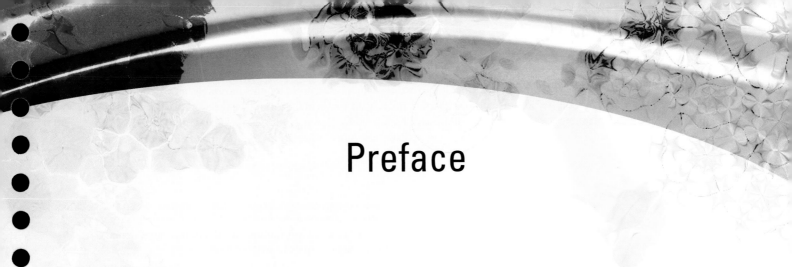

Preface

Dentistry is a dynamic profession, and this edition of the textbook continues to display how the profession functions as a health care system while being a business for profit. The business office in today's modern dental practice functions as a highly technological facility and with the use of skilled personnel, can increase service to the patient while being a highly productive component of the dental practice.

BACKGROUND

This textbook evolved from a course team taught by the authors of the first edition, Jerry Crowe Patt and Betty Ladley Finkbeiner. When Jerry retired, Charles Finkbeiner, Betty's spouse, assumed the second author's role, as they team-taught a practice management course at Washtenaw Community College in Ann Arbor, Michigan. The resultant benefits of two faculty members with working experience in both dentistry and business continue to be evident in this 7th Edition.

AUDIENCE

This textbook is intended to be used by dentists, dental students, dental assistants, and dental hygienists as a primer and reference guide for the new employee in the dental business office. For the newly practicing dentist this textbook is an excellent resource on how to set up the business office and select staff, equipment, and supplies to maintain this vital part of the practice. For the inexperienced person this book provides a broad overview of the dental business operation, as well as technical information about patient charts, tooth nomenclature, insurance billing information, ethics, and infection control as it relates to the business office. For the more experienced employee this book becomes an adjunct reference for those times when one may be needed.

IMPORTANCE TO THE PROFESSION

The authors believe that the business office needs to take its rightful place in the dental practice; that is, it should not be just the "front office," but rather a place where communication, organization, and skillful management concepts can enhance the success of the practice. This textbook provides suggested answers and comments for new employees to use in patient communication when they otherwise might appear not know how to respond to a patient. It also provides working solutions to many of the common day-to-day tasks in the business office.

ORGANIZATION

The book introduces the reader first to the concepts of the business of dentistry as a service profession, dental team and patient management, legal and ethical issues, technology in the office, and design and equipment placement in the office. Chapters within the second portion of the book discuss communication, the key to patient success, include document management and storage, as well as written communication and telecommunication. The third section of the book introduces business office systems that include appointment management, recall, inventory, dental insurance, accounts receivable, and accounts payable. The final section of the book places emphasis on the dental assistant in the workplace and aids in the planning and management of a career path. The back pages of the book provide the reader easy access to grammar, numbers, prefixes and suffixes, common abbreviations, and dental terminology – common points of reference.

KEY FEATURES

- *Comprehensive Coverage:* This textbook covers all aspects of the business of managing a dental practice, information that is vital to its success. Although the emphasis is often on the administrative dental assistant, all members of the dental team are highlighted in specific areas.
- *Practice Management Software:* Screen shots throughout the book supplement text discussions and paperwork examples to illustrate how processes and procedures can be properly and efficiently performed through the use of practice management software. Examples are provided from EagleSoft, one of the most widely used programs in dental offices.
- *Expert Authorship:* Betty Ladley Finkbeiner is a leading authority in dental assisting education, with many years of experience and many publications to her credit. She has been writing this text for more than 30 years. Charles Finkbeiner is an experienced instructor in the areas of business and computer information systems. Their combined experience and teamwork provide students with the tools they need to become successful members of the dental office team.
- *Need-to-Know Content:* Some highlights include the following:
  - Foundational chapters present truly practical discussions of ethics and legal issues.
  - Patient and staff communication resolutions are highlighted throughout.
  - A broad overview is provided for the application of infection control concepts related to the business office.
  - Chapters incorporate information on a wide spectrum of practices involving documentation and technology to suit the needs of a variety of office settings.
- *Art Program:* Chapters incorporate plenty of illustrations to supplement text descriptions with examples of paperwork, office software, technology, and processes.
- *Key Terminology:* Key terms are bolded throughout the text, with definitions provided in a listing at the end of each chapter to help familiarize readers with unfamiliar new vocabulary.
- *Learning Activities:* End-of-chapter exercises involve a mixture of review questions and those that encourage readers to assimilate chapter information and learn to think critically about day-to-day office situations.
- *Summary Tables and Boxes:* Concepts are summarized throughout chapters in boxes and tables, calling readers' attention to important nuggets of information and providing easy-to-read recaps of text discussions that serve as useful review and study tools.
- *Chapter Outlines and Objectives:* Each chapter begins with an outline of content to be presented and listing of learning outcomes, setting the stage for chapter coverage and serving as checkpoints readers can use for reference or study.
- *Spiral Binding:* The spiral makes for easy lay-flat reading and improves the use of the book as an office reference.

NEW TO THIS EDITION

- *Focus on the Paperless Dental Office:* Emphasis throughout is placed on the use of the computer as a replacement for paper records, although plenty of hard-copy document examples are included for those offices that have not yet made this switch completely.
- *Emphasis on Technology:* Chapters incorporate information on the latest technology used in dentistry so that readers remain current with the increasingly important role of electronics.
- *Updated Art Program:* Many new illustrations help readers visualize current paperwork, new technologies, and plenty of examples that demonstrate the efficiencies that can be realized through the use of practice management software.
- *New Content:* Additions include the following:
  - Updated management styles
  - New management concepts in organizational culture

- Electronic banking and payroll
- Tax forms
- Updated infection control concepts
- Updated insurance management techniques
- *New Design:* A two-column format makes for easier reading and also helps ensure that the book is smaller and more easily portable for students.

ANCILLARIES

Student Workbook

A new accompanying workbook provides practical exercises as well as those that promote critical thinking. A CD-ROM of the latest version EagleSoft practice management software is provided in the back of the workbook, and original exercises are included throughout.

Evolve Website

A companion Evolve website has been created specifically for this book and can be accessed directly at http://evolve.elsevier.com/Finkbeiner/practice. Resources are available for free to all students and for instructors who have adopted the book.

Instructor Resources
- *Test Bank:* Approximately 350 objective-style questions – multiple-choice, true/false, and matching – with accompanying rationales for correct answers and page-number references for remediation
- *Image Collection:* All the book's images available for download into PowerPoint or other presentation formats
- *PowerPoint Presentations:* Lecture slides for each chapter
- *Critical Thinking Exercises:* Mini-case scenarios followed by thought questions that deal with typical office situations and dilemmas
- *Instructor's Resource Manual:* A detailed chapter outline, listing of key terms, learning activities, bibliographical citations, related websites for each chapter, along with answers to the workbook questions and activities

Student Resources
- *Exclusive EagleSoft Screen Shot Exercises:* Scenarios that incorporate actual screen shots from the EagleSoft program and are followed by questions and instant feedback for student practice
- *Working Forms:* Office-ready forms and templates
- *Glossary Exercises:* Crossword puzzles created from chapter key terms and from dental vocabulary
- *Image Identification:* Drag-and-drop exercises to reinforce the types of technology used in today's dental business office
- *Content Updates:* Central site for posting of new or updated information to keep the book current

Betty Ladley Finkbeiner
Charles Allan Finkbeiner

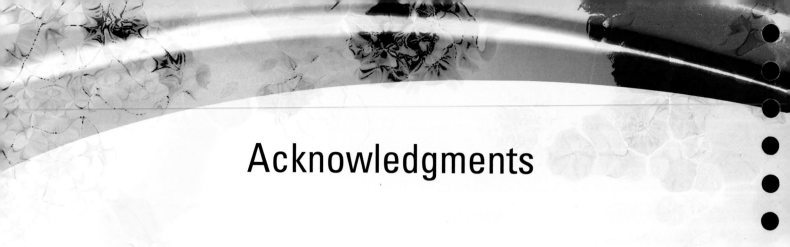

Acknowledgments

This seventh edition has brought new meaning to communication technology. As the authors prepared the manuscript, we did so with major use of a variety of communication tools. The wide use of e-mail and digital photography made this edition much easier to transmit materials. However, it was not the Internet or the technology that made the job so successful, but rather the people behind these systems. This book has evolved into its published state with the tremendous support of the staff behind the scenes at Elsevier, including Executive Editor John Dolan and Managing Editor Kristin Hebberd. Production guidance and support was provided by Project Manager Marquita Parker and Designer Charlie Seibel.

The authors have been supported by many professionals who have lent their expertise to this edition. For support during this time, we thank our friends who were always listening to our latest challenges and to our professional colleagues who provided us with materials to enhance the textbook and ancillary materials. To Linda Stakley, Betty's former administrative assistant, we thank you for resolving so many of our Word document problems; to Dr. Joseph M. Ellis for his ever-present support; to Kathy Weber and Kristina Sprague at Washtenaw Community College and Carol Chapman of Edison College for providing their educational expertise; to Pamela Zarkowski, from the University of Detroit Mercy for her legal expertise; to Becky Nagy for assistance with the insurance chapter; to Mary Govoni and Linda Collins for input on the infection control and patient records chapters, respectively and to Kim McQueen, Marybeth Poleck, and Helen Park with Patterson Office Supplies, for their assistance with the artwork for the documents, communications, appointment management, and recall chapters.

Lastly, we owe a debt of gratitude to the staff at EagleSoft, A Patterson Company, for making it possible to include the interactive CD-ROM that accompanies every copy of the workbook. We extend our sincere appreciation to Jana Berghoff, Corporate Technology Marketing Manager with Patterson Dental, for her support from the project's inception and her steady advice and guidance through publication.

Betty Ladley Finkbeiner
Charles Allan Finkbeiner

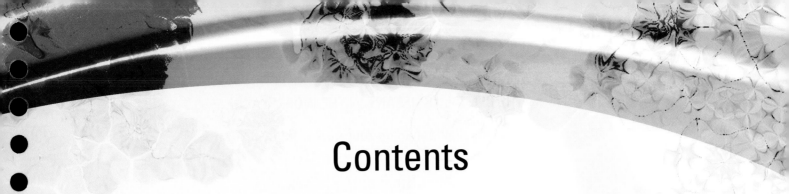

Contents

PART I

DENTISTRY AS A BUSINESS

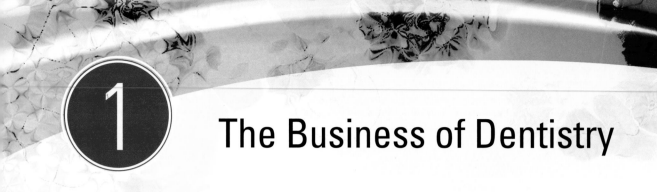

The Business of Dentistry

LEARNING OUTCOMES

- Define glossary terms.
- Explain the dual role of dentistry as a business and a healthcare service.
- Describe the importance of patient service.
- Define organizational culture.
- Describe common organizational cultures that could exist in a dental practice.
- Define communication.
- Differentiate between leadership and management.
- Identify common leadership traits.
- Describe management responsibilities.
- List characteristics necessary for establishing relationships.

The administrative professional's role in the dental office of the twenty-first century is one that will continue to change and be ever-challenging. Although projections by futurists tell us that nearly all purchases will be made virtually and that numerous jobs will be transferred from people to virtual programmers, a phenomenon known as intelligence sourcing, or I sourcing, the dental practice will remain a people-oriented health profession. The person assigned to the administrative role in the dental office must have the ability to achieve the mission of the practice, increase productivity, demonstrate skills in computer technology, and effectively use the most important asset of the practice—its human resources. Indeed this is a time of exploding technology, both in the business office and in clinical treatment areas within the practice. Dentistry as a business must face the same issues as other healthcare and business systems and realize that the world is changing. There is diversity in race, ethnicity, gender, and age, and today's dental professional must be able to address these issues.

Dentistry is a healthcare profession that has a twofold role: (1) to provide healthcare service and (2) to make a profit as a small business. As a healthcare service, dentistry provides quality care for the patient, following standards of care established by governmental agencies and the profession itself. As a healthcare profession, dentistry embraces the following objectives:

- Promote optimal oral health in a culturally sensitive manner.
- Provide oral health education.
- Promote prevention.
- Emulate the highest standards of patient-centered care.
- Acquire the most advanced knowledge and skills to meet the changing needs of a diverse patient population.
- Exhibit a willingness to share knowledge.
- Participate in professional activities.

As a business, an enterprise in which one is engaged to achieve a livelihood, the dental practice must meet the following criteria:

- Practice ethically.
- Operate efficiently.
- Operate safely.
- Be productive.
- Utilize technology.
- Create a profit.

For years dentists have referred to the business office as the *front office*. This terminology serves to decrease the importance of this area of the practice. After all, there is no "back office." Dentists refer to other areas of the dental practice according to the work that takes place in them. The clinical areas of the office are referred to as treatment, laboratory, hygiene, or radiographic rooms. The business office should assume its rightful name, since all business activities of the practice take place there, including financial transactions, patient and staff communication, appointment management, recall, inventory, insurance management, and records maintenance.

The traditional education of the dentist has placed great emphasis on developing a highly competent diagnostician and clinician but has often left a noticeable void in the area of practice management. Dentistry in the twenty-first century faces an ever-changing population, a culturally diverse workforce and patient clientele, heightened consumer rights, changing economy, increased state and federal regulations, an aging population, managed care, satellite offices, expanding group practices, and redefinition of dental assistant and dental hygienist utilization and credentialing. Futuristic-thinking dental practitioners will embrace change as a lifelong, ongoing process for the individual and the practice. The successful dental practice will be led by individuals who look at all situations as opportunities to create excitement and enthusiasm in meeting new challenges. These individuals will realize that technology alone cannot drive the practice, but that employees are a major asset. Therefore a greater emphasis must be placed on practice leadership and management. The administrative assistant or business office manager becomes a vital professional by maintaining records, implementing business systems, managing business operations, and maintaining communication (transmitting information from one person to another) among the dentist, the staff, the patient, and the community.

As modern dentists accept the roles of dentist and entrepreneur, they accept the responsibility of delegating expanded intraoral duties to the appropriate clinical assistants and dental hygienists, more extraoral duties to the laboratory technician, and additional responsibility to the administrative assistant or business manager.

DENTISTRY AS A SERVICE PROFESSION

In the twenty-first century it is evident that the industrial age that dominated the society of our parents and grandparents has given way to a service-oriented age, and dentistry is a major healthcare service. Dental treatment may be the objective for a patient; however, the dental staff must be constantly aware that when patients come to the office to seek treatment or perhaps a restoration (a tangible product), they are also seeking the most important product—service—an intangible product in the form of care. Service is a system of accommodating or providing assistance to another person.

Patients remain with a dental practice only if they are satisfied with the services rendered. Figure 1-1 illustrates the many "ifs" the dental staff will encounter in the retention of a patient in its practice. It is important to remember that patients have choices. If patients choose to come to the office from either a recommendation or random selection, and if they are satisfied with the treatment and care, they may return. If patients are still satisfied at the return visit, they may continue to return. However, if there is dissatisfaction at any stage of the service, patients may opt not to return to the office.

The basis for patient retention is communication, the ability to understand and be understood. A patient seldom leaves a dental practice because of dissatisfaction with the margins of his or her composite restoration. However, the patient may leave because a staff member made it difficult to obtain a completed insurance claim form, was too busy to listen to a concern, made frequent errors on statements, or didn't communicate the treatment plan in advance.

> **PRACTICE NOTE**
> The basis for patient retention is communication.

Service is not a result of clinical and cognitive skills, but rather attitudinal skills that evolve into a commitment to the welfare of others. Box 1-1 lists a variety of activities that indicate a service-oriented office.

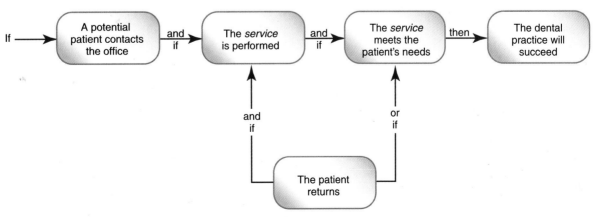

Figure 1-1 The service concept.

Activities That Promote Service

- Maintaining regularly scheduled office hours
- Providing emergency care during the dentist's absence
- Maintaining the appointment schedule without delays
- Maintaining professional ethics
- Practicing quality care
- Recognizing the patient's needs
- Taking time to listen to the patient's concerns
- Respecting the patient's right to choice
- Informing patients of alternative treatment plans
- Allaying fears
- Hiring qualified employees
- Assigning only legally delegable duties to qualified staff
- Seeking staff input in decision making
- Encouraging an environment of caring
- Updating procedural techniques, equipment, and office decor regularly
- Maintaining office equipment
- Maintaining professional skills routinely
- Operating safely
- Maintaining quality assurance
- Attending risk-management seminars
- Participating in community services
- Being genuine and honest

ORGANIZATIONAL CULTURE

The term organizational culture has become well-known in business. Many authors have defined organizational culture, but perhaps for the purpose of dental management it can best be defined as something that an organization or dental practice "is" rather than what it "has." Organizational culture comprises the attitudes, experiences, beliefs, and values of an organization. It has been defined as the "specific collection of values and norms that are shared by people and groups in an organization and that control the way they interact with each other and with others outside the organization or dental practice." Some authors even add to this definition the physical being of the organization; dress codes; and office arrangement and design.

Organizational culture can become very complex. However, the following list describes common organizational cultures that could be applied to a dental practice:

- A *power culture* concentrates on power among a few. Control radiates from the center like a web. Power cultures have few rules and little bureaucracy; swift decisions can ensue. This could be compared with former leadership styles such as authoritarian.
- In the *role culture*, people have clearly delegated authorities within a highly defined structure. Typically these organizations form hierarchical bureaucracies. Power derives from a person's position and little scope exists for expert power.
- In the *task culture,* teams are formed to solve particular problems. Power derives from expertise so long as a team requires expertise. These cultures often feature multiple reporting lines of a matrix structure.

- A *person culture* exists when all individuals believe themselves superior to the organization. Survival can become difficult for such organizations, because the concept of an organization suggests that a group of like-minded individuals pursue the organization goals. Some professional partnerships, such as dentistry, can operate as person cultures, because each partner brings a particular expertise and clientele to the office.
- The *work-hard/play-hard culture* is characterized by few risks being taken, all with rapid feedback. This is typical in large organizations, which strive for high-quality customer/client service. It is often characterized by team meetings, jargon, and buzzwords.
- The *bet-your-company culture* is one in which big stakes decisions are taken, but it may be years before the results are known. This does not apply directly to dentistry perhaps, except in situations of large corporate clinics.
- The *process culture* occurs in organizations where there is little or no feedback. People become bogged down with how things are done, not with what is achieved. This is often associated with bureaucracies. Although it is easy to criticize these cultures for being overly cautious or bogged down in red tape, they do produce consistent results, which is ideal in public services for example. This type of culture could apply to public dental clinics.
- The *blame culture* cultivates distrust and fear. People blame each other to avoid being reprimanded or put down, and this results in no new ideas or personal initiative because people don't want to risk being wrong. This type of culture can be fatal to a dental practice staff.
- *Multidirectional culture* cultivates minimized cross-department communication and cooperation. Loyalty is to specific groups or departments. Each department becomes a clique and is often critical of other departments, which in turn create a lot of gossip. This type of culture could exist in a large clinic or dental school with multiple departments.
- A *live-and-let-live culture* spurns complacency. It manifests mental stagnation and low creativity. Staff members in this culture have little future vision and have given up on their passion. There is average cooperation and communication and things do get done, but they do not grow. People in this culture have developed personal relationships and decided who to stay away from; there is not much left to learn.
- In a *leadership-enriched culture*, people view the organization as an extension of themselves. They feel good about what they personally achieve through the organization, and this promotes exceptional cooperation. Individual goals are aligned with goals of the practice and people do what it takes to make things happen. As a group, the organization is more like family, providing personal fulfillment that often transcends ego so that people are consistently bringing out the best in each other. In this culture every individual in the organization wants to do a good job. This is an ideal culture to promote in a dental practice. In dentistry it is likely that a multifaceted culture could develop, such as the leadership-enriched combined with the task culture.

What does organizational culture mean for the new employee looking at a prospective job? It is not easy to identify the type of culture during an hour's interview, but if a working interview is possible, the type of culture may soon be identified; see if the "hum" is there that fits with individual values, beliefs, attitudes, and emotions.

LEADERSHIP AND MANAGEMENT IN THE TWENTY-FIRST CENTURY

Traditionally the dentist may have managed the office in an authoritative, free-rein, or participatory type of leadership style. Today the effective leader or manager must have skills in change mastery, technology, and virtual office systems that extend beyond the local domain.

Leadership and management are related but different in concept and definition. The leader in a dental practice is commonly the dentist. The manager is often the administrative assistant. However, to be a good leader one must possess the characteristics of a manager, and the manager may find a situation in which he or she must assume a leadership role.

To be an effective leader a person must possess a set of personal traits as described in the following discussion.

Live by a Set of Values

In today's dental practice ethical behavior is the acceptable behavior. The difficult task at hand is how this ethical behavior survives in the entire practice. The leader of the dental practice, the dentist employer, must work within the office to identify and define those principles of ethics and acceptable behavior and ensure that they are carried out during routine daily practice. Effective leaders often must make difficult decisions to stand on their values and understand that the set of values they identify for the practice must begin at the top and permeate throughout all levels of the practice.

Build a Shared Vision

The ethical dental office has a visionary leader and may even have more than one. This person(s), the dentist, must be able to build on the shared vision and involve employees at all levels. It is wise for the dentist to determine a practice mission statement that speaks to the way the practice is to be managed and the role of the staff and the patients. Chapter 3 shows a sample of an office policy that is distributed to patients in which this mission statement defines the practice.

Building an organizational vision means that employees at all levels must be involved. An effective leader works with the staff to determine how the practice vision and individual goals and objectives meet the vision of the practice. As this vision takes shape the leader and employees need to determine the following:
- What are the dental practice's values? What values should it have? Does some modification need to be made?
- What contributions should the dental practice make to the community? Which staff members should be involved?

- Who are the patients? What are the demographics and needs of these individuals?
- What is the dental practice's reputation? What reputation should it have? Are changes needed in this reputation?
- How do people work together within the practice?

Maintain Commitment to Service

A dentist has made a commitment to service when choosing dentistry as a career. Sometimes this commitment can be overshadowed by the need to make a profit and build a career for oneself. There can be a successful balance if the dentist, as a leader, understands how a successful business can be achieved and at the same time makes a commitment to help people grow in the work place. Thus the commitment to service is not only to serve the patients, but to help the staff to grow.

Empower Others

Power is the capacity to influence others. Power can flow in any direction within the dental practice and can apply to an individual or a group. Empowerment can be defined as "putting power where it is needed." When taking the following actions an effective leader empowers the staff:
- Provide employees with access to information that will help them increase their productivity and effectiveness.
- Allow staff members to take on more responsibility, including assignment of all legal tasks delegated in a given state.
- Allow staff members to have a voice in decision making.

Empowered employees feel a sense of ownership in the practice and become confident in their job. They are enthusiastic and are responsible for getting their jobs done efficiently. Usually empowered employees are happier individuals; they feel they are part of the practice and enjoy the job's rewards.

The empowered leader has a basic trust in people; and believes the staff is good, honest, and trustworthy. This leader believes that the staff will accomplish more if given the right resources and responsibility to accomplish the assigned tasks.

Reward Risk Taking

Leaders of successful dental practices are willing to seek new answers to problems, try new approaches, utilize technology, and be flexible. Successful dentists know that not all risk taking is successful, but they are willing to take calculated risks, knowing that the status quo can also result in failure. This type of leader encourages the staff to take some risks also. For instance, one of the staff may be considering taking an online educational program to become a registered dental assistant. The dentist encourages the assistant to do this, but the employee is fearful of failure. The assistant indicates she has children at home, has never taken such a course online, and is unsure she will succeed. She must take a risk. The dentist employer needs to reward this risk taking. Encouragement to take such a course on the part of the dentist, and then rewarding this risk-taking employee with increased responsibility and compensation can ensure a confident employee. Keys to successful risk taking include the following:

- Trust in one's own abilities.
- Be open-minded.
- Overcome the fear of mistakes.
- Develop support teams.

Manage Chaos

A good leader can sort out a chaotic situation and move on to a desired outcome. Crises occur in the daily routine of the dental office. The effective leader can quickly move in and practice the art of meeting individuals where they are in a conflict situation and move them forward to bring about desired outcomes.

Know How to Follow

A good leader is also a good follower. The effective leader knows the importance of stepping back and being a follower when a situation demands it. A good leader also has trust in others, and knows that they can be leaders also, if given the proper opportunities and training.

Today's Leader

The leader in the dental office today must embrace trust, a willingness to understand change, humility, commitment, focus, compassion, integrity, peacemaking, and endurance (Box 1-2).

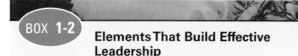

BOX 1-2   Elements That Build Effective Leadership

- *Trust* promotes good relationships and confidence with the staff, as expanded duties are delegated to clinical staff and advanced management techniques are assigned to business staff.
- *A willingness to understand change* and recognize that disruptions are inevitable is part of effective leadership, with the willingness to shift gears to pave the way for change.
- *Humility* is a focus on being open, teachable, and flexible.
- *Commitment* seeks to develop vision and values in a leader and moves leaders to stand for something greater.
- *Focus* gives leaders the ability to achieve and direct their time and energy to important goals and objectives.
- *Compassion* is the desire to understand and care for others, such as staff, family, patients, or community.
- *Integrity* demands that leaders be responsible for seeking to create quality assurance in their service for patients, as well as in all their relationships.
- *Peacemaking* leaders bring calmness to the office by listening, learning from others, and seeking good solutions rather than making quick decisions.
- *Endurance* refers to courage, perseverance, and strength when situations, people, or the environment become chaotic or difficult.

As a business, the dentist/leader of the twenty-first century strives to achieve practice goals by:

- Considering long-term over short-term results
- Stressing effectiveness over efficiency alone
- Thinking strategically rather than operationally
- Being proactive rather than reactive to situations
- Being driven by plans rather than problems

Members of an effective dental office cannot think and act independently. Marketing service in a dental practice means considering human, financial, and technical resources in a world-wide market. Patients seen in the dental office come from diverse backgrounds and present complex and diverse treatment options. Likewise the dental materials and technology used in all facets of the office come from a worldwide market. The dental office of this century must be a virtual office that not only serves the local community, but also recognizes its role in the global community.

PERSONAL CHARACTERISTICS OF AN EFFECTIVE LEADER

Generally the first contact a patient has with the office is with a staff person in the business office, administrative assistant, or office manager. It is difficult to identify a job today that does not include interaction with people. Whether you have a job in education, custodial services, law, science, religion, office technology, or architecture, you will find that productivity is greatly enhanced by an ability to communicate. In fact it is difficult to find any job today in which communication is not important. It has been found that 80 percent of the people who fail at their jobs do so not because of a lack of technical skills, but because they do not relate well with people.

One's attitude either gives the patient a positive impression or convinces her or him to seek dental care elsewhere. Whether communicating with patients, staff, or friends, basic "people skills" must be developed for successful communication. In addition to the elements found in a leader discussed earlier in this chapter, the office manager must have skills that include self-confidence, genuineness, enthusiasm, assertiveness, honesty, acceptance of others, the ability to be a good listener, and a willingness to be a team player.

Self-Confidence

Self-confidence is the ability to believe one can do a job well. To have self-confidence, a person must accept herself or himself. This requires a healthy mental personal picture and accentuation of positive attributes. Having self-confidence means identifying strengths and building on them, and accepting weaknesses and not dwelling on them.

An administrative assistant with self-confidence assumes responsibility, adapts to change, accepts challenges, and provides input in decision making. For instance, administrative assistants who are self-confident initiate marketing needs, make suggestions for changes, and implement new procedures without hesitation, confident that they know what is going on. They are willing to take risks and are able to recommend changes in a routine or procedure with the confidence that the idea is worthwhile and merits consideration.

Genuineness

Being genuine means being oneself. A person who is genuine is sincere and straightforward. This is important when dealing with people in a healthcare profession. A genuine caring person is not afraid to reach out and touch someone. Placing a hand on a shoulder of a frightened patient or holding a frightened child's hand (Figure 1-2) shows caring and displays a genuine concern for another person's feelings. It requires putting oneself in the patient's place, and showing the kind of concern one would like to receive.

Patients feel comfortable with a genuinely caring administrative assistant and are likely to open up and share their innermost feelings. When patients express fear or frustration, an assistant with genuine concern says, "I'm sorry to hear you feel this way. Is there anything I can do to help you?" Patients may simply need a person to listen, a friendly smile, or a comforting pat on the shoulder.

Acceptance of a Culturally Diverse Population

Today's administrative assistant must communicate with people who speak English as a second language. It may be necessary to use another dictionary or reference such as *Spanish Terminology for the Dental Team* if an interpreter is not available. Such references aid in communicating with patients to determine basic information for clinical and financial records as well as clinical questions.

Each person's values are established from his or her background and previous experience. To accept others one must be willing to accept them as worthy human beings without a desire to change them to fit into a preconceived value system. Accept them for what they are, not for what they "ought" to be. Communication is often difficult when a person acts or appears "different" than what is perceived as the norm. For instance, when a patient with a prosthesis replacing his or her right arm visits the office, the prosthesis may attract attention, and a staff member may even stare at the device. The focus is on the disability, not the patient. In the healthcare profession, it is important to concentrate on seeing the patient, not the disability.

Enthusiasm

Being enthusiastic means being interested in work, being expressive, and leaving problems at home. Being enthusiastic does not mean being a phony or a constant chatterbox, but having a sincere interest in work and the greater world. A dental assistant who is enthusiastic about work is likely to read professional journals, seek knowledge about new technology or specific areas of interest, participate in community activities or professional organizations, and become an involved professional. To be enthusiastic one must act enthusiastically.

PRACTICE NOTE
To be enthusiastic, you must act enthusiastic.

An enthusiastic dental assistant takes time to learn about the patients and their interests. When patients ask questions, the dental assistant seeks the answers. An enthusiastic dental assistant is happy to get to work, enjoys sharing others' experiences, appreciates good humor, and is not totally exhausted at the end of the day. Enthusiastic people have a positive outlook on life.

Assertiveness

Being assertive does not mean being aggressive. An assertive person is bold and enterprising in a nonhostile manner. An administrative assistant is often called on to assume new responsibilities and must take the initiative to get the job done. Consider this situation. Staff members in the office where the administrative assistant has been employed for 3 years have been complaining about salaries, often among themselves at lunchtime. Everyone feels awkward about discussing it with the dentist because they are not sure what to say. An assertive person will take the initiative to research salaries in areas that represent comparable responsibilities, determine the production and value of each staff member, and present the data to the dentist in a nonthreatening manner. To be assertive often requires tact, initiative, and willingness to take a risk.

Effective Listening

Listening is more than hearing. A good listener hears not only the facts, but also the feeling behind the facts. Good listening is a combination of hearing what a person says and becoming involved with the person who is talking. Sometimes a hearing

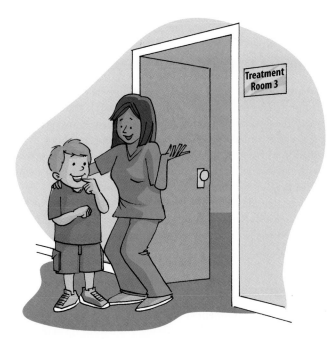
Figure 1-2 An arm resting on a child's shoulder displays caring.

loss or preoccupation with one's own problems, goals, or feelings can make it difficult to hear what is really communicated. In a busy dental office, what the patient is really saying may be ignored because a staff member is too preoccupied with work, deadlines, or future activities to listen effectively to the patient's needs. Often only what one wants to hear or has time to hear is actually heard.

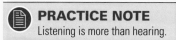

> ### PRACTICE NOTE
> Listening is more than hearing.

Sometimes a listener forgets to listen with the eyes. To see what a person is saying; it is necessary to look at the speaker when he or she is talking (Figure 1-3). When observing a person's body language, facial expressions, gestures, and posture, which all give clues to that person's feelings, are also observed. Consequently it is possible to hear what people are saying by observing the emotions they display.

In reflective listening the listener absorbs what has been said, reflects on it, and restates or paraphrases the feeling or content of the message in a way that demonstrates understanding and acceptance. This type of listening is beneficial to a healthcare professional as both dentist and patient interact to create a better understanding of the situation. A scenario in a dental office might go something like the following:

> *Patient:* "I just don't know whether to have a porcelain crown on this front tooth or not. My family has always accepted me like this, but every time I have my picture taken I always worry that this gray tooth will show, so I keep my mouth closed."
> *Assistant:* "You have considered having the crown done, but sometimes feel you shouldn't do it?"
> *Patient:* "Uh, huh."

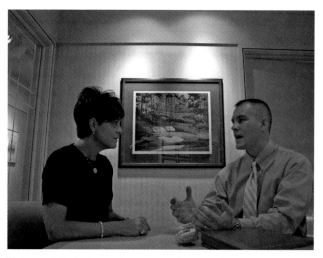

Figure 1-3 A dentist listens with his eyes during a consultation with a patient. (Courtesy Shane McDowell, DMD [Snyder McDowell LLC] and Staci DiRoma, Fort Myers, FL.)

The assistant has restated the basic statement of the patient. The message was in her own words and wasn't judgmental. When correctly paraphrased, the speaker generally responds in the affirmative. If not, the paraphrase needs to be restated until the message is received clearly.

Another form of this listening style and paraphrasing is as follows:

> *Dentist employer:* "I don't understand why we haven't received the new impression material that we ordered."
> *Assistant:* "Do I hear you saying that you think maybe I didn't place the order?"
> *Dentist employer:* "No, I was just wondering if maybe the supply house isn't stocking that material."

This conversation could have ended with the dentist's original statement, in which the assistant became upset, thinking there was a hidden meaning. Instead the assistant queried the dentist to determine what the statement really meant and then realized the true meaning of the statement.

At first using these techniques may seem cumbersome or artificial. Try them and practice them, and soon the benefits of reflective listening will become clear. Good listening skills require that a listener understands a person before speaking. Such action results in improved relations with patients and staff, and may result in fewer conflicts.

Recognition of Others' Needs

All people need some form of recognition. Office colleagues need friendship, recognition, and a desire to feel they are valued for their contribution to the team's success. This doesn't mean that office colleagues have to socialize outside the office. It simply means that they should be willing to work cooperatively together to accomplish the objectives of the practice. Ignoring another person's needs does not facilitate good interpersonal relations.

Sense of Humor

A dental office can be a stressful setting for staff members who clamor to meet the demands of the daily schedule and the patient who is filled with fear about potential treatment. How one interprets a crisis situation, however, is more important. Look at the situation with a sense of humor, and lighten up. However, always be careful to laugh at the situation and not at the person. Patients and colleagues should not be made the brunt of jokes.

Consider adding humor to the office with cartoons on the bulletin board. Remember that humor lessens conflict and eases tension and is perhaps the best medicine prescribed in any dental office.

Willingness to Be a Team Player

Dentistry is a team-oriented business. Building a team is a simple concept when it is realized that teams are made up of individuals with diverse skills and talents. Each team member must have clearly defined skills that need to be identified and measured against the skills of other team members. Once a person realizes his or her role on the team and how best to accomplish specific tasks, achieving team goals can be accomplished and eagerly anticipated. Offices that are committed to building a team can achieve results more effectively than offices in which each individual works independently.

KEY TERMS

Business—An enterprise in which one is engaged to achieve a livelihood.

Communication—The process of transmitting information from one person to another.

Dentistry—A healthcare profession concerned with the care of the teeth and surrounding tissues, including prevention and elimination of decay, replacement of missing teeth and structures, esthetics, and correction of malocclusion.

Intelligence sourcing (I-sourcing)—Transferring jobs from people to virtual programmers.

Leadership—The method of influencing others for good, rousing others to action and inspiring them to become the best they can be, as a group works together toward a common goal.

Management—The act or art of leading a team to accomplish goals and objectives while using skill, care, and tactful behavior.

Organizational culture—The sum of the attitudes, experiences, beliefs, and values of an organization. It is the specific collection of values and norms that are shared by people and groups in an organization and that control the way they interact with each other and those outside the organization or dental practice.

Service—In dentistry, the process of providing quality care for patients while following standards of care established by governmental agencies and the profession itself.

LEARNING ACTIVITIES

1. Define organizational culture and explain how it affects the function of a dental practice.
2. Explain the role of a leader and a manager in a dental practice.
3. Describe common organizational cultures that could exist in a dental practice.
4. Describe situations in a dental office that are more effective when performed as a team.

Please refer to the student workbook for additional learning activities

BIBLIOGRAPHY

Alvesson M, Sveningsson S: *Changing organizational culture: cultural change work in progress*, New York, 2008, Routledge.

Bruch H, Wass DL, Covey SR et al: *Habits of highly effective managers*, ed 2, New York, 2009, Simon & Schuster.

Fulton-Calkins PJ: *The administrative professional*, ed 13, Mason, OH, 2007, Thomson South-Western.

Jacobson T: What it takes to be an effective leader, *Canadian Manager Winter*, 2002.

Keyton J: *Communication and organizational culture*, Thousand Oaks, CA, 2005, Sage Publications.

Giuliani R: *Leadership through the age*, New York, 2002, Miramax Books.

McNamara C: *Field guide to leadership and supervision*, Minneapolis, 2002, Authenticity Consulting.

Mosby: *Spanish terminology for the dental team*, ed 2, St Louis, 2011, Mosby.

Schein EH: *Organizational culture and leadership*, ed 3, San Francisco, 2004, Josey-Bass.

Thill JV, Bovée CL: *Excellence in business communication*, ed 5, Upper Saddle River, NJ, 2002, Prentice-Hall.

Please visit http://evolve.elsevier.com/Finkibeiner/practice for additional practice activities.

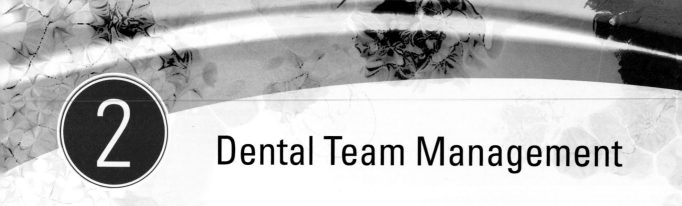

2 Dental Team Management

LEARNING OUTCOMES

- Define glossary terms.
- Determine goals and objectives for a dental practice.
- Explain business etiquette.
- List duties of an administrative assistant.
- Identify the five *R*s of good management.
- Identify functions of an administrative assistant.
- Identify characteristics of an effective administrative assistant.
- Manage interpersonal communications of staff and dentist.
- Explain employee empowerment.
- Discuss the procedures for conducting a staff meeting.
- Explain the importance of hiring a skilled administrative assistant.
- Define *time management*.
- Describe how to manage time efficiently.
- Explain the purpose of an office procedural manual.
- Identify components of an office procedural manual.
- Describe recruitment and hiring practices.
- Describe the contents of a personnel policy in an office procedural manual.
- Explain the use of pre-employment testing.
- Describe new employee orientation.
- Manage staff conflict.

ESTABLISHING PRACTICE GOALS AND OBJECTIVES

Before opening a dental practice, the dentist should define a practice philosophy, establish specific objectives, and determine a mission statement for the practice. A lack of goals and objectives results in lack of direction for the dentist and staff and may result in poor relationships with patients. As the practice grows, these goals and objectives will need to be revised and the mission statement updated. It is vital that the dentist in a healthcare practice seek input from the staff when establishing these objectives.

A common sequence for establishing objectives includes the following steps:

- *Develop a practice philosophy.* The dentist identifies in a broad statement the basic concepts about patient care, business management, auxiliary utilization, health and safety, and continuing education for the practice.
- *Develop practice objectives.* In this stage, each broad goal is broken into a series of specific objectives for the practice. These objectives should be specific positive action statements that indicate the expected results.

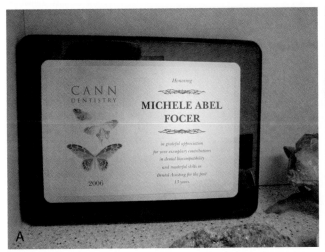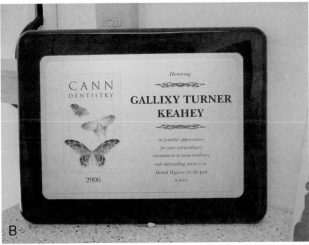

Figure 2-1 A certificate of recognition awarded to a dental assistant **A,** and a dental hygienist **B,** for team excellence in the practice. (Courtesy Roberta D. Cann, DMD, Cann Dentistry, Atlanta.)

- *Determine a mission statement.* This is a statement that speaks to the way the practice is to be managed and the role of the staff and the patients. It is provided to the staff and the patients for an understanding of the mission of the practice.
- *Develop practice policies.* These are statements of basic policy that will affect both staff members and patients. These statements may be covered by broad headings, followed by specific policies. It is wise to share these with the patients as shown in the office policy in Chapter 3 and with the staff as shown in the procedural manual later in this chapter.
- *Develop procedural policies.* Each broad statement can be broken down again into specific objectives and further defined into specific tasks for all of the common office procedures. A result of this effort will be most valuable when inserted in the procedural manual.
- *Develop business principles.* These objectives place emphasis on the actual business activities of the office. Here the dentist outlines in numeric terms the budget process for the practice and procedures for managing business activities.
- *Develop a practice standard.* It is necessary for the dentist to identify a quality standard that defines a self-performance level and performance level expected of the staff. The dentist should provide for the staff an explanation of how this standard is to be maintained. Plans should be made about how to periodically validate that this practice standard is being met.

    As a dentist and staff work through the development of objectives for the practice, these objectives become rules by which the office is managed. As the practice expands and new technology is developed, it will be necessary to review and revise these goals and objectives. Most important in participatory management is the involvement of the entire dental team in the development of these objectives.
- *Develop a staff recognition program.* As stated, the staff is the greatest asset a dentist can have in the office. Specific guidelines should be established for hiring a qualified staff,

selecting a wide range of creative benefits, and establishing a competitive salary scale that reflects productivity and cost-of-living increases. Most employees work hard if they are compensated well and recognized for their efforts. However, a common complaint of dental assistants is lack of recognition. An employee must be given challenging responsibilities, and salaries must be commensurate with the accomplishment of these responsibilities. Frequent thank-yous help to improve rapport, but don't overlook profit sharing, gift certificates, and travel as real incentives in a recognition program. A certificate displayed in the treatment room as shown in Figure 2-1 illustrates one method of staff recognition for outstanding performance.

BUSINESS OFFICE ETIQUETTE

Office etiquette refers to business manners. Rules that applied to social graces 25 years ago or even 10 years ago may no longer work in our society. Many former rules of etiquette were formal and rigid and often do not apply to the more casual lifestyles of today's society. Yet in a professional business office, the fact still remains that one's actions and behavior are observed by clients, patients, visitors, and those who have the potential to promote.

For a dentist employer, the potential for practice growth and patient acceptance depends on the etiquette of the staff. Good manners can lead to promotions over equally qualified persons with less poise; create a self-confident, successful, professional person; help professionals handle their superiors; and lessen awkwardness among people. They are essential to building good relationships. Specific applications of etiquette are applied to different phases of business activities in many of the ensuing chapters.

Etiquette or the application of good manners can be applied to daily interactions with each member of the staff as well as all of the patients. Good etiquette must be practiced on a daily basis, and it cannot simply be turned on and off when

---

BOX 2-1

Tips for Professional Etiquette in the Dental Office

- Determine the office code of behavior.
- Extend a friendly greeting to coworkers each day.
- Make introductions when individuals are not acquainted.
- Extend friendly greetings to people who enter the office; stand when you greet the person.
- Introduce yourself.
- Extend a cordial "thank you" or "goodbye" when someone leaves the office for the day.
- Maintain good relations with your peers.
- Learn how to handle your rivals with tact.
- Be a team player.
- Avoid becoming a do-gooder who seeks constant recognition.
- When conflict exists, learn to mend fences.
- Dress and act professionally when representing the office at conferences or seminars.
- Use correct grammar; pronounce words correctly; expand your vocabulary.

- Explain technical terms in understandable language without being demeaning.
- Make patients feel important; discuss issues of interest to them.
- Introduce yourself to a new patient; shake hands heartily to extend a warm welcome.
- If a person is engaged in a conversation with another person, avoid standing within hearing range. If you wish to talk to one of them, leave the area and return later.
- Don't eat or drink in front of patients.
- Say "thank-you" when a patient or staff member is helpful, has cooperated during treatment, or has complimented you.
- Send thank-you notes for referrals or other thoughtful acts.
- Respect the patient's and colleague's privacy.
- If the telephone rings while you are talking to another person, excuse yourself to answer it. If a lengthy conversation is expected, ask the caller if you can return the call; then complete the business with the patient.

---

patients are around. The statement "Good manners begin at home," can be adapted to the dental office by remembering that good manners begin with the staff. The failure to promote good manners with each other can be detrimental. Employers subconsciously take the pulse of relationships among their employees and staff, and if such readings reveal poor relationships among the staff and patients, action needs to be taken to modify this behavior to ensure the success of the practice. Furthermore, as discussed later in this chapter, poor relationships relate directly to productivity. Box 2-1 lists several suggestions for implementing good professional business etiquette.

THE SHIFTING ROLE OF THE ADMINISTRATIVE ASSISTANT

For many years the administrative assistant's role has been defined by various terms, including *secretary, receptionist, business assistant*, and even *front-desk person*. Many of these titles are still used today, but the changing role of this important staff person shifts the title to a more appropriate one of *administrative assistant*. The duties of the **administrative assistant** are varied and may be assigned at different levels. As the dental team expands, the dentist is likely to delegate more management duties to the administrative assistant. In a large dental practice, a dentist may employ several staff members in the business office, each with separate responsibilities as an administrative assistant, receptionist, insurance manager, and data clerk. However, in a smaller practice, these duties may be delegated to one person. The administrative assistant title in this text refers to the person whose primary responsibility involves business activities of the dental office. In general, the duties of an administrative assistant include many of the tasks identified in Box 2-2.

STAFF MANAGEMENT

The term *management* was defined in Chapter 1, but now as this chapter looks more specifically at the business office, realize that management in the dental office may be defined as the process of getting things accomplished with and through people, by guiding and motivating their efforts toward common objectives.

Some people say, "Managers are born, not made." However, **managers** can nurture their natural skills into sound management skills through experience, effort, and learning. As a person advances into an administrative position, he or she will make mistakes, but remember that learning comes from mistakes as well as successes.

The Five *R*s of Management

Successful management can be attributed to five basic *R*s: responsibility, respect, rapport, recognition, and remuneration.

 PRACTICE NOTE

Individuals can nurture their natural skills into sound management skills through experience, effort, and learning.

An employee should be delegated all tasks that are legally delegable and for which he or she is properly qualified. Employees cannot work to achieve their maximum productivity if they feel they are not given responsibility for which they are answerable. *Responsibility* denotes duty or obligation. It also denotes follow-through and completion of a project. An employee who is to become a valuable member of the dental health team must be delegated responsibility. If responsibility is withheld, then it is assumed that the administrative assistant or employer does not

BOX 2-2   Basic Job Responsibilities of the Administrative Assistant

Maintain Patient and Staff Relations

- Schedule appointments.
- Set up meetings and conferences.
- Obtain information for and maintain all patient clinical and financial records.
- Prepare consultation materials.
- Communicate both verbally and in writing with patients and staff both within and outside the office.
- Administer computer networks.
- Set up and administer financial arrangements with patients and other parties.
- Maintain recall and inventory systems.
- Implement marketing strategies.
- Design office manuals and pamphlets.
- Arrange for and conduct staff meetings and other conferences.
- Solve day-to-day problems within the role of the administrative professional.
- Provide support for patients and professional staff.
- Make travel arrangements.
- Implement state and federal regulations.
- Initiate job advertisements, interview, and make recommendations on the employment of office personnel.
- Set up training and evaluation processes for employees.
- Organize, assign, and evaluate workloads.
- Arrange for risk management and OSHA seminars.
- Supervise appropriate office support staff.

Operate Electronic Office Equipment

- Use telecommunication technology, including the telephone, voicemail, e-mail, and facsimile.
- Manage web sites.
- Help to upgrade and recommend office software.
- Provide computer and software training.

Manage Records

- Manage patient records including clinical charts, insurance forms, laboratory requisitions, HIPAA forms, and other financial and clinical data.
- Maintain employee records.
- Maintain OSHA records.
- Maintain MSDS forms.
- Prepare state and federal forms.
- Maintain an accounts payable system.
- Utilize a credit bureau and collection agency.
- Order and receive supplies and verify invoices.

Manage Mail

- Manage incoming and outgoing mail.
- Maintain an e-mail system.
- Maintain USPS mail.

---

feel the employee is capable of the task, and concern should be given for retaining this employee.

Respect is consideration or esteem given to another person. Each member of the dental health team must respect the others' education, skills, and values. To not have respect indicates a lack of confidence and again reflects a poor attitude toward another person's capabilities. Each member has a major role on the team and should possess expert skills and credentials that warrant respect.

Rapport is a mutual trust or emotional relationship that exists among the office staff members. Each dentist sets the tone for the rapport in the office. A good rapport in the office is effused to the patients who recognize how well the team members work together during tense times and how they enjoy each other's professional friendship.

Recognition is achievement. A person can be recognized for a task well done or for special achievements. Recognition can come in the form of verbal praise or a sign placed in the office recognizing employment and credentials.

Remuneration is a monetary recognition of achievement. Most employees say that they are willing to work hard if they are compensated for their efforts. Remuneration should be based on education, merit performance, longevity, and cost of living. Dentist employers who affirm that their employees have worked with them for many years, with repeated job satisfaction reviews, are those who delegate responsibility; create good rapport in the office; respect, trust, and recognize their employees; and provide compensation commensurate to other small business and allied health employment.

Functions of an Administrative Assistant

The basic functions of an administrative assistant in a dental office are shown in the schematic drawing in Figure 2-2. Some assistants may interpret this diagram to mean that their job is "a vicious circle." In actuality many of these functions overlap, and the basis for each depends on planning. Sound planning before beginning an activity may eliminate the need for crisis management, or handling one crisis after another.

Planning is identifying what is to be done in the future. The goals and objectives discussed earlier are vital to planning. The administrative assistant will be involved in long-range planning as well as daily planning.

Organizing is determining how the work will be divided and accomplished by members of the dental team. After procedures have been identified and tasks enumerated for each procedure, the administrative assistant is required to assign the duties to specific staff members. It is essential that the dentist give this authority to the administrative assistant. Without this authority, the administrative assistant cannot manage effectively.

Staffing includes the recruiting, selecting, orienting, promoting, paying, and rewarding of employees. Cooperation between staff members will be necessary as new employees are integrated into each technical area of the office. Staffing also involves

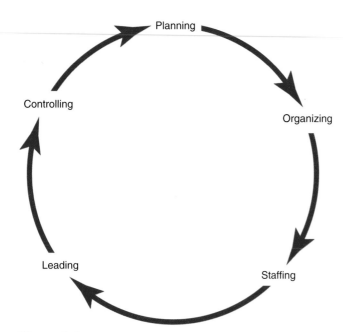

Figure 2-2 Functions of an administrative assistant.

instructing, evaluating, and educating employees and providing opportunities for their future development. Additionally the business administrative assistant is responsible for recommendations of an appropriate system of pay and benefit package.

Leading involves directing, guiding, and supervising the staff in the performance of their duties and responsibilities. It consists of exercising leadership; communicating ideas, orders, and instructions; and motivating employees to perform their work effectively and efficiently. This is really the "people" function of management.

Controlling is the function of management that deals with determining whether or not the plans are being achieved and, when necessary, making decisions to modify the plans to achieve the specific objective.

Basic Skills of an Administrative Assistant

At this point one may wonder what basic skills are required to function as an administrative assistant and perform the administrative role effectively. Although many skills are needed, a few of the most important ones are the following:

- Conceptual skills
- Human relations skills
- Administrative skills
- Technical skills

The relative importance of these skills varies according to the type of office; the type of practice, whether it is a specialty or general practice; the job being performed; and the staff being managed.

Conceptual skills involve the ability to acquire, analyze, and interpret information in a logical manner. These skills help to put an idea or concept into perspective and perceive how this idea would affect the whole practice.

Human relations skills aid in understanding people and allow effective interaction with them. These skills are vital in a health profession and involve communication, motivation, and an ability to lead.

> **PRACTICE NOTE**
> Human relations skills aid you in understanding people and allow you to interact with them.

Administrative skills are those that help you to use all of the other skills effectively in performing administrative functions. These include the ability to establish and follow policies and procedures, process paperwork in an organized manner, and coordinate activities in the office.

Technical skills include understanding and being able to supervise effectively the specific processes, practices, and techniques required of specific jobs in the business office. This is the use of all of the knowledge of dentistry and business that allows the performance of day-to-day operations in the office.

The Ethical Administrative Assistant

In addition to the basic skills the administrative assistant should possess, the professional attitude and ethics of this person have a significant influence on the staff. The following suggestions may identify some attributes of an ethical, caring administrative assistant:

- *Respect the dentist and the practice concepts.* Being respectful of a dentist employer means not circumventing him or her with issues or concerns. If an administrative assistant has an idea to improve the practice, discuss it with the employer. If there are problems with a task or staff person, share these concerns. Believe in the dentist and the practice, and support the objectives that have been defined. If a person stays in a practice in which unethical conduct occurs, he or she is essentially supporting this type of practice; thus, one's personal ethics become questionable.
- *Be a good listener.* Listen with the eyes; hear what the other person is saying; ask questions; and restate the ideas to be sure to understand the person's message.
- *Maintain frequent communication.* For people to follow someone, they must know who that person is, what he or she represents and can do, as well as his or her vision. To do this, tell and show them. Disseminate ideas in meetings and in day-to-day interactions with the staff. Cultivate relationships outside the office, to have a network of contacts from which to draw information when a task is to be done. As an administrative assistant, written and verbal communication must be continuous and supportive. Take time to communicate positive responses to the staff. The attitude presented to others affects their performance both positively and negatively. Let the staff know that you possess the skills and knowledge to lead them in their daily workload and that you, too, are capable of performing the tasks that you assign. Frequent communication does not relate to staff interaction only. It must be practiced with patients. They must understand relevant issues

that relate to their dental care and must receive frequent communication from and about the office.

- *Utilize feedback.* Recognize nonverbal cues; use feedback as a positive source of communication; and transmit feedback between management and staff.
- *Make ethical decisions.* Gather facts and analyze problems; develop alternatives; determine ethical issues involved; brainstorm with staff members; determine what actions should be taken and if they are practical; and evaluate the results of decision making.
- *Avoid unnecessary delays in decision making.* Sound decisions should be made as soon as possible; if conflicts go unresolved, greater problems may be created.
- *Delegate authority.* Show confidence in the staff members by allowing them to assume responsibility; provide freedom for them to work.
- *Identify constraints within which work must be done.* Establish time limits on production needs; allow staff members to develop their own approaches within the defined framework.
- *Exercise self-control.* Emotional outbursts don't lead to constructive management; don't "talk down" to staff members.
- *Make time available to staff.* Don't be too busy to listen to a staff person. This doesn't mean dropping everything to listen, but rather making time available for staff input.
- *Respect diversity.* The ethical administrative assistant must understand that the world is diverse and will continue to become even more diverse in the future. This means that the administrative assistant must respect diversity of all people, whether it is in ethnicity, race, gender, or age.
- *Build and develop strong followers.* One of the hallmarks of a successful administrative assistant is to surround oneself with action-oriented, dedicated followers. By showing confidence in the followers' abilities, providing challenging assignments, and being genuinely concerned, the administrative assistant garners respect, loyalty, and commitment while inspiring high-quality performance. In essence, the administrative assistant makes it easier to delegate and free himself or herself to devote more energy to issues that require his or her time. The key in this characteristic is for the administrative assistant to be genuine and honest in delegation and simply not delegate duties that have no challenge or are not recognized.
- *Be visible.* An administrative assistant cannot hide behind a desk and be a leader. There is nothing arrogant or inappropriate about letting others know what the administrative assistant and other members of the staff have accomplished. Share a complimentary memo with the staff or patients when significant achievements have been made. Participate and encourage staff members to participate in activities that place the people and the office in the spotlight. Be cautious not to take on too much. However, complete what is taken on with quality and panache.
- *Learn from mistakes.* Everyone makes mistakes, so don't agonize over them. Find ways to avoid making the same mistake again. Avoid assigning the blame to others. Some individuals consistently blame others for their mistakes. This characteristic does not make a good administrative assistant. Leadership is about accepting the mistake, moving forward, and not wallowing in the past.

- *Expand the leadership role.* An administrative assistant or office manager must extend the leadership role beyond the dental office. Make an effort to become involved in other professional or business groups that will provide valuable information for the office and offer the opportunity to place the office in the spotlight.

STAFF COMMUNICATION

Communication is an essential element in management and becomes a vital link in establishing a meaningful relationship among the administrative assistant, the dentist, other members of the staff, and the patient. The basic definition of communication is to understand and be understood by another person. Bob Adams states in his book, *Streetwise Managing People: Lead Your Staff to Peak Performance*, that "Quality Communication = Positive Interaction." When an office staff employs positive, constructive communication, it is sending a consistent message. The relative success of a dental practice is measured by the ability of the staff members to communicate with each other and the patient.

Communicating with staff members is in many ways like communicating with patients. Information is being transmitted with another person; and therefore understanding. However, the difference in communication with staff members is that the status of the persons involved has changed and the channels of communication may be more complex. To achieve quality communication, consider following the simple steps suggested in Box 2-3.

Channels of Communication

As a dental practice increases in size, the channels of communication become more complicated. Formal and informal communication exists. A formal communication channel is dictated by the type of management that exists in the practice. Formal communication may be downward, upward, or horizontal.

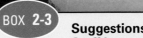

BOX 2-3 **Suggestions for Creating Positive Staff Interactions**

- Help others to be right, not wrong.
- Whenever possible, have fun.
- Be enthusiastic.
- Seek ways for new ideas to work, not reasons why they won't.
- Be bold and courageous; take chances.
- Help others achieve success.
- Maintain a positive mental attitude.
- Maintain confidentiality.
- Verify information given to you before you repeat what you hear; avoid gossip.
- Speak positively about others whenever the opportunity arises.
- Say "thank you" for kind gestures or a job well done.
- Express a happy attitude in your nonverbal communication.
- If you don't have anything positive to say, don't say anything.

Downward communication is exemplified when a dentist issues an order, or mandate, that is disseminated to the staff member at the next level. The basic channel is shown in Figure 2-3. A more complex system, as shown in Figure 2-4, illustrates an office as it increases in staff size, including several dentists and auxiliaries. Downward communication includes instructions, explanations, and communication that aid the employee in performing work.

Upward channels of communication are vital in a formal setting. Employees should be free to express attitudes and feelings. This type of communication reverses the flow of information in Figures 2-3 and 2-4, and is generally of a reporting nature.

It may include suggestions, complaints, or grievances. A lack of upward communication may result in dissatisfied employees.

Horizontal communication is essential for a larger organization. This type of communication involves transmittal of information from one department to another. This type of communication exists within large offices, clinics, hospitals, and dental schools.

Informal channels of communication can also be referred to as the "grapevine." This form of communication is often feared by administrative assistants but, if handled effectively, can provide the assistant with insight into staff emotions. Frequently the grapevine carries rumors, personal interpretations, or distorted

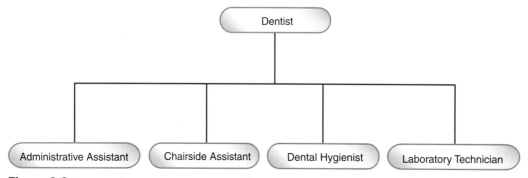

Figure 2-3 Downward communication as exemplified in a traditional dental practice.

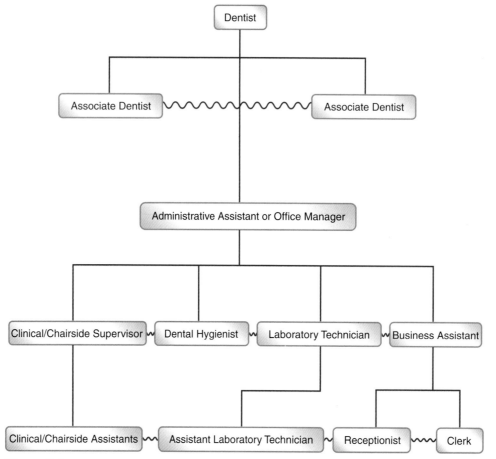

Figure 2-4 Downward and horizontal communication shown in an organizational chart of a group practice. Note that the levels of the dentists may vary according to the organization of the practice.

information. Fear often causes an active grapevine. It becomes the responsibility of the administrative assistant to listen to the grapevine and eliminate rumors by explaining the true facts. Thus the administrative assistant develops skill in handling tension created by the grapevine.

Empowering Employees

In Chapter 1, *empowerment* was defined as follows

> Just as the dentist leader has empowered the administrative assistant or office manager, this person should also provide the staff working in the business office the power and authority to accomplish office objectives.

The dentist who gives employees the power, ability, and permission to accomplish office objectives and perform legal tasks independently will have the edge over the competition. To be successful, the dentist must be able and willing to recognize the value that each employee brings to the office. In Bob Adams' book, *Streetwise Managing People: Lead Your Staff to Peak Performance*, the author declares that "empowered employees attempt to work above and beyond their anticipated capabilities." He recommends that to empower employees, an environment must be created in which the staff does the following:

- Behaves as an owner of the job and company
- Behaves in a responsible manner
- Sees the consequences of the work they do
- Knows how they are doing and how they are valued in the practice
- Is included in determining solutions to problems
- Has direct input into the way in which the work they do is done
- Spends a good deal of time smiling
- Asks others if they need help

 PRACTICE NOTE
To be successful, the dentist must be able and willing to recognize the value that each employee brings to the office.

Many concepts that Adams introduces seem to show common sense. When applied to a dental practice, these concepts seem to fit like a glove. Box 2-4 lists concepts that can be adapted easily to any dental practice to empower each member of the staff to become a meaningful member of the dental team.

Conducting a Staff Meeting

Two types of staff meetings commonly occur in the dental office: (1) morning "huddle" meetings and (2) routine team or staff meetings, which occur at least monthly.

The "huddle" meeting occurs once a day, most often in the morning, before the day begins. It lasts about 10 to 15 minutes, reviewing all of the patients for the day, preventive and restorative work that needs to be done, emergency times, patient concerns, and any radiographs to be taken. During

---

BOX 2-4   Concepts to Empower Employees

- Create a communication process that is complete, consistent, and clearly understood by all members of the staff.
- Ensure that all employees understand what is expected of them in their respective job positions.
- Provide each employee with the appropriate training, information, and materials to successfully accomplish their job duties.
- Clearly define and establish evaluation instruments for the responsibilities for each job.
- Create controls that are guidelines that allow flexibility.
- Encourage and practice behaviors that promote encouragement, support, and clear feedback to employees.
- Encourage and promote a sense of responsibility in each employee.
- Encourage and promote continuing education and credentialing.
- Create opportunities for staff members to work together in teams.
- Make it easy for people praise each other. Make the office one that recognizes and acknowledges praiseworthy actions.
- Listen to employees at all times. Make the office systems listen to the employees.
- Trust the employees.

---

this time patient management problems can be addressed, staff assignments can be made for assorted expanded duties, and business activities reviewed. Some office staff expand this meeting to twice a day and review the morning patients before beginning the afternoon assignments. Such meetings provide the opportunity to adequately prepare for patient treatment and ensure that the entire team is tuned in to rendering patient care.

Regularly scheduled staff or team meetings should become a routine part of the dental practice and should occur at least once a month. They are an effective means of keeping communication channels open. The staff meeting provides an opportunity to define and review the goals for the practice and help to motivate the staff. Although criticism may be part of a staff meeting, such a meeting should not be designed as a gripe session. The time and length of the staff meeting will vary according to the needs of the staff. Some offices schedule an hour per week or month, others close the office for a half or a full day for a retreat session, and still others find luncheon or breakfast meetings effective.

 PRACTICE NOTE
The staff meeting provides an opportunity to define and review the goals for the practice.

An agenda may be used in planning a staff meeting. The agenda, combined with the list of rules in Box 2-5, expedites the business objectives of the staff meeting.

Managing Conflict

Some administrative assistants become defensive and irritated when confronted with a complaint. Some individuals feel that a complaint is a personal reflection. Conflicts are normal between an administrative assistant and an employee or between

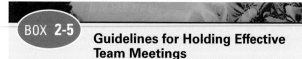

BOX 2-5   Guidelines for Holding Effective Team Meetings

- Notify each staff member of the time and place of the staff meeting. The use of e-mail will ensure that all parties are sent the information.
- Request a return reply for attendance.
- Determine the priority of agenda items.
- Obtain suggestions for these items from the staff members.
- Provide a copy of the agenda to each staff member, and adhere to the agenda items.
- Review accomplishments.
- Determine goals and needs for change.
- Establish a method for accomplishing these goals.
- Review outcomes of the meeting.
- Provide keyboarded minutes to the staff.
- Maintain a strict meeting schedule.
- Don't allow one person to monopolize the meeting.
- Don't turn the meeting into a gripe session.

a patient and a member of the staff; however, concern should be raised if numerous complaints arise, because this may indicate a serious problem.

Regardless of the nature of the complaint, the administrative assistant should review the details of the complaint and seek to resolve the problem quickly. Steps in resolving the problem might include the following:

- *Make time available* as soon as possible to discuss the problem. A delay may result in additional conflict or may be interpreted to mean that the administrative assistant is not interested in listening to the problem.
- *Listen patiently* to all the issues, keeping an open mind. The administrative assistant can gain the staff member's confidence by encouraging the person to talk and indicating that there is an intention to provide fair treatment.
- *Determine the real issue.* Frequently a complaint is made about a problem, when in reality a deeper concern is the real issue. For example, a person may be complaining about unfair work assignments, when actually the source of the problem is a personality clash between two staff members.
- *Exercise self-control.* Avoid arguments or expressions of personality conflicts between the complaining parties. Emotional outbursts generally do not lead to constructive resolution of the problem. Should this result, it is wise to terminate the meeting until a future meeting can be scheduled and the problem can be discussed in a calm manner.
- *Avoid a delay in decision making.* A dental office is a relatively small business organization, and allowing a conflict to go unresolved can cause undue stress on the entire staff. If it is necessary to delay a decision, let the persons involved know the status of the problem.
- *Maintain a record.* Documentation of meetings or discussions is helpful should future conflict arise over the same problem. It is impossible to recall all of the issues about an incident; therefore, information should be retained in the employee file or appropriate area for future reference.

It is not easy to resolve conflict. Most of us wish to avoid it. However, conflict will arise whenever two or more people are working together. As an administrative assistant, try to be fair and objective. If these suggestions are followed, at least an attempt to resolve the complaint in a professional manner will have been made; this may avoid minor conflicts that can escalate into major crises.

Barriers to Staff Communication

Barriers that exist in patient communication are prejudice, poor listening, preoccupation, impatience, and even impaired hearing. These barriers all exist within the staff. Additional barriers, such as status or position, resistance to change and new ideas, or attitudes about work, compound communication difficulties with coworkers. Because these barriers exist, administrative assistants should never assume that the message being sent will be received as it was intended. They should be aware of potential misinterpretations and work to overcome barriers to improve channels of communication with the staff.

Periodically the staff should evaluate its exchange of information and determine if all channels of communication are open to everyone. During a staff meeting, an agenda item might be the completion of a questionnaire that would indicate each staff member's feelings about office communication.

ADVANTAGES OF HIRING A SKILLED ADMINISTRATIVE ASSISTANT

A dentist today can ill afford the risk of hiring inexperienced personnel to manage the business office. In addition to having a broad knowledge of dentistry, the administrative assistant should be curious, highly organized, and able to accept responsibility and make decisions, as well as have an understanding of computers and other automated business equipment, possess skills in management, and communicate with people.

Few statistics are available, but it seems that in the past dentists have hired persons with a little knowledge of dentistry and minimal experience, or they have promoted chairside/clinical assistants to administrative assistants. Because administrative assistants need a broad background in dentistry, it appears that the last arrangement would have a distinct advantage if the assistant were willing to accept the transition. Many dentists today are hiring administrative assistants with a strong background in business and providing a rigorous training program in dental terminology and concepts. If the clinical assistant is transitioned to the administrative role this will require the clinical assistant become more involved in the financial systems of the office. The administrative assistant today is responsible for a myriad of dental, financial, and governmental forms. Therefore, a strong business background is highly desirable. Regardless through which door the administrative assistant arrives in this position it is desirable to hire a person with education in both business and dental assisting. In the past the Dental Assistant National Board (DANB) offered a specialty examination for Certified Dental Practice Management Assistant (CDPMA) but this certification is no longer available. The advantages of hiring an educated administrative assistant are listed in Box 2-6.

BOX 2-6 Advantages of Hiring an Educated Administrative Assistant

An educated administrative assistant has the following attributes:

- Understands basic dental terminology
- Understands interpersonal communication
- Understands clinical data
- Is able to transpose clinical data to financial data
- Is able to explain treatment procedures to a patient
- Can promote or sell dental care
- Understands the consequences of dental neglect
- Practices infection-control procedures
- Implements OSHA regulations
- Understands appointment sequencing for various dental procedures
- Is able to manage emergency procedures
- Is less likely to make common errors

TIME MANAGEMENT

Learning to Use Time Efficiently

A vital aspect of the job as an administrative assistant is **time management**. There is more to working efficiently than just knowing how to perform a specific task. Administrative assistants also need to know when to perform each task, how to choose which job to do first, and how long each project will take. Understanding the relationship of time to production is also important. All of these together make up time management.

Much research has been done over the years on time and motion studies in the dental treatment room. These studies have resulted in the dental profession implementing the concepts of four-handed dentistry and the utilization of a chairside/clinical assistant to increase productivity and reduce stress. Less emphasis has been placed on production in the dental business office. However, much can be learned from the research general business has done on time management. Remember, although dentistry is a healthcare system, it is still a small business and has profit as its objective. Thus time management is a vital component in the dental practice.

Time management in the dental business office involves planning, scheduling work, and avoiding wasted time. The behaviors that waste time in the business office are failing to plan and budget time, giving in to interruptions, failing to follow through and complete a task, slowness in reading and making decisions, performing unnecessary work, and failing to delegate. Other time wasters are lack of privacy and desk clutter. Solutions to many common time wasters are suggested in Box 2-7.

To determine the effectiveness of one's own time management, assess the way work is currently being performed. Determine ways to use time more effectively, or confirm that time is already being used efficiently. Evaluation of time management is an ongoing process and can be done routinely by recording the way time is currently being spent; analyzing how time is spent; determining what activities can be adjusted to make a worker more effective; scheduling activities daily, weekly, monthly, and long range; and adhering to the schedule. Efficient time management requires organizing individual tasks, maintaining daily schedules, analyzing daily tasks, scheduling major projects, establishing deadlines, and organizing workflow.

Maintaining Daily Schedules

To efficiently maintain a daily schedule, it is necessary to use a calendar of activities and tasks and a "to-do" list, determine priorities, show flexibility, use free time, and review the schedule with the dentist.

The use of a calendar and personal appointment book as well as the office appointment book is necessary in maintaining a daily schedule. A desk or electronic calendar provides a method for keeping track of the daily schedule and is used for short- and long-range scheduling. Make entries neatly if done manually, be consistent in making entries, and avoid making confidential entries if an electronic calendar is used that is accessible to others.

A to-do list should provide a summary of all pending tasks, not just those to be done on a specific day. This list need not include routine daily tasks, such as opening and closing the office or opening mail. Delete each task upon completion, and transfer tasks not completed to a list for the following day.

BOX 2-7 Solutions to Eliminate Time Wasters

Time Waster	Solution
• Lack of goals	• Prepare a to-do list and use it.
• Telephone interruptions	• Use an answering machine or voicemail during specified work times.
• Procrastination	• Do it first!
• Feeling tired, stressed, or irritable	• Schedule a thorough physical examination; develop a wellness plan; enroll in a stress-management course.
• Lack of future plans	• Develop short- and long-range goals.
• Disorganized work area	• Purchase organizers; put away work when finished; don't begin a new project until one is complete.
• Accepting too many jobs	• Learn to say no!
• Waiting for information/return calls	• Use an answering machine or voicemail.
• Incomplete work	• Plan time to finish projects with no interruptions.
• Socializing with coworkers	• Avoid the situations; restrict others from too much socializing.
• Unnecessary work	• Analyze the task; eliminate it if not necessary.

Determine priorities by ranking each task on the list by its priority or its level of urgency and importance. Items on the list can be ranked as: (1) tasks that must be completed immediately, (2) tasks that must be completed that day, and (3) tasks that must be done whenever there is time.

Be flexible in making plans for the day, because emergencies arise and new priority tasks will be identified. For instance, the dentist may need the administrative assistant to produce an important document immediately that was not on the list. At this point, it may be necessary to seek help from other staff members to complete other pressing tasks. With total team effort, a reprioritizing of previously identified tasks can be accomplished quickly to meet unplanned needs.

In addition to the routine to-do list, another list could be kept that details various tasks that should be completed when time permits. Such a list provides tasks to do when there is a slow time or when there are no patients scheduled.

DESIGNING A PROCEDURAL MANUAL

The procedural manual is a valuable instrument in maintaining maximum efficiency in the dental office while providing a means of communication. It includes the dentist's philosophy of the practice and defines the job responsibilities for each team member. The manual also states in specific detail the technique to be implemented for each procedure in both the business and clinical areas of the office. Although the manual should be written under the direction of the dentist, each member of the team should contribute equally in the development of the manual to provide a total team effort. This manual should be made available to each staff member and may be posted for the staff on the computer at the in-house public site.

The following list of guidelines provides subjects to be included in an office procedural manual. Purchase basic office manual formats and add inserts for the dentist's philosophy and specific duties relating to the practice. Templates are also available for manuals in Microsoft Office Templates online. Individual tabs can be made as needed.

Guidelines for a Procedural Manual

I. Statement of purpose or objective of the manual
II. Statement of philosophy for the practice
III. Table of contents
IV. Office communications
    A. Vocabulary
    B. Telecommunications
    C. Reception techniques
    D. Written communication
    E. Patient education
    F. Confidentiality
V. Staff policies
    A. Conduct
    B. Grooming and appearance
    C. Dress codes: clinical and business office attire
    D. Staff meetings
        1. Daily
        2. Regular
    E. Use of office phones for personal need
    F. Personal cell phone usage
VI. Employment policies
    A. Probationary period
    B. Promotion
    C. Hours of work
    D. Overtime
    E. Holidays
    F. Vacations
    G. Absences and leaves
    H. Salaries
    I. Insurance
    J. Additional benefits
    K. Termination of employment
    L. Personal telephone calls and personal mail
VII. Office records
    A. Infection control
        1. Clinical
        2. Records handling
    B. Patient records
    C. OSHA records
    D. Material Safety Data Sheets (MSDSs)
    E. Employee records
    F. Transfer of records
    G. Accounts receivable
    H. Accounts payable
    I. Filing
VIII. Infection-control policy
    A. OSHA guidelines
    B. Health risk categories
    C. Nomenclature
    D. Disinfection and sterilization guidelines
    E. Waste management
    F. Medical history procedures
    G. Universal precautions
    H. Preventive vaccinations
IX. Clinical procedures
    A. Emergencies
    B. Tray setups
    C. Sterilization
    D. Prescriptions
    E. Inventory system
X. Continuing education
XI. Professional organizations

Writing a Personnel Policy

As part of the office procedural manual, a well-defined personnel policy must be established. A fair and equitable personnel policy may help to eliminate conflicts that could arise among team members. The material in Box 2-8 illustrates a suggested personnel policy. This policy may be altered to satisfy the needs of an individual office.

BOX 2-8   Personnel Policies for the Office of Joseph W. Lake, DDS, and Ashley M. Lake, DDS

Probationary Period

Your first 3 months will be considered a probationary period, during which Drs. Joseph and Ashley Lake will see how you progress with the new work. During this period your employment may be terminated without notice. The dentist will create a Merit Rating Report at the termination of the probationary period and quarterly thereafter. This report will be used as the basis for salary increases and promotions.

Promotion

Your demonstrated ability to perform your job well, your attendance and punctuality record, and your relationships with employees will all have a bearing on your opportunities for promotion and advancement in salary. Any outside courses of study that result in skills in addition to those noted on your application will be added to your record to ensure complete information when reviewing your record for advancement. All employees will be reviewed every 6 months.

Hours of Work

The office is open from 8:00 AM to 5:00 PM Monday and Wednesday, and 8:00 AM to 9:00 PM on Tuesday and Thursday. On Fridays the office is closed. Lunch hour is from 12:00 PM to 1:00 PM. The basic week totals 35 working hours that will be assigned by each dentist.

Overtime

Overtime salary is paid for units of ½ hour. Fractions of less than ½ hour of overtime are not reported. If your salary is less than $3520 per month, compensation for work authorized by the dentist in excess of 35 hours is at the rate of time and one half beyond 35 hours in any week, or for work on Saturdays, Sundays, and holidays.

Staff meetings are held daily before seeing patients. You are expected to attend each of these meetings to plan for the day's activities. Each month, at an announced time, a staff meeting is held for a minimum of 1 hour to plan for practice development. All staff must be in attendance unless otherwise excused.

Holidays

You will have the following legal holidays with pay: New Year's Day, Memorial Day, Independence Day, Labor Day, Thanksgiving Day, and Christmas Day. When the office is closed for a religious holiday or other holiday, an announcement will be made in advance.

Vacations

Requests for vacation time in excess of 1 day must be made 30 days in advance. You will be entitled to 2 weeks of vacation after completing 12 months of continuous employment, and 4 weeks of vacation after 10 years of employment. A legal holiday that falls within the vacation period adds 1 day to your vacation. When a vacation falls within a vacation period, salary will be paid in advance to the latest regular salary payment date falling within the vacation period.

Absences and Leaves

Regular attendance and punctuality are necessary for smooth functioning of the dental office, and your record in this respect will be considered in determining your advancement and salary adjustment. However, there are certain absences that are unavoidable and for which provision will

be made. In each case, the dentists should be notified in advance when possible, or before 7:30 AM on the day of your absence. If you fail to make proper notification, the unadvised absence will be counted as absence without salary.

Sick Leave for Your Own Confining Illness

When absence is for your own illness, salary is paid for up to 1 day for each month of employment, cumulative to 30 days. If you need sick leave in addition to the above, such a request should be made to Dr. Lake for additional time without pay.

Court Duty

If you are required to serve as a juror or witness, your absence is considered as a leave with salary.

Death in the Immediate Family

If there is a death in your immediate family, up to 3 days of leave may be granted with salary.

Leave of Absence for Other Reasons

If you request a leave of absence for other reasons or for a longer period than is provided with salary, various factors will be taken into consideration, including your previous work and attendance records, the length of leave you are requesting, the work needs of the office, and any other pertinent factors.

Salaries

Payment of your salary is by check on a weekly basis, covering salary through Wednesday of the current week. Salary checks are distributed each Friday. Salary increases are considered every 6 months. The quality of your work, the amount of responsibility you assume, your attendance and punctuality records, your attitude toward the staff and patients, and your length of service are factors that enter into the consideration. Deductions from salary regularly include withholding tax and Social Security. Deductions for group insurance, hospital care, and other benefits are made only on written request.

Insurance

To help provide security in times of sickness and hospitalization, health insurance is available as follows: membership in a group health insurance plan is available to all those employed up to 1 year on a payroll deduction basis.

Staff members may select this insurance at their own expense for the first 12 months of employment. Deductions for hospital care are made the first payday of each month. At the end of 12 months, Dr. Lake will pay this coverage upon a successful merit rating evaluation. Coverage of your spouse and dependent children under 19 years of age may be included in your hospital care contract.

Social Security is provided through payments by you and Dr. Lake to the U.S. government. Your share of the cost is deducted from each salary payment.

Additional Benefits

In addition to regular salary increases, the members of the staff are eligible for several additional benefits.

(Continued)

BOX 2-8   **Personnel Policies for the Office of Joseph W. Lake, DDS, and Ashley M. Lake, DDS—cont'd**

Uniform Stipend

Dr. Lake will provide a uniform stipend as follows:

- Chairside or clinical assistants/hygienists will wear surgical scrubs with outer laboratory coats provided by the office, for which all laundry will be provided. At the end of 6 months of successful employment, Dr. Lake will issue an additional stipend to the Central Uniform Shop for the cost of shoes.
- Administrative assistants will receive a dress stipend not to exceed $1200 at the end of 6 months. At the end of 12 months, an additional dress/uniform stipend will be issued not to exceed $2000. Thereafter a stipend will be issued annually not to exceed $2750.

Professional Organizations

At the end of 12 months of successful employment, the dues of your professional organization will be paid by Dr. Lake. The statement and proof of membership must be submitted to Dr. Lake for payment.

Education and Travel

You are encouraged to increase your skills at all times. To ensure your exposure to current changes in dentistry, Dr. Lake will provide the following benefits: After 6 months of employment, payment not in excess of $450 for any educational seminar; after 12 months of employment, 3 days absence with pay and $1200 applicable to coursework or educational travel; after 5 years of employment, 5 days absence with pay and $2500 applicable to coursework or educational travel.

Profit Sharing

After completion of 2 full years of successful employment, Dr. Lake will provide the following profit-sharing bonus to each staff member: 2% of total business in excess of $125,000, plus 2% of total receipts in excess of $125,000.

Infection-Control Policy

An effective infection-control program has been implemented in the office for the protection of staff members, patients, and family members. It is recommended that you adhere to the *Infection Control Policy Handbook* and that you are aware of all updates of this manual as they occur. The cost of Hepatitis B vaccine and TB vaccine will be covered by the office.

It is highly recommended that you receive other protective vaccines for childhood diseases not previously contracted. You will be compensated for such immunization. Each employee is expected to follow the basic guidelines of the OSHA bloodborne pathogens standard as follows:

- A written exposure control plan must be updated annually.
- Use standard precautions.
- Consideration, implementation, and use of safer needles and sharps
- Use of engineering and work practice controls, using appropriate personal protective equipment (ppe) such as gloves, face and eye protection, and gowns.
- Use of labels and color coding for sharps disposal boxes and proper containers for regulated waste, contaminated laundry, and other specimens.
- Employee training
- Decontamination of surfaces
- Recommended decontamination and processing of all dental instruments and equipment

Termination of Employment
Resignation

You are asked to give 2 weeks written notice of resignation. If you have been employed for 6 months or more and you resign during the vacation period having given 2 weeks notice, you will be compensated for your vacation according to the vacation schedule.

Release

If you are released from your position for reasons other than misconduct, in which case no notice is given, you will have notice or salary in lieu of notice as follows: If you have been employed for at least 6 but less than 12 months, 1 week; If you have been employed for 13 months or more, 2 weeks.

Personal Telephone Calls and Personal Mail/E-Mail

Telephone traffic is heavy at the Joseph W. Lake, DDS, and Ashley M. Lake, DDS, practice. Personal telephone calls affect the workload in two ways: They prohibit incoming calls from patients, and they take time from your job. Limit the number of personal calls, and receive incoming calls only in an emergency. Personal cell phones should be turned off or set on "silent" mode during office hours. Similarly the volume of mail is heavy at the office; therefore, do not use the office address for personal mail/e-mail.

HIRING PRACTICES

Writing a Job Description

A current, accurate job description should exist for each position in the dental office. These job descriptions aid employees in telling prospective employees what will be expected of them on the job and assist in training new staff members.

To write a job description, a job analysis must be done. A job analysis involves observing the employee and gathering information about the job. List the tasks that make up the job, and determine the skills, personality characteristics, and educational background needed for the employee to per-form this job satisfactorily. The staff then reviews the job description. It is revised as necessary and placed in the procedural manual. An outline for a job description is shown in Figure 2-5.

Writing a Job Advertisement

The content of an advertisement for new staff members should be the result of a well-thought-out job description. List the skills the person is expected to have, require a resumé, and identify attractive features of the job such as benefits, salary, and working conditions. To attract highly qualified candidates, the advertisement cannot be a mundane, brief statement seeking

Job Title _____
You will report to _____

GENERAL OBJECTIVES:

The administrative assistant will manage the day-to-day activities of the business office. This person will be responsible for maintaining office documents, patient, employee, and governmental records; scheduling patients; interviewing and managing staff; managing accounts receivable and payable; managing inventory and recall systems; operating electronic office equipment; and maintaining various types of telecommunications systems.

SPECIFIC OBJECTIVES:

Maintain office documents
- Select and complete patient clinical records
- Manage insurance claim forms
- Establish and maintain a recall system
- Maintain employee records
- Complete and maintain governmental forms

Maintain an accounts receivable system
- Maintain accounts receivable activity
- Prepare bank deposits
- Prepare statements
- Follow up delinquent accounts

Perform accounts payable activities
- Verify invoices with monthly statements
- Write checks
- Reconcile the bank statement
- Prepare materials for the accountant

Supervise staff personnel
- Prepare job descriptions
- Interview and screen potential employees
- Determine staff needs and schedules
- Orient new staff
- Evaluate staff

Perform support duties
- Establish equipment maintenance program
- Plan for update and risk management seminars
- Implement state and federal regulations
- Help support staff as needed

JOB CRITERIA:

Education
- Certified/Registered Dental Assistant, Certified Dental Office Manager, or a minimum of 5 years experience in business management
- Knowledge of electronic office automation
- Formal business courses
- Knowledge or experience in management

Personal requirements
- Must be able to work with any employee and be able to resolve conflicts between employees
- Must be able to discuss all dental/financial needs with patients and be objective and pleasant to them
- Must be able to cooperate with other dental office staff personnel
- Must be able to work with the doctor and convey needs to the staff in a participatory manner

SALARY:

$40,000 - $69,500 plus benefits
Salary based on the salary chart in the office procedure manual

Date prepared: 01/25/--

Figure 2-5 A sample job description.

inexperienced people. Periodically look at the classified ads in the local paper for ideas in other allied health professions. Compare the two advertisements in Figures 2-6 and 2-7. Which advertisement presents a greater challenge for a prospective employee? The ad seeking an inexperienced person will probably get more response, but this isn't a contest to get the largest response. The procedure of advertising should seek to screen potential candidates. A request for an educated person cuts down on potential training costs for the dentist and can ensure a minimal level of education.

Interviewing Prospective Employees

Part of the management role for the administrative assistant may be interviewing applicants for a position on the staff. This is an important responsibility and requires a great deal of skill. The suggestions in Box 2-9 may aid you when conducting an interview.

Legal Considerations in Hiring

There are several legal factors to be considered in hiring an employee. These include application forms, citizenship status, and testing.

An employer must ensure that application forms avoid any questions regarding race or ethnic background. Furthermore, each applicant who completes an application form must be provided with the same type of form. Be certain that the application form used in the office does not violate any state requirements. For example, a state may deem it unlawful to use a lie-detector test. Thus, such a question on an application asking the applicant to take a lie detector test could be in violation of state law.

It is illegal to discriminate against any individual (other than an alien not authorized to work in the United States) in hiring, discharging, recruiting, or referring for a fee because of that individual's national origin or citizenship

Registered Dental Assistant who is ambitious and skilled in ergonomic four-handed dentistry. Duties require clinical, laboratory, and business office management skills in a general practice. Must have expanded functions credential. Attractive salary and benefits. Write to: Joseph W. Lake, D.D.S., 611 Main St. S.E., Grand Rapids, MI 49502

Figure 2-6 A sample newspaper advertisement.

Dental Office Administrative Assistant: Interested in an exciting position you find in a large, diverse, professional office? A group dental practice is expanding its clinical facilities. Position demands strong supervisory skills, ability to work effectively under pressure, use good judgment, and be able to accept responsibility. Forward your resume to: Box #2589, Grand Rapids News, Grand Rapids, MI 49502

Figure 2-7 A sample blind advertisement.

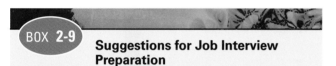

BOX 2-9 Suggestions for Job Interview Preparation

- Perform a task analysis of the proposed job.
- Determine the competencies needed to fulfill the job requirements.
- Prepare a well-defined job description.
- Have the applicant complete a job application.
- Determine how to measure an applicant's ability. Tests may be utilized to measure certain abilities, such as keyboarding speed and accuracy.
- Explain the requirements of the job completely.
- Determine key questions to ask in the interview.
- Review reactions toward the applicant. Were you comfortable? Was the applicant an active participant in the conversation? Was the individual shy or domineering?
- Make accurate observations about the applicant's answers, grammar, and nonverbal cues during the interview. Use a check-off form to ensure that each candidate is evaluated on the same basis.
- Record evaluations as soon as the interview is completed to assure that you don't forget the responses.
- Investigate references the applicant has provided. This confirms the accuracy of the applicant's statements.

status. It is illegal to discriminate against work-eligible individuals. It is in violation of federal law to hire an unauthorized (illegal) alien. An employer must require proof of an applicant's legal status, and the Immigration and Naturalization Service (INS) Form I-9 (Employment Eligibility Verification form) must be filled out before employment. Documents accepted for verification are listed on the Lists of Acceptable Documents available on the Form I-9 web site at www.formi9.com. See Figure 2-8

for a sample of the I-9 Form and the Lists of Acceptable Documents to establish employment eligibility.

Preemployment Testing

A variety of employment testing may include standardized tests, polygraph tests, and drug and alcohol tests. Although a small dental office seldom uses all these tests, it is possible that an institution or larger corporation with dental facilities may take advantage of them all.

Businesses such as a dental practice may legally use professionally developed standardized tests to verify knowledge, aptitude, and skills during a selection process. Tests used to screen applicants can become discriminatory when they serve to disqualify members of a minority culture who are unfamiliar with the language or concepts but are fully qualified for the job. Dentistry can avail itself of standardized tests developed by the Dental Assistants National Board and various state regulatory agencies. To create a new test when many such tests already exist can place a practitioner at potential legal risks.

Many private sector employers are considering drug and alcohol testing as a pre-employment requirement. The main type of test is a urinalysis, which is likely to be part of a pre-employment physical examination.

An employer refusing to hire someone with AIDS violates federal and state disability discrimination laws. Protection under Title VII of the 1964 Civil Rights Act has been extended to disabled persons, including those infected with the AIDS virus or who have tested positive for the HIV virus. An employer probably would not be justified in refusing to hire an individual with AIDS, unless the employer could establish that the prospective employee would endanger the health and safety of others. This issue is controversial for the dental care profession and must be met with a thorough understanding of both legal and ethical ramifications.

Conducting an Interview

Before conducting an interview, gather all of the information about each candidate, develop an outline of questions, and determine the physical setting for the interview. Often a neutral location such as a lounge or conference room will make the candidate feel more at ease.

As the interview begins, establish rapport with the candidate with a personal introduction, and create a sense of pleasantness with the candidate. Explain the purpose of the interview, and generate a relaxed atmosphere. During the interview motivate the candidate to participate.

The main part of the interview consists of asking questions, listening to responses, answering questions, and providing a transition from one discussion topic to another. Gain confidence in questioning the applicant to reflect each facet of the individual's background. Ask questions such as, "Tell me about your previous job experiences," "What is your attitude toward your previous working experience?" or "What do you feel your strengths and weaknesses are for the position available in this office?"

Common types of questions asked during an interview include direct, indirect, and hypothetical. The direct question generally elicits an expected response. An indirect question does not imply a yes or no response. The following examples illustrate the differences in these types of questions.

Direct: "Would you be opposed to traveling to a satellite office?"
Indirect: "How would you feel about traveling to a satellite office?"

A hypothetical question describes an actual situation and elicits a response from the candidate, as follows:

OMB No. 1615-0047; Expires 06/30/09

Department of Homeland Security
U.S. Citizenship and Immigration Services

Form I-9, Employment Eligibility Verification

Read instructions carefully before completing this form. The instructions must be available during completion of this form.

ANTI-DISCRIMINATION NOTICE: It is illegal to discriminate against work-authorized individuals. Employers CANNOT specify which document(s) they will accept from an employee. The refusal to hire an individual because the documents have a future expiration date may also constitute illegal discrimination.

Section 1. Employee Information and Verification *(To be completed and signed by employee at the time employment begins.)*

Print Name: Last	First	Middle Initial	Maiden Name
Address *(Street Name and Number)*		Apt. #	Date of Birth *(month/day/year)*
City	State	Zip Code	Social Security #

I am aware that federal law provides for imprisonment and/or fines for false statements or use of false documents in connection with the completion of this form.

I attest, under penalty of perjury, that I am (check one of the following):
- ☐ A citizen of the United States
- ☐ A noncitizen national of the United States (see instructions)
- ☐ A lawful permanent resident (Alien #) ______
- ☐ An alien authorized to work (Alien # or Admission #) ______ until (expiration date, if applicable - *month/day/year*)

Employee's Signature | Date *(month/day/year)*

Preparer and/or Translator Certification *(To be completed and signed if Section 1 is prepared by a person other than the employee.) I attest, under penalty of perjury, that I have assisted in the completion of this form and that to the best of my knowledge the information is true and correct.*

Preparer's/Translator's Signature | Print Name

Address *(Street Name and Number, City, State, Zip Code)* | Date *(month/day/year)*

Section 2. Employer Review and Verification *(To be completed and signed by employer. Examine one document from List A OR examine one document from List B and one from List C, as listed on the reverse of this form, and record the title, number, and expiration date, if any, of the document(s).)*

	List A	OR	List B	AND	List C
Document title:	______		______		______
Issuing authority:	______		______		______
Document #:	______		______		______
Expiration Date *(if any)*:	______		______		______
Document #:	______				
Expiration Date *(if any)*:	______				

CERTIFICATION: I attest, under penalty of perjury, that I have examined the document(s) presented by the above-named employee, that the above-listed document(s) appear to be genuine and to relate to the employee named, that the employee began employment on *(month/day/year)* ______ **and that to the best of my knowledge the employee is authorized to work in the United States. (State employment agencies may omit the date the employee began employment.)**

Signature of Employer or Authorized Representative | Print Name | Title

Business or Organization Name and Address *(Street Name and Number, City, State, Zip Code)* | Date *(month/day/year)*

Section 3. Updating and Reverification *(To be completed and signed by employer.)*

A. New Name *(if applicable)* | B. Date of Rehire *(month/day/year) (if applicable)*

C. If employee's previous grant of work authorization has expired, provide the information below for the document that establishes current employment authorization.

Document Title: ______ Document #: ______ Expiration Date *(if any)*: ______

I attest, under penalty of perjury, that to the best of my knowledge, this employee is authorized to work in the United States, and if the employee presented document(s), the document(s) I have examined appear to be genuine and to relate to the individual.

Signature of Employer or Authorized Representative | Date *(month/day/year)*

Form I-9 (Rev. 02/02/09) N Page 4

Figure 2-8 Federal Employment Eligibility Verification form (I-9). (From U.S. Citizen and Immigration Services, Department of Homeland Security, Washington, DC.)

(Continued)

LISTS OF ACCEPTABLE DOCUMENTS
All documents must be unexpired

LIST A	LIST B	LIST C
Documents that Establish Both Identity and Employment Authorization OR	Documents that Establish Identity AND	Documents that Establish Employment Authorization
1. U.S. Passport or U.S. Passport Card	1. Driver's license or ID card issued by a State or outlying possession of the United States provided it contains a photograph or information such as name, date of birth, gender, height, eye color, and address	1. Social Security Account Number card other than one that specifies on the face that the issuance of the card does not authorize employment in the United States
2. Permanent Resident Card or Alien Registration Receipt Card (Form I-551)		
3. Foreign passport that contains a temporary I-551 stamp or temporary I-551 printed notation on a machine-readable immigrant visa	2. ID card issued by federal, state or local government agencies or entities, provided it contains a photograph or information such as name, date of birth, gender, height, eye color, and address	2. Certification of Birth Abroad issued by the Department of State (Form FS-545)
4. Employment Authorization Document that contains a photograph (Form I-766)	3. School ID card with a photograph	3. Certification of Report of Birth issued by the Department of State (Form DS-1350)
	4. Voter's registration card	4. Original or certified copy of birth certificate issued by a State, county, municipal authority, or territory of the United States bearing an official seal
5. In the case of a nonimmigrant alien authorized to work for a specific employer incident to status, a foreign passport with Form I-94 or Form I-94A bearing the same name as the passport and containing an endorsement of the alien's nonimmigrant status, as long as the period of endorsement has not yet expired and the proposed employment is not in conflict with any restrictions or limitations identified on the form	5. U.S. Military card or draft record	
	6. Military dependent's ID card	5. Native American tribal document
	7. U.S. Coast Guard Merchant Mariner Card	
	8. Native American tribal document	6. U.S. Citizen ID Card (Form I-197)
	9. Driver's license issued by a Canadian government authority	
	For persons under age 18 who are unable to present a document listed above:	7. Identification Card for Use of Resident Citizen in the United States (Form I-179)
6. Passport from the Federated States of Micronesia (FSM) or the Republic of the Marshall Islands (RMI) with Form I-94 or Form I-94A indicating nonimmigrant admission under the Compact of Free Association Between the United States and the FSM or RMI	10. School record or report card	8. Employment authorization document issued by the Department of Homeland Security
	11. Clinic, doctor, or hospital record	
	12. Day-care or nursery school record	

Illustrations of many of these documents appear in Part 8 of the Handbook for Employers (M-274)

Form I-9 (Rev. 02/02/09) N Page 5

Figure 2-8, cont'd (From U.S. Citizen and Immigration Services, Department of Homeland Security, Washington, DC.)

Hypothetical: "If one of our patients told you he refused to pay an account because he didn't like the way he was treated, how would you respond?"

This type of question is valuable because it is as close as the interviewer will get to observing the candidate's behavior.

During the discussion the interviewer has two major functions: to gather information about the candidate's qualifications for the job in a nondiscriminatory manner, and to convey information to the candidate about the office and specific job responsibilities. By keeping questions and discussion relevant to the job, the first task will be achieved. The first task requires awareness of certain legal considerations related to interviewing. Rules of thumb for asking interview questions are shown in Box 2-10. Guidelines by the U.S. Department of Labor and the U.S. Equal Employment

---

BOX 2-10

Three Rules of Thumb for Interviewing

When asking interview questions, consider these rules of thumb:
1. Ask only for information that you intend to use to make hiring decisions.
2. Know how you will use the information to make a decision.
3. Recognize that it is difficult to defend the practice of seeking information that you do not use.

Opportunity Commission (EEOC) prohibit discriminatory hiring based on race, creed, color, gender, national origin, handicap, or age. Questions related to any of these as well as marital status, children, ownership of a house or car, credit rating, or type of military discharge can also be considered discriminatory. Questions that should and should not be asked during an interview include many of those shown in Box 2-11, and topics that should be avoided are listed in Box 2-12. The second task of the interview can be met if all of the following areas are included:

- Specific job responsibilities
- Orientation procedures
- Opportunities for advancement
- Management procedures
- Professional responsibilities
- Work hours, salary, and fringe benefits

Concluding an Interview

The conclusion of the interview is a good opportunity for the applicant to tour the office. This is a good time, if convenient, for the rest of the staff to meet the candidate. Inform the applicant of the plans for arriving at a decision and a date by which the decision will be made. Factors to avoid in making a decision are listed in Box 2-13.

Once all of the candidates have been interviewed and the decision made about each, the person to be hired should be contacted promptly. A letter of confirmation should be sent to the new employee stating the conditions of employment; that is, wages, hours, promotions, beginning date, and other conditions agreed on during previous discussions. The letter should identify probationary periods, which allow either party to terminate employment within an established period of time without fear of penalty. It is wise to have the employee sign the letter. A copy is then retained by the employee and a copy is placed in the employee file. A letter should also be sent to candidates not being hired, and their applications may remain on file if desired.

New Employee Training

A well-organized dental team provides a smooth transition for the new employee into the practice. The time frame for the new employee to become well established in the office will vary according to the individual office. The many activities involved in new employee training include the following:

- Describe how the practice is run and what standards are required of the staff.
- Explain the organizational chart and job descriptions.
- Complete employee documents, including federal and state tax forms.
- Review procedural techniques.
- Allow time for observation, but let the skills and responsibilities of the new employee be used as soon as possible.

BOX 2-11 Questions to Ask and Not to Ask During an Interview

Do Ask

- What was your absentee record at your prior place of employment?
- Do you know of any reason (for example, transportation) why you would be unable to get to work on time and on a regular basis?
- Are you available to work overtime?
- We are looking for employees with a commitment to this position. Are there any reasons why you might not stay with us?
- What are your career objectives?
- Do you foresee any reasons why you could not be assigned to a branch or satellite office?
- Where do you see yourself in 5 years?

Don't Ask

- Where were you born?
- Where and when did you graduate from high school?
- Do you have any handicaps?
- What religious holidays do you practice?
- Are you married?
- Do you plan to have children? How many?
- Do you own a home?
- Do you own a car?
- Do you have any debts?
- Can you provide three credit references?
- Is your spouse likely to be transferred?
- Is your spouse from this area?
- How old are you?
- How do you feel about working with members of a different race?
- What language(s) do your parents speak?

BOX 2-12 Topics to Avoid During the Interview Process

- Arrest records
- Marital status
- Maiden name
- Spouse's name
- Spouse's education
- Spouse's income
- Form of birth control
- Child care arrangements
- Lawsuits or legal complaints
- Ownership of car or residence
- Loans
- Insurance claims
- National origin
- Mother's maiden name
- Place of birth
- Disabilities
- Weight
- Age
- Date of high school graduation
- Religion
- Social organizations

BOX 2-13 Factors to Avoid in Making Staff Selections

In making a selection or recommendation for hiring a staff person, avoid making assumptions such as the following:

- The dentist or staff members might prefer employees of certain ethnic or racial origins.
- Those who come in contact with your employees might not want to deal with women or minorities.
- Coworkers might object.
- The job might involve unusual working conditions that would disqualify the applicant.

- Identify areas of strengths and weaknesses. Positive reinforcement is necessary to create confidence. However, poor performance should be altered to avoid reinforcement of less-than-quality work. It is easier to correct poor performance early in training rather than later, when it seriously affects office production.
- Provide additional training beyond the educational experiences already achieved. This may be accomplished within the office or may require a more formal setting in a nearby school.
- Evaluate the performance of the new employee regularly. This allows changes to be made in performance and provides the staff person with knowledge of his or her status.
- Review progress with adequate promotion via benefits or a pay increase.

- Terminate an employee if substandard performance continues. If all efforts to improve the employee's performance have failed, it is wise to terminate the employee promptly rather than continue with substandard performance.

KEY TERMS

Administrative assistant—A person whose role is often defined as secretary, receptionist, business assistant, or "front-desk person," and whose responsibilities include the day-to-day management of the dental practice.

Communication—The ability to understand and be understood.

Manager—A term often used to refer to an administrative assistant.

Time management—The ability to prioritize tasks, determine how long each project will take, and work effectively in managing time to production.

1. Write job descriptions for a chairside/clinical assistant, administrative assistant, and dental hygienist. What tasks should be identified for each of these jobs in a job analysis? Review classified advertisements in a local paper.
2. Compare the content of ads in various health occupations. What characteristics appeal to you in these ads? Why?

3. Create an interview outline that lists the sequence of events of an interview.
4. Develop a series of questions that will determine a candidate's skills for a job.

Please refer to the student workbook for additional learning activities.

BIBLIOGRAPHY

Adams B: *Streetwise managing people: lead your staff to peak performance,* Holbrook, Mass, 1998, Adams Media Corporation.

Fulton-Calkins PJ: *The administrative professional,* ed 13, Mason, Ohio, 2007, Thomson South-Western.

Hastings W, Potter R: *Trust me,* Colorado Springs, 2004, WaterBrook Press.

Ishimoto C: Unlocking teamwork potential, *Dental Economics,* 99 (September): 1, 2007.

McNamara C: *Field guide to leadership and supervision in business,* Minneapolis, 2002, Authenticity Consulting.

Miles L: *Dynamic dentistry: practice management tools and strategy for breakthrough success,* Virginia Beach, VA, 2003, Link Publishing.

Perkins PS: *The art and science of communication: tools for effective communication in the workplace,* New York, 2008, John Wiley & Sons.

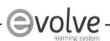

Please visit http://evolve.elsevier.com/Finkibeiner/practice for additional practice activities.

3 Patient Management

LEARNING OUTCOMES

- Define glossary terms.
- Understand patient needs.
- Explain the special needs of patients.
- Identify barriers to communication.
- Recognize nonverbal cues.
- Manage interpersonal communication in the reception area.
- Design an office policy statement.
- Explain marketing techniques in dentistry.
- Describe external and internal marketing.
- Understand patient rights.

People are an essential part of the dental practice. The most important person in a dental practice is the patient. Never overlook the fact that each patient has a different background and different needs. Therefore, while communicating with patients, it is important to recognize each as an individual with specific needs and determine how to be sensitive to those needs. Remember that dentistry is a helping profession. Not only must every effort be made to alleviate patients' discomfort, but patients must be taught to help themselves.

UNDERSTANDING PATIENT NEEDS

Each person who comes in contact with patients should have an understanding of the basic drives involved in motivating patients. Unless the dentist and staff have a basic understanding of these drives, they will become discouraged after numerous attempts fail to motivate patients to appreciate good dental health and quality dentistry.

With concern for humanism in this healthcare profession, it seems appropriate to be aware of the contributions of two humanistic psychologists, Abraham Maslow and Carl Rogers.

 PRACTICE NOTE
The most important person in a dental practice is the patient.

Maslow's Hierarchy of Needs

Dr. Abraham Maslow has described a **hierarchy of needs** (Figure 3-1) that aids in understanding how a person's needs motivate his or her behavior. Maslow identified the following five basic levels of needs ranging from basic biological needs to complex social or psychological drives:

1. *Physiological or biological:* These are bodily needs, and they are the first to be satisfied. You must satisfy these physical needs, or you won't live long enough to satisfy any social or

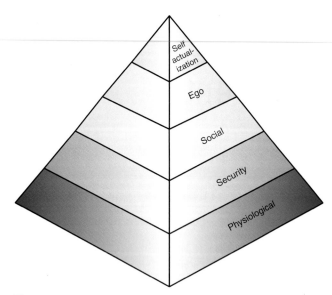

Figure 3-1 Maslow's hierarchy of needs.

psychological needs. If you are healthy, eat regularly, and are housed adequately, you can advance to the next level of the hierarchy with a sense of well-being.

2. *Safety or security needs:* Once the basic biological needs are met, you are ready for the second level of the hierarchy. This level allows you to explore your environment. Just as small children begin to explore their environment once their food and comfort needs have been met, you as an adult begin to explore. This is the level at which you feel safe and free from danger, threats, or other deprivation. If you have a job that is nonthreatening and live in a safe environment, you will feel secure and will be able to advance to the next level.

3. *Social or love needs:* Once you are secure in your environment, you can advance to the level of social interaction. The poet John Donne wrote, "No man is an island, complete to itself." Donne realized that to be human means to interact with others. At this level on the hierarchy, Maslow realized the to need to interact with others with whom you share similar beliefs and who provide you with reinforcement to continue your social relationships. This love or social inter-action gives you confidence to advance to the next level on the hierarchy.

4. *Esteem needs:* From interaction with others at the previous level, you will generate goals for yourself. Your peers often consider these needs as ego needs that relate to your self-esteem, reputation, and recognition. Here you look forward to achieving your goals, and from accomplishment you will receive self-esteem. Typically the self-satisfaction you receive from accomplishing these goals provides an impetus to establish new goals and begin the cycle again.

5. *Self-actualization:* Self-actualized people are motivated by the need to grow. To achieve this need, you must have achieved self-esteem and have confidence in yourself. Later in life, Maslow expanded his thoughts on the self-actualized person and explained that to achieve this level people must be relatively free of illness, sufficiently satisfied in their basic needs, positively using their capacities, and motivated by some existing or sought-after personal values. A person at this level often wants to help others achieve their goals by teaching them lessons he or she learned in the earlier stages. Some people never reach this level because they have not aspired to its recognition.

Relating this hierarchy to dentistry means getting to know the patients and the individuals with whom one is associated. Before a dentist can motivate a patient to accept a certain type of dental treatment, it must be understood where the patient is on the hierarchy of needs.

To help realize the application of these needs to dentistry, consider this situation. One of the practice's patients is a bank president who is respected for his civic activities and has a warm, loving family and a fine home. The patient develops severe pain in the maxillary anterior area. The pain is sudden, sharp, and excruciating. It is difficult for him to eat, and there is a great deal of swelling in his upper lip. This person has dropped from perhaps a self-esteem level to the physiological, and the den-tist must satisfy this physiological need immediately before attempting to suggest any further treatment.

Setting up payment plans for a patient often exposes a con-flict of needs. A patient must ensure that basic needs of food, housing, and clothing are met, yet there may be a desire to meet social needs by improving appearance with some form of den-tal treatment. A conflict arises in the decision-making process when the patient is confronted with conflict on how to satisfy all of these needs with a specified income. The dentist and staff must make an effort to determine the patient's needs, realize the patient's potential conflict, and consider presenting an alterna-tive treatment plan so the patient has some options.

This theory need not only apply to relationships with patients. It also can be applied to interactions among staff members. The dentist, assistant, and hygienist all have the same needs, and each is concerned, like the patient, about security today and in the future. Often conflict arises when a person becomes fixed at one level. There may appear to be no change in motivation, and the person remains unchanged in his or her perspective. This is evidenced often when a person has an inter-est in making money or increasing social status without regard for other people's levels of motivation.

Perhaps one of the best lessons to be learned from Maslow's theory is that an individual has a choice in determining his or her behavior. Although basic physiological and environmen-tal needs have a strong influence, an individual makes choices voluntarily.

Rogers' Client-Centered Therapy

Dr. Carl Rogers, another humanistic psychologist, believed that "it is the client who knows what hurts, what directions to go, what problems are crucial, what experiences have been deeply buried." Rogers also suggests accepting the patient or other person as a genuine person with his or her own set of values and goals, and that these people must be treated with "uncon-ditional positive regard." **Client-centered therapy** assumes that patients know how they feel, what they want, and their priorities. Applied to dentistry, this philosophy encourages listening to the patient. Further, this concept suggests respecting patients as human beings, not just numbers, case studies, or research projects. These people have needs, and their desires should not be repressed. The combined concepts of Maslow and Rogers provide the groundwork for a humanistic, caring attitude, which should be a requisite for all healthcare providers.

BARRIERS TO PATIENT COMMUNICATION

Common Obstacles

Often practitioners are unable to communicate with patients because barriers have been established. One of the first barriers that may be created is prejudging a patient. A dentist may hesitate to present an extensive treatment to a patient because of the way the patient dresses or the type of car he or she drives. As a result, the patient is never told about alternative forms of treatment because his or her economic status has been prejudged. Often a person with a disability is prejudged. When a patient who has an artificial limb, is in a wheelchair, or has a visible birthmark on the face enters the dental office, frequently the first noticeable feature is the disability. If this patient is with a spouse or another person, the patient may go unnoticed while questions are directed to the accompanying person. As a dental healthcare worker, it is important to treat people with disabilities as any other patients and direct all communication to that person.

Another barrier occurs when one hears but does not *listen*. A dental professional should never be too busy to listen with understanding to a patient. Don't just listen to the words. Listen to the *meaning* of the words and the feeling behind the meaning. Before presenting a personal point of view, be able to restate what has been said to the patient's satisfaction. This may sound easy, but is not. Often people are too eager to present their own point of view and fail to understand the real meaning of what the patient is attempting to say. What is the patient really saying when he or she says, "I think I'll wait to have that treatment done"? If the dental professional responds, "Oh, that's okay, Mrs. Gates, I understand," he or she won't find out what the patient is really saying, and may cut off communication. The patient may really be saying, "I'm scared," "I can't afford it," or "I don't like the way you treat me." The best way to arrive at the real meaning is to continue the dialogue until the patient's true feelings are discerned. The following example demonstrates this idea:

Assistant: "Mrs. Romano, do you feel you want to wait with the treatment?"
Patient: "Yes."
Assistant: "Do you want to wait because you are too busy now?" (*The patient may say yes and terminate the conversation at this point, or the conversation may continue.*) If yes, reply; "Mrs. Romano, we understand busy schedules and do value

your time. We can custom design your appointments just as we design a personalized treatment plan. Why don't we take a look at your schedule and see if we can work together to find time for your treatment?"
Patient: If the patient had responded, "No, it's just that I don't know if I should spend that much money as I have so many other expenses right now.."
Assistant: Then reply, "Mrs. Romano, we know how budgets can be stretched today and we can work with you to help you afford this investment, which is going to pay dividends over the next 10 to 20 years." At this point explain the financial arrangements that can be made in the office.

Notice in this dialogue the assistant offered a solution to the problem so that it could be discussed further.

However, the dialogue may have continued along different lines, such as the following example:

Patient: The patient may have responded, "Well, it's not that I can't afford it. I guess what it boils down to is that I've never had that type of treatment, and I'm not certain what it's going to involve."
Assistant: "In other words, you don't understand the procedure?"
Patient: "Yes, I guess that's it. I'm really a bit skeptical about what's going to happen." (*The hidden meaning becomes evident.*)

In this case, the assistant rephrased what the patient said to arrive at the real meaning.

A third barrier is preoccupation. During daily routines many demands are placed on one's time, and it is easy to begin to suddenly think about other activities while trying to communicate with a patient. Everyone has been in that position at one time or another. A patient is trying to explain why an appointment time is not convenient, and suddenly the dental professional realizes that she or he hasn't heard a word that was said because of concentration on another problem. This often happens in an office that is understaffed. Each staff member has so much work to accomplish that listening to a patient sometimes just becomes an additional burden. Unfortunately patients are quick to recognize such preoccupation and may suddenly stop talking or eventually may even stop coming into the dental office. This type of situation re-emphasizes the service model illustrated in Chapter 1. As mentioned, the patient is the most important person in the office and should be given complete attention.

Unawareness of importance, impatience, and even hearing loss are barriers to communication. How important the problem is to a patient may not be realized, and the patient's concern may simply be ignored as a whim. Likewise, one may inadvertently become impatient with a chatty young child or an older person who is slow. Furthermore, it is possible not to hear everything a person says because of an unrealized hearing loss.

It is not beneficial just to know about these barriers. The dental professional must be willing to evaluate him or herself.

Before each contact with a patient, decide to ignore extraneous activities, and be willing to listen and understand a patient's problem before offering a solution.

Recognizing Nonverbal Cues

Many books have been written in recent years defining and guiding the reader to recognize nonverbal communication cues. Nonverbal cues refer to the gestures and body movements a person makes in a given situation.

Every member of the dental staff should have some awareness of this area. Just as a "picture is worth a thousand words," so a gesture can give meaning to a person's inner feelings. Nonverbal communication provides feedback on the patient's reactions.

The alert assistant is able to pick up these cues and interpret them while communicating with a patient. Care should be taken not to be misled by one gesture. A series of gestures generally give a more realistic indication of a person's attitude. A dental office presents many opportunities to use and to receive nonverbal cues.

Nervousness

A patient who enters the reception room and sits down, locking the ankles together and clenching the hands, may be expressing fear by holding back emotions (Figure 3-2). This may occur in the dental chair when a person clenches the armrests and locks the ankles together (Figure 3-3). When the patient relaxes, he or she will automatically unlock the ankles.

Defensiveness

A patient or staff member may use a gesture of crossed arms and clenched fists as signals to indicate disagreement or defensiveness. This gesture may even indicate the person has withdrawn from the conversation (Figure 3-4). This may occur when a patient is being ignored by the dentist and assistant as they communicate with each other (Figure 3-5).

Touching

An assistant has many opportunities to use this gesture, which indicates caring or interest in the child (Figure 3-6). A hand on a small child's shoulder may show concern, or an arm around the shoulder of a senior citizen may give reassurance (Figure 3-7).

Openness

During a consultation with a patient, a dentist should express openness rather than assume an authoritative posture behind a desk. Having the patient seated beside the desk removes this barrier and allows the dentist an opportunity for more open gestures, as in Figure 3-8.

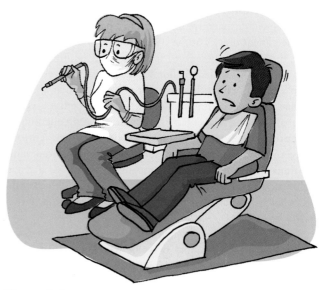

Figure 3-3 A patient displaying nervousness in the dental chair.

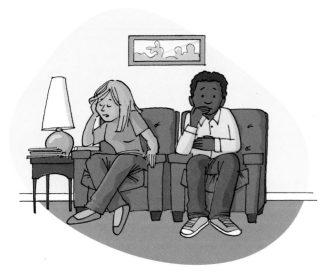

Figure 3-2 The difference between a bored patient and a "scared-to-death" patient.

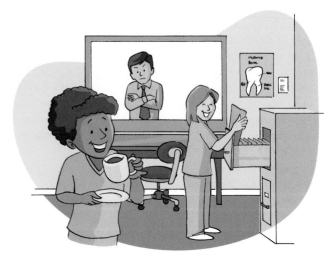

Figure 3-4 A patient who is being ignored, crossing his arms defensively.

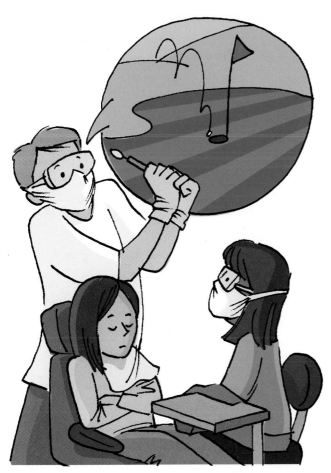

Figure 3-5 A dentist and an assistant ignoring a patient.

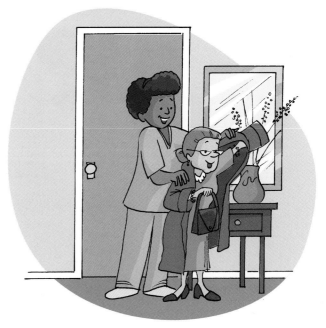

Figure 3-7 Assisting an older adult patient with her coat indicates caring.

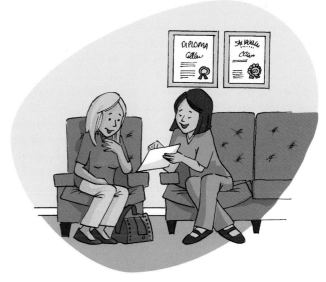

Figure 3-8 A dentist in consultation with a patient.

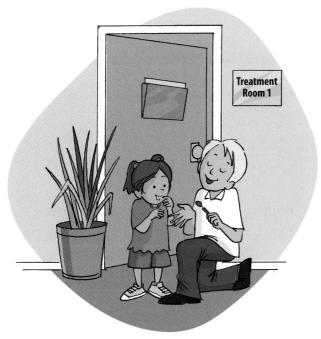

Figure 3-6 An assistant displaying caring by showing interest in child.

Embarrassment

A patient's hand covering the mouth may indicate a wish to avoid the embarrassment of exposing an unsightly oral condition. A similar signal may be tightening of the upper lip to conceal the teeth (Figure 3-9).

Many more nonverbal cues exist. It is vital to become aware of the meaning of these valuable tools in communication. No one tool or technique will assure successful communications. Communication is based on a leader who has well-defined goals and a staff working as a team. These efforts, combined with a sincere interest in satisfying a patient's needs, provide a successful communication system in the dental office.

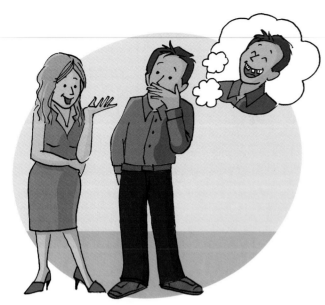

Figure 3-9 A patient covering his mouth to indicate embarrassment.

IMPROVING VERBAL IMAGES

A health professional has an obligation to allay fears and comfort patients. The most obvious way of accomplishing these tasks is to create a good image in the patient's mind. In a dental office eliminate the use of words or phrases that conjure a negative thought. For instance, when a clinical assistant says, "This won't hurt," the patient has been told there is a possibility it will "hurt." If the assistant had said, "We will make you as comfortable as possible," or "You may feel this," the patient would know the assistant is there to help him or her be comfortable. Terms and phrases frequently used in a dental office are discussed in greater detail in Chapter 10. Try replacing discomforting terms or phrases with words that create a more positive environment. Also use language the patient will understand when discussing treatment.

THE PATIENT

As mentioned, the most important person in the dental office is the patient. Although it is obvious that dentistry is a business, it should never be forgotten that it is first a healthcare profession. A great deal is expected of a patient: following directions, keeping appointments, and paying the fee promptly. In return, dental professionals must take time to recognize the patient as a person and realize that the patient has special needs and inherent rights.

 PRACTICE NOTE
A health professional has an obligation to allay fears and comfort patients.

Patient Rights

The phrase *patient rights* is much used today. The result has been action on the part of most healthcare professions to design *A Patient's Bill of Rights.* It is unfortunate that in some healthcare

---

> **BOX 3-1** **Patient Rights**
>
> Patients in a dental practice are entitled to:
> - Be treated with adequate, appropriate, compassionate care at all times and under all circumstances
> - Be treated without discrimination based on race, religion, color, national origin, gender, age, handicap, marital status, sexual preference, or source of payment
> - Be informed of all aspects of treatment
> - Be informed of appointment and fee schedules
> - Be able to review the patient financial and clinical records
> - Obtain a thorough evaluation of their needs
> - Be treated as a partner in care and decision making related to treatment planning
> - Receive current information about treatment and be assured of quality treatment
> - Be able to refuse treatment to the extent provided by law and be informed of the medical/dental consequences of that refusal
> - Expect confidentiality of all records pertinent to their dental care
> - Be informed if the dentist participates in different third-party payment plans
> - Request and expect appropriate referrals for consultation
> - Be taught how to maintain good oral health for a lifetime
> - Receive treatment that will prevent future dental or oral disease
> - Expect continuity of treatment
> - Be charged a fair and equitable fee
> - Have appointment schedules and times maintained
> - Be treated by a staff of professionals who maintain good health and hygiene
> - Be respected for requesting a second opinion
> - Be respected as a human being who has feelings and needs

agencies the care has become so impersonal that it is necessary for a professional association or agency to formally document the things that are naturally considered **patients' rights**. Some healthcare workers see this action as confirmation of a patient's inherent rights, not the result of a lack of consideration.

As society becomes increasingly concerned with individual rights, members of the dental healthcare team cannot afford to neglect patient rights. The dental professional must be considerate of the patient as a human being rather than as just as a subject of a dental procedure. Take time to recognize the patient as a person and consider the list of rights in Box 3-1 as rights of the patient, not as threats to the profession of dentistry.

Managing the Patient's Special Needs

Many patients with special needs enter a dental practice. Some of these were reviewed earlier, during the discussion of barriers to communication. A patient who is physically or psychologically disabled or challenged, an older adult, a child, a single parent, or a homeless person may visit the office for various types of treatment. Both of the terms *physically challenged* and *disabled* are acceptable today. Although *physically challenged* is used less, it should be realized that not all persons may be disabled.

The Americans with Disabilities Act of 1990, commonly known as the ADA, sets specific guidelines for businesses. Several issues regarding structural design of a building are discussed in Chapter 6. Other factors in this law require the dentist not to discriminate against a person who needs dental care. For most disabled persons, if they can get into a treatment room, they can receive treatment. Perhaps the biggest problem a dentist faces in treating a challenged patient is when the patient can't mentally or physically cooperate. For example, a dentist faces several compromises when a patient has cerebral palsy and the mouth is uncontrollably moving, or is a quadriplegic whose high neck injuries make moving from a wheelchair to a dental chair dangerous. Even though there are some dental treatments that can be done in a wheelchair, the law allows a dentist to make referrals for the patient's safety.

It may be necessary to make a special effort in communication with some patients. For instance, if the disabilities include vision or hearing impairments or the patient uses a wheelchair or walker, it may be necessary to take special care when communicating. The dental professional may need to stand in front of patients who have hearing difficulty when talking to ensure that they are able to read the lips. For patients with poor vision, the dental professional may need to read questions or have a guardian review materials that require a response, such as a health questionnaire. For people using wheelchairs, walkers, or crutches, it may be necessary to take extra time when asking them to move about, or it may even be necessary to go to them directly with forms that need to be signed.

Recognizing Abuse

Abuse is evident in many forms in today's society, most commonly child and adult abuse. Each year more than 3 million children are abused or neglected by caregivers, relatives, or strangers. More than 1000 children die annually as a result of this abuse. Child abuse may be classified as physical, sexual, emotional, or overall neglect. Adults, those who are elderly and dependent on others for care, as well as people from a volatile relationship, may also be victims of abuse.

Dentists are faced with abuse in two ways. The forensic dentist may be presented with a postmortem case of a victim who has bite marks or tooth marks. In addition, a dentist may treat victims of abuse in the office.

Abused children or adults may show overall signs of neglect, abnormal fears or neuroses, or evidence of extraoral or intraoral anomalies such as bite marks, scars, lacerations, fractured teeth, burns, and bruises of varying colors on exposed areas of the body.

The dentist has an obligation to examine the patient thoroughly, ask reasonable questions about existing conditions, and document the injuries on the dental record. Reports of suspected abuse should be made to the state or county social services office. In most states, failure to report suspected abuse is a misdemeanor.

RECEPTION ROOM TECHNIQUES

Because the duties of the administrative assistant include many facets of communication, continual awareness of communication barriers is necessary.

The impression that the administrative assistant makes on patients is usually lasting and, of course, should be favorable. Remember to represent the dentist and the practice; a patient who feels comfortable with the administrative assistant will probably feel comfortable with the dentist.

The Role of the Receptionist

The receptionist will be the first person to greet patients as they enter the office. The receptionist should appear neat and professional. In many business offices today, the administrative assistant wears professional businesslike clothing rather than a uniform. The receptionist should be certain that his or her clothing or uniform is clean, shoes are well-polished, and hair neatly styled. The positive image created as a receptionist indicates a clean and well-organized office The image portrayed in this role must remain with the patient, so this is no place to try out new clothing styles, experiment with garish jewelry, visible tattoos, or wear facial and oral piercings.

As the patient enters the office, the receptionist should be seated, acknowledge the patient immediately with a pleasant smile and cheerful "hello," and call him or her by name. Everyone likes the feeling of being known and recognized. Even though the receptionist may be busy with a telephone call, at least look up and smile. This will inform patients that the receptionist is aware of their presence.

Reception Room Appeal

A bright, cheerful, and pleasantly decorated office usually makes a favorable impression on the patient. If the room appears to have a warm and friendly atmosphere, the patient will relax. (Design of the reception room for the patient's comfort is discussed in Chapter 6.) Offering a cup of coffee, tea, or other beverage may put the patient at ease.

Reading material in the reception room should be current and geared toward a wide variety of interests. A good selection might include gourmet cooking, sports, travel, community and world news, and health magazines. Recipe cards can be placed in an attractive holder (Figure 3-10) to aid patients in copying information from magazines and assorted health-related cookbooks (Figure 3-11). This will prevent them from tearing pages from books and magazines. Avoid dirty carpet, frayed furniture, and unsightly plants. Also, children's books, as well as quiet games and toys, should be available. An area designated as a children's play area is helpful. If background music is played in the office, be sure to select music that has a soothing effect rather than loud rock or heavy concert music.

Waiting Patients

One of the responsibilities of the receptionist is to keep patients informed of delays or indicate the waiting time. Unexpected delays or emergencies should be explained honestly. Be careful not to make excuses or say that the dentist is running late (Figure 3-12). Be honest about the length of time the patient will have to wait to be seen.

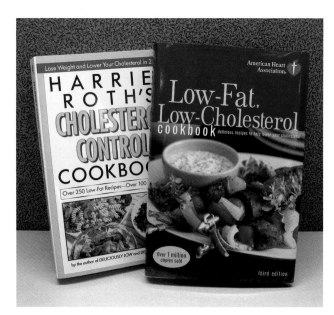

Figure 3-10 A recipe card for copying information from magazines.

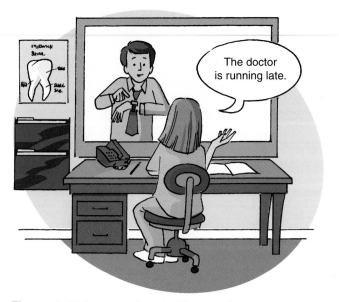

Figure 3-12 Team members should avoid telling patients that the dentist is running late, but instead should be honest about the expected wait time.

Often a new practitioner neglects to establish an office policy, only to be confronted with misunderstandings with patients at a later date. The office policy should be implemented when the office is first opened and revised as the practice grows and changes. However, such a policy can be integrated into an established practice with minimal effort.

Contents of an Office Policy

Each practice has its own specific needs, but every policy should include the following elements:

- *Philosophy:* This is a statement of the dentist's attitude toward the practice of dentistry and, more specifically, the moral and ethical obligation to the patient. It is in this section that the dentist can make a statement about how the practice is unique and what gives it something special that will attract and retain patients.
- *Office hours:* Although these may occasionally vary, specific hours should be listed for the patient's benefit. It is advisable to inform patients of times available for emergency appointments. This will avoid a congested schedule and unnecessary calls at inconvenient times.
- *Appointment control:* A statement should be included designating the person who controls appointment making. It should also be noted that patients are seen by appointment only to discourage "drop ins." A broken appointment policy should be included in the office policy and adhered to consistently.
- *Payment policy:* The dentist should outline specific acceptable payment plans. These plans should be described in detail, and the person responsible for implementing them should be identified. Finally a statement should be made regarding parental responsibility for the treatment of minors.
- *Hygiene:* The value of hygiene, self-care, and preventive dentistry through the periodic recall system should be emphasized.

Figure 3-11 Cookbooks related to health.

OFFICE POLICY

The **office policy** brochure is the key to establishing communication and understanding between the patient and the office staff. The office policy should be a written statement of the dentist's philosophy, mission statement, and policies, defining the responsibilities of both the patient and the dental office staff. It is given to a new patient at the first visit and serves not only as an informational device but also as a good public relations tool. Some of the policies in this brochure may be included in the office web site if one is available.

The system used in the office should be explained thoroughly to each patient.

- *Attitude toward children:* The roles of the dentist, staff, and parent in the treatment of children must be explained. The preparation of a child before treatment and management of the parent and child during treatment should be well defined to avoid future conflicts.
- *Auxiliary use:* The dentist has the responsibility to define the relationship of each staff member to patients, thus explaining the value of team dentistry for quality care and maximum efficiency. The dentist should identify the credentials and responsibilities of each staff member.
- *Infection-control policies:* Such policies can be explained to assure patients that the latest barrier techniques and most current preventive concepts are being used for their protection.
- *Quality assurance:* This is an explanation of efforts taken to ensure that procedures and techniques used in the office are routinely evaluated to maintain good quality.

- *Staff continuing education:* This explains the efforts the dentist makes to continuously update himself or herself and the staff in life support, infection control, and other technological advances.
- *Office data:* The dentist's name, address, phone number, fax, and e-mail address should appear on the cover or be easy to find within the policy for the patient's convenience.

Designing an Office Policy Statement

The administrative assistant can be invaluable to the dentist in designing the office policy statement. Once the basic policy has been established, the assistant makes the final draft and aids in designing several styles for final selection. The final style is the dentist's choice, but should be attractive, well-organized, brief, and sized to be easily handled by patients. Many offices prefer to use a professional printer to achieve a professional-looking pamphlet. In Figure 3-13, the policy has

---

Welcome to our office...

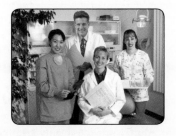

Joseph W. Lake, DDS
Ashley M. Lake, DDS

611 Main Street, SE
Grand Rapids, MI 49502
Phone: 616-101-9575
Fax: 616-101-9999
e-mail: office@dapc.com

INITIAL EXAMINATION...

Each patient that we have the privilege to serve is entitled to and will receive a thorough examination. This examination includes necessary x-rays, diagnostic models, and an oral examination as required to make an accurate analysis of your mouth. An estimate of the fee involved will be given.

OFFICE HOURS...

Office hours are from 8 to 12 and 1 to 5 on Monday and Wednesday and 9 to 12 and 1 to 7 on Tuesday and Thursday. There are no office hours on Friday or Saturday, though on those days a recorder will answer your call, take messages, and refer you to an on-call doctor.

APPOINTMENTS...

The administrative assistant has complete charge of appointments in the office. We will reserve a time that is convenient for you. We will make every effort to keep our schedule on time.

When a change of appointment is necessary, 24 hours advance notice is required.

EMERGENCY TIME...

Time is specifically reserved for emergency care at 10:15 A.M. and 3:45 P.M. We will treat your immediate problem and re-schedule you for further necessary treatment.

MINORS...

Parental approval of the dental treatment is necessary. Parents are requested to wait in the reception room except for consultation.

Small children are more receptive to dental care in the morning. We will request cooperation in having them excused from school.

Figure 3-13 An example of an office policy intended to be printed on heavy letter-sized paper and folded in half.

(Continued)

PAYMENT POLICIES...

When extensive treatment is necessary, an estimate of the fee will be presented before services are rendered. The administrative assistant will explain our payment policies and make financial arrangements that are mutually satisfactory.

The fee for treatment requiring a single office visit is payable at the conclusion of the appointment. Other treatment is billed monthly and payable upon receipt of the statement.

Please feel free to make inquiries about our fees, or your dental treatment. You will find the staff most capable, sympathetic, and courteous in providing this information.

Our fees are related directly to the cost of office operation and to strict attention to office efficiency.

INFECTION CONTROL POLICY...

In this office we use a variety of barrier techniques for your individual protection. These techniques include gloves, masks, protective eye shields and coverings, protective clothing, and when necessary specialized intra-oral devices. Our staff regularly attends meetings on safety standards and we implement all of the latest OSHA standards and recommendations of the American Dental Association.

DENTAL STAFF...

The administrative and clinical assistants in this office are Certified or Registered Dental Assistants and they are highly skilled in the areas of office management and clinical assisting. The administrative assistant is in charge of all payment arrangements, insurance forms, billing, and appointment scheduling. The clinical assistants are the doctor's operative assistants and with the utilization of these skilled assistants is able to increase efficiency in treatment, thus enabling you to receive complete and thorough dentistry.

While all assistants may assume responsibility for patient education, the Registered Dental Hygienist is in charge of dietary analysis and the oral prophylaxis. After the defective areas are charted, the doctor will do a complete oral examination. The extensive education and experience of our hygienist establishes this professional as an authority in the field of oral hygiene.

PERIODIC EXAMINATION...

We share the desire of all of our patients to minimize the need for extensive dental treatment. This can only be done by regular examinations which detect dental disease before it becomes extensive.

At the conclusion of your treatment, you will be placed on our Preventive Recall Program, which requests you to return at a specified time for a re-examination. Your current dental treatment will be inspected, your home care program reviewed, and your teeth cleaned and polished.

The goal of this program is to:
• Maintain your attractive appearance
• Provide good dental comfort and health
• Prevent unnecessary loss of teeth

• • •

To keep abreast of new techniques, our staff enrolls in four to eight days of continuing education each year. During the time that the doctor and the staff attend meetings, a recorder will direct you to a colleague who will take emergency calls for this office.

Our office is always receptive to suggestions that might be useful to improve our services to you.

Figure 3-13, cont'd

been designed to be printed on both sides of heavy 8½-×-11-inch bond paper folded in half. A simpler, less expensive statement printed on office letterhead is shown in Figure 3-14. Remember that the office policy has two primary purposes: It is a practice builder, and it informs the patient about office procedures and the dentist's philosophy. When it achieves both purposes, the office policy becomes a valuable public relations device.

MARKETING

When advertising was first legalized in 1977 by action of the Supreme Court, many dentists perceived this action to be demeaning to the profession. Today, dentists across the country have come to realize that in a competitive, consumer-oriented society, they must become involved in **marketing** to increase their practice loads. No matter how one attempts to change it, marketing is advertising, and all dentists practice some form of advertising.

Marketing Skills

Marketing should be a natural habit that is practiced at all times. Team members must work together to educate patients about the practice and procedures, provide quality treatment in a comfortable, safe environment, offer outstanding customer service, and make patients want to tell their family and friends about their great dentist and staff. To market a dental practice effectively, the staff needs a specific set of skills that will aid them in promoting the practice.

Office Trademark

The dentist needs to verbalize an identity. What makes the practice different? Large corporations such as 3M, Sony, Starbucks, Microsoft, and Amazon all have an identity. For instance, a dentist might sum up the office identity by using words such as *thorough, caring,* or *leading edge*. The word *thorough* denotes that each patient will be given quality time. *Caring* suggests old-fashioned commitment to the

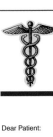

Dental Associates, PC

Joseph W. Lake, DDS – Ashley M. Lake, DDS

Dear Patient:

On behalf of the staff and myself, I welcome you to our office. You are important to us. We pride ourselves in making dentistry a pleasant experience for our patients. You can always expect to be treated as a guest when visiting us.

It is our desire to provide the most thorough and efficient treatment possible. Complete oral health care comprises not only the elimination of existing dental disease but also the prevention of future disease. Except in emergency cases, new adult patients receive a thorough dental examination consisting of the following:

1. Record of medical/dental history
2. Visual mouth examination
3. Complete x-ray examination
4. Prophylaxis (preventive cleaning)
5. Any other diagnostic aids necessary to render a thorough diagnosis
6. Oral hygiene instructions

The requirements for children vary according to age and dental needs.

After the examination is completed, an appointment will be made to discuss the conditions present and the most thorough treatment plans for you. Also at this visit, appointments will be scheduled, estimated fees given, payment plans presented, and all financial arrangements completed. The practice depends upon reimbursement from patients for the costs incurred in their care and financial responsibility on the part of the patient must be determined before treatment. If you require a consultant at this time, we require that he or she accompany you for this important appointment. The responsible adult must be present at a consultation involving children.

We sincerely believe that one of the most important services that we have to offer is a plan for preventive dentistry. All patients are notified at periodic intervals for preventive examinations and the oral prophylaxis.

Except for emergency cases, you may expect us to be on time. Likewise, we will expect the same courtesy. Should it be necessary for you to reschedule an appointment, we require 24 hours notice, except in case of an emergency. This allows us to use your reserved time for another patient.

It is our hope that your dental visits will be prompt and pleasant so that in the future you will want to help increase our fine family of patients through your recommendations.

To continue improving our service, we invite your comments and suggestions at all times.

Sincerely,

Joseph W. Lake, DDS

611 Main Street, SE – Grand Rapids, MI 49502 Phone: 616.101.9575 Fax: 616.101.9999
E-mail: office@dapc.com or Visit us at: www.Lakedental.com

Figure 3-14 An example of an office policy statement printed on letterhead.

patient, regardless of business pressure. The phrase *leading edge* indicates that the dentist and staff are progressive and keep abreast of new materials and techniques. These messages must be driven home at every opportunity. For instance, when a patient contacts the office for the first appointment, the administrative assistant can take the opportunity to promote the thoroughness of the practice. Instead of first asking what time of day is most convenient, he or she can start the conversation with "Mrs. Timmon, let me be the first to welcome you to Dr. Lake's practice. She is a very caring and thorough dentist who takes time to be current with all of the leading technology and materials. I promise you that all members of our team will go out of our way to provide you with dental care and to make your visits pleasant."

Enthusiastic Attitude

The single most important characteristic in a staff member is an enthusiastic attitude. The employee with an enthusiastic attitude shows up for work every day on time, is willing to help others, maintains a cheery disposition all day, and ensures that patients come first. This enthusiastic attitude means the "no whining" rule is always in place, because whining is contagious. The enthusiastic attitude means the patient's problems come first and personal problems are kept to oneself or shared with a friend in private.

 PRACTICE NOTE
The single most important characteristic in a staff member is an enthusiastic attitude.

Seizing Opportunities

There are many ways to get the word out about a practice. For instance, when a new patient makes an appointment, say, "Mrs. Timmons, we are looking forward to seeing you at 3 PM on Wednesday. By the way, would you like to make an appointment for any other members of the family at this time?" This is also a good opportunity to refer them to the office web site, giving them directions on how to reach the web site, and suggesting they look at it thoroughly because it contains information about the staff and the educational goals of the office, as well as directions to the office.

Practice Ambassadors

Each member of the staff is expected to be an ambassador to the practice. Each staff member should be provided with his or her own business cards, and should promote the practice to family and friends. It may even be possible to suggest that the office be used after hours for community group meetings if office space is adequate. When a new staff member joins a practice, the dentist should prepare an announcement that can be sent to the new team member's circle of family, friends, or other professional associates.

Internal Marketing

Marketing can be divided into two forms, internal and external. Internal marketing is what one does within the office to retain patients. Internal marketing is that "first impression." It is how the patient perceives that the dental staff is caring and enjoys the work; it is the patient's feeling that the dentist is willing to listen to his or her individual dental problem. Internal marketing is how patients are retained once they have been attracted to the practice.

As mentioned in Chapter 2, one of the most important assets a dentist has in an office is the dental staff. When the staff members are committed to the practice, highly motivated, and enthusiastic, they become the impetus to a successful internal marketing program. Look at Figure 3-15, and note that most of

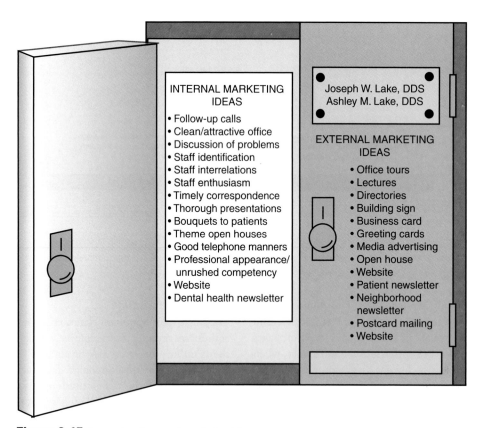

INTERNAL MARKETING IDEAS
- Follow-up calls
- Clean/attractive office
- Discussion of problems
- Staff identification
- Staff interrelations
- Staff enthusiasm
- Timely correspondence
- Thorough presentations
- Bouquets to patients
- Theme open houses
- Good telephone manners
- Professional appearance/ unrushed competency
- Website
- Dental health newsletter

Joseph W. Lake, DDS
Ashley M. Lake, DDS

EXTERNAL MARKETING IDEAS
- Office tours
- Lectures
- Directories
- Building sign
- Business card
- Greeting cards
- Media advertising
- Open house
- Website
- Patient newsletter
- Neighborhood newsletter
- Postcard mailing
- Website

Figure 3-15 Internal and external marketing ideas.

the ideas for internal marketing for patient retention are staff-oriented. Staff members should be given specialized duties in which they perform well as part of an internal marketing program. For instance, a staff person who writes well could manage written communication, whereas another who has a good understanding of insurance could explain insurance benefits to patients.

Patients who know that the dentist and staff care about them and don't consider them merely case numbers or blank checks will return to the practice and, more important, will refer friends and colleagues.

External Marketing

Some dentists view external marketing with skepticism, but if used, it must be presented in an ethical form. The key to successful external marketing is to determine prospective patients and the best method to attract them. The dentist must identify his or her objectives, define the strengths of the practice, determine the budget, and review all the sources for external advertising. Some forms of such marketing can be as simple as offering lectures to local organizations or as complex as media advertising. A review of Figure 3-15 illustrates other potential sources of external marketing. When using any source of advertising, the dentist must realize that the results will not be immediate, and that a consistent and repetitive message must be directed to prospective patients to obtain results.

Today the dental office staff can design a web page (Figure 3-16) about the practice and be able to reach prospective new patients, and welcome and educate them and their families through the professional web site. The dentist is able to promote the practice and provide resources to inform patients of all of the professional services. Patient education software can be included in the web site, to provide explanations and satisfy a current or prospective patients' questions about specific procedures. It is common for the dentist to hire an outside agency to set up the web site to ensure maximum contact as well as provide a professional image.

The most important factor to remember in any form of marketing is to produce what you claim. No matter where or how much the dentist advertises, if quality dental care is not delivered in a caring, sensitive manner, the patient will not return. A good motto for a dentist to remember is, "You may attract them, but you won't keep them."

Newsletters as Marketing Devices

Today, as dentistry seeks to address the consumer market, newsletters have become a major asset for the dental practice. Newsletters may be considered for the internal market by sending them to current patients, or for the external market by sending a newsletter to the nearby community addressed to the resident at the given address. If done ethically, with concern for the values of the community and the education of the public, this form of marketing can be a valuable tool.

Automated systems in the dental office make it easier to incorporate marketing procedures into the dental business. Some dentists prefer to produce their own newsletters, but this can be a costly and time-consuming practice. Today there are several companies that provide this service to the dental practice, as shown in Figures 3-17 and 3-18. Such services can provide customized educational articles and photos that can be personalized for the individual office. Such a newsletter can promote the practice as well as establish rapport with existing patients and the community. Most companies provide mailing services for the office.

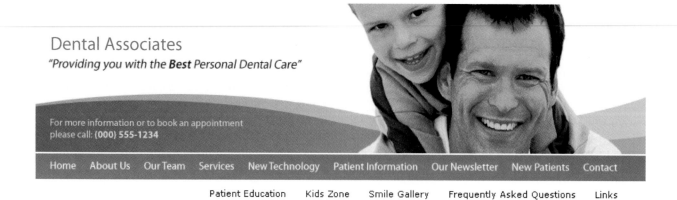

Dental Associates
*"Providing you with the **Best** Personal Dental Care"*

For more information or to book an appointment
please call: **(000) 555-1234**

Home   About Us   Our Team   Services   New Technology   Patient Information   Our Newsletter   New Patients   Contact

Patient Education   Kids Zone   Smile Gallery   Frequently Asked Questions   Links

Welcome to Main Street Dental

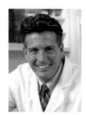

"We are proud to offer state-of-the-art dentistry for your whole family in a caring, welcoming environment."

- Dr. Joseph W. Lake

I am happy to inform you that our office is currently accepting new patients, and is offering a special no-charge introductory consultation to you as a special "welcome" to our practice!

Please talk to us about any dental concerns or questions that you may have, whether it relates to general dental hygiene or cosmetic improvement.

Call us today! We look forward to seeing you soon!

Office Hours

Monday through Thursday
9:00 a.m. - 7:00 p.m.

Friday
8:00 a.m. - 1:00 p.m.

Saturday
9:00 a.m. - 1:00 p.m.

How to find us

611 Main Street, S.E
Grand Rapids, MI 49502
616.101.9575

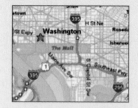

CLICK TO VIEW MAP

Site Maintained by Market Connections

Figure 3-16 An example of a web page for internal or external marketing. (Courtesy Market Connections, Inc., www.dentalhealthnews.org, Toronto, Ontario, Canada.)

Dental Health News™

Compliments of Dental Associates, PC

News from the office of:

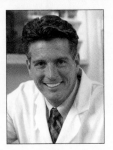

Dr. Joseph W. Lake

Many people finally have time to play catch-up over the summer months, whether it's catching up with friends and family, catching up to some overdue vacation time or just catching up with a "to do" list that's been lengthening over the year. Is a visit to our office on your list?

When you look at our article "Open Wide For The Inside Story", you'll realize just how important it is to stay on top of your dental health, for the sake of your overall general health. If you have any questions on this topic or on any other dental issues, we would be happy to talk them over with you!

Enjoy your summer plans, and we'll look forward to catching up with you soon.

All the best,

Joseph W. Lake

Dr. Joseph W. Lake and Team

CALMING YOUR DENTAL FEAR FACTOR

IF THE MERE THOUGHT OF VISITING A DENTIST CAUSES YOUR HEART TO POUND AND YOUR PALMS TO SWEAT, REST ASSURED THAT YOU'RE NOT ALONE!

There are no hard statistics on it, but it's estimated that millions of North Americans are so fearful of going to the dentist that they simply don't go. And of course, the trouble with dental problems is that they don't go away if you ignore them.

We encourage you to share your anxieties with us. Getting your concerns out in the open will let us adapt any treatments to your needs. In addition to open communication, try these tips too:

• Set aside a stress-free time for your appointment – don't try to squeeze it in between other meetings you're rushing to get to.

• Avoid taking any stimulants – coffee or cola for instance – before your appointment.

• When preparing for a dental procedure, let us know if you'd prefer to sit up or lie down in the chair. This often makes a big difference in people's comfort levels.

• Before we start anything, let's also agree on a signal, such as raising your hand, if you need to take a break.

• Feel free to bring a blanket from home, especially if you'll be in the office for an extended procedure. It may sound funny, but you'd be surprised at how comforting it can be.

• Bring an iPod or some other personal music device with your favorite tunes, to distract you from the noise of the office.

• Use deep breathing exercises, or relaxation techniques like those taught in yoga.

Some patients steer clear of the dentist because they think we might chastise them for neglecting their mouths for so long. If you fear my reaction to the condition of your teeth and gums, please relax. My job isn't to judge you and your dental history, it's to bring your mouth back to health and to restore your smile. And believe me, your smile can be fixed, no matter how bad you think it is!

GEN

Dental Associates, PC. 611 Main Street SE, Grand Rapids, MI 49502   **(616) 101-9575**

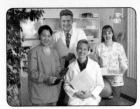

Christine *Dental Hygienist*
Dr. Joseph W. Lake, DDS
Dr. Ashley M. Lake, DDS
Jennifer Ellis *Patient Coordinator*

Joseph W. Lake, DDS
Ashley M. Lake, DDS

611 Main Street, SE
Grand Rapids, MI 49502

Phone: (616) 101-9575
Fax: (616) 101-9999

E-Mail: office@dapc.com
Website: www.Lakedental.com

Our Services Include:
• General Dentistry
• Emergency Dental Care
• Bad Breath Advice and Treatment
• Tooth Whitening
• Cosmetic Dentistry
• Denture Fittings
• Dental Implants
• Bonding & Veneers
• Crowns & Bridges

PAGE 1

Figure 3-17 An example of a dental practice newsletter, which can be used as a marketing tool to help promote the business. (Courtesy Market Connections, Inc., www.dentalhealthnews.org, Toronto, Ontario, Canada.)

Dental Associates

Compliments of Dental Associates, PC

Greetings from your Neighborhood Dentist!

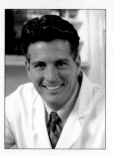

Dr. Joseph W. Lake
611 Main Street, SE
Grand Rapids, MI 49502

Phone: (616) 101-9575
Fax: (616) 101-9999

E-Mail: office@dapc.com
Website: www.Lakedental.com

Our Services Include:

- General Dentistry
- Cosmetic Dentistry
- Emergency Dental Care
- Tooth Whitening
- Bonding & Veneers
- Crowns & Bridges
- Denture Fittings
- Dental Implants
- Most Insurance Plans accepted
-   welcomed

New Patients Welcome!

a Perfectly HealtHy sMile!

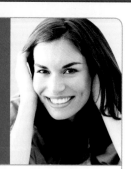

While achieving healthy smiles is our number one priority for our patients, we recognize that the emphasis on having a "perfect"- looking smile is also a highly desired goal for many men and women today.

According to some, the perfect masculine smile has square teeth, with the edges of the teeth following a straight line, while a feminine smile involves more rounded teeth, with the edges of the top teeth following the lower lip line, creating more curvature.

Overall, the standard for straight teeth is that they should be equally spaced and symmetrical, and they should line up with the teeth on the opposite jaw. Proper tooth positioning includes teeth that are vertical, with no protrusions or angles. A lot of emphasis is put on the front teeth from the perspective of general appearance, but it's important not to forget about the back teeth, the molars, as they must be healthy and positioned correctly in order to bear the work of chewing and grinding food, to relieve wear and tear on the front teeth.

Teeth whitening is a popular cosmetic enhancement. While it's true that whiter teeth can project an attractive, younger image, it's important to make sure that your gums and teeth are healthy before starting any whitening process. If you have sensitive teeth and gums, receding gums or perhaps some restorations in your mouth, it's especially important to have your mouth checked before agreeing to any type of teeth whitening.

Healthy gums and teeth are a prerequisite to any kind of cosmetic smile enhancement. However, sometimes improved oral health can be linked to something that is considered a cosmetic enhancement. For example, you may want to straighten your teeth for a more attractive smile, but on a more practical level, it's harder to clean cavity-causing plaque from between crowded or crooked teeth. A malocclusion can even cause headaches, so you'll want to look into options to fix your teeth for both an attractive smile and improved general health.

 PLEASE ASK US TO EXPLAIN ALL THE OPTIONS AVAILABLE, TO CREATE YOUR OWN "PERFECT" SMILE!

Dental Associates, PC· 611 Main Street SE, Grand Rapids, MI 49502   (616) 101-9575

Resident
1234 North Rd.
City, State 01234-5678

92024-5508

Figure 3-18 Several companies provide newsletter services to dental practices. Shown here is a detachable address label that patients or prospective patients can send directly back to the dental office. (Courtesy Market Connections, Inc., www.dentalhealthnews.org, Toronto, Ontario, Canada.)

KEY TERMS

Client-centered therapy—A form of therapy that when applied to dentistry encourages listening to patients to learn about their feelings, desires, and priorities.

Hierarchy of needs—Five basic levels of needs described by Abraham Maslow, which are used to aid in understanding how a person's needs motivate behavior. They are physiological, safety or security, social or love, esteem, and self-actualization.

Marketing—Marketing is a form of advertising, and in dentistry it is what one does within the office to retain patients.

Nonverbal cues—Gestures and body movements a person makes in a given situation to denote a feeling.

Office policy—A form of written communication that identifies the dentist's philosophy and policies and defines the responsibilities of the patient and dental staff.

Patients' rights—Inherent rights of a patient to be informed of services being performed, the cost, and the consequences of such treatment.

LEARNING ACTIVITIES

1. Identify and give examples of barriers in communication.
2. Describe the duties of a receptionist in communicating with patients and putting them at ease.
3. Explain Maslow's Hierarchy of Needs and Carl Rogers' client-centered therapy as they relate to dentistry.
4. What is marketing?
5. List five rights of the patient that should be considered during a treatment procedure.

Please refer to the student workbook for additional learning activities.

BIBLIOGRAPHY

Bernstein DA, Nash PW: *Essentials of psychology*, ed 2, Boston, 2002, Houghton Mifflin.

Frazier GL: *Connecting with customers*, ed 2, Upper Saddle River, NJ, 2004, Prentice Hall.

Fulton-Calkins PJ: *The administrative professional*, ed 13, Mason, Ohio, 2007.

Griffin J, et al: *How to say it at work: power words, phrases, and communication*, Upper Saddle River, NJ, 2008, Prentice Hall.

Locker KO, Kyo Kaczmarek S: *Business communication: building critical skills*, ed 2, New York, 2003, Irwin/McGraw-Hill.

McNamara C: *Field guide to leadership and supervision in business*, Minneapolis, 2002, Authenticity Consulting.

Miles L: *Dynamic dentistry: practice management tools and strategy for breakthrough success*, Virginia Beach, Va, 2003, Link Publishing.

Perkins PS: *The art and science of communication: tools for effective communication in the workplace*, New York, 2008, John Wiley & Sons.

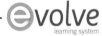
learning system

Please visit http://evolve.elsevier.com/Finkibeiner/practice for additional practice activities.

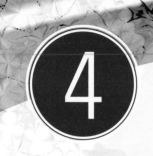

Legal and Ethical Issues in the Dental Business Office

CHAPTER OUTLINE

Definition of Law
    Law Relative to Dentistry
    Classifications of Law
Crimes and Torts
    Overview and Definitions
    Litigation
Dental Practice Act
Professional Standards
Code of Ethics
    American Dental Association Principles of Ethics and Code
        of Professional Conduct
    American Dental Assistants Association Principles of Ethics
    American Association of Dental Office Managers (AMDOM)
Ethical and Legal Considerations for the Administrative Assistant
    Vigilance
    Assignment of Duties
Consent
    Informed Consent
    Implied Consent
    Informed Refusal
Managed Care
Risk Management Programs
Abandonment
Fraud
Records Management
Defamation of Character
Negligence
Invasion of Privacy
Good Samaritan Law
Americans with Disabilities Act
Computer Security
Twelve Steps to Making Ethical Decisions

LEARNING OUTCOMES

- Define glossary terms.
- Explain the impact of ethics and law on the dental business office.
- Differentiate between the various types of law that affect the practice of dentistry.
- Explain various types of consent.
- Describe situations in the dental business office that would lead to potential litigation.
- Describe the code of ethics of professional dental organizations.
- Identify 12 steps in making ethical decisions.

Each day dental professionals are faced with issues involving the legal requirements and standards of care, voluntary and involuntary, in the delivery of dental treatment. The **dental practice act** of each state defines the requirements necessary to practice dentistry and the scope of dental practice for that particular state. Standards for dental care may arise from both **common law** (judicial decisions) and statutory law (enacted by a legislative body), such as the state dental practice act. The dental

professional is governed also by voluntary standards, such as the principles of ethics, developed and implemented by the dental profession itself. Both legal and voluntary requirements and standards are implemented for the protection of society and, ultimately, the patient. This process of regulation is illustrated in Figure 4-1.

An administrative assistant practicing in a dental office today needs to have an understanding of the effect of law on the dental

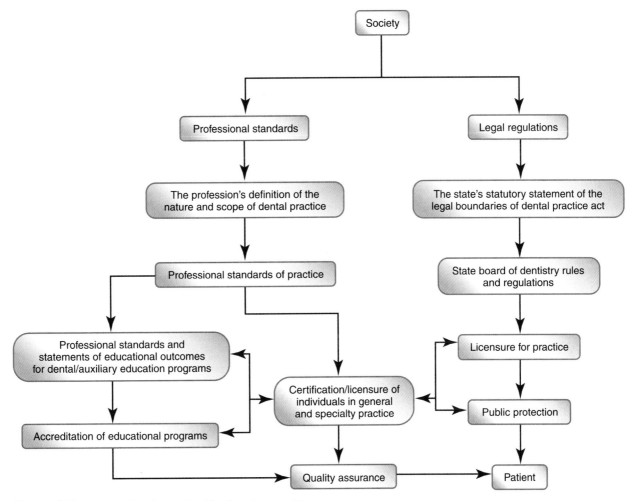

Figure 4-1 Diagram of professional and legal regulations of dentistry.

practice and an awareness of its importance on his or her performance of daily duties. Further, each member of a professional organization should be familiar with the code of ethics for its professional group and its colleagues.

Membership in a professional organization is voluntary, and thus the standards of these organizations are considered voluntary. However, these standards are used as guidelines in peer review. Professional organizations continually reassess the functions of their standards and the qualifications of their members. The standards of professional health organizations reflect the assessment of the need for dental care and the public's expectations for dentistry and its professional staff to appropriately meet those needs. Examples of voluntary standards are illustrated in the profession's code of ethics, professional standards for accreditation of educational programs, standards for credentialing, and standards of various service organizations. Legal standards for dental care are determined through common law and result in standards such as the Informed Consent Doctrine, which is discussed later in this chapter. Legislative action through the Dental Practice Act establishes the legal requirements and scope of the practice within the state. This action establishes education, credentialing, and licensure requirements for the dentist and any dental auxiliaries recognized in the state dental practice act.

Copies of the principles of ethics for any of the dental professional organizations may be obtained from their national offices or official web sites. To obtain a copy of the state dental practice act, contact an individual state's board of dentistry. Some states have the dental practice act online for easy access or downloading. A *State Fact Booklet* may also be purchased from the Dental Assisting National Board (DANB) web site, available at www.DANB.org.

DEFINITION OF LAW

Law consists of enforceable rules governing relationships among individuals and between individuals and their society. A broad definition of the law implies that there must be established rules, such as constitutions, statutes, administrative agency rules, and judicial decisions. Rules of law must be enforceable and establish limits of conduct for governments and individuals in society.

Law Relative to Dentistry

In many states the board of dentistry is an administrative agency at the state level. The executive officers of an administrative agency perform specific functions, including enforcing laws within their agency. The state boards have the power to make rules and regulations that conform to enacted laws, such as the dental practice act. Rules and regulations adopted by the board are components of the body of law referred to as administrative laws. State statutes must conform to the state's constitution and the federal constitution. The dental practice act is an example of state statutory law.

Classifications of Law

Law can be divided into two classifications: (1) civil and (2) criminal. Civil law relates to duties between persons or between citizens and their government. Criminal law deals with wrongs committed against the public as a whole.

In a civil case, one party (the plaintiff) tries to correct an interference with his or her interest by another party (the defendant). The defendant may have failed to comply with a duty or otherwise breached an acceptable standard of conduct. The defendant may be required to pay for the damages caused by failure to comply with that duty. In criminal law, the interests of society are at stake and the government may seek to impose a penalty, such as a fine or imprisonment, on the guilty person.

CRIMES AND TORTS

Overview and Definitions

A crime is a wrongdoing against the public at large, and is prosecuted by a public official. In most cases when a crime is committed, there is intent to do wrong. However, a person or entity that breaks certain laws may be guilty of a crime whether there was intent or not. Criminal liability typically involves both the performance of a prohibited act and a specified state of mind or intent on the part of the actor. In some cases, the omission of an act can be a crime if the person or entity has a legal duty to perform the act, such as failure to file a federal income tax return.

A crime can be classified as a misdemeanor or a felony. A misdemeanor is less serious than a felony and is punishable by a fine or imprisonment up to one year. A felony is a more serious crime and generally is punishable by imprisonment for longer period of time.

A tort is a civil wrongdoing. It is an interference with a recognized interest or a breach of a legal duty owed by a defendant to a plaintiff. The plaintiff in most instances must show that the defendant's action or omission was a cause of loss or harm to the plaintiff. A tort is generally resolved through a civil trial with a monetary settlement for damages. Included in torts are the areas of negligence, assault and battery, infliction of mental distress, defamation, and fraud.

Torts may be intentional or unintentional acts of wrongdoing. If intentional, this means that the person committing the tort intended to commit the wrongful act. Intentional torts for which a dental assistant could be held liable include assault and battery, defamation of character, invasion of privacy, immoral conduct, and fraud.

Unintentional torts do not require a particular mental state. Failure to exercise a standard of care, such as performing a treatment that a reasonably prudent professional would perform in similar circumstances, is an example of an unintentional tort. Thus, even if a dental professional neither wishes to bring about the consequences of the act, nor believes that they will occur, negligence may be alleged whereby someone suffers injury because another failed to live up to a particular standard of care. Questions relating to the failure to exercise a standard of care must be answered. The following four elements make up the unintentional tort of negligence:

1. Was there a duty to follow a standard of care?
2. Was this duty breached?
3. Did the plaintiff suffer injury?
4. Was the injury a direct result of that breach of duty?

PRACTICE NOTE
Failure to exercise a standard of care, performing treatment that a reasonably prudent professional would perform in similar circumstances, is an example of an unintentional tort.

Strict liability is an unintentional tort. It relates to a person being liable for actions regardless of the care exercised and for damages or injuries caused by the act. Negligence is the performance of an act that a reasonably careful person under similar circumstances would not do, or the failure to perform an act that a reasonably careful person would do under similar circumstances. Professionals usually consider malpractice a form of negligence, but it can mean, in a broader sense, any wrongdoing by a professional. Malpractice can refer to any professional misconduct, evil practice, or illegal or immoral conduct, not just negligence. Malpractice can be either unintentional or intentional. Box 4-1 contains a list of negligent acts that might occur in a dental office.

PRACTICE NOTE
Professionals usually consider malpractice as a form of negligence, but it can mean, in a broader sense, any wrongdoing by a professional.

Litigation

Litigation is the process of a lawsuit. A lawsuit is a legal action in a court. The person or party that institutes the suit in court is the plaintiff. The person being accused of the wrongdoing is the defendant.

During malpractice litigation, the patient may be the plaintiff. The dentist or person who is being sued is the defendant. It is likely that other individuals in the dental office, such as a dentist associate, dental assistant, or dental hygienist, might be named as a defendant, fact witness, or an expert witness in the legal proceedings. A fact witness, when placed under oath, must provide only firsthand knowledge, not hearsay. In such testimony, the fact witness describes what he or she saw or did during a specific act. For instance, if the fact witness is being

BOX 4-1 Negligent Acts That Could Occur in a Dental Office

- Abandonment
- Burns
- Mistaken identity
- Foreign objects left in a patient after surgical procedures
- Use of defective equipment
- Failure to observe patient reactions and take appropriate action
- Medication errors
- Drug administration errors
- Failure to take an adequate history
- Failure to exercise good judgment
- Failure to communicate
- Loss of or damage to patient's personal property
- Failure to obtain informed consent
- Disease transmission

questioned about the administration of a local anesthetic for a patient, the witness may be asked if he or she was told what type of anesthetic to prepare, if he or she prepared the anesthetic and passed it to the dentist, how much anesthetic was administered to the patient, and what the patient's reaction was after the anesthetic was administered. If the fact witness only received the directions and prepared the anesthetic for the setup, but did not participate in its administration, only the initial questions can be answered. To describe any further action not observed would be inappropriate and may be considered speculation or hearsay.

An **expert witness** is called to testify and explain to the judge and jury what happened based on the patient's record and to offer an opinion as to whether or not the dental care, as administered, met acceptable standards. Standards may vary by state. Often a dentist may be called as an expert witness to testify in malpractice litigation because of his or her educational background and strong clinical expertise. A strong knowledge of dental law and dental standards, as well as an understanding of malpractice liability, is beneficial in such cases.

DENTAL PRACTICE ACT

The legal requirements necessary to practice dentistry as well as the scope of what can be practiced are developed through legislative action within the state and are identified in the state dental practice act. This act defines the minimum educational standards, requirements for credentialing, and criteria for license revocation or suspension for a dentist, dental hygienist, and in several states the dental assistant. Other legal requirements are enacted by the government in the form of rules and regulations and, like the dental practice act, also regulate the practice of dentistry. An example of a government agency that creates requirements that affect the practice of dentistry is the state Department of Labor.

A state dental practice act is not frequently changed. However, as changes take place in technology and standards of dental care are modified, it may be necessary to apply new rules and regulations to the state dental practice act. An administrative assistant should regularly obtain a copy of any changes in the dental practice act or new rules and regulations and retain it on file.

Many state dental practice acts define conditions under which a dental assistant or dental hygienist may perform specific duties. Each state provides a list of definitions within the law, and the descriptive language may vary significantly from state to state. Examples of such terminology include patient of record, assignment, and supervision. **Patient of record** refers to a patient who has been examined and diagnosed by a licensed dentist and whose treatment has been planned by that dentist. **Assignment** commonly refers to the dentist assigning a specific procedure to a dental assistant or dental hygienist that is to be performed on a designated patient of record. For certain procedures, the dentist does not need to be physically present in the office or in the treatment room at the time the procedure is being performed. **Supervision** refers to the conditions under which a patient of record may be treated by an assistant or hygienist and the protocol to be followed after the treatment is rendered. One type of supervision is referred to as *direct supervision* and generally means that the dentist has designated a patient of record on whom services are to be performed and has described the procedure to be performed. The dentist examines the patient before prescribing the procedures to be performed and again on completion of the procedure. Under the definition of direct supervision, the dentist generally must be physically present in the office at the time the procedures are being performed.

It is important to remember that the legal standards within a dental law are for the protection of the general public, and interpretations of requirements for the protection of the general public may differ in each state. Terminology used in various dental practice acts may vary from state to state. The term *assignment* may be used in one dental practice act; however, in another state the term *general supervision* may have a similar or identical description to assignment. It is important to carefully read all definitions and descriptions found in a dental practice act to completely understand scope of practice and supervisory requirements.

PROFESSIONAL STANDARDS

Over the last half century, the dental assisting profession has taken several steps to ensure the competence of its practitioners in such areas as the credentialing process. *Credentialing* is a generic term that refers to the ways in which professionals can measure and maintain their competence.

The processes used in credentialing include accreditation, certification, and licensure. Accreditation generally is the process by which an entity or educational program is evaluated and recognized by an outside agency for having attained a predetermined set of standards. These standards are identified by the professional and educational organization, including peer groups. In dentistry, the Commission on Dental Accreditation of the American Dental Association is responsible for accrediting educational programs in dentistry, dental assisting, dental hygiene, and dental laboratory technology. When a program is accredited by the American Dental Association's (ADA) Commission on Dental Accreditation (CODA), the program makes public its accreditation status. Such accreditation validates that a specific educational program has met a set of standards to address the needs of the profession and the public. In many instances a criterion for obtaining a credential such as certification or licensure is contingent on successful completion of an ADA-accredited educational program.

National certification in dental assisting is a voluntary procedure and may be achieved through the DANB. This organization provides credentialing for the clinical dental assistant, the orthodontic assistant, and the administrative assistant as described in Chapter 2. The process of credentialing requires prerequisites involving education and clinical experiences and measures whether the person has met certain criteria established by the nongovernmental organization for the dental assisting profession.

Licensure is the credential granted to a candidate by the state after the candidate has provided appropriate documentation indicating the candidate has met the state's designated requirements to practice in the profession. Generally this license is granted after the person has met certain educational requirements and has successfully completed some form of designated state testing, such as a clinical or written examination. Licensure is intended to protect the consumer and is designed for the clinical dental assistant who has direct patient care responsibilities.

CODE OF ETHICS

Ethics is a branch of philosophy and is a systematic, intellectual approach to the standards of behavior. The purpose of a professional code of ethics is to help members of the profession achieve high levels of behavior through moral consciousness, decision making, and practice by members of the profession. Ethics in daily professional practice challenges a practitioner to differentiate between right and wrong. Morals are considered voluntary personal commitments to a set of values. Values are the standards used for decision making that endure over a significant period of time. The expected behaviors of the dental professional are based on a set of standards derived from aspired acceptable behaviors. Every health professional must realize that there is right and wrong and that there is no right way to do a wrong thing.

American Dental Association Principles of Ethics and Code of Professional Conduct

Each organized group within the profession of dentistry, including the ADA, ADAA (American Dental Assistants Association), and ADHA (American Dental Hygienists' Association), has developed a code of ethics for its members. The codes are based on ethical principles that reflect a concern for the patient's protection during all aspects of care.

 PRACTICE NOTE
There is no right way to do a wrong thing.

Dentistry as a profession enjoys a certain right of independence, in decision making and self-governance, as a result of the training and education of its members. However this right carries with it an obligation to maintain quality standards and be responsible to one's patients and peers. This right does not allow a member of the profession to disregard professional standards or laws governing the practice of dentistry. The profession's primary goal is to provide quality care to patients in a competent and timely manner. To maintain high standards of care, the dental professional can continue to improve the quality of care through education, training, research, and adherence to a stringent code of ethics and professional conduct. The *ADA Principles of Ethics and Code of Professional Conduct* can be found at the ADA web site, http://www.ada.org/prof/prac/law/code/index.asp. This document identifies five basic categories of ethics and professional conduct for a dentist. An overview of these principles is included in Box 4-2.

American Dental Assistants Association Principles of Ethics

Like the ADA, the ADAA has addressed the issue of ethics by preparing the following statement as the principles of ethics for its members:

> Each individual involved in the practice of dentistry assumes the obligation of maintaining and enriching the profession. Each member may choose to meet this obligation according to the dictates of personal conscience based on the needs of the human beings the profession of dentistry is committed to serve. The spirit of the Golden Rule is the basic guiding principle of this concept. The member must strive at all times to maintain confidentiality and exhibit respect for the dentist/employer. The member shall refrain from performing any professional service that is prohibited by state law and has the obligation to prove competence prior to providing services to any patient. The member shall constantly strive to upgrade and expand technical skills for the benefit of the employer and the consumer public. The member should additionally seek to sustain and improve the local organization, state association, and the ADAA by active participation and personal commitment. More information can be found at the website www.dentalassist.org/.

American Association of Dental Office Managers (AMDOM)

This is a relatively new organization that has been created for dental office managers "and practice administrators". This organization deals with specific issues related to the dental business office and makes special efforts to ensure that its members maintain confidentiality. More information may be found at the web site www.dentalmanagers.com.

BOX 4-2   Overview of ADA Principles of Ethics and Code of Professional Conduct

SECTION 1—Principle: Patient Autonomy ("self-governance")

The dentist has a duty to respect the patient's rights to self-determination and confidentiality.

This principle expresses the concept that professionals have a duty to treat the patient according to the patient's desires, within the bounds of accepted treatment, and to protect the patient's confidentiality. Under this principle, the dentist's primary obligations include involving patients in treatment decisions in a meaningful way, with due consideration being given to the patient's needs, desires, and abilities, and safeguarding the patient's privacy.

SECTION 2—Principle: Nonmaleficence ("do no harm")

The dentist has a duty to refrain from harming the patient.

This principle expresses the concept that professionals have a duty to protect the patient from harm. Under this principle, the dentist's primary obligations include keeping knowledge and skills current, knowing one's own limitations and when to refer to a specialist or other professional, and knowing when and under what circumstances delegation of patient care to auxiliaries is appropriate.

SECTION 3—Principle: Beneficence ("do good")

The dentist has a duty to promote the patient's welfare.

This principle expresses the concept that professionals have a duty to act for the benefit of others. Under this principle, the dentist's primary obligation is service to the patient and the public at large. The most important aspect of this obligation is the competent and timely delivery of dental care within the bounds of clinical circumstances presented by the patient, with due consideration being given to the needs, desires, and values of the patient. The same ethical considerations apply whether the dentist engages in fee-for-service, managed care, or other practice arrangement. Dentists may choose to enter into contracts governing the provision of care to a group of patients; however, contract obligations do not excuse dentists from their ethical duty to put the patient's welfare first.*

SECTION 4—Principle: Justice ("fairness")

The dentist has a duty to treat people fairly.

This principle expresses the concept that professionals have a duty to be fair in their dealings with patients, colleagues, and society. Under this principle, the dentist's primary obligations include dealing with people justly and delivering dental care without prejudice. In its broadest sense, this principle expresses the concept that the dental professional should actively seek allies throughout society on specific activities that will help improve access to care for all.

SECTION 5—Principle: Veracity ("truthfulness")

The dentist has a duty to communicate truthfully.

This principle expresses the concept that professionals have a duty to be honest and trustworthy in their dealings with people. Under this principle, the dentist's primary obligations include respecting the position of trust inherent in the dentist–patient relationship, communicating truthfully and without deception, and maintaining intellectual integrity. Codes of professional conduct can be found for each section in the Principles of Ethics and Code of Professional Conduct handbook (an ADA publication), or on the ADA web site, available at http://www.ada.org/prof/prac/law/code/index.asp.

ETHICAL AND LEGAL CONSIDERATIONS FOR THE ADMINISTRATIVE ASSISTANT

Vigilance

Each day the dental professional is confronted with ethical and legal decisions. The basis for each of these decisions may change as laws and societal influences affect the delivery of dental care. As mentioned, each member of the dental profession must constantly be vigilant of the changes taking place in laws affecting dentistry. Even though the administrative assistant has contact with the clinical areas of the office, emphasis in this text is placed on only those areas that directly relate to activities of the dental administrative assistant. Box 4-3 lists those activities that the administrative assistant may encounter that could lead to potential litigation. The following discussion provides the administrative assistant with a practical understanding of various issues. These situations also should provoke one's critical-thinking processes to consider other situations that might be common to a dental practice.

Assignment of Duties

As described in the section on the state dental practice act, it is the responsibility of the licensed dentist to assign specific procedures to dental auxiliaries. If a duty that is illegal within

BOX 4-3   Common Business Activities That Lead to Potential Litigation

- Making false accusations about another person in verbal or written communication
- Providing another party or agency with confidential information without patient consent
- Entering inaccurate data on patient records
- Duplicating copyrighted material without permission
- Using unauthorized software
- Gaining illegal access to computer data
- Maliciously or deliberately damaging data in a computer
- Falsely entering data on insurance claims
- Failing to follow federal or state disease transmission or waste management regulations
- Failing to maintain accurate local, state, or federal governmental records

the state is assigned to the dental assistant, the dentist is liable for this illegal action. Further, if a dental assistant performs a procedure that is not legally delegable to be performed by the assistant; the assistant is liable for such action.

Several factors should be considered in the issue of assignment. First, before an employee is hired, copies of appropriate documentation for appropriate credentials should be reviewed to assure

> **PRACTICE NOTE**
> If a duty that is not legal within the state is assigned to the dental assistant, the dentist is liable for this illegal action.

the person does indeed have the specified credentials. This may include transcripts, certificates of completion or other licenses. Second, the administrative assistant or office manager must be responsible for retaining on file current copies of all employee credentials. In some states this may include current licenses, reported from required background checks or CPR certification. Third, the employer–employee relationship often creates conflict in such assignments. An assistant may feel that if a dentist assigns a task, it must be performed because the dentist is an authority figure, or the assistant may feel that his or her job will be jeopardized if the assignment is not carried out. To perform a task that is not legally delegable or for which an assistant is not qualified or has no credentials simply because it was assigned by the dentist can place the assistant in a position of a potential allegation of negligence.

CONSENT

Consent is the voluntary acceptance or agreement to what is planned or done by another person. To examine or treat a patient without consent constitutes an unauthorized touching and makes the person committing the act guilty of battery. Battery is contact with someone that may result in bodily harm or offensive touching. Two forms of consent exist in the delivery of dental care: *informed* and *implied*.

> **PRACTICE NOTE**
> Consent is the voluntary acceptance or agreement to what is planned or done by another person.

Informed Consent

Informed consent is a concept that has evolved for decades in courts and legislatures to assist patients in determining the care they find acceptable. It has resulted in more disclosure on the part of the provider to allow the patient to make an informed decision. The basis for the concept of informed consent is that every adult of sound mind has the right to determine what can and cannot be done with his or her body. For that person to make a proper judgment, he or she must be given information by the healthcare provider. The patient must be given enough information about the proposed treatment, in understandable language, to make an intelligent decision as to whether to proceed with the treatment. Moreover, the patient must have ample opportunity to ask questions and have them answered.

In general courts and legislatures have defined specific elements that describe informed consent. These elements state that consent must be given freely; treatment and diagnosis must be described in understandable language; risks, benefits, and estimate of success of treatment must be described; prognosis if no treatment is elected and alternative treatment plans must be

explained; and the patient must be given the right to ask questions and have them answered.

It is important to remember that if these conditions are not met the courts may conclude that the patient did not consent to the procedure and therefore the dentist may be liable for actions such as battery or negligence (depending on the individual state).

For consent to be legally valid, it must be informed and given freely, and the patient must be an adult of sound mind. Patients under the influence of alcohol, drugs, or severe stress may not have sufficient mental capacity to grant permission for treatment. When a dentist treats a minor, only the parent or guardian of the minor may grant consent. This excludes grandparents, caregivers, and siblings. However, parents may authorize another party to grant consent for treatment during the parents' absence. Such authorization must be signed before treatment consent. Even with this documentation, it is suggested to confirm telephone consent with a parent if someone other than the parent accompanies the child.

An emancipated minor is someone who has not reached the age of majority, but because of circumstances, can provide consent. This may include a young woman who has children of her own, not living with her parents and receiving no financial support from her parents. A variety of consent forms are available and should be used during all invasive procedures.

Specialty practices such as endodontics and oral surgery have forms designed specifically for their specialties. Figure 4-2 shows an example of a common form for a general practice. These forms must be signed, dated, and retained in the patient record. It is not recommended to have the patient sign an informed consent form that gives the provider permission to "perform any and all procedures." This violates the intent of the concept of informed consent and the patient's right to have adequate and appropriate information when making a decision about a specific recommendation or treatment option.

Implied Consent

Other agreements that flow automatically from the relationship between the patient and the dental professional fall under the category of implied consent. These agreements trigger responsibilities that work in two ways; those that the dentist owes to the patient, and those that the patient owes to the dentist. Accepting a patient for treatment implies that the dentist agrees to accept certain responsibilities for that patient's dental care. Likewise if a patient agrees to accept treatment by the dentist, it is considered that the patient assumes certain responsibilities. Boxes 4-4 and 4-5 list implied responsibilities for each of these parties.

Informed Refusal

A patient may decline a recommended procedure or referral from a dentist. Examples include refusal of radiographs, periodontal care, fluoride treatments, or referral to a specialist or physician. An office should document this refusal for recommended care in writing. The informed refusal process parallels the principles found in informed consent. An informed refusal form should

PATIENT'S NAME: _____   DATE:_____

TIME:_____ (A.M.) (P.M.)

I HEREBY AUTHORIZE DR._____ AND HIS/HER ASSOCIATES AT _____
_____ TO PERFORM UPON ME OR THE NAMED PATIENT THE FOLLOWING
PROCEDURE(S): _____
_____ (EXPLAIN IN PLAIN ENGLISH).

DR. _____ HAS FULLY EXPLAINED TO ME THE PURPOSE OF THE PROCEDURE(S) AND HAS ALSO
INFORMED ME OF EXPECTED BENEFITS AND COMPLICATIONS (FROM KNOWN AND UNKNOWN CAUSES), ATTENDANT
DISCOMFORTS AND RISKS THAT MAY ARISE, AS WELL AS POSSIBLE ALTERNATIVES TO THE PROPOSED TREATMENT, INCLUDING
NO TREATMENT. THE ATTENDANT RISKS OF NO TREATMENT HAVE ALSO BEEN DISCUSSED. I HAVE BEEN GIVEN AN
OPPORTUNITY TO ASK QUESTIONS, AND ALL MY QUESTIONS HAVE BEEN ANSWERED FULLY AND SATISFACTORILY. I
ACKNOWLEDGE THAT NO GUARANTEES OR ASSURANCES HAVE BEEN MADE TO ME CONCERNING THE RESULTS INTENDED
FROM THE PROCEDURE(S).

I UNDERSTAND THAT DURING THE COURSE OF THE PROCEDURE(S), UNFORESEEN CONDITIONS MAY ARISE WHICH
NECESSITATE PROCEDURES DIFFERENT FROM THOSE CONTEMPLATED. I, THEREFORE, CONSENT TO THE PERFORMANCE OF
ADDITIONAL PROCEDURE(S) WHICH THE ABOVE-NAMED DENTIST OR HIS/HER ASSOCIATES MAY CONSIDER NECESSARY.

I ALSO UNDERSTAND THE FINANCIAL OBLIGATION ATTACHED TO THIS PROCEDURE AND AGREE TO COMPLY AS LISTED BELOW:
AMOUNT DUE _____ TO BE PAID IN _____ MONTHLY PAYMENTS OF $_____ STARTING _____.
BALANCE TO BE PAID IN FULL BY _____.

I UNDERSTAND THAT I AM RESPONSIBLE FOR ALL FEES REGARDLESS OF INSURANCE COVERAGE. I ALSO UNDERSTAND THAT AS
TREATMENT PROGRESSES THE ABOVE FEES MAY HAVE TO BE ADJUSTED, BUT THAT I WILL BE INFORMED OF THESE
ADJUSTMENTS AND HOW THEY WILL AFFECT MY PAYMENT PLAN. IN THE EVENT THAT MY PAYMENTS ARE NOT RECEIVED WITHIN
30 DAYS OF THEIR DUE DATE, I AGREE TO PAY ALL COSTS OF COLLECTIONS, INCLUDING, BUT NOT LIMITED TO, REASONABLE
ATTORNEY'S FEES.

I CONFIRM THAT I HAVE READ AND FULLY UNDERSTAND THE ABOVE AND THAT ALL BLANK SPACES HAVE BEEN COMPLETED
PRIOR TO MY SIGNING.

I HEREBY CONSENT TO THE PROPOSED DENTAL TREATMENT.

_____   _____
SIGNATURE OF PATIENT OR PARENT/GUARDIAN IF MINOR   DATE

_____   _____
INTERPRETER (IF USED)   DATE

_____   _____
SIGNATURE OF WITNESS   DATE

DENTIST CERTIFICATION:
I HEREBY CERTIFY THAT I HAVE EXPLAINED THE NATURE, PURPOSE, BENEFITS, RISKS OF, AND ALTERNATIVES (INCLUDING NO
TREATMENT AND ATTENDANT RISKS), TO THE PROPOSED PROCEDURE(S). I HAVE OFFERED ANSWERS TO ANY QUESTIONS AND
HAVE FULLY ANSWERED ALL SUCH QUESTIONS. I BELIEVE THAT THE PATIENT/PARENT/GUARDIAN FULLY UNDERSTANDS WHAT I
HAVE EXPLAINED AND ANSWERED.

DENTIST'S SIGNATURE _____

PRINT NAME _____ DATE _____
Item 051-5742/27005 Patterson Office Supplies 800-637-1140

PATIENT NUMBER

CONSENT TO DENTAL TREATMENT

Figure 4-2 Informed consent form. (Courtesy Patterson Office Supplies, Champaign, IL.)

include the specifically recommended procedures, the potential risks (both oral and general health) by declining the procedure, and an opportunity for the patient to ask and have their questions answered. The dentist, the patient, and a witness, such as the administrative assistant, should sign the form. The date should be recorded. If an allegation of negligence occurs, the informed refusal may assist in the defense of the dentist. Not all courts recognize informed refusal, but should be considered as a method to document patient refusal.

MANAGED CARE

Managed care refers to a cost containment system of healthcare insurance that may direct use of health benefits by restricting the type, level, and frequency of treatment; limiting access to care to certain entities or practitioners; and basing the level of reimbursement for services on a capitation or other risk basis. Limitations imposed by managed care companies generally are directed at payment for services, but the policies may also limit the actual services received by a patient.

In this way managed care systems raise several legal and ethical issues for the dentist and healthcare professional. Patients may ask dentists to render only the treatment that is covered by the insurance plan, rather than the necessary treatment. Insurance companies are profit driven and may not sufficiently consider the healthcare professional's responsibilities. Capitated plans can cause an ethical dilemma for a dentist when, for example, a dentist is paid for patient care whether or not it is provided, because it is obvious that it is not in the dentist's short-term economic interest

BOX 4-4 Implied Duties Owed by the Dentist to the Patient

- Use reasonable care in the provision of services as measured against acceptable standards set by other practitioners with similar training in a similar community.
- Be properly licensed and registered, and meet all other legal requirements to engage in the practice of dentistry.
- Obtain an accurate health (medical and dental) history of the patient before a diagnosis is made and treatment is begun.
- Employ competent personnel and provide for their proper supervision.
- Maintain a level of knowledge in keeping with current advances in the profession.
- Use methods that are acceptable to at least a respectable minority of similar practitioners in the community.
- Refrain from performing experimental procedures.
- Obtain informed consent from the patient before instituting an examination or treatment.
- Refrain from abandoning the patient, and ensure that care is available in emergency situations.
- Charge a reasonable fee (by community standards) for services.
- Refrain from exceeding the scope of practice authorized by your license or permitting those acting under your direction to engage in unlawful acts.
- Keep the patient informed of his or her progress.
- Refrain from undertaking any procedure for which you are not qualified.
- Complete care in a timely manner.
- Keep accurate records of the treatment rendered to the patient.
- Maintain confidentiality of information.
- Inform the patient of any untoward occurrences in the course of treatment.
- Make appropriate referrals, and request necessary consultations.
- Comply with all laws regulating the practice of dentistry.
- Practice in a manner consistent with the codes of ethics of the profession.
- Use universal precautions in the treatment of all patients.

BOX 4-5 Implied Duties Owed by the Patient to the Dentist

- Cooperate in your care by following home care or other reasonable instructions, taking prescribed medications, and showing up for recalls.
- Keep appointments, and notify the office of cancellations or appointment delays.
- Provide honest answers to questions asked on the history form and by the dentist and office personnel.
- Notify the office staff or dentist of any change in health status.
- Pay a reasonable fee for the service if no fee is agreed on in writing or orally.
- Remit the fee for services within a reasonable time.

to provide that care. Further, if certain care is not reimbursed, a patient may forgo needed treatment because of financial concerns. For the patient's interest to be protected, the dentist must be relied on to adhere to both legal and ethical principles.

RISK MANAGEMENT PROGRAMS

A dental professional teaches preventive concepts to patients with a firm conviction that such practice will prevent future disease. This concept can be applied to prevention of malpractice claims. Most dental societies, organizations, and institutions are taking an active role in providing seminars and programs in risk management. The dental administrative assistant commonly assumes the responsibility for scheduling risk management seminars and maintaining records of such attendance.

Risk management programs primarily show where dentists have been found liable in the past and try to teach dentists how to avoid exposing themselves to such liability. Often these programs accomplish this goal by reviewing real cases where dentists have been successfully sued. This method has a great impact on the dentists and auxiliaries. Risk management programs aid the dental professional in identifying, analyzing, and dealing with risks in the dental office.

Risk management programs generally include information on operating safety, product safety, quality assurance, and waste disposal. Operating safety programs emphasize methods of operating in an environment that ensures the safety of the patient, staff, and visitors. Programs about product safety update the dental team on the use of current materials and equipment and methods of evaluation and maintenance of these products. Quality assurance programs provide information on evaluating all systems used in the care of a patient. Waste disposal programs provide the most current information on disposing of medical and dental wastes. Risk management programs can also provide suggestions about appropriate communication and record keeping strategies to protect all members of the dental team. Risk management education combined with competent practice can be great insurance to the dental professional for avoiding potential litigation.

ABANDONMENT

Abandonment is defined as the severance of a professional relationship with a patient who is still in need of dental care and proper transfers or referrals. Although this legal concept primarily affects the dentist, the administrative assistant should be aware of its existence and aid the dentist in ensuring that no patient is abandoned in midtreatment.

An example of abandonment might arise when a dentist who has been in practice for many years is suddenly diagnosed with a terminal illness. Many patients are in midtreatment stages, and it appears that the dentist will be unable to resume work immediately. The future is uncertain for the dental practice. In this situation, arrangements must be made by the dentist and his or her family or staff to provide treatment for the patients. It may be necessary to hire a dentist for interim professional coverage of the patients or provide the names of dentists who are willing to accept the patients into their practices. The practice may ultimately need to be sold to another dentist. The administrative assistant plays a major role in this situation, because patients should be informed of the transition. Further information on patient care must be provided or transferred to the new treating dentists in an efficient manner. When informing patients of such changes, the administrative assistant must tell patients where their dental records are located. Patients should be given a reasonable period of time, typically 30 to 60 days, to contact the office to have their records transferred elsewhere if they do not wish to be seen by the new dentist. The administrative assistant should also ensure that the transfer of information meets federal and state law requirements on patient records, including meeting privacy requirements. Be certain to refer to the latest privacy guidelines by the Health Insurance Portability and Accountability Act of 1996 (HIPAA) for legal protocol.

Another potential abandonment situation could occur when a patient in the practice has been very irritating. For example, a patient may have failed to keep multiple appointments or give advance notification for broken appointments. The dentist may become very distressed with the patient and state that the patient is no longer desired in the practice.

To refuse to treat this patient is abandonment. Therefore the administrative assistant must inform the patient in writing why the dentist is no longer able to treat him or her. A letter should be sent informing the patient that the relationship with the dental office and patient is being terminated. The letter should clearly state that if the patient needs a referral in the geographical area, he or she may contact the local dental society (include the name, address, and phone number of the dental society). The letter should also include a statement indicating that the dentist is willing to provide emergency care, including treatment for pain and infection, for a period of time, such as 30 days from the date of the letter. This notification of a period of time is very important so that the patient is not "abandoned" and has adequate time to identify another provider. The letter should be sent by certified mail with a return receipt requested. A copy of the letter and the returned receipt should be retained in the patient record. It would be prudent for the dentist to have a written policy on this issue. The policy should be posted or otherwise communicated to all patients so that there are no surprises, and liability is mitigated, when a patient receives such a letter.

The administrative assistant should be cautious about talking with patients once a letter is sent. Frequently a patient will call the office and seek an additional explanation or attempt to return to the office. If a decision is made to terminate a patient, the office should not waver in its decision and only repeat the objective information found in the letter. For example, if the dentist chose to terminate the patient because the patient was uncooperative in care, that reason is the only one that should be provided with any further explanation. Additional explanation is unnecessary because it may provide the patient with information that could be misinterpreted and lead to patient accusations of discrimination or defamation.

FRAUD

Fraud is a deception that is deliberately practiced to secure unfair or unlawful gain. One of the most common practices of fraud is in the obtaining of fees through third-party payments by misrepresentation.

An example of a fraudulent action occurs when a patient has insurance coverage from July 1 of the past year until June 30 of the current year, after which time the patient would no longer receive this benefit. The patient had maximum benefit coverage of $1200 for the year and to date had only used $450 of the benefit. Toward the end of June, it was determined that the patient needed a fixed bridge. The patient was informed of the fee for the bridge. The patient was further informed that after June 30 the services would not be covered and that she would be responsible for payment. The patient argued that it was the responsibility of the dentist to alter the date on the claim form, since she still had a $700 available benefit and in the future would bring her business to the dentist.

It is fraud to change the date on the claim form to indicate that the bridge was inserted before June 30 when indeed the bridge would not be inserted until mid-July. Although efforts might be made to complete the case prior to the deadline, a common solution is to explain to the patient that she is asking you to commit fraud. At this point the patient will usually refrain and apologize.

Another example of a fraudulent act occurs when a patient's dental fee is covered by two insurance carriers requiring the coordination of benefits. The claim forms are processed. A check is received from the primary carrier for the correct amount of money. However, when a check is received from the secondary carrier, the amount is in excess of the fee and it appears the carrier has paid as a primary carrier. Consequently there is extra money received. The assistant enters the fee as it should have been on the patient's financial record but enters the entire check into the deposit, leaving an excess of funds in the account.

To prevent this situation the administrative assistant should have informed the insurance carrier immediately after the check in excess of the correct payment was received. It is possible to enter the check into a deposit, but then a check for the amount of overpayment must be written and returned to the insurance carrier with the appropriate information concerning the overpayment. The return of the overpayment should be documented in the appropriate financial record section of the patient's chart or file.

RECORDS MANAGEMENT

Nothing can be more valuable in defending against potential litigation than adequate records. These are a vital responsibility of the administrative assistant. Although discussed in other areas of this text, the importance of including complete and thorough information in a patient's record cannot be overemphasized. You should record not only the exact date, type of treatment, materials used, complications, and special notations about the treatment but also any untoward incidents regarding patient comments or reactions. Signatures of the treating operator(s) and recorder must be included. Remember that the better the documentation is, the less the legal risk will be.

Any irregularities or unusual incidents occurring between patients, employees, and employers should also be documented. All employee reports need to be retained in employee records.

Such documentation might include narratives of episodes of accidental needle punctures. These incidents require a report that includes the name of the employee, the name of the patient being treated, and the date and time of the injury. Other incidents that may warrant documentation might include unusual behavior on the part of a patient or a verbal confrontation between staff members. Thorough, accurate, and objective documentation is your best defense in litigation.

DEFAMATION OF CHARACTER

Defamation of character is the communication of false information to a third party about a person that results in injury to that person's reputation. Such communication can be verbal (slander) or written (libel). The false statement could be about a person's product, business, profession, or title to property. A dental professional should make statements about a patient or other professional only as it relates to the rendering of dental care and only to other dental care providers involved in that care.

NEGLIGENCE

Negligence is an act of omission (neglecting to do something that a reasonably prudent person would do) or commission (doing something that a reasonably prudent person would not do). To prove negligence, it is necessary to prove that there has been a breach of duty owed, including deviation from the standard of care. In a dental negligence case, it is often necessary to provide expert testimony. To prove negligence, the plaintiff must show that there is an obligation to provide care according to a specified standard; that there was failure to meet that standard; that the failure to meet the standard led to injury; and that there was in fact an actual injury to the patient.

Although most often this action involves direct patient care, indirect patient care can also be a basis for finding negligence. Therefore by the way of example, the administrative assistant who may be assigned to such tasks as sterilization or other supportive clinical tasks should be aware that negligence can occur as a result of activities that do not involve direct contact with the patient.

The Health Care Quality Improvement Act of 1986 authorized creation by the federal government of a National Practitioner Data Bank (NPDB) as a central repository to collect and release information on professional competence and conduct. The repository includes information on paid malpractice claims and adverse reports of healthcare licensees. In most states, when a dentist is found negligent, the adverse act is reported to the NPDB. The administrative assistant may review this act and research the NPDB at the web site www.npdb-hipdb.com// index.html.

INVASION OF PRIVACY

Invasion of privacy is a tort that refers to a number of wrongs involving the use of otherwise private information. As relevant here, tort may involve the publishing or otherwise making known or using information relating to the private life or affairs of a person without that person's approval or permission; prying into private affairs; or appropriating the plaintiff's identity for commercial use.

When an insurance company employee contacts an administrative assistant to clarify information about a patient on a claim form, the potential for invasion of privacy is present. The insurance clerk asks for verification of data from the patient's chart, specifically the date of birth of the child patient and the father's name and social security number. The administrative assistant offers to fax this to the insurance company. To save time, the assistant simply transfers a copy of the entire patient record, including information about a communicable disease. This action has now placed the patient record in a setting not requested nor otherwise authorized by the patient. Thus the patient's privacy has been violated.

The administrative assistant should have requested that the incomplete form be returned to the dental office or that a written request for information clarification be made by the insurance company. Only the information requested should have been provided, and it should have been reviewed to be certain the information was part of the claim form that the patient had signed.

Another potential invasion of privacy situation could occur when an administrative assistant is having difficulty collecting an account in a dental office. The patient had failed to make payment on the account of $3000 for the past 12 months. During a private conversation about the account, the patient informed the administrative assistant that her business was about to enter bankruptcy, and that her spouse had just been diagnosed with schizophrenia and was recovering from a serious alcohol dependency. During a discussion with a friend who worked in a local business, the assistant shared the story about the patient, who was a well-known member of the community.

Disparaging remarks and personal information about the patient were passed on to the listener. The story came back to the patient, and the source of information was traced to the assistant.

To prevent this situation, all staff must recognize that any information a patient gives to the dental staff remains confidential within the office. No information about a patient should be shared outside the office. When a patient requests a transfer of records of dental treatment, a signed authorization to transfer should be completed by the patient. The administrative assistant, once again, must adhere to the regulations of the HIPAA.

GOOD SAMARITAN LAW

In the last two to three decades, every state in the United States has passed some form of legislation that grants immunity for acts performed by a person who renders care in an emergency situation. This concept, called the *Good Samaritan* law, was considered necessary to create an incentive for healthcare providers to provide medical assistance to the injured in cases of automobile accidents or other disasters without the fear of possible litigation. This law is intended for individuals who do not seek compensation but rather are solely interested in providing care to the injured in a caring, safe manner, with no intent to do bodily harm. This law does not provide protection for a negligent healthcare provider who is being compensated for services.

AMERICANS WITH DISABILITIES ACT

In 1990, the federal government enacted legislation to ensure that persons with some degree of disability are not discriminated against. The **Americans with Disabilities Act** (AwDA), not to be confused with the ADA (American Dental Association), affects the dental office in the area of prohibitions against employment discrimination and by requiring facilities be accessible to physically and mentally compromised patients. This law identifies five categories of persons who are protected from discrimination. The categories protect individuals who have a physical or mental impairment that substantially limits one or more major life activities, those who have a record of such impairment, and those who are regarded as having such impairment. The categories include the following:

1. Persons whose physical or mental impairment substantially limits one or more major life activities, such as seeing, hearing, speaking, walking, breathing, performing manual tasks, learning, caring for oneself, or working. Included in this category are persons who have disabling conditions such as AIDS, HIV infections, heart disease, diabetes, cancer, learning disabilities, and mental retardation.
2. Persons who have a record of impairment, such as a history of heart disease or mental illness.
3. Persons who, while fully functional and not actually disabled, are regarded as having such an impairment owing to severe disfigurement.
4. Persons who are discriminated against because they have a known association or relationship with a disabled individual.
5. Persons who currently participate in or who have completed a drug or alcohol rehabilitation program.

Box 4-6 shows a list of titles that describe the provisions of the AwDA. This federal mandate is aimed at the elimination of discrimination against individuals with disabilities and clearly defines enforceable standards. Attention should be given to Title III and Title V, as they relate to the dental office. It is important for the office manager to obtain a copy of this act for the office and routinely update the office policies as required. The address for the Office of Americans with Disabilities is available at www.usdoj.gov/crt/ada/adahom1.htm.

COMPUTER SECURITY

The administrative assistant may be exposed to potential activities that would cause illegal or unethical activity while using a computer. **Computer security** refers to safeguards that are implemented to prevent and detect unauthorized access or deliberate damage to a computer system and data. A computer crime is the use of a computer to commit an illegal act.

In a dental office, the most common activity that would violate computer integrity is software theft, or piracy. Some people make an illegal copy of a disk or tape instead of paying for an authorized copy. Software theft is a violation of copyright law and is a crime. For large users, such as dental schools or other healthcare institutions, most software companies provide a site license and multiple copy discounts.

Although most dental offices use personal computers rather than a mainframe, the potential for gaining unauthorized access to data can still exist. If a dental assistant inadvertently gains access on the computer to unauthorized or confidential data, that person should exit the file including this data and report to the appropriate supervisor that a confidential file was accidentally entered. However, to make changes in a confidential file without authorized permission constitutes an unethical and possibly illegal act. Refer to the HIPAA standards in Chapter 7 to ensure information integrity.

TWELVE STEPS TO MAKING ETHICAL DECISIONS

The administrative assistant has much to consider when carrying out routine duties in the dental business office. During all activities, consider questions about the tasks being performed. Routinely review the questions in Box 4-7.

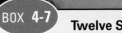

BOX 4-7 Twelve Steps to Making Ethical Decisions

1. Is the task I am performing legally delegable to me?
2. Do I have the necessary credentials to perform this task?
3. Am I physically and emotionally competent to perform this task?
4. Am I performing this procedure in a safe working environment that meets OSHA standards?
5. Has the patient been informed about his or her treatment?
6. Am I respecting the patient's right to privacy and confidentiality?
7. Do I maintain complete and accurate records, and have I documented special problems arising with patients, employees, or an employer?
8. Do I maintain professional liability insurance?
9. Do I participate in risk management programs?
10. Am I willing to maintain appropriate standards at the risk of losing a job when confronted with a lack of ethics or legal responsibility on the part of an employer or fellow employee?
11. Do I maintain current knowledge of changes in reporting methods and occupational safety required by the Dental Practice Act?
12. Do I actively participate in my professional organization and contribute to community dental health?

BOX 4-6 Provisions of the Americans with Disabilities Act

Title I — Prohibits discriminating employment policies

Title II — Prohibits discrimination against disabled persons in the use of public transportation.

Title III — Requires that public accommodations operated by private entities do not discriminate against persons with disabilities

Title IV — Prohibits discrimination against disabled individuals in the area of communication, especially hearing-impaired and speech-impaired individuals.

Title V — Contains miscellaneous provisions regarding the continued viability of other state or federal laws that provide disabled persons with equal or greater rights than the act. Specifically, this section prohibits state or local governments from discriminating against individuals with disabilities.

KEY TERMS

Abandonment—The severance of a professional relationship with a patient who is still in need of dental care and attention without giving adequate notice to the patient.

Americans with Disabilities Act (AwDA)—A federal law that affects the dental office by prohibiting employee discrimination and by requiring facilities to be accessible to physically and mentally compromised patients.

Assignment—Refers to the dentist assigning to a dental assistant or dental hygienist a specific procedure that is to be performed on a designated patient of record.

Beneficence—The principle of ethics that refers to "doing good." The dentist has a duty to promote the patient's welfare.

Civil law—Law that relates to duties between persons or between citizens and their government.

Common law—Law that relates to judicial decisions.

Computer security—Refers to illegal or unethical use of computer software either by theft or piracy.

Consent—Voluntary acceptance or agreement to what is planned or done by another person.

Crime—A wrongdoing against the public at large that is prosecuted by a public official.

Criminal law—Law that refers to wrongs committed against the public as a whole.

Defamation of character—Communication of false information to a third party about a person that results in injury to that person's reputation.

Defendant—The person or party that is being sued in a lawsuit.

Dental Practice Act—The law in each state that defines the scope of dental practice and the requirements that are necessary to practice dentistry.

Ethics—Branch of philosophy that identifies a systematic, intellectual approach to the standards of behavior.

Expert witness—A witness who is called to testify and explain what happened based on the patient's record and to offer an opinion as to whether the dental care, as administered, met acceptable standards.

Fact witness—A witness who describes what he or she saw or did during a specific act.

Felony—A serious crime that is punishable by imprisonment, generally for more than 1 year.

Fraud—A deliberately practiced deception that is committed to secure unfair or unlawful gain.

Informed consent—Consent for treatment that is given by a patient of sound mind after being informed in understandable language about such treatment by the healthcare provider.

Invasion of privacy—Publishing, making known, or using information relating to the private life or affairs of a person without that person's approval or permission.

Justice—The concept of fairness and integrity.

Lawsuit—A legal action in court.

Litigation—The judicial process used in a lawsuit.

Malpractice—Intentional or unintentional professional misconduct, evil practice, or illegal or immoral conduct.

Managed care—A cost containment system that directs utilization of health benefits by restricting the type, level, and frequency of treatment; limiting access to care; and controlling the level of reimbursement for services.

Misdemeanor—A crime of a less serious nature than a felony.

National Practitioner Data Bank (NPDB)—An agency that was implemented as a central repository for information about paid malpractice claims and adverse reports of healthcare licensees.

Nonmaleficence—Refers to the "do no harm" clause in the principle of ethics. The dentist has a duty to refrain from harming the patient.

Negligence—An act of omission (neglecting to do something that a reasonably prudent person would do) or commission (doing something that a reasonably prudent person would not do).

Patient of record—A patient who has been examined and diagnosed by a licensed dentist and whose treatment has been planned by that dentist.

Plaintiff—The person or party that institutes a lawsuit.

Standard of care—Treatment that a reasonably prudent professional would perform in similar circumstances.

Supervision—Refers to the conditions under which a patient of record may be treated by an assistant or hygienist and the protocol to be followed after the treatment is rendered.

Tort—A civil wrongdoing that is a breach of legal duty owed to the plaintiff by the defendant and that must be the primary cause of harm to the plaintiff.

LEARNING ACTIVITIES

1. Explain the application of the two forms of consent that apply to the delivery of dental care.
2. What four questions should be asked to determine an unintentional tort of negligence in dental care?
3. Identify 10 steps that should be followed when making ethical decisions.
4. Identify 10 implied duties that a dentist owes a patient.
5. List five business office activities that could lead to potential litigation.

Please refer to the student workbook for additional learning activities.

Bibliography

ADA principles of ethics and code of professional conduct, (revised) Chicago, 2008, American Dental Association.

D'cruz L, Legal aspects of general dentist practice, St. Louis, 2006, Mosby.

Davison JA: *Legal and ethical considerations for dental hygienists and assistants,* St Louis, 2000, Mosby.

Lantz M, Zarkowski P: Can ethics be taught?, *J Mich Dent Assoc* September, 2008.

State fact booklet, Chicago, 2009, Dental Assisting National Board.

Recommended Web Sites

www.danb.org
State-specific dental assistant information
www.npdb-hipdb.com/index.html
www.usdoj.gov/crt/ada/adahom1.htm
www.ada.org/prof/prac/law/code/index.asp

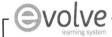

Please visit http://evolve.elsevier.com/Finkibeiner/practice for additional practice activities.

5

Technology in the Business Office

CHAPTER OUTLINE

Information Systems
    Hardware
    Software
    Data
    Personnel
    Procedures
Operations and Information System
    Information Processing Cycle
    Parts of a Computer
Profitability of the Information System
Software Selection
Integrated Applications
    Clinical Records Applications
    Establishing Procedures in Computerization
Summary of Technology in the Business Office

LEARNING OUTCOMES

- Define glossary terms.
- Differentiate between a manual office and an office using technology.
- List types of electronic office equipment used in technology.
- Describe the elements of information systems.
- Explain the four operations of a computer.
- Explain how technology can be used to increase profitability.
- Describe the application of technology to a dental practice.
- Explain the purpose of a feasibility study.
- Explain the difference between general and specific task software.
- Discuss dental software, word processing, electronic spreadsheet, database, graphics, and Internet software.
- List guidelines to follow when selecting software.
- Explain why implementing a change to a computer system is important to all staff members.

The use of modern technology in dentistry today helps the staff to be productive and the dentist remain on the cutting edge. Technology in the office is the application of computers and associated electronic equipment to prepare and distribute information. Indeed the computer has made an impact on the profession of dentistry and is used routinely in the clinical and business applications of the office. The dental staff should expect their duties as well as the way they work to change from time to time. The need for high productivity and quality performance means that all Dental Health Care Workers (DHCWs) must be willing to change work methods and adapt to this change.

Few businesses today can avoid the explosion in the need for more information. The prudent selection of technology equipment is a major component of dental office productivity and efficiency. Presently there are millions of electronic workstations in all types of offices in the United States, and the numbers are growing. In fact office automation using the Internet has been called the "primary way to do business in a high-tech world." Some form of computer usage is now installed in more than 90% of dental offices in North America. The electronic office is a workplace in which sophisticated computers and other electronic equipment carry out many of the office's routine tasks and provide more

options for gathering, processing, displaying, and storing information. Some applications of technology in the business office are outlined in Box 5-1.

The technological revolution that led to the information age has had a profound effect on the business office. The use of electronic office technology in the dental business office allows the staff to be more organized and efficient. It can help to automate routine office tasks, improve cash flow, and increase accuracy. Today a patient in a general practice can have a radiograph digitally processed and transferred to the oral surgeon before the patient even leaves the general dentist's office. This concept can be likened to the application of four-handed dentistry in the clinical setting, because both result in improved patient care, increased productivity, and reduction of stress on the dental staff.

INFORMATION SYSTEMS

An information system is a collection of elements that provide accurate, timely, and useful information. To understand the procedure of an information system, the administrative assistant must understand basic terminology related to this concept. A glossary of terms and definitions helps the novice

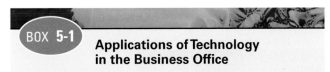

BOX 5-1 Applications of Technology in the Business Office

- Electronic charting
- Computerized scheduling
- Online office procedures manuals
- Addition of progress notes to online records
- Automated insurance claims
- Purchase of supplies from online supply warehouses
- Telemarketing with web pages
- E-mailing to staff and patients
- Enrollment in online college courses
- Provision of a means for continuing education
- Allowance for "virtual group practices" where solo practitioners share one set of records
- Consultation with experts from all over the world

BOX 5-2 Information System Terminology

Storage Term	Approximate Number of Bytes
Kilobyte (KB)	1 Thousand
Megabyte (MB)	1 Million
Gigabyte (GB)	1 Billion
Terabyte (TB)	1 Trillion
Petabyte (PB)	1 Quadrillion
Exabyte (EB)	1 Quintillion
Zettabyte (ZB)	1 Sextillion
Yottabyte (YB)	1 Septillion

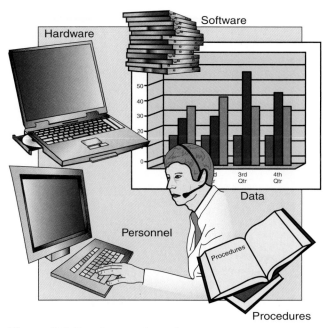

Figure 5-1 Five elements of an information system.

understand the terminology of the modern electronic office and is useful in selecting contemporary office equipment. Box 5-2 contains a detailed list of basic information system terms.

Figure 5-1 depicts the five elements that make up the information system:

1. Hardware (the equipment)
2. Software (programs)
3. Data
4. Personnel
5. Procedures

Hardware

Hardware is the information system's physical equipment. The central piece of hardware in the information system is the computer (Figure 5-2). A computer is a device that electronically accepts data, processes the data arithmetically and logically, produces output from the processing, and stores the result for future use.

Other technologies prevalent in the business office today include telephone systems with the capacity for voicemail or paging, voice equipment, fax (facsimile) machines, copy machines, calculators, dental imagers, scanners, and digital

cameras (Box 5-3). The notebook/laptop computer is becoming popular with dentists as they seek to work on office business outside the office. Technology can help enhance productivity and customer service within a dental practice, as follows:

- Voicemail allows both incoming and outgoing telephone messages to be recorded and processed.
- Pagers carried by members of the office staff allow them to be signaled when needed.
- Voice equipment records voice sounds as input for a voice-activated system or for later transcription, for referral letters or for recording information to be transferred to the clinical records, or to record research reports, minutes of a staff meeting, or the summary of a conference.
- Fax machines send and receive documents or other graphic images over the telephone systems or the Internet.
- Copy machines reproduce letters, pages from magazines and books, charts and drawings, financial reports, clinical records, and statements from the patients' ledger cards. (See Box 5-4 and Figure 5-3 for features of copiers.)
- Calculators found in computer software or those purchased separately are a great help to assistants with many routine duties that require mathematical skill. Except for the computer calculators, many are inexpensive enough to be sold at department and discount stores and also at office machine dealers. The price of a calculator is not determined entirely by the number of its functions, although this is an important factor. The types of components and materials used to produce the machine also affect the price (Box 5-5 and Figure 5-4).
- Digital cameras or intraoral cameras allow images to become part of the patient record. Data are stored, and a hard copy of the intraoral condition can be printed. Cosmetic imagers are capable of displaying proposed changes that will result from specific treatment.

(Text continued on p. 65.)

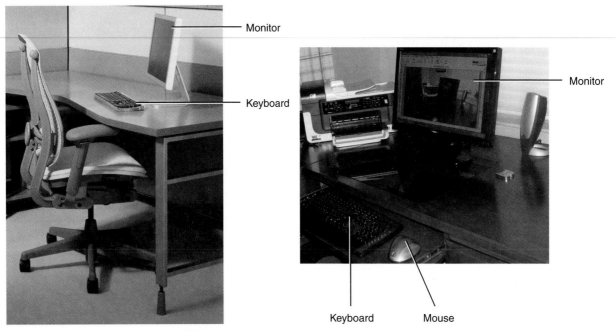

Figure 5-2 Components of a microcomputer. (*Left*, Courtesy Herman Miller, Inc., Zeeland, MI.)

BOX 5-3

Selected Technology Terms

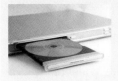

CD/DVD Drives: Most computers come with a 48× or higher speed CD-ROM drive that can read CDs. If planning to write music, audio files, and documents on a CD or DVD, then consider upgrading to a CD-R or CD-RW. An even better alternative is to upgrade to a DVD+R/+RW combination drive. It allows reading DVDs and CDs and writing data on (burn) a DVD or CD. A DVD has a capacity of at least 4.7 GB versus the 650-MB capacity of a CD. See the following table for DVD, BD, and HD DVD storage capacities.

Sides	Layers	DVD-ROM	BD-ROM	HD DVD-ROM
1	1	4.7 GB	25 GB	15 GB
1	2	8.5 GB	50 GB	30 GB
2	1	9.4 GB	50 GB	30 GB
2	2	17 GB	100 GB	60 GB

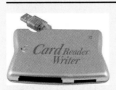

Card Reader/Writer: A card reader/writer is useful for transferring data directly to and from a removable flash memory card, such as the ones used in a camera or music player. Make sure the card reader/writer can read from and write to the flash memory cards that are used.

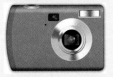

Digital Camera: Consider an inexpensive point-and-shoot digital camera. They are small enough to carry around, usually operate automatically in terms of lighting and focus, and contain storage cards for storing photographs. A 1.3- to 2.2-megapixal camera with an 8- or 16-MB storage card is fine for creating images to use on the Web or send via e-mail.

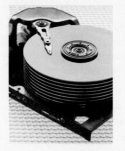

Hard Disk: It is recommended to buy a computer with 40 to 60 GB if your primary interests are browsing the Web and using e-mail and Office Suite–type applications; 60 to 80 GB to also edit digital photographs; 80 to 100 GB to edit digital video or manipulate large audio files even occasionally; and 100 to 160 GB to edit digital video, movies, or photography often, store audio files and music, or are a power user.

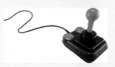

Joystick/Wheel: If the computer is used to play games, then purchase a joystick or wheel. These devices, especially the more expensive ones, provide for realistic game play with force feedback, programmable buttons, and specialized levers and wheels.

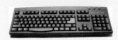

Keyboard: The keyboard is one of the more important devices used to communicate with the computer. For this reason, make sure the keyboard purchased has 101 to 105 keys, is comfortable, easy to use, and has a USB connection. A wireless keyboard should be considered, especially if there is a small desk area.

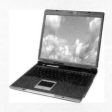

Laptop/Notebook Computer: Portable personal computer designed to fit on a user's lap.

BOX 5-3 Selected Technology Terms—cont'd

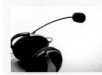

Microphone: To record audio or use speech recognition to enter text and commands, purchase a close-talk headset with gain adjustment support.

Modem: Most computers come with a modem so the telephone line can be used to dial out and access the Internet. Some modems also have fax capabilities. The modem chosen should be rated at 56 kbp.

Monitor: The monitor is where documents are viewed, e-mail messages are read, and pictures are observed. A minimum of a 17-in. screen is recommended, but if planning to use the computer for graphic design or game playing, then purchase a 19- or 21-in. monitor. The LCD flat panel monitor should be considered, especially if space is an issue. A touch-screen monitor may be used in some areas; this allows the user to interact by touching areas of the screen without using the mouse.

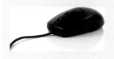

Mouse: The mouse is used constantly with the computer. For this reason, spend a few extra dollars, if necessary, and purchase a mouse with an optical sensor and USB connection. The optical sensor replaces the need for a mouse ball, which means that a mouse pad is not needed. For a PC, make sure the mouse has a wheel, which acts as a third button in addition to the top two buttons on the left and right. An ergonomic design is also important because the hand is on the mouse most of the time when using the computer. A wireless mouse should be considered to eliminate the cord and allow the assistant work at short distances from the computer.

Network Card: If planning to connect to a network or use broadband (cable or DSL) to connect to the Internet, then purchase a network card. Broadband connections require a 10/100 PCI Ethernet network card.

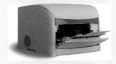

Printer: The two basic printer choices are ink jet and laser. Color ink jet printers cost from $50 to $300 on average. Laser printers cost from $300 to $2000. In general the cheaper the printer, the lower the resolution and speed, and the more often the ink cartridge or toner must be changed. Laser printers print faster and with a higher quality than an ink jet, and their toner on average costs less. If color is desired, then go with a high-end ink jet printer to ensure quality of print. Duty cycle (the number of pages that will be printed each month) also should be a determining factor. If the duty cycle is on the low end—hundreds of pages per month—then stay with a high-end ink jet printer, rather than purchasing a laser printer. If planning to print photographs taken with a digital camera, then purchase a photo printer. A photo printer is a dye-sublimation printer or an ink jet printer with higher resolution and features that allow printing quality photographs.

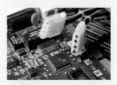
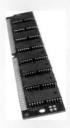

Processor: For a PC a 2.0 GHz Intel or AMD processor is more than enough processor power for home and small office/home office users. Game home, large business, and power users should upgrade to faster processors.

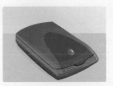

RAM: RAM (random access memory) plays a vital role in the speed of the computer. Make sure the computer purchased has at least 1 GB of RAM. If there is extra money to invest in the computer, consider increasing the RAM. The extra money for RAM will be well spent.

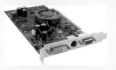

Scanner: The most popular scanner purchased with a computer today is the flatbed scanner. When evaluating a flatbed scanner, check the color depth and resolution. Do not buy anything less than a color depth of 48 bits and a resolution of 1200 × 2400 dpi. The higher the color depth, the more accurate the color. A higher resolution picks up the more subtle gradations of color.

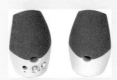

Sound Card: Most sound cards today support the Sound Blaster and General MIDI standards and should be capable of recording and playing digital audio. If planning to turn the computer into an entertainment system or for game home use, then spend the extra money and upgrade from the standard sound card.

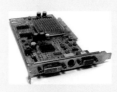

Speakers: Purchasing a good sound card, quality speakers, and a separate subwoofer that amplifies the bass frequencies of the speakers can turn the computer into a premium stereo system.

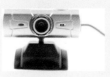

Video Graphics Card: Most standard video cards satisfy the monitor display needs of home and small office users. If the purchaser is a game home user or graphic designer, upgrade to a higher quality video card. The higher refresh rate will further enhance the display of games, graphics, and movies.

PC Video Camera: A PC video camera is a small camera used to capture and display live video (in some cases with sound), primarily on a Web page. A PC video camera also can capture, edit, and share video and still photos. The camera sits on the monitor or desk. Recommended minimum specifications include 640 × 480 resolution, a video with a rate of 30 frames per second, and a USB 2.0 or FireWire connection.

(Continued)

BOX 5-3 Selected Technology Terms—cont'd

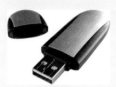

USB Flash (Jump) Drive: If different computers are used and access to the same data and information is needed, then this portable miniature storage device that can fit on a key chain is ideal. USB flash drive capacity varies from 128 MB to 4 GB.

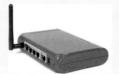

Wireless LAN Access Point: A Wireless LAN (local area network) Access Point allows networking several computers, so they can share files and access the Internet through a single cable modem or DSL connection. Each device connected requires a wireless card. A wireless LAN Access Point can offer range of operation up to several hundred feet, so be sure the device has a high-powered antenna.

Data from Shelly GB, Cashman TJ, Vermaat ME: *Discovering computers: fundamentals edition*, Boston, 2004, Course Technology.
Photos copyright 2009 JupiterImages Corporation.

BOX 5-4 Features to Consider When Selecting or Using Copiers

- Style of copiers—tabletop size or stand-alone floor models
- Volume of work to be done—low-volume, mid-volume, high-volume
- Quality of copy desired—clear and sharp
- Selection of paper size for reports, ledger cards, and letters
- Ability to reproduce from a colored original or colored ink
- Speed and output—number of copies per minute
- Capability to make copies on regular office forms and paper
- Availability of outside copying business to handle a large volume of documents (such as a new office policy) or other specialized copying services

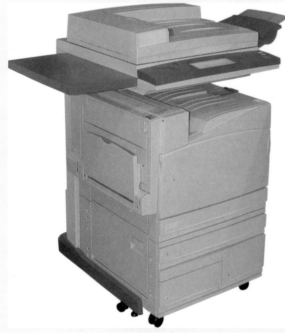

Figure 5-3 Multi-task machine. Performs four functions in one—a true multi-task machine: color printer, scanner, plain-paper FAX, and copier. (Copyright 2009 JupiterImages Corporation.)

BOX 5-5 Features to Consider When Selecting a Calculator

- Type of display
- Printing capabilities
- Quality of keyboard
- Type of batteries: On portable models, are they easily obtained? Are they throwaway or rechargeable?
- The durability of components and materials. Factors other than cost will influence the selection of a calculator.
- Ease of operation: The calculator should allow for the basic computations of addition, subtraction, multiplication, and division. Some machines can solve difficult trigonometry problems that only an accomplished mathematician could answer accurately.
- Decimal functions: A fixed decimal restricts the number of decimals; a floating decimal puts no restriction on the position of the decimal point.
- Repeat and constant operations: This feature allows the operator to add or subtract a series of identical numbers by depressing the *add* or *subtract* function key repeatedly.
- Memory register: Figures can be added to or subtracted from and are available until the register is cleared.

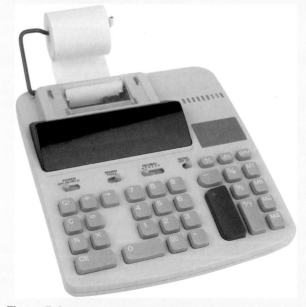

Figure 5-4 Calculator. (Copyright 2009 JupiterImages Corporation.)

- Scanners input text or graphical data directly into computer storage. Any of these devices may be directly connected to the computer system and provide a centralized source for information. Chapter 10 includes detailed descriptions of telecommunications systems and techniques.
- Laptop/notebook computers enable the dentist and/or staff to work outside the office at meetings or conferences and stay in contact with the office via e-mail or the Internet.

Software

The computer system is directed by a series of instructions called a *computer program*, or **software**, which directs the sequence of operations the system is to perform. Software in the dental office might include general purpose software, such as word processors, spreadsheets, or **database** systems; or it may include software specifically designed for dental practice management. Software may be provided with the computer system or be purchased as individual or bundled packages. A typical desktop window is shown in Figure 5-5.

Data

Data refers to the facts or figures that the information system needs to produce accurate and timely information. Data are the raw material of the information system and are manipulated or processed by the computer to produce the finished product/information. For instance, the administrative assistant enters data such as fees, treatment rendered, and payments on a financial record. The finished product can result in a statement or an insurance claim form. If the data are incorrect, the resulting information will be incorrect: "garbage in, garbage out." The term **byte** is roughly equivalent to one character of text. For example, typing the letters *a, b,* and *c* requires three bytes of storage. Data is measured in the storage terms shown in Box 5-2.

Personnel

In some larger computer installations, properly trained data processing personnel are required to operate and maintain the information system. However, in most dental practices the administrative assistant is responsible for the accuracy of both the input and output of the information system as well as the setup and maintenance. When a system is installed in an office, most system vendors provide a training session for the staff. As updated versions are released, seminars on system operations are offered. Most software suppliers offer ongoing telephone- or Internet-based support options on a monthly or yearly basis.

Procedures

Procedures are the written documentation or policies that help maintain the information system efficiently. Specialized manuals can be assembled, or these procedures may be included in the office procedures manual described in Chapter 2.

PRACTICE NOTE
If any of the elements—hardware, software, data, personnel, or procedures—are missing or flawed, the entire information system may be affected.

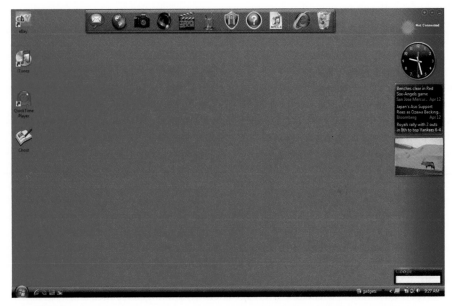

Figure 5-5 Parts of a typical desktop window.

OPERATIONS AND INFORMATION SYSTEM

Information Processing Cycle

Regardless of the computer that is selected for business office use, computers are capable of performing four general operations known as the *information processing cycle*. These four operations are (1) input, (2) process, (3) output, and (4) storage. By using these four processes, the computer will process the data into information.

Parts of a Computer

Input Device

The most common means of entering information and instructions into the computer is the keyboard (Figures 5-6 and 5-7). Special keys may include a numeric keypad, cursor control keys, and function keys. In addition to the keyboard, a host of other data collection devices include the mouse or trackball, touch screens, graphic input devices, scanners, and voice input. These devices may input data directly without any keystrokes.

Processor

The processor is the controlling unit of the system that contains the electronic circuitry to manipulate data. This unit is known as the **central processing unit** (**CPU**; see Figure 5-6), and it directs and controls all of the computer's activities. As the data are accepted from the input device, the data are processed according to the program. The program is a series of instructions directing the computer to perform a sequence of tasks. The number of programs and data that can be stored in the processing unit depends on the main memory of the system. The memory capacity of computers varies, but the computer has a fixed memory capacity.

Output Device

The printer and the monitor are the two most commonly used output devices (see Figure 5-6). If a paper copy (hard copy) is needed, the computer will be directed to print a copy. When no permanent record is needed, the output is displayed on the monitor (soft copy).

The laser printer, often called an **intelligent printer**, shapes characters through the use of light (laser beams). The intelligent printer is able to collate, stack, and place images on both sides of the paper. The cost of these printers has decreased and so they now produce multiple copies more economically. Terminals are classified as dumb terminals or intelligent terminals. **Dumb terminals** depend on the system to which they are connected for memory and processing circuitry. **Intelligent terminals** have their own processing capabilities (see Figure 5-7).

Storage Media

Auxiliary storage is used to store data and programs that are not being processed on the computer. Types of storage include hard disk, disk, zip disk, tape cartridge, compact disk, and jump or flash drive and external hard drives (Figure 5-8). The hard disk is a rigid metal disk coated with magnetic material that makes it suitable for recording and storing data. Zip disks are similar to floppy disks but can hold over 100 times more data. Disks, tape cartridges, and external hard drives are used primarily for backup purposes. The optical compact disk system uses a laser to burn microscopic holes on the surface of a hard plastic disk. The most popular optical disk formats used for data storage are the recordable compact disk (CD-R/DVD-R) and rewritable compact disk (CD-RW/DVD-RW), which can hold even more data than a zip disk. Another small optical disk format used for storage is the CD-ROM, which stands for compact disk read-only memory. Most software is distributed on the CD-ROM format. Another type of storage becoming more popular are jump or flash drives, which are portable storage devices that plug directly into computers, hold large amounts of data and do not require any type of disk.

PROFITABILITY OF THE INFORMATION SYSTEM

All of the high-tech equipment available today will not make the private dental office, clinic, or dental laboratory more efficient if proper procedures are not followed before investing in the information system. Before the office acquires new equipment or updates equipment of any kind, the needs of the office should be identified (Box 5-6). The major categories of equipment that should be considered include computers dedicated to such tasks as word processing, records management, insurance management, and accounting; scanners, copying machines; calculators; and dictation/transcription equipment. Other specific types of equipment used to handle mail and telephone systems are discussed within the content of specific chapters of this book.

 PRACTICE NOTE

All of the high-tech equipment available today will not make the private dental office, clinic, or dental laboratory more efficient if proper procedures are not followed before investing in the information system.

A **feasibility study** is one of the most reliable ways to determine what type of updates the computer in the practice needs and if new technologies are needed. This study can be conducted within the office by a vendor (usually an equipment manufacturer), an organization, or a qualified individual (such as the administrative assistant). A feasibility study must involve everyone who will use the system and other support staff. Some factors to consider when doing the feasibility study include (1) type and size of the practice, (2) cost, (3) changes in the practice since the initial computer purchase (4) ability of the staff, and (5) training requirements. Investing in a new computer is unwise if it is to be a billing machine or not improve the current system.

Once the need for a new or modified system has been established, it will be time to begin selecting equipment and software modifications, setting up the procedures for using the equipment, training personnel, and entering or transferring data from one system to another.

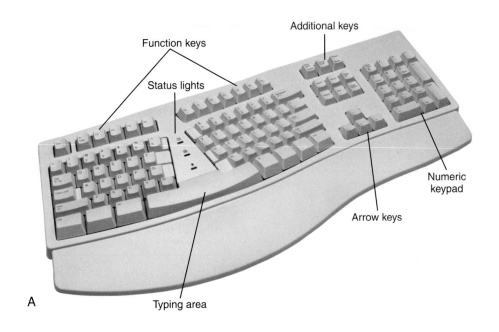

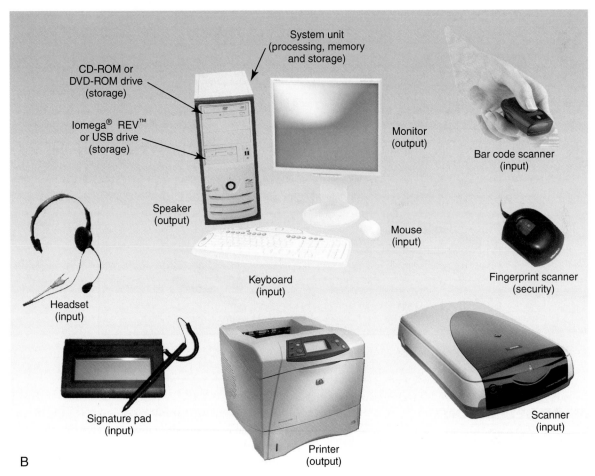

Figure 5-6 A, Computer keyboard. **B,** Computer system. (**B,** Courtesy Patterson Office Supplies, Champaign, IL.)

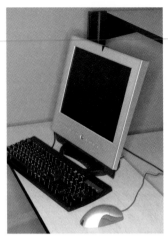

Figure 5-7 Workstation—keyboard and monitor. (Copyright 2009 JupiterImages Corporation.)

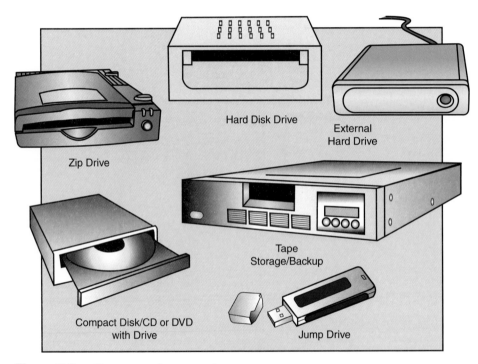

Figure 5-8 Different types of storage media.

SOFTWARE SELECTION

The first part of the chapter can be used as a guideline in selecting the hardware components of the information system for the office needs, with the help of equipment manufacturers. The next task is the selection of software. Software is the computer program(s) written to meet specific user needs. Remember that some software companies sell both hardware and software. This is good, because the company is aware of the requirements of the software and can enable the user to select the appropriate hardware to support the chosen software.

Selecting software that will perform the jobs specific to a particular office is important. Software is available that performs general tasks such as word processing, spreadsheets, database, graphics, electronic, and desktop publishing. Practice management software is available that can support all the previous mentioned tasks and can also perform specific tasks for dental offices, including account reports, patient reports, patient history, transactions, prescription history, insurance claim processing, appointment scheduling, treatment planning, summary reports, billing and aging receivables, referral tracking, income analysis, recall, and inventory management. Figures 5-9 through

5-21 include illustrations of some of the various screens that can be accessed in a commonly used software system, as follows:

- The *patient information screen* (Figure 5-9) includes comprehensive patient information.
- The *patient accounts screen* (Figure 5-10) includes accounts receivable information. A variety of payment and remittance information is found on this screen including the minimum monthly payment, date of the last statement, current account balance, and outstanding insurance or budget plan balances.
- The *patient master report* (Figure 5-11) can be filtered or sorted using different criteria, such as patient zip codes, birthdays, phone numbers, insurance coverage, and more.
- The *prescription window* (Figure 5-12) enumerates the patient medication history.
- The *transaction entry screen* (see Figure 5-13 on p. 71) is a window with the ADA window showing the ADA codes for the completed treatment.
- The *claim transaction window* (see Figure 5-14 on p. 71) is the portion of practice management software that handles claims processing. It tracks all open claims, keeps track of what was submitted on each claim, and allows for the electronic submission of claims.

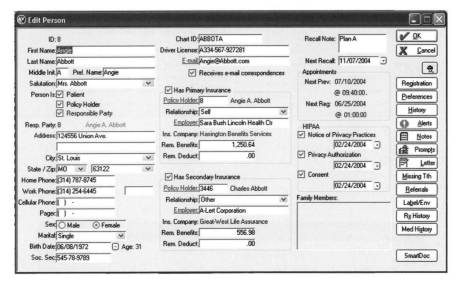

Figure 5-9 Patient information screen. (Courtesy Patterson Dental, St. Paul, MN.)

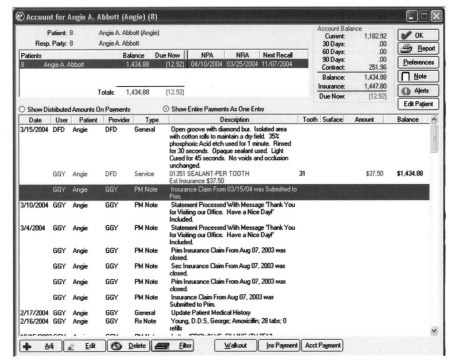

Figure 5-10 Patient accounts screen. (Courtesy Patterson Dental, St. Paul, MN.)

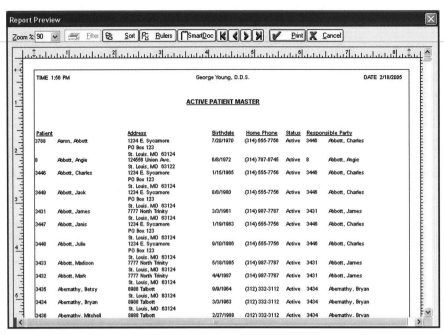

Figure 5-11 The patient master report can be filtered or sorted using a variety of criteria—patient zip code, birthday, phone number, insurance status, and more. (Courtesy Patterson Dental, St. Paul, MN.)

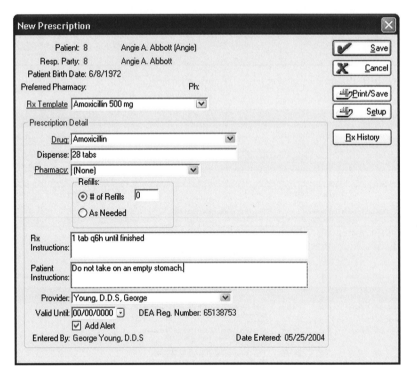

Figure 5-12 Prescription window. (Courtesy Patterson Dental, St. Paul, MN.)

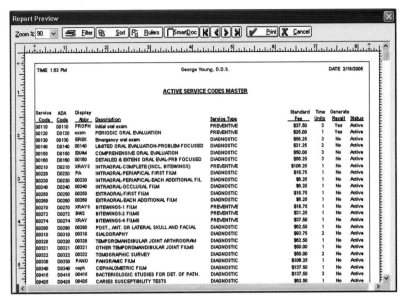

Figure 5-13 Service codes list with American Dental Association (ADA). (Courtesy Patterson Dental, St. Paul, MN.)

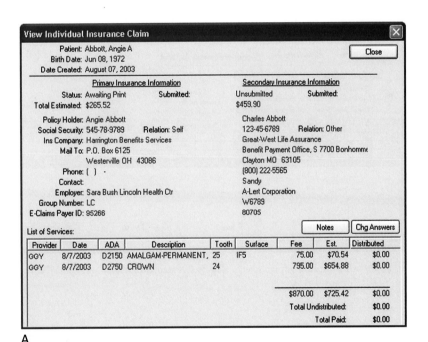

A

Figure 5-14 Claim transaction window. **A,** Claims view. (Courtesy Patterson Dental, St. Paul, MN.)

(Continued)

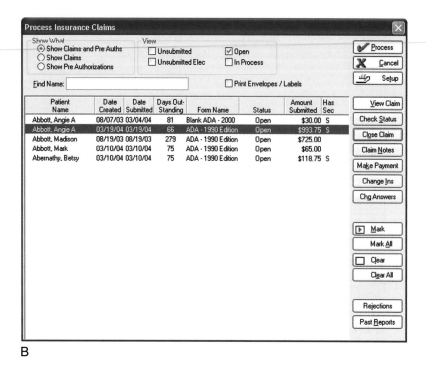

B

Figure 5-14, cont'd **B,** Process in claim. (Courtesy Patterson Dental, St. Paul, MN.)

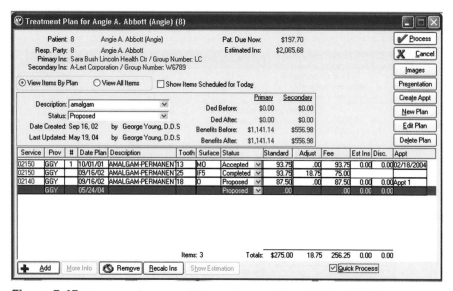

Figure 5-15 Treatment plan screen. (Courtesy Patterson Dental, St. Paul, MN.)

- The *treatment plan screen* (Figure 5-15) enables the production of a treatment plan for the patient and tracks all of the planned treatment to completion.
- The *daily appointment screen* (Figure 5-16) indicates various treatment rooms.
- The *schedule versus goal screen* allows the viewing of a provider's scheduled appointments versus the goal for each day (Figure 5-17).
- The *family recall* feature (see Figure 5-18 on p. 74) can pull up everyone in a family and identify the exam due date.

- The *tickler file* (see Figure 5-19 on p. 74) is provided in the appointment section of the program to collect and store information on patients who have missed, canceled, or broken appointments. It allows for easy tracking of patients who need to be contacted to reschedule.
- *Clinical charting* (see Figure 5-20 on p. 75) can be done in the treatment room using a graphic format. Charting can be done in a basic format or may include complex charts for periodontics and other specialty areas. X-rays from the patient's chart can even be e-mailed to another dentist for evaluation.

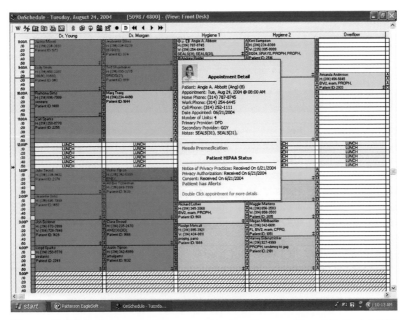

Figure 5-16 Daily appointment screen. (Courtesy Patterson Dental, St. Paul, MN.)

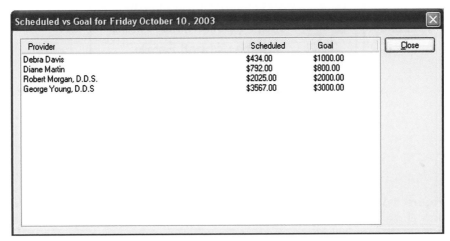

Figure 5-17 Schedule versus goal screen. (Courtesy Patterson Dental, St. Paul, MN.)

- The *day sheet report* (see Figure 5-21 on p. 76) summarizes practice activity for a period of time.
- *Annual graphic reports* are generated to illustrate categorical treatment production (see Figure 5-22 on p. 76).

Appropriate selection of a software package is extremely important. For the software to be effective, the computer functions must be applicable to the specific dental practice. Stored data and information must be usable and easily accessible. The required applications should be presented to the vendor rather than asking the vendor what the dental practice should do. To be more specific, take a routine accounts receivable task and have the vendor explain how it would be processed with that company's equipment and software. Inquire how different procedures (e.g., billing, payments, appointment notification) can be combined. Another option is starting with basic software packages, such as insurance estimating and billing, appointment tracking treat-

ment planning, marketing, and payroll. It is strongly recommended that an office make sure that the software can provide all that they will need going forward. If an office will someday want to use digital x-ray it is very important that the software have that option available when the office needs it.

The preceding text illustrates a sampling of dental software, all of which help to improve cash flow and increase productivity. The list goes on, however. The word processing function is also invaluable to the dental practice and can be integrated with the information system to improve communications with the patients. The computer, when used to produce welcome letters, treatment letters, and special greetings, can be a very effective marketing tool.

When word processing software is used on the computer, the document is prepared electronically and the text is entered on the computer keyboard in the same manner as on a typewriter. As the text is entered, it is displayed on the screen (monitor)

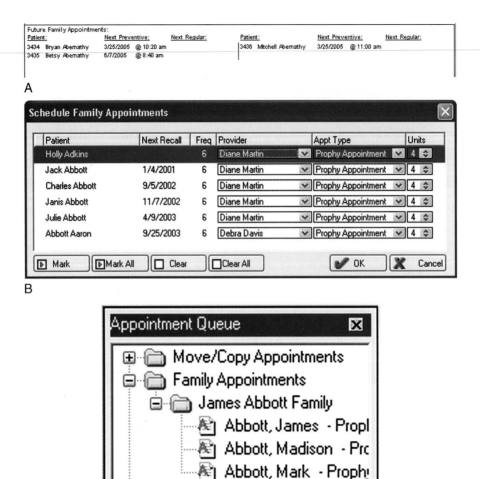

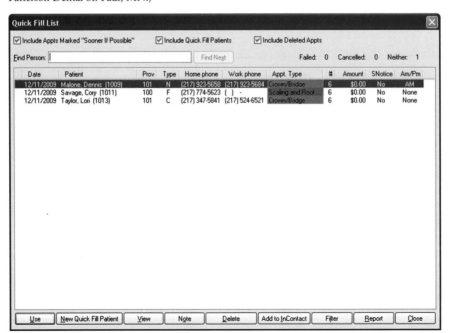

Figure 5-18 Family recall. **A,** Future dates of family member appointments. **B,** Next recall dates of each person in family group. **C,** Appointment query screen for a family. (Courtesy Patterson Dental St. Paul, MN.)

Figure 5-19 Tickler file. (Courtesy Patterson Dental, St. Paul, MN.)

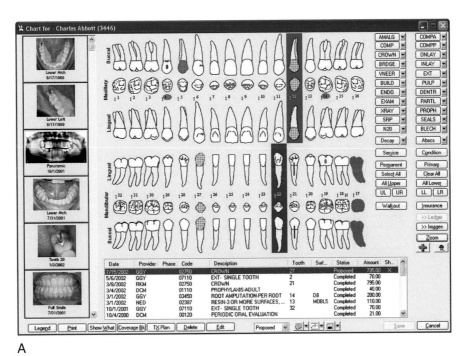

A

B

Figure 5-20 Clinical charting. **A,** Presentation manager. **B,** Chart e-mail screen. (Courtesy Patterson Dental, St. Paul, MN.)

and stored in the computer's memory. This is an electronic format, and it is easy to edit a document by making changes in the text. Text can be corrected by using a backspace or delete key. Words, sentences, paragraphs, or pages may be added or deleted from a document. Text can be moved from one section to another. The document is formatted according to individual specifications. For example, margins, type style, double or single spacing, underlining, boldface or italics, and page length are determined by the user. When the document is finalized and all corrections made, a command is made to have the document printed. More than one copy can be printed, and each copy is an original. These documents are stored in the computer's memory, and can be used again in the original text or edited and brought up to date.

Many word processing packages include other features such as spell check, grammar check, and a thesaurus. Some spell check software enables you to add words common to your specific dental practice.

TIME 12:24 PM   Patton Dental Services   DATE 12/11/2009

DAY SHEET
Today

Type	Production	Collections	Adjustments	A.R. Impact
Services:	$3,330.50	...	...	$3,330.50
Deleted Services:	$0.00	...	...	$0.00
Taxes:	$0.00	...	...	$0.00
Deleted Taxes	$0.00	...	...	$0.00
Discounts:	$0.00	...	...	$0.00
Deleted Discounts:	$0.00	...	...	$0.00
Returned Checks:	$0.00	$0.00	$0.00	$0.00
Returned Check Service Charges:	$0.00	$0.00	$0.00	$0.00
Debit Adjustments	$0.00	$0.00	$1.00	$1.00
Finance Charges:	$0.00	$0.00	$0.00	$0.00
Billing Charges	$0.00	$0.00	$0.00	$0.00
Deleted Debits	$0.00	$0.00	$0.00	$0.00
Cash Payments:	...	$0.00	...	$0.00
Check Payments:	...	$475.80	...	($475.80)
Other Payments	...	$0.00	...	$0.00
Credit Adjustments:	$0.00	$0.00	$0.00	$0.00
Deleted Credits	$0.00	$0.00	$0.00	$0.00
Write Offs:	$0.00	$0.00	$0.00	$0.00
Totals:	$3,330.50	$475.80	$1.00	

Beginning A.R. $0.00
Change in A.R. $2,855.70
Ending A.R. $2,855.70

System Summary For Activity Today

Total Payments	$475.80	Less Trans Pmts:	$475.80*	Total Production	$3,330.50
Total Walkouts	$3,330.50**	Less Est. Ins:	$2,158.30****	Total Collection:	$475.80
Payments Made On Walkouts	$424.60			Collection Ratio	14.29%
Walkout Collection Ratio	12.75%***		19.67%*****		
Patients Seen	14			Patients Seen	14
Total Production	$3,330.50			Total Collection:	$475.80
Avg. Production Per Visit	$237.89			Avg. Collection Per Visit	$33.99

* Total of Payments made today less those from prior days that were deleted & recreated today due to transferring patients with history.
** Total of Services + Taxes - Discounts from the above totals less any service amounts that were both entered and deleted within this period
*** Total of Payments Made On Walkouts divided by Total Walkouts within this peri
**** Total Walkouts less any estimated insurance calculated on those walkouts. This amount does not change when the claims these are on are close
***** Total of Payments Made On Walkouts divided by Total Walkouts less estimated insurance within this peri

Figure 5-21 Summary of activities. (Courtesy Patterson Dental, St. Paul, MN.)

Word processing software can be a very productive tool for the dental practice and should be selected wisely. Box 5-7 lists common features of word processing software packages.

An **electronic spreadsheet** software package allows the user to organize numeric data in a worksheet or table format.

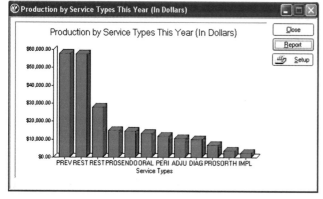

Figure 5-22 Provider report of actual production by service. (Courtesy Patterson Dental, St. Paul, MN.)

The user enters the data into the formula that has been typed in specific rows and columns, known as *cells*. As the data are entered into the proper cells, the electronic calculations are performed automatically. Daily postings and updates can be made very easily. An electronic spreadsheet's ability to recalculate data makes this an invaluable tool for business office management.

A graphics software package allows the user to create graphs from numeric data; this is sometimes part of the spreadsheet software package. The most common forms of graphics are pie charts, line diagrams charts, and bar charts (see Figure 5-22). Graphs are good management tools for reviewing information and helping to communicate information more effectively. A popular graph is used in periodontal charting. In Figure 5-23 is an example of an automated periodontal probe system that records, stores, and prints the data in a readable form for the dentist or hygienist to review with the patient. When using graphics in a presentation, select the type of graph that is most appropriate for your purpose. Don't try to present too much information, use few words, be consistent, and keep the graphics simple.

BOX 5-7   Common Features of Word Processors

Insert	Function keys	Spelling and grammar
Insert character(s)	Control keys	Thesaurus
Insert word(s)	Status line	Track changes
Insert line(s)	Line	Merge documents
Insert document(s)	Column	Letters and mailings
Insert graphics	Format	Table
Insert pictures	Top and bottom margins	Insert
Delete	Left and right margins	Delete
Delete character(s)	Tab stops	Sort
Delete word(s)	Single and double spacing	Printing
Delete sentence(s)	Move	Print columns
Delete paragraph(s)	Move sentence(s)	Subscripts
Delete page(s)	Move paragraph(s)	Superscripts
Delete entire document	Move blocks	Underline
Keyboard and Screen Control Printing	Search and Replace	Boldface
Cursor movement	Search to specific text	Headers
Page up and down	Search and replace word	Footers
Word wrap	Search and replace character strings	Page numbering
Upper- and lower-case display	Tools	Document title

INTEGRATED APPLICATIONS

Today most dental software integrates electronic spreadsheets and word processing into the software. As stated, choosing the right software for the specific need of the dental practice can be difficult. The information in Box 5-8 should help. The computer and software selection process requires a great deal of thought and time, so make the selection carefully. Everyone will have to live with the decision that is made.

Clinical Records Applications

Although it may appear that the bulk of record management is generated only in the business office, one cannot overlook the computer as a communication tool between the treatment room and business office. A variety of charting systems allows a clinical assistant to enter data directly on a keyboard at chairside, which then provides a printout in the business office. An example of this system is shown in the periodontal examination and charting system in Figure 5-23. Systems are available for patient histories, general and specialty charting, and treatment completed. Such a system also eliminates record contamination, because barrier covers may be placed over the keyboard and the chances of disease transmission through record management are decreased.

Establishing Procedures in Computerization

There are times in the office when it is necessary to modify or change an existing system. Resistance to change can be expected if employees are not made aware of and involved in the change. The early planning stages is the best time to begin

BOX 5-8   Guidelines for Choosing the Right Software

1. Determine the needs of the dental practice—type of practice, size of practice, ability of staff, cost, and training required for the doctor and support staff.
2. Select a vendor who is reputable and provides fast and efficient support when there are questions.
   - Ask about other dental practices that use the system.
   - How many systems has the vendor installed within the geographic area?
   - Are the insurance forms that are processed through the system accepted by participating insurance companies?
   - Does the system provide for electronic claim form filing?
3. Determine what the software is to do—process insurance claims, improve billing, improve practice management, improve office efficiency and auditing, track delinquent accounts, compute monthly finance charges, or aid in communications as a marketing device?
4. Identify what type of backup system is available in case of computer failure.
5. Establish how security is managed.
6. Determine the type of training available from the vendor. Systems are available that have tutorial software. Some software uses online instructions for the learner.

communicating with other staff members. Their cooperation and support will be gained if they are made aware of the new system's advantages. The staff needs to know that the workload may need to be modified during the update or change and will be distributed to more than one individual, so that it lessens the workload.

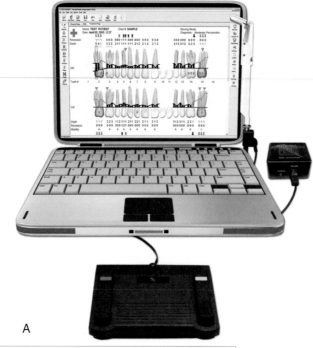

A

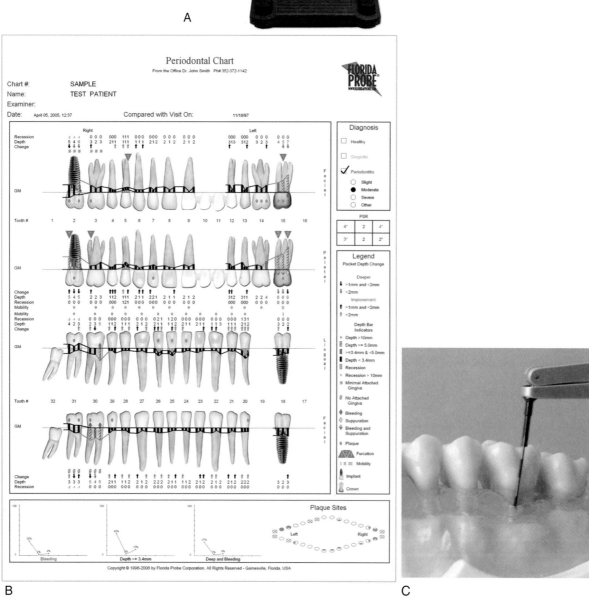

B

C

Figure 5-23 A, The Florida Probe Periodontal Exam and Charting System provides highly accurate and repeatable periodontal measurements with superior charting capabilities. The system requires only a single operator and records, stores, and prints the examination automatically. (Courtesy The Florida Probe, Inc., Gainesville, FL.) **B,** Samples of the periodontal charts automatically produced by the Florida Probe system. **C,** Objective measurements of pocket depth and gingival recession from the CEJ are ensured by the probe's constant 15-g pressure.

Establishing procedures is necessary to make sure that work flows smoothly through the entire process—from origination to completion. Probably it will be necessary to update the procedures manual for computer tasks and then hold staff meetings to train the staff in the use of the new hardware or software, depending on the changes being made. A manual provides detailed information about how various tasks are completed and by whom, as well as the purpose of each task.

Software manuals that are provided with the software should be carefully evaluated. If the documentation and instructions are difficult to follow and understand, the individual will not use the system properly and efficiently. Consequently demonstrations and regular staff meetings help in solving any confusion or conflict that may arise using the new system.

SUMMARY OF TECHNOLOGY IN THE BUSINESS OFFICE

A computer's primary advantage is the accuracy and quality of its end product, but without proper management and usage, the computer becomes a costly investment with poor returns. A well-planned information system helps make the office more efficient, and the combination of an experienced staff and high technology equipment will result in higher productivity, better patient relations, and a happier staff.

KEY TERMS

Byte—The basic unit of measurement of information storage in computer science Eight bits that are grouped together as a unit. A byte provides enough different combinations of 0s and 1s to represent 256 individual characters.

Central processing unit (CPU)—The electronic component on a computer's motherboard that interprets and carries out the basic instructions that operate the computer.

Computer—An electronic device that operates under the control of instructions stored in its own memory, that can accept data, process the data according to specified rules, produce results, and store the results for future use.

Data—A collection of unprocessed items, which can include text, numbers, images, audio, and video.

Database—A structured collection of records or data that is stored in a computer system. The structure is achieved by organizing the data according to a database model.

Dumb terminal—A terminal that cannot function as an independent device because is has not processing power.

Electronic office—A term used to describe the increasing use of computer-based information technology in office work.

Electronic spreadsheet—Application software that allows the user to organize data in rows and columns and to perform calculations on the data.

Feasibility study—An analysis of business practices that is one of the most reliable ways to determine what type of updates the computer in the practice needs and if new technologies are needed.

Hardware—The electric, electronic, and mechanical components contained in a computer. Information system The hardware, software, data, people, and procedures that a computer requires to generate information.

Information system—A collection of elements that provide acurate, timely, and useful information.

Intelligent printer—The laser printer, often called an intelligent printer, shapes characters through the use of light (laser beams). The intelligent printer is able to collate, stack, and place images on both sides of the paper.

Intelligent terminal—One of two types of terminals. Unlike the dumb terminal, this terminal has its own processing capabilities.

Internet—Worldwide collection of networks that connects millions of business, government agencies, educational institutions and individuals.

Shredder—An device used to electronically shred documents and paper in order to guard against identity theft and strengthen the office's document confidentiality policies.

Software—A series of instructions that tells a computer what to do and how to do it.

NOTE: Please refer to Box 5-3 for additional technology-related terms and accompanying images.

LEARNING ACTIVITIES

1. Describe the importance of an information system to dentistry.
2. List and explain the operations a computer can perform.
3. Describe how a feasibility study aids in determining the need for automation.
4. Describe computer software.
5. Explain the difference between general- and specific-task software.

Please refer to the student workbook for additional learning activities.

BIBLIOGRAPHY

Fulton-Calkins PJ: *The administrative professional*, ed 13, Mason, OH, 2007, Thomson South-Western.

Heiert CL: Computer use by dentists and dental team members, *J Am Dent Assoc* 128:91, 1997.

Lavine L: Proper positioning of monitors, *Dent Econ* 94(11):102, 2004.

Shelly GB, et al: *Discovering computers: complete 2009*, Boston, 2008, Course Technology.

RECOMMENDED WEB SITES

www.floridaprobe.com
www.pattersondental.com
www.dentistryiq.com

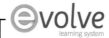

Please visit http://evolve.elsevier.com/Finkibeiner/practice for additional practice activities.

6

Office Design and Equipment Placement

LEARNING OUTCOMES

- Define glossary terms.
- Define ergonomics as it applies to the dental business office.
- Describe classifications of motion.
- Describe the implementation of time and motion in a dental business office.
- Describe seasonal affective disorder.
- Explain the effect of the Americans with Disabilities Act on office design.
- Explain a work triangle as it relates to the dental business office.
- Identify criteria for reception room design.
- Identify criteria for business office design.
- Describe factors involved in office design that relate to the Americans with Disabilities Act.
- Describe the arrangement of common business equipment.

At some point in one's career it is likely that he or she will be asked to help design, remodel, or improve the efficiency of the dental business office. These responsibilities demand an understanding of the principles of motion economy and the placement of office equipment to create an environment in which a person can work smarter and not harder.

In the past more emphasis was placed on the design of the dental treatment rooms than the design of the business office. However, planning of the business office workspace is equally important. This area should be ergonomically designed so that the business staff can perform its tasks with the greatest efficiency. **Ergonomics** is the science that studies the relationship between people and their work environments. Interrelated physical and psychological factors are involved in the creation of a stress-free work environment. By understanding the abilities that people have and their work patterns, it is possible to design work environments that conform to the abilities and work needs of the employee. The appropriate use of ergonomics can make the job more productive and efficient and can reduce work-related discomfort and injuries.

PHYSICAL ENVIRONMENT

Physiological factors include color, lighting, acoustics, heating and air conditioning, space, and furniture and equipment. Color plays a major role in how a patient perceives a practice and in the staff's health, productivity, and morale. An attractive, cheerful, and efficient office inspires confidence in the staff and comfort in the patient. A drab, dirty, or untidy office can create an attitude of doubt or mistrust. The use of light and dark colors can be effectively used and may vary according to geographic location. Some decorators work with dark colors for walls, but use lighter accent colors to downplay the dark base color. Designers today can effectively use a variety of color palettes to enhance an office and make it warm and comfortable for both the patients and staff. Dental offices no longer need to present a stark, sterile image. A comfortable patient is a happier patient. Moreover, staff productivity is likely to be greater in a pleasant working environment. Many office plans are available; the one chosen should reflect the dentist's personality and satisfy the needs of the staff and patients.

 PRACTICE NOTE
Ergonomics is the study of the effects of the work environment on health and well-being.

PRACTICE NOTE
An attractive, cheerful, and efficient office inspires confidence in the staff and comfort in the patient.

Office Design and the Americans with Disabilities Act

For years patients have had difficulty gaining access to dental treatment rooms because of poorly designed offices. The Americans with Disabilities Act of 1990 has affected the design of dental offices in patient treatment. Special attention should be directed to this act to ensure that the office design complies with state and federal guidelines. The Justice Department issues accessibility specifications for offices, but some states have even stricter standards. Accessibility features must be incorporated into renovations of a building, and those features must be accessible from elsewhere in the building. For example, making a lobby bathroom accessible to a wheelchair patient is not adequate if the patient cannot get to the lobby. Wider hallways enable a patient in a wheelchair to easily access treatment rooms and other areas of the office (Figure 6-1). Box 6-1 presents a list of recommendations for designing a barrier-free office.

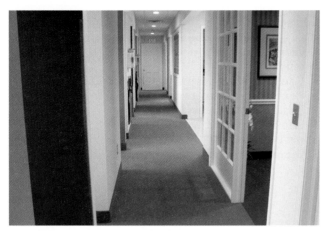

Figure 6-1 A hallway made wider to the specifications of the Americans with Disabilities Act enables a patient in a wheelchair to easily access treatment rooms. (Courtesy Joseph Ellis, DDS, and Lisa Tartaglione, DDS, Grand Rapids, MI.)

The government estimates that the cost of incorporating accessibility features into new construction is less than 1% of construction costs. Because remodeling existing buildings usually is more costly, the requirements for them are less stringent. Currently the law requires only "reasonable modifications" that are "readily achievable," both terms that may lead to litigation. Further information on any part of the Americans with Disabilities Act is available from the sources listed in Box 6-2. Also visit www.ada.gov or www.access-board.gov.

Seasonal Affective Disorder

In geographic locations in which there are extremes of sunshine and darkness, patients or staff may be affected by seasonal affective disorder (SAD). Sunlight serves to keep the body's internal circadian clock in sync, so a person is alert and awake in the day and ready to sleep at night. A person's health, mood, and behavior can be affected when the quality and quantity of sunlight are lessened. A direct consequence of SAD can be winter depression or sleep disorders.

Many companies provide lighting systems to overcome SAD. If staff members are affected by SAD, it may be worth the investment to increase the health of the staff. Most of the lights are designed for the brightness needed for light therapy. With a brightness level of 10,000 lux at 18 to 24 inches, these lights have been proved to be a fast and effective light therapy at a comfortable distance. Most lights are easy to use and safe (no harmful UV rays).

Design of the Reception Room

The **reception room** (the term *waiting room* has a negative connotation) is the gateway to the dental office and provides the patient's first impression of the dentist. A warm atmosphere can be created in the reception room, furnishing a comfortable "living room" environment. The office should reflect the theme originating in the reception room (Figure 6-2).

BOX 6-1   Design Features of a Barrier-Free Office

The following modifications for creating a barrier-free environment comply with the Americans with Disabilities Act:
- Designate handicapped parking areas.
- Install sidewalk and curb access to accommodate wheelchairs or other devices.
- Install access ramps to building and office areas.
- Widen doors and doorways to accommodate wheelchairs and other devices.
- Install raised letters and Braille on elevator controls.
- Provide visual and sound alarms.
- Install grab bars.
- Install raised toilet seats and wider stalls.
- Make paper towel dispensers accessible.
- Install paper cup dispensers at existing water fountains.
- Eliminate plush, low-density carpeting.

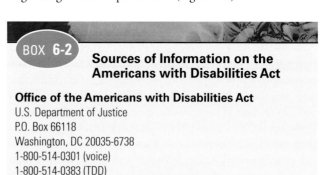

BOX 6-2   Sources of Information on the Americans with Disabilities Act

Office of the Americans with Disabilities Act
U.S. Department of Justice
P.O. Box 66118
Washington, DC 20035-6738
1-800-514-0301 (voice)
1-800-514-0383 (TDD)
Internet web site (ADA home page): www.ada.gov

Architectural and Transportation Barriers Compliance Board
1111 18th Street NW, Suite 501
Washington, DC 20036
1-800-872-2253 (voice)
1-800-993-2822 (TDD)
Electronic bulletin board: 202-272-5448
Internet web site: www.access-board.gov

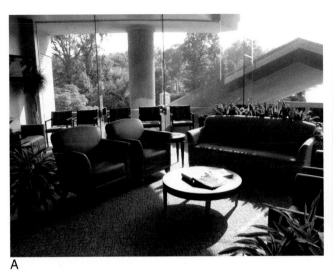
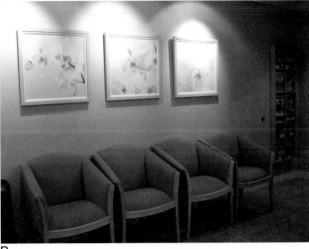

A   B

Figure 6-2 A, The reception room of a dental office reflects the theme of the practice. Open areas allow a patient personal space as well as work areas. (Courtesy Dr. Roy A. Smith, Birmingham, AL.) **B,** A reception room with comfortable chairs provides adequate seating space. (Courtesy Roberta D. Cann, DMD, Atlanta, GA.)

Patients should be able to check in with the administrative assistant at the desk as soon as they arrive. For privacy, patients should have access to a restroom off the reception room, and appropriate signs should direct them to this area.

Seating in the reception room varies from office to office, depending on individual practice styles. A general rule is to provide two seats for each dental chair in a general practice. High-volume practices, such as orthodontics or pediatrics, require three or four seats per dental chair, whereas an oral surgery or endodontic practice needs only one or two seats per chair.

Seating space is an important consideration. People generally do not like to have others sitting too close to them. When completing forms or other business activities, a person needs some privacy. Comfort should be the major concern when selecting furniture for this area. It needs to be sturdy but not too formal or too casual. Low, cushiony couches and armless chairs are sometimes difficult for even an agile person to get out of and even more difficult for an older adult or arthritic patient. Figure 6-2, *B*, illustrates comfortable armchairs with a sturdy base.

 PRACTICE NOTE
The reception room is the gateway to the dental office and provides the patient's first impression of the dentist.

Special amenities are a thoughtful gesture, such as a desk-height table with an electrical outlet that makes it convenient for businesspeople or students to bring laptop computers to use while waiting. A self-serve coffee or juice bar is a considerate gesture toward busy patients. These amenities send a message that the dentist respects the patient's time and wants to make the office a friendly place to visit (Box 6-3 and Figures 6-3 and 6-4).

Business Office Work Triangle

The design of the business office can be likened to the design of a kitchen in one's home. A kitchen design starts with the "work triangle." The triangle keeps the three primary work centers or zones in close proximity, eliminating wasted effort and time. The triangle in a kitchen is measured from the center of the sink to the center of the refrigerator to the center of the cooktop. Likewise the design of a business office can take into consideration three main zones in its design; the reception zone, the intraoffice communication center, and the work area zone. A good rule of thumb would be to measure the distance from the center of the reception zone, to the center of the communications zone, and then to the work zone to ensure that the perimeter of the triangle does not exceed 26 feet. This distance should be uninterrupted by traffic or cabinetry. By limiting the distance between these three zones, the business office staff can be efficient and yet reduce the stress of walking long distances.

Zones, also known as *work centers*, complement the work triangle. By planning zones within the triangle, one can ensure that different tasks can be carried out without collisions. In the reception zone of the triangle there should be adequate space to meet and greet patients and make appointments. In the intraoffice communication zone, the administrative assistant should be able to manage the telephone; access a computer for appointments, clinical data, financial records, or other information; as well as communicate with the clinical areas. The work zone maintains space to prepare, file or copy records, use the fax, or perform other activities that require counter space or file access to work. Figure 6-5 illustrates an example of a work triangle.

Design of the Business Office

The business office work space should provide a healthful, enjoyable environment that minimizes disruption and distraction. The business office should be centrally located between the reception

BOX 6-3 — Keys to Creating a Comfortable Reception Room

- A soft warning bell or chimes should announce the patient's arrival in the reception area.
- The patient's arrival should be acknowledged immediately. A clear glass window affords privacy, yet allows the administrative assistant to see all the activity in the reception room. Today many offices are designed with open barrier free reception areas. Whether a window or barrier free opening is used, it commonly is 44 inches from the floor and a minimum of 36 × 36 inches. A barrier-free environment can be created with the open concept. A desk area for physically challenged patients is positioned 27 to 29 inches from the floor.
- Coat racks should be convenient for both children and adults. A nearby bench benefits older adults, small children, and anyone putting on boots.
- Magazine racks can be placed on a wall or table for patient convenience (see Figure 6-3).
- If necessary, a small children's corner can be included (Figure 6-4). In many specialty offices, such as orthodontics or pediatric dentistry, an office theme can be created.
- The style and number of seats and tables depend on the patients' requirements. A combination of sofas and chairs also provides a comfortable seating arrangement. Chairs should be of a height and depth that afford easy seating and exiting.
- An automatic air freshener eliminates "dental" odors, and cordial "no smoking" signs can be posted at the entrance and in the reception room.
- An adjoining restroom eliminates trips to the inner office.
- Wood paneling, fabric, textured wallpaper, antiques, live plants, artwork, and mirrors add warmth to the reception room and reflect the dentist's personality.
- Signs directing patients to various rooms should be large and easy for all patients to read.
- Lighting intensity and color should be adequate for easy reading of printed materials in any part of the room.

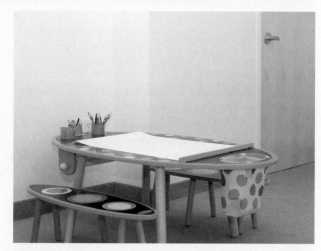

Figure 6-4 A dedicated space for children to play can contribute to comfort and convenience in the reception area. (Copyright 2007 Cora Reed, Cora Reed Photography, Denver, CO. Image from BigStockPhoto.com)

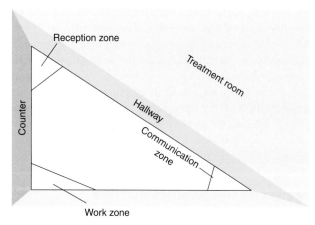

Figure 6-3 A reception area with a magazine rack accessible to children and adults.

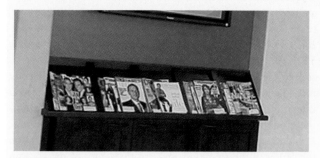

Figure 6-5 Business office work triangle designed to include the reception, intraoffice communication, and work zones within a 26-foot perimeter.

room and the dental treatment rooms. This central location is convenient for the patient and allows the administrative assistant to be aware of the activities in the office. Figure 6-6 illustrates two different floor plans that use a central location for the business office. The first is an example of a small dental offices; the second is a basic floor plan for a team concept that uses advanced functions dental staff. The factors involved in designing a business office work environment are motion economy, space planning, health issues, safety, and security. The following suggestions should be considered:

- The administrative assistant or receptionist should be seated facing the reception room.
- Two desk heights ensure comfort and efficiency. The keyboard level should be approximately 27 inches, and the writing level about 29 inches (Figure 6-7). Twenty inches is an adequate depth for most working areas. A depth over 30 inches is excessive; it makes reaching inconvenient and reduces the amount of floor space in the office.

- A counter approximately 44 inches high provides a writing area for patients and privacy for the assistant and for documents on the desk (see Figure 6-7).
- The business office clock should be out of view of patients in the reception room.
- Central controls for an intercom system should be integrated with the telephone or mounted on the wall as a separate unit within easy reach of the assistant (Figure 6-8). Auxiliary units should be connected with the private office, laboratory, and treatment rooms.
- Master controls for the music system, heating, cooling, and lighting also should be located in the business office. Labeling these controls prevents accidental shutoff of any of the utilities.
- Lateral or open files (Figure 6-9), at a depth of 18 inches, require less space than vertical files. These files are supplied in 30-, 36-, and 42-inch widths with two to five drawers.
- Cupboard space is necessary for storage of paper and supplies.
- Small compartmentalized areas above the desk provide easy access to items such as appointment cards and telephone message pads.
- Telephones should be installed at each workstation and should be made hands free whenever possible.
- Desk drawers should have full suspension for maximum use.
- Inserts and dividers in drawers aid in organization of materials.
- A small area adjacent to the business office set up for private calls and conversations with patients is convenient and can be used for completion of insurance forms.

Many of these criteria have been incorporated into the design of the business office shown in Figure 6-7.

PRINCIPLES OF TIME AND MOTION

When determining the placement of office equipment and supplies, the principles of time and motion should be considered. **Time and motion** refers to the amount of time and degree of motion required to perform a given task. This principle is as important in the business office as in the dental treatment rooms. Many studies and much research have gone into minimizing the amount of time and motion it takes to perform basic chairside tasks. However, these principles have not always been applied to the dental business office. Because the dentist seldom spends time in the business office, the staff's suggestions should be considered when designing the area. Before positioning equipment and supplies, staff members should determine the most common tasks and routinely used materials and should attempt to classify the motions used during those tasks.

In the early 1950s, researchers at the University of Alabama classified motions according to the amount of energy required to perform various chairside tasks. These **classifications of motion** systems (Box 6-4) can also be applied to the business office. The administrative assistant should try to use only Class I, II, and III motions, which require the least amount of energy and reduce stress.

To improve motion economy, it is often necessary to eliminate unnecessary steps or tasks, rearrange equipment and materials, organize procedures, simplify tasks, and evaluate the outcomes. The principles of motion economy (Box 6-5) can aid in accomplishing each of these goals, thereby reducing stress and increasing productivity in the practice.

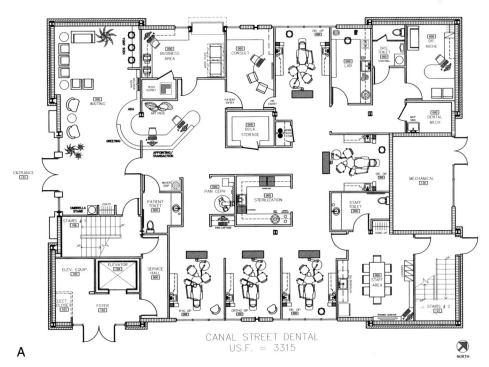

A

Figure 6-6 Sample dentist office designs. **A,** A small office designed for efficiency and patient comfort includes all the basic rooms and also provides openness.

(Continued)

FLOOR PLAN

1 PATIENT ENTRY	10 TOILET ROOM	20 CLEAN LAB
2 RECEPTION	11 PAN-CEPH	21 MESSY LAB
3 TOILET ROOM	12 OPERATORY	22 STAFF ENTRY
4 APPOINTMENTS	13 DIGITAL SCANNING	23 CHANGING
5 FRONT DESK	14 HYG. COORD. STAND UP	24 STAFF TOILET
6 OFFICE MANAGER	15 HYGIENE STORAGE	25 STAFF LOUNGE
7 BUSINESS AREA	16 STERILIZATION	26 DR.'S OFFICE
8 CONSULT #1	17 DOCTOR STORAGE	27 DR.'S TOILET
9 CONSULT #2	18 DENTAL MECHANICAL	28 COURTYARD
	19 CENTRAL COMPUTERS	29 TRELLIS

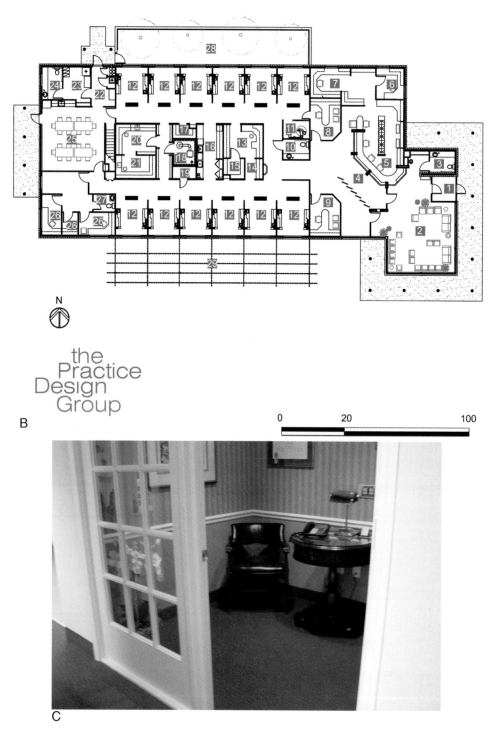

the Practice Design Group

B

0   20   100

C

Figure 6-6, cont'd B, This multi-dentist office suite includes an open concept, multiple treatment and hygiene rooms as well as a larger reception area; it also provides patient privacy. **C,** Consultation room adjacent to the business office provides privacy for the patient and dentist. (**A** and **B,** Courtesy PDGFazio Design Group, Austin, TX, **C,** Courtesy Joseph Ellis, DDS and Lisa Tartaglione, DDS, Grand Rapids, MI.)

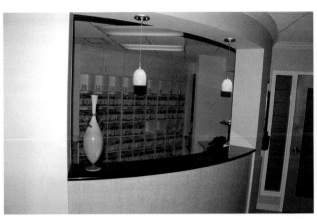
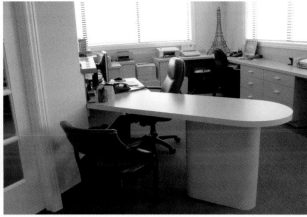

Figure 6-7 Counter space in the business office allows the patient a comfortable position for business transactions. (*Left*, Courtesy Roberta D. Cann, DMD Atlanta, GA. *Right*, Courtesy Joseph Ellis DDS and Lisa Tartaglione, DDS Grand Rapids, MI.

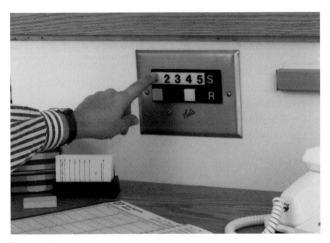

Figure 6-8 A wall-mounted nonverbal intercom system places controls within easy reach of the assistant. (Courtesy Theta Corp., Niagara Falls, NY.)

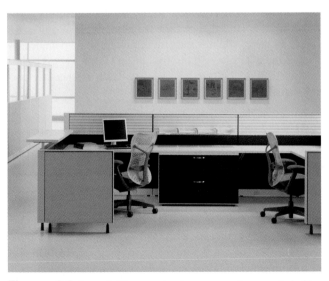

Figure 6-9 Lateral files require less space than vertical files. (Courtesy Herman Miller, Inc., Zeeland, MI.)

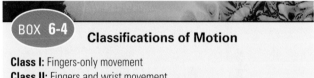

BOX **6-4**   **Classifications of Motion**

Class I: Fingers-only movement
Class II: Fingers and wrist movement
Class III: Fingers, wrist, and elbow movement
Class IV: Fingers, wrist, elbow, and shoulder movement
Class V: Arm extension and twisting of the torso

BOX **6-5**   **Applying the Principles of Motion Economy in the Business Office**

- Position materials as close to the point of use as possible.
- Use motions that require the least amount of movement.
- Minimize the number of materials to be used for a given procedure.
- Use smooth, continuous motions, not zigzag motions.
- Organize materials in a logical sequence of use.
- Position materials and equipment in advance whenever possible.
- Use ergonomically designed stools or chairs to provide good posture and body support.
- Use body motions that require the least amount of time.
- Minimize the number of eye movements.
- Provide lighting that eliminates shadows in work areas.
- Avoid abrupt contrasts in room lighting to minimize eyestrain.
- Position computer monitors to allow for line of sight to screen within 10 to 40 degrees horizontal.
- Provide work areas that are elbow level or 1 to 2 inches lower.

BODY POSITIONING

Basic Principles

The administrative assistant must consider proper seating arrangements during routine daily activities. When possible, all activities should be performed in a seated position to avoid undue stress on the neck, back, and legs. A chair with a broad base, four or five casters, and a well-padded seat and back support is helpful (Figure 6-10). Improper posture while standing or sitting can lead to fatigue, which in turn affects productivity. The suggestions presented in Box 6-6 can help ensure the greatest comfort and efficiency.

Figure 6-11 illustrates proper seated posture while using a computer with a tabletop monitor. An alternative position for the computer monitor is to recess it beneath the desk as shown in Figure 6-11, *B*. The schematic drawing in Figure 6-11, *C* illustrates the positioning of a person in an ergonomic chair using the recessed monitor.

Tilt and glare are both factors in monitor placement. When the recessed monitor position is used, it is necessary to follow the manufacturer's recommended position to avoid any neck problems. Two side benefits of recessed monitor placement are the elimination of the patient observing the monitor screen and additional space made available on the desktop.

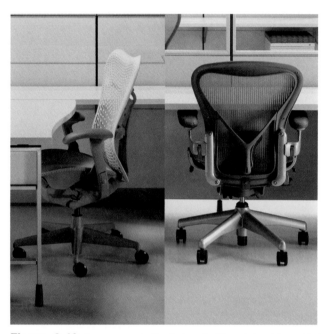

Figure 6-10 An ergonomically designed office chair with padded seating and proper back support promotes productivity. (Courtesy Herman Miller, Inc. Zeeland, MI.)

BOX 6-6   **Ergonomically Correct Body Positioning**

- When a person is seated, the thighs should be parallel to the floor, the lower legs vertical, and the feet firmly on the floor.
- When a person is using a keyboard, the arms should be positioned so that the forearms and wrists are as horizontal as possible.
- The eye to computer screen distance should be 16 to 24 inches.
- The keyboard should tilt 0 to 25 degrees.
- The back and neck should be erect, and the upper arms perpendicular to the floor.
- The buttocks should be well supported on the chair seat, which should be 16 to 19 inches from the floor.

Persons who have used this system often wonder why they have always used the desktop monitor. For further information on this system, refer to the web site for Nova Desks later in this chapter. Refer to Box 6-6 for recommendations for desk height and foot clearance using any of these systems. Much of the success of an office may be attributed to its efficiency and productivity without loss or waste. Again, the goal in ergonomic body positioning should be to work smarter and not harder.

Health and Safety Issues

A variety of factors can affect the health and safety of business office personnel. For example, spending hours each day looking at a computer screen can result in eyestrain and fatigue. Repetitive keyboarding can lead to wrist discomfort and possibly carpal tunnel syndrome, although use of an ergonomically designed keyboard (Figure 6-12) can help reduce this stress. The following tips can help reduce fatigue and eyestrain when working at a computer:

- Make sure the screen is neither too dark nor too bright.
- If you are using the computer continuously, take a 10- to 15-minute break every two or three hours.
- Use good posture.
- Stand up every half hour.
- Periodically look away from the screen for a few minutes.
- Use an ergonomically designed mouse, such as a track ball.
- Use an ergonomically designed chair.
- Consider a recessed monitor system.

Safety hazards can exist in the dental business office. In 1970 the Occupational Safety and Health Act was passed to ensure that workers in the United States have a safe working environment. Much has been discussed in terms of the relation of this act to the dental treatment room, but often the impact on the business area is overlooked. The Occupational Safety and Health Administration (OSHA) requires employers to provide a hazard-free work environment, that is, one without recognized dangers that can cause death, injury, or illness. Box 6-7 presents a list of hazards that might be found in business offices. Of course, in dental and medical offices, this list is compounded by the possibility of disease transmission (see Chapter 17). The lists in Boxes 6-7 and 6-8 can be used periodically to check for possible hazards.

SELECTING OFFICE SUPPLIES

When first setting up a business office, determining what supplies will be needed may be an overwhelming task. Many dental suppliers assist in stocking the clinical area, but they seldom consider the "nuts and bolts" of the business office. Box 6-9 presents a basic list of the various forms and office supplies needed in a dental business office. Most office supply companies can assist you, and a variety of stationery suppliers can provide samples of stationery and forms. A walk through a favorite office supply discount store can be fascinating, but buy only the supplies most needed, not one of everything available.

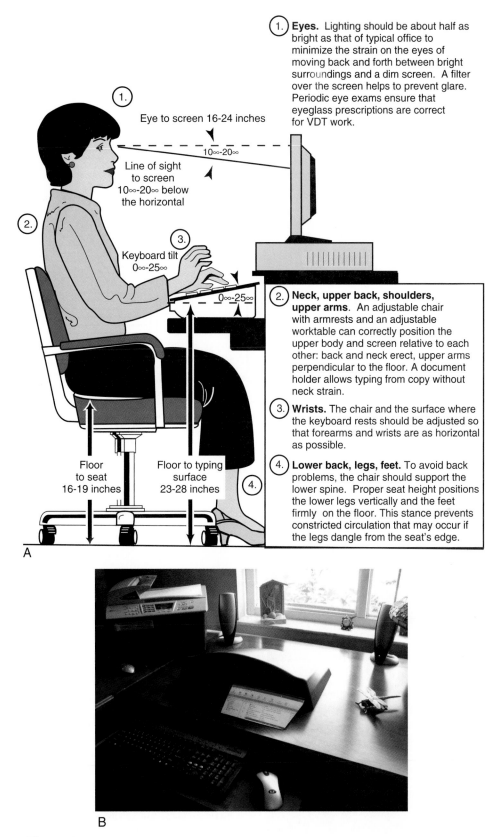

1. **Eyes.** Lighting should be about half as bright as that of typical office to minimize the strain on the eyes of moving back and forth between bright surroundings and a dim screen. A filter over the screen helps to prevent glare. Periodic eye exams ensure that eyeglass prescriptions are correct for VDT work.

Eye to screen 16-24 inches

Line of sight to screen 10∞-20∞ below the horizontal

Keyboard tilt 0∞-25∞

2. **Neck, upper back, shoulders, upper arms.** An adjustable chair with armrests and an adjustable worktable can correctly position the upper body and screen relative to each other: back and neck erect, upper arms perpendicular to the floor. A document holder allows typing from copy without neck strain.

3. **Wrists.** The chair and the surface where the keyboard rests should be adjusted so that forearms and wrists are as horizontal as possible.

4. **Lower back, legs, feet.** To avoid back problems, the chair should support the lower spine. Proper seat height positions the lower legs vertically and the feet firmly on the floor. This stance prevents constricted circulation that may occur if the legs dangle from the seat's edge.

Floor to seat 16-19 inches

Floor to typing surface 23-28 inches

A

B

Figure 6-11 **A,** Posture and positioning in relation to equipment promotes high-level productivity. **B,** Recessed monitor provides ergonomic positioning and increased work surface on the desk.

(Continued)

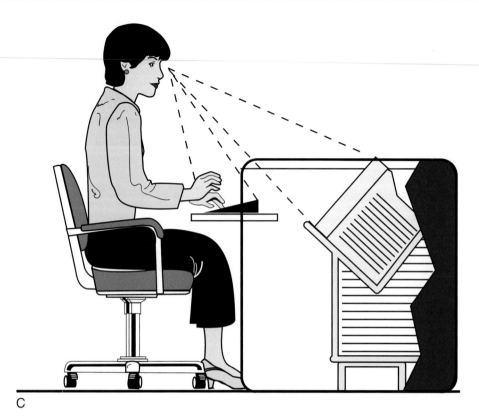

Figure 6-11, cont'd C, A schematic illustrates the ergonomic position of an operator using a Nova Station.

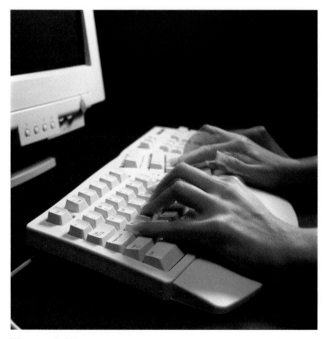

Figure 6-12 An ergonomic keyboard reduces overuse stress on the wrist. (Copyright 2009 JupiterImages Corporation.)

BOX 6-7   **Potential Hazards**

- Frayed or loose telephone cords or electrical wires
- Wires loosely secured to the floor
- Improperly grounded wall or floor switches
- Use of improper electric current to electronic equipment
- Spilled beverages or food on the floor
- Paper cutters, knives, or spindle files
- Loose floor covering on the stairs or floor
- Wearing of jewelry that can be caught in electronic equipment such as copiers
- Open files or drawers

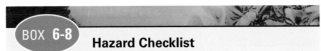

BOX 6-8 **Hazard Checklist**

The following points should be evaluated routinely to ensure that safety measures have been observed:

- Floor coverings are durable and in good repair.
- Floor surfaces in clinical areas are hard and uncarpeted.
- Antislip protection is available on smooth floor surfaces.
- Electrical equipment and cords are in safe operating condition.
- Employees have been trained in proper operation of equipment.
- Only one drawer of a file cabinet is opened at a time.
- Office furniture has no sharp edges but does have stable arms and legs.
- The locations of eyewash areas are posted in laboratory and clinical areas.
- First aid kits are well stocked and readily accessible.
- *No smoking* signs are posted in visible locations.
- All guidelines on infection control from the Occupational Safety and Health Administration (OSHA) are followed and are posted in visible locations.
- Hazard information is posted and available for all employees.

BOX 6-9 **Basic Office Supplies**

General Supplies

Ballpoint pens
Calendar and calendar holder
Clear tape with dispenser
Double edged tape with dispenser
Erasers
Felt-tip markers
Hole puncher; three-hole puncher
Label maker
Letter opener
Masking tape
Paper clips (small and large)
Paper shredder
Pen holder
Pencil sharpener
Pencil tray
Pens and pencils
Rubber bands
Rubber stamps and pad
Ruler
Scissors
Stapler, staples, staple remover
Utility tray (for paper clips, pens, pencils, and other small items)
Wastebasket

Paper Supplies

Adhesive notes
Assorted envelopes (e.g., coin, large and special mailing services envelopes)
Business cards

Copy paper (assorted sizes)
Drug reference
Fax paper
File folders
File folder labels
File guides
Index cards
Index tabs
Letterhead (second sheets)
Letterhead and envelopes
Medical and dental dictionaries
Message reply forms
Note pads
Plain white paper
Preprinted office forms
Report covers
Ring binders
Ruled letter- and legal-size writing pads
Standard dictionary
Storage cartons
Telephone message pads

Appointment Management Supplies

Appointment book (optional if not computerized)
Appointment cards
Appointment schedule forms (optional if not computerized)
Replacement sheets for appointment book (optional if not computerized)
Work or school excuse forms

(Continued)

BOX 6-9 Basic Office Supplies—cont'd

Clinical Forms

Clinical charts with assorted forms
Colored filing labels
Consent forms
File guides
Health alert labels
Health questionnaire forms
HIPAA forms
Laboratory requisition forms
Patient file envelopes and folders
Prescription pads
Referral forms
Registration forms
Update forms
OSHA reporting forms
Safety management forms

Financial Record Forms

Application for Employer Identification Number (SS-4)
Bank deposit slips
Bookkeeping forms (optional if not computerized)

Checkbook and replacement checks
Citizenship Eligibility Form (I-9)
Employee's Withholding Allowance Certificate Form (W-4)
Employer's quarterly tax return form (941)
Employer's annual federal unemployment tax return form (940)
Insurance claim forms
Ledger cards and forms (optional if not computerized)
Payroll forms
Statements
Transmittal of income and tax statements form (W-3)
Wage and tax statement form (W-2)

Microcomputer Supplies

Disks
Cleaning materials
Disk cases
Disk labels
Disk mailers
Mouse pad
Printer ink
Toner cartridges

NOTE: When available, ergonomically designed supplies and materials should be purchased.

LEARNING ACTIVITIES

1. List eight suggestions for the design of a reception room.
2. Discuss 10 factors to consider when designing a business office.
3. Describe the impact of the Americans with Disabilities Act on a dental practice.
4. Describe the concept of time and motion as it applies to a dental business office.
5. List six tips that will help reduce fatigue and eyestrain when working at a computer.

Please refer to the student workbook for additional learning activities.

KEY TERMS

Classifications of motion—Referring to the amount of energy it takes to perform various tasks.

Ergonomics—The science that studies the relationship between people and their work environment.

Reception room—This room is the gateway to the dental office and provides the patient's first impression of the dentist.

Time and motion—Referring to the amount of time and the extent of motion it takes to perform a given task.

BIBLIOGRAPHY

BIFMA Ergonomics guideline, Effingham, IL, 2008 Nova. Available at www.novadesk.com.

Fulton-Calkins PJ: *The administrative professional*, ed 13, Mason, OH, 2007, Thomson South-Western.

RECOMMENDED WEB SITES

www.access-board.gov
www.ada.gov
http://sad.com
www.novadesk.com

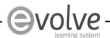

Please visit http://evolve.elsevier.com/Finkibeiner/practice for additional practice activities.

PART II

COMMUNICATION MANAGEMENT

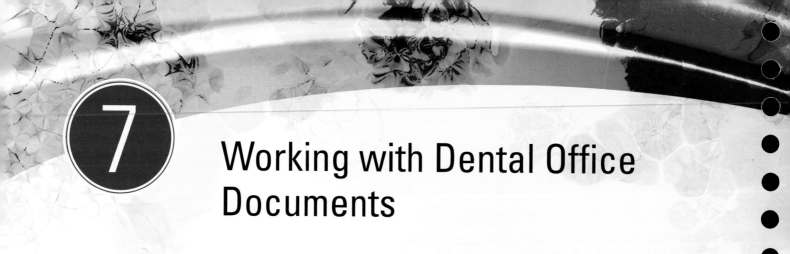

7

Working with Dental Office Documents

CHAPTER OUTLINE

Health Insurance Portability and Accountability Act
Overview of a Records Management System
Categories of Records
    Vital Records
    Important Records
    Useful Records
    Nonessential Records
Types of Patient Records
    Clinical Record
    Clinical Chart
    Patient Sign-in Sheets
    Entering Data on a Clinical Chart
    Types of Clinical Data Entries
    Charting Symbols and Abbreviations
    Records Retention
    Records Transfer
    Records Maintenance
    Occupational Safety and Health Administration Records

LEARNING OUTCOMES

- Define glossary terms.
- Define *HIPAA*.
- Describe how to implement HIPAA regulations in the dental office record management system.
- Identify the types of records maintained in a dental office.
- Categorize the various types of records.
- Distinguish between active and inactive records.
- List the components of a clinical record.
- Describe the function of the components of a clinical record.
- Explain the rules for data entry on patient records.
- Explain the use of symbols and abbreviations in clinical records.
- List the components of patient financial records.
- Identify various types of records required by the Occupational Safety and Health Administration (OSHA) that must be maintained in a dental office.
- Identify the various types of employee records.
- Explain the importance of maintaining accurate records.
- Describe methods of records retention and transfer

Although every dental professional dreams of a paperless office, an office cannot operate without records. Thus when reality strikes one generally concludes that it is not possible to achieve this longed-for dream. There is also the human nature side of a potential paperless office. Some dentists could easily manage with a totally paperless office and yet there are those who must have a paper record to hold onto for each activity.

The dental office is inundated with a plethora of records and forms, all needed as part of the total dental business practice. These records are kept so that the people in the office can refer to the information later or use it to complete another task. A records management system will help store and retrieve records efficiently and keep the files current. The administrative assistant is required to maintain clinical, financial, employee, state, and federal records. Failure to perform any of these tasks can be a costly experience for the dental practitioner. Therefore, the administrative assistant who can pay routine special attention to detail in maintaining all types of records becomes an immeasurable asset to the dental practice.

HEALTH INSURANCE PORTABILITY AND ACCOUNTABILITY ACT

The **Health Insurance Portability and Accountability Act** (HIPAA) of 1996, which became effective in April 2003, has significantly affected the dental profession in a number of ways.

Administrative simplification provisions of the Health Insurance Portability and Accountability Act of 1996 (HIPAA) have affected the dental profession. These provisions require national standards for electronic healthcare transactions. Dentists who transmit health information in an electronic transaction are required to use a standard format. Plans and providers who do not use electronic standards can use the Employee Retirement Security Act (ERISA) healthcare clearinghouse to comply with the requirement. Providers' paper transactions are not subject to this requirement. Primarily the most affected area in the dental office is the area of transmission of dental claim forms, which is reviewed in Chapter 14. However, as one begins to study the management of patient records, the impact of privacy is one of primary concern.

HIPAA laws may seem daunting at first. However, the purpose is to protect and enhance patient rights; therefore, it is a positive action because everyone is a patient at one time or another. Protecting health information is the right thing to do, and it promotes safe practice for everyone on the dental team, especially the patient. It is also good risk management, helping each dental professional to prevent potential litigation. Security regulations, which the Department of Health and Human Services released under HIPAA, were conceived to protect electronic patient health information. Protected patient health information is anything that ties a patient's name or Social Security number to that person's health, health care, or payment for health care, such as radiographs, charts, or invoices. Each dental professional should become familiar with state as well as federal laws, as these laws are often more stringent than federal laws.

The American Dental Association (ADA) and most state dental associations have done an excellent job of providing its members with the necessary tools for the implementation of HIPAA. The ADA and state dental associations as well as many dental office stationers provide a HIPAA Security Tool Kit as shown in Figure 7-1. This kit contains most of the forms needed for privacy practices, including the following:

- The Notice of Privacy Practices form (Figure 7-2) presents information that the dental professional is required to give patients regarding the office's privacy practices. This form may need to be changed to reflect the dental practice's particular privacy polices or stricter state laws. The name of the practice may be on the notice, and it must be given to each

patient at the date of the first service. In addition, the notice may be posted in a clear and prominent location in the office that is visible to any patient seeking service. Boxes 7-1 and 7-2 provide checklists for managing the privacy and security of patient records.

- Acknowledgement of Receipt of Notice of Privacy Practices (see Figure 7-3 on p. 100) is the form the patient signs to acknowledge that he or she has received a copy of the Notice of Privacy Practices. If the patient refuses to sign the form, the administrative assistant can indicate that an attempt was made to have the patient sign in the *in-office* section on the form. The patient may also opt to sign a separate refusal form that may then be placed in the record.
- Business Associate Contract Terms is a contract form that satisfies the obligation under the HIPAA and its implementing regulations issued by the U.S. Department of Health and Human Services (see Figure 7-4 on p. 101). This form ensures the integrity and confidentiality of protected health information that a business associate may create or receive for or from the dental practice. Other forms such as the Health Information Access-Response/Delay, Complaint, and Staff Review of Policies and Procedures, are available in the ADA manual or from the state dental society. In order to ensure that records are maintained for patients, a preprinted chart label can provide information about important HIPAA information for patient files (see Figure 7-5 on p. 101).

OVERVIEW OF A RECORDS MANAGEMENT SYSTEM

A dental office operates on information; it is created, processed, stored, printed, and distributed in many forms to various sites. Therefore, the dental administrative assistant must establish a logical, functional system for storing and retrieving information. A **record** is data in forms such as text, numbers, images, or voice that is kept for future reference. In a dental office this comes in the form of clinical, financial, radiographic, and photographic forms. **Records management** or an **information management** system refers to a set of procedures used to organize, store, retrieve, remove and dispose of records. Records have a life cycle, which begins with inception and ends with disposition (see Figure 7-6 on p. 102). The life cycle proceeds as follows:

PRACTICE NOTE
Records have a life cycle that begins with creation and ends with disposition.

- *Creation:* This is the origination of the data. In the case of a patient record, creation begins with the completion of a patient registration form and health questionnaire. At the time of creation, a decision is made as to what information must be retained and the format of the record. If the patient is to continue treatment with the office, a

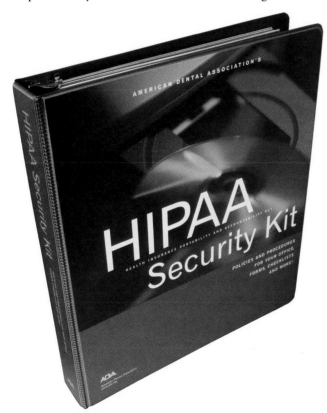

Figure 7-1 HIPAA Security Kit. (Courtesy American Dental Association, Chicago, IL.)

NOTICE OF PRIVACY PRACTICES

THIS NOTICE DESCRIBES HOW MEDICAL INFORMATION ABOUT YOU MAY BE USED AND DISCLOSED AND HOW YOU CAN GET ACCESS TO THIS INFORMATION. PLEASE REVIEW IT CAREFULLY.

This practice is required, by law, to maintain the privacy and confidentiality of your protected health information and to provide our patients with notice of our legal duties and privacy practices with respect to your protected health information.

Disclosure of Your Health Care Information

Treatment
We may disclose your health care information to other health care professionals within our practice for the purpose of treatment, payment or health care operations. (example)

> "On occasion, it may be necessary to seek consultation regarding your condition from other health care providers associated with this practice."

> "It is our policy to provide a substitute health care provider, authorized by this practice, to provide assessment and/or treatment to our patients, without advanced notice, in the event of your primary health care provider's absence due to vacation, sickness, or other emergency situation."

Payment
We may disclose your health information to your insurance provider for the purpose of payment or health care operations. (example)

> "As a courtesy to our patients, we will submit an itemized billing statement to your insurance carrier for the purpose of payment to this practice for health care services rendered. If you pay for your health care services personally, we will, as a courtesy, provide an itemized billing to your insurance carrier for the purpose of reimbursement to you. The billing statement contains medical information, including diagnosis, date of injury or condition, and codes which describe the health care services received."

Workers' Compensation
We may disclose your health information as necessary to comply with State Workers' Compensation Laws.

Emergencies
We may disclose your health information to notify or assist in notifying a family member, or another person responsible for your care, about your medical condition or in the event of an emergency or of your death.

Public Health
As required by law, we may disclose your health information to public health authorities for purposes related to: preventing or controlling disease, injury or disability, reporting child abuse or neglect, reporting domestic violence, reporting to the Food and Drug Administration problems with products and reactions to medications, and reporting disease or infection exposure.

Page 1

©H.J. Ross Company, Inc. 2002, 2003 HIPAA Interactive-All Rights Reserved   ITEM 066-6305/18252 © JULY2003

Figure 7-2 Notice of Privacy Practices form. (Courtesy Patterson Office Supplies, Champaign, IL.)

permanent record usually is started on paper or the data are entered into the computer. If the person is a transient patient, the form for recording the data may be different from the standard form, and the record may not be stored with the active clinical charts.

- *Distribution:* In this stage, the information may be distributed manually or electronically. It includes sending the patient's clinical record to the dentist for diagnosis once the record has been completed.
- *Use:* The dentist evaluates the data and makes a diagnosis or refers the data to an appropriate location for maintenance.
- *Maintenance:* This stage of the cycle involves determining if the data or information should be retained. If it is to be retained, the administrative assistant must decide the best way to store it for easy retrieval and how long it should be stored. If the patient is to be seen again and become a patient of record, the clinical record is filed alphabetically either electronically or in a file folder and envelope in

a protected file. Some components of the record, such as notes the dentist may have made during evaluation, probably could be destroyed and only the pertinent data kept.

- *Disposition:* At this stage it must be determined if the record should be destroyed because it no longer has value to the office or if it should be stored permanently as an important document. The clinical record is vital and must be retained for a period consistent with the state statute of limitations. Electronic data can be transferred to disks for storage. Paper records, which have no backup, must be kept in a safe, dry area.

CATEGORIES OF RECORDS

The administrative assistant must decide which records to keep, how to organize and store them, how long they legally must be retained, and when to dispose of them. In general, records can be categorized as *vital, important, useful,* or *nonessential,* and as *active* or *inactive.*

BOX 7-1   HIPAA Privacy Checklist

The purpose of the HIPAA Privacy Rules is to safeguard the privacy of patients' confidential health information.

Develop
- Written privacy policy and procedures*
- Notice of Privacy Practices (This must be posted.)*
- Acknowledgement of Receipt of Notice of Privacy Practices (Patients must sign this form.)*

Designate
- Privacy officer to oversee enforcement of the privacy procedures
- Contact person to receive complaints and answer questions

Evaluate
- Relationships with business associates, such as consultants, technology/computer support personnel, accountants and other business/service people or companies that have access to your patient's protected health information.
- Sign business associates agreements with individuals or companies that meet these criteria.*

Provide
- Employee training on the provisions of the HIPAA Privacy Rules*

Document
- All employee training and any violations of the privacy policies by employees

Courtesy Mary Govoni, CDA, RDA, RDH, MBA, Clinical Dynamics, Okemos, MI (www. marygovoni.com).
*An excellent resource for templates for these items is the American Dental Association's HIPAA Privacy Kit, available at www.ada.org or a dental stationary supply house.

Vital Records

Vital records are essential documents that cannot be replaced. These include patient clinical and financial records and the office's corporate charter and deed, mortgage, or bill of sale. These records should be kept in a fireproof theft-proof vault or safe, and copies often are kept in a protected, offsite location.

 PRACTICE NOTE
Vital records are essential documents that cannot be replaced.

Important Records

Important records are extremely valuable to the operation of the office, but they are not vital. They include accounts payable and receivable, invoices, canceled checks, inventory and payroll records, and other federal regulatory records. Such records may be needed for a tax audit or if a question arises about a financial transaction. Important records generally should be retained for 5 to 7 years. Most offices keep them for about 7 years or in accordance with federal or state regulations.

BOX 7-2   HIPAA Security Checklist

The purpose of the HIPAA Security Rules is to safeguard the confidentiality and integrity of electronic data regarding patients and their protected health information.

Develop
- Written security policy and procedures*

Designate
- A security officer to oversee enforcement of the security procedures and protocols

Evaluate
- Security risks that might allow unauthorized access to electronic data
- Methods used to back up and store electronic data

Provide
- Employee training on the provisions of the HIPAA Security Rules*
- Access control measures (unique passwords) for all employees who access electronic data

Document
- All employee training and any violations of the privacy policies by employees.
- Periodic system audit reviews—audit trail reports to check for unauthorized access to electronic data

Courtesy Mary Govoni, CDA, RDA, RDH, MBA, Clinical Dynamics, Okemos, MI (www. marygovoni.com).
*An excellent resource for templates for these items is the American Dental Association's HIPAA Security Kit, or a dental stationary supply house.

Useful Records

Useful records include employment applications, expired insurance policies, petty cash vouchers, bank reconciliations, and general correspondence. This category is difficult to define, because one office may consider a document useful, whereas another might find it indispensable. These records usually are retained for 1 to 3 years. Before discarding a document, it is always wise to check with the dentist or other staff members to see if it is still needed.

Nonessential Records

Nonessential records are the documents that lie around, have little importance, and take up space. They include such items as notes to you, reminders of meetings, outdated announcements, and pamphlets. Common sense dictates when these materials may be discarded.

TYPES OF PATIENT RECORDS

Patient records generally fall into two categories, clinical and financial. A recall system is another type of record that is retained separate from the clinical chart but that could be considered a type of clinical record. Clinical records are reviewed in this chapter; financial records are discussed in Chapter 15.

ACKNOWLEDGEMENT OF RECEIPT OF NOTICE

As required by the Privacy Regulations, I hereby acknowledge that I have received a current copy of this practice's "NOTICE OF PRIVACY PRACTICES", revision date _____ .

As required by the Privacy Regulations, _____ from

Name of Staff Member

this practice has explained the "NOTICE OF PRIVACY PRACTICES" to my satisfaction.

As required by the Privacy Regulations, I am aware that this practice has included a provision that it reserves the right to change the terms of its notice and to make the new notice provisions effective for all protected health information that it maintains.

Requests:

☐ I wish to file a "Request for Restriction" of my Protected Health Information.

☐ I wish to file a "Request for Alternative Communications" of my Protected Health Information.

☐ I wish to object to the following in the "Notice of Privacy Practices":

_____

_____

I understand that this office may change their Notice of Privacy Practices and is not required to honor the terms of the original/previous version(s).

_____   _____
            Signature   Date

_____
            Print Name

_____

(OFFICE USE ONLY)

Signed form received by: _____ Date: _____

Good faith effort to obtain receipt: (Describe) _____

_____

_____

©H.J. Ross Company, Inc. 2002, 2003 HIPAA Interactive-All Rights Reserved   ITEM 066-6289/18243 © JULY2003

Figure 7-3 Acknowledgement of Receipt of Notice of Privacy Practices. (Courtesy Patterson Office Supplies, Champaign, IL.)

Clinical Record

The **clinical record** is a collection of all the information about the patient's dental treatment. Although each patient's clinical record is used during dental treatment, updating and maintaining this record is the administrative assistant's responsibility. Success in maintaining clinical records requires cooperation and efficiency from each member of the dental healthcare team.

Accurate clinical records are vital for several reasons, as follows:

- In treatment of the patient, clinical records serve as a road map. They contain the patient's history and outline future treatment.
- In a malpractice suit, the dental record is legally admissible as evidence. It can be used for or against the dentist.
- In third-party payment plans, the dental consultants representing the carrier may review the clinical chart and other parts of the clinical record to determine if services have been rendered adequately.

- The record acts as verification of treatment rendered for Internal Revenue Service purposes.
- Components of the clinical records are vital in forensic odontology, the field of dentistry concerned with identification of individuals based on dental evidence.

A patient's clinical record commonly has the following components:

- Patient file envelope or folder
- Registration form
- Health history and update forms
- HIPAA acknowledgment form
- Clinical chart or examination form
- Progress notes form
- Dental diagnosis, treatment plan, and estimate sheet
- Medication history and prescription forms
- Laboratory requisitions
- Consent forms

**AUTHORIZATION TO USE OR DISCLOSE
PROTECTED HEALTH INFORMATION**

Patient Name:_____

Address: _____

Date of Birth: _____ Date of Request: _____

As required by the Privacy Regulations, this practice may not use or disclose your protected health information except as provided in our Notice of Privacy Practices without your authorization.

I hereby authorize this office and any of its employees to use or disclose my Patient Health Information to the following person(s), entity(s), or business associates of this office:

_____

Patient Health Information authorized to be disclosed:

_____
_____

For the specific purpose of (describe in detail)

_____
_____

Effective dates for this authorization: _____/_____/_____ through _____/_____/_____
This authorization will expire at the end of the above period.

I understand that the information disclosed above may be re-disclosed to additional parties and no longer protected for reasons beyond your control.

I understand I have the right to:

1. Revoke this authorization by sending written notice to this office and that revocation will not affect this office's previous reliance on the uses or disclosure pursuant to this authorization.

2. Knowledge of any remuneration involved due to any marketing activity as allowed by this authorization, and as a result of this authorization.

3. Inspect a copy of the Patient Health Information being used or disclosed under federal law.

4. Refuse to sign this authorization.

5. Receive a copy of this authorization.

6. Restrict what is disclosed with this authorization.

I also understand that if I do not sign this document, it will not condition my treatment, payment, enrollment in a health plan, or eligibility for benefits whether or not I provide authorization to use or disclose protected Patient Health Information.

_____   _____
Signature of Patient or Patient's Authorized Representative   Date

_____   _____
Authorized Signature of Facility   Date

Figure 7-4 Preprinted HIPAA Record of Disclosures forms for patient charts. (Courtesy Patterson Office Supplies, Champaign, IL.)

HIPAA Requirements

Privacy Policy: **By:**
☐ Given to Patient   _____
☐ Signed Acknowledgment Received   _____
Disclosure Authorization on File:
☐ Disclosure Authorization on File   _____
☐ Restriction Request on File   _____
☐ Other _____   _____

Figure 7-5 Preprinted label for patient's chart to affirm HIPAA requirements are met. (Courtesy Patterson Office Supplies, Champaign, IL.)

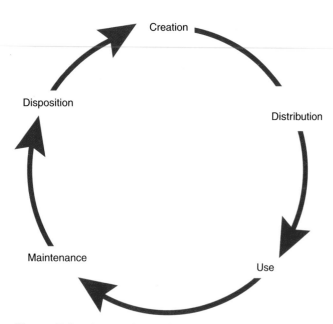

Figure 7-6 Life cycle of a record.

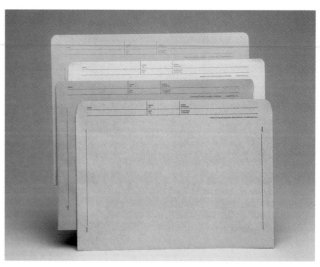

Figure 7-7 Patient file envelopes. (Courtesy Patterson Office Supplies, Champaign, IL.)

- Consultation and referral reports
- Letters
- Postal receipts
- Treatment record/progress notes
- Radiographs
- Copies of laboratory tests

Bulkier materials, such as diagnostic models, generally are stored in an area other than the business office. A cross-reference on the patient record makes these materials easier to locate. Although the dentist chooses the components of the clinical record, staff members' opinions are important when selecting the forms because the staff members must maintain them. With more dental practices moving toward computerized systems, patient records and files are changing. More of the data will be stored in the computer, and the need for paper copies of these documents will decline.

Patient File Envelope or Folder

In most dental practices, use of an 8½ × 11-inch file envelope or folder guards against misplacement of records. In practices in which patients are seen by the dentist only or do not return on a regular basis, such as in an oral surgeon's office, a smaller envelope (5 × 8 inches) may be desirable, or the envelope may be eliminated. File envelopes may be plain or color-coded. They are supplied in a preprinted format with spaces for patient information, including the patient's name, address, and telephone number (Figure 7-7). This type of envelope is widely used and satisfies the needs of many practices.

Another very common type of storage for patient records is an end-tab file folder with one or two two-hole fasteners (Figure 7-8 A,B). This type of folder requires the use of vertical-style records. The folders generally have a reinforced tab for easy label placement. They also are precut for quick insertion of a two-hole file fastener. Options include folders with pockets and

diagonal cuts and expandable folders. Other auxiliary aids for these records include the hole punch, perm-clip fasteners, and polyvinyl pockets to hold small materials such as radiographs and CDs (see Figure 7-8 C,D).

Whether folders or envelopes are used, some form of color-coding is necessary to make sorting, storing, and retrieval easier. Color-coding can be done as an alphabetical system or, in a group practice, can be categorized by dentist. In addition to the traditional label (Figure 7-9), either an alpha or numeric label system can be used to sort the records. Year aging labels can be used to identify inactive patient records that may need to be purged from the active storage system (Figure 7-10 A,B). In Figure 7-10, C, the letter T is the first letter of the patient's last name, and H is the first letter of the patient's first name. The two-digit number indicates the year of the patient's last visit to the office.

Patient Registration and Health History Forms

Although they are often combined, these two forms contain two different types of data. They should be retained because they provide more detailed information about the patient. Stock forms are available from dental forms suppliers. Custom forms can be designed by most companies and these will address the special needs of the office. Some forms are available to address questions such as, "May we leave a message on you're answering machine at the phone number you have given?" or "May we contact you at a cell phone number or text message you?" If there are other questions desired for the office, talk with the supplier and for a nominal price these can be modified to meet the office's needs. Most supply companies provide patient forms in English and Spanish versions for use in various areas of the country. Many offices with Spanish-speaking patients have both forms available.

The **patient registration form** contains general information such as addresses and telephone numbers, as well as employment and insurance information. Figure 7-11 on p. 105 presents two

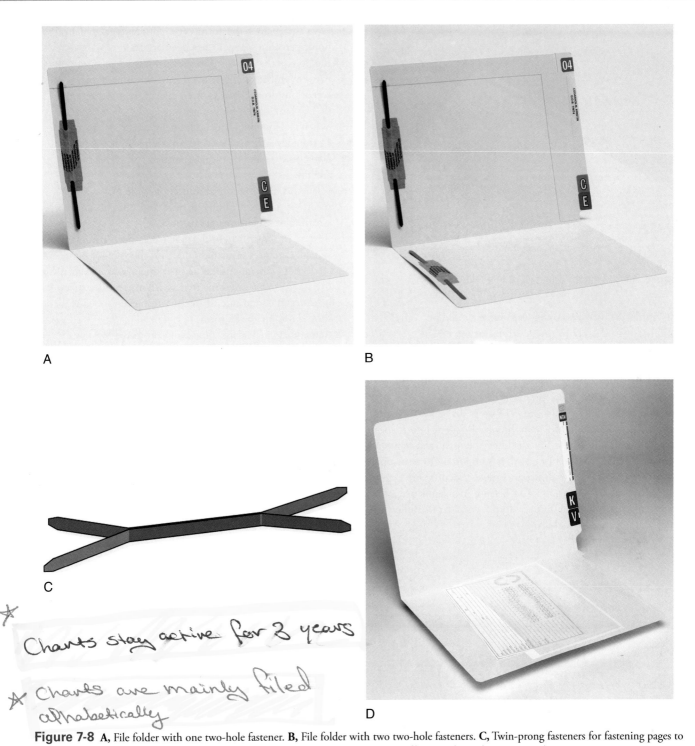

A

B

C

D

Charts stay active for 3 years

Charts are mainly filed alphabetically

Figure 7-8 **A,** File folder with one two-hole fastener. **B,** File folder with two two-hole fasteners. **C,** Twin-prong fasteners for fastening pages to either side of a file folder. **D,** Polyvinyl pocket. (**A** through **D** Courtesy Patterson Office Supplies, Champaign, IL.)

common types of registration forms. This form enables the staff members to become better acquainted with the patient and can provide information for third-party payments and credit checks. Incomplete information on this form can complicate account collection later. Experienced business managers know that an account properly opened is half collected.

Each patient should fill out a **health history form** (see Figure 7-12 on p. 106) and date and sign it. If the dentist prefers to ask these questions in person, the patient should verify the answers recorded and sign the form. Figure 7-13 on p. 107 shows a combination health history and adult registration form. Figure 7-14 on p. 108 shows the pediatric version of this form. With children, the health history form should be completed by a parent or guardian, not by the child or a baby sitter. Make sure no nicknames are used and that all data are accurate, because this information is used later to complete insurance forms.

The patient's history should be reviewed when the person returns for treatment if several months have elapsed since the

Figure 7-9 Traditional name label on file folder.

last visit. A **health history update form** should be completed periodically to keep both the health history (see Figure 7-15, *A* on p. 109) and the personal information (see Figure 7-15, *B* on p. 109) current. The patient should sign and date this form.

Many types of patient registration and health history forms are available. For example, the form in Figure 7-16 on p. 110 can be used for children. Figure 7-17 on p. 111 shows a short-form style, which combines an abbreviated patient information form and health history form, which may be used for a transient patient. Regardless of the form used, it is important to remember that a current, accurate health history serves as a preventive measure in patient treatment and as a defense in malpractice suits. When collecting the data on these forms, consider the following points:

- Give the patient the form on a clipboard to which a ball-point pen (not a pencil) has been attached.
- Do not ask the questions in the business office. Some answers may be embarrassing if overheard by other patients in the reception room. Patients often give more information if they do not have to respond orally.
- When making appointments for new patients, ask them to arrive 15 minutes early to allow time for completion of these forms.
- Make sure a parent or legal guardian completes the form for a child.
- Keep the information absolutely confidential. The patient record is not for public review and should not become a feature of lunchtime gossip.
- Review the form to ensure that it has been completed and signed. Patients may avoid questions they do not understand or do not want to answer. If the patient says, "I don't think this question has anything to do with my teeth," explain how it relates to dental care. If the question cannot be justified, it should not be on the form.

Remember, a person's privacy is protected by law. Several questions on forms shown as examples may be considered discriminatory or in violation of a patient's rights. Consequently the administrative assistant must be aware of the state laws that protect a person's rights and change the form to accommodate these rights. As legal changes occur, most suppliers try to produce forms that are in accord with the laws protecting patient rights.

Clinical Chart

A wide selection of dental charts is available for use in the dental office. Obviously, the needs of specialty practices are different from those of a general practice, and several choices are

(Text continued on p. 112)

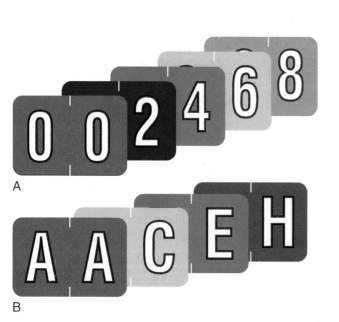

A

B

C

Figure 7-10 A, Numeric and year aging labels on a clinical chart. **B,** Alpha and year aging labels on a clinical chart. **C,** Record indicating first letter of the last name, the first letter of the first name, and year of the last treatment. (Courtesy Patterson Office Supplies, Champaign, IL.)

Welcome

Thank you for selecting our dental healthcare team!
We will strive to provide you with the best possible dental care.
To help us meet all your dental healthcare needs, please fill out this form completely in ink. If you have any questions or need assistance, please ask us - we will be happy to help.

Patient # ____
SS#/SIN ____

Patient Information (CONFIDENTIAL)

Date ____
Name ____ Birthdate ____ Home Phone ____
Address ____ City ____ State/Prov. ____ Zip/P.C. ____
Email ____ Cell Phone ____
Check Appropriate Box: ☐ Minor ☐ Single ☐ Married ☐ Divorced ☐ Widowed ☐ Separated
If Student, Name of School/College ____ City ____ State/Prov. ____ ☐ Full Time ☐ Part Time
Patient or Parent/Guardian's Employer ____ Work Phone ____
Business Address ____ City ____ State/Prov. ____ Zip/P.C. ____
Spouse or Parent/Guardian's Name ____ Employer ____ Work Phone ____
Whom may we thank for referring you? ____
Person to contact in case of emergency ____ Phone ____

Responsible Party

Name of Person Responsible for this Account ____ Relationship to Patient ____
Address ____ Home Phone ____
Email ____ Cell Phone ____
Driver's License# ____ Birthdate ____ Financial Institution ____
Employer ____ Work Phone ____ SS#/SIN ____
Is this person currently a patient in our office? ☐ Yes ☐ No
For your convenience, we offer the following methods of payment. Please check the option you prefer. Payment in full at each appointment.
☐ Cash ☐ Personal Check Credit Card ☐ VISA ☐ MasterCard ☐ I wish to discuss the office's payment policy.

Insurance Information

Name of Insured ____ Relationship to Patient ____
Birthdate ____ SS#/SIN ____ Date Employed ____
Name of Employer ____ Union or Local # ____ Work Phone ____
Address of Employer ____ City ____ State/Prov. ____ Zip/P.C. ____
Insurance Company ____ Group # ____ Policy/ID # ____
Ins. Co. Address ____ City ____ State/Prov. ____ Zip/P.C. ____
How much is your deductible? ____ How much have you used? ____ Max. annual benefit ____

DO YOU HAVE ANY ADDITIONAL INSURANCE? ☐ Yes ☐ No IF YES, COMPLETE THE FOLLOWING:

Name of Insured ____ Relationship to Patient ____
Birthdate ____ SS#/SIN ____ Date Employed ____
Name of Employer ____ Union or Local # ____ Work Phone ____
Address of Employer ____ City ____ State/Prov. ____ Zip/P.C. ____
Insurance Company ____ Group # ____ Policy/ID # ____
Ins. Co. Address ____ City ____ State/Prov. ____ Zip/P.C. ____
How much is your deductible? ____ How much have you used? ____ Max. annual benefit ____

Over Please

A

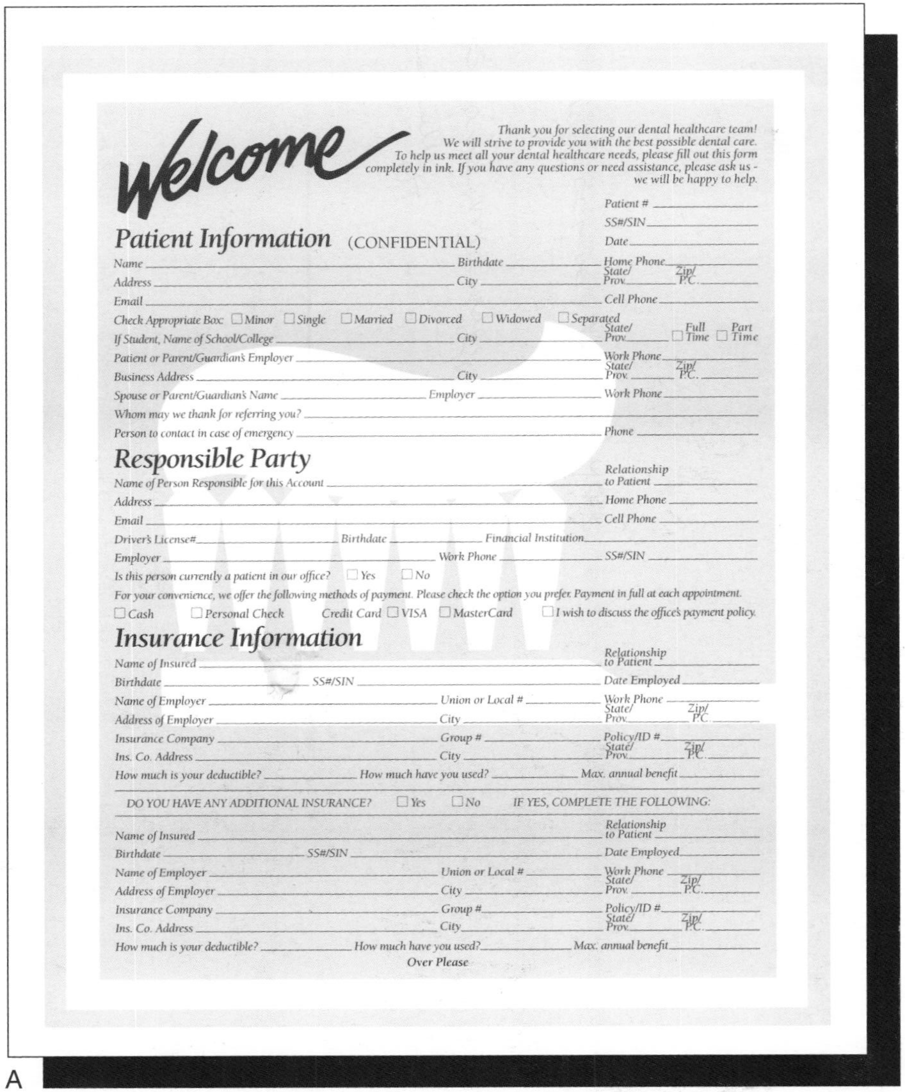

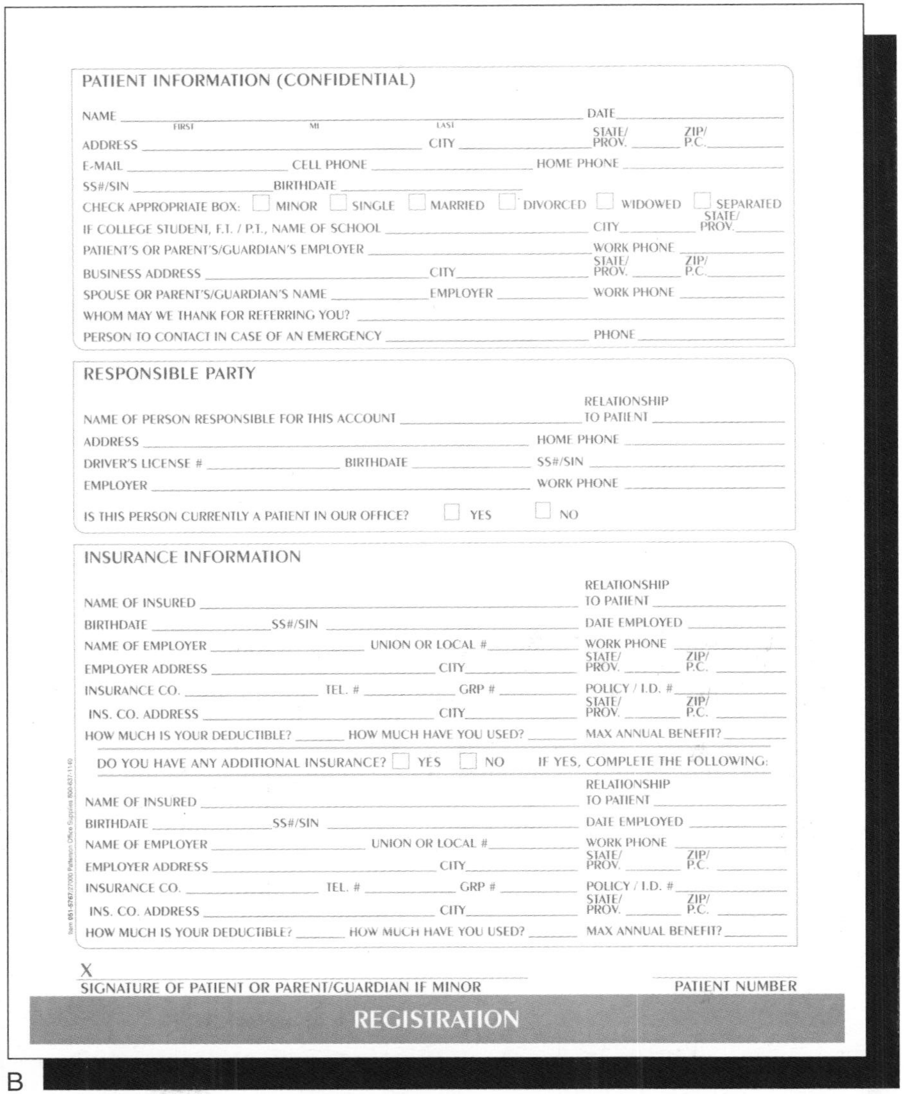

PATIENT INFORMATION (CONFIDENTIAL)

NAME ____ (FIRST) ____ (MI) ____ (LAST) ____ DATE ____
ADDRESS ____ CITY ____ STATE/PROV. ____ ZIP/P.C. ____
E-MAIL ____ CELL PHONE ____ HOME PHONE ____
SS#/SIN ____ BIRTHDATE ____
CHECK APPROPRIATE BOX: ☐ MINOR ☐ SINGLE ☐ MARRIED ☐ DIVORCED ☐ WIDOWED ☐ SEPARATED
IF COLLEGE STUDENT, F.T. / P.T., NAME OF SCHOOL ____ CITY ____ STATE/PROV. ____
PATIENT'S OR PARENT'S/GUARDIAN'S EMPLOYER ____ WORK PHONE ____
BUSINESS ADDRESS ____ CITY ____ STATE/PROV. ____ ZIP/P.C. ____
SPOUSE OR PARENT'S/GUARDIAN'S NAME ____ EMPLOYER ____ WORK PHONE ____
WHOM MAY WE THANK FOR REFERRING YOU? ____
PERSON TO CONTACT IN CASE OF AN EMERGENCY ____ PHONE ____

RESPONSIBLE PARTY

NAME OF PERSON RESPONSIBLE FOR THIS ACCOUNT ____ RELATIONSHIP TO PATIENT ____
ADDRESS ____ HOME PHONE ____
DRIVER'S LICENSE # ____ BIRTHDATE ____ SS#/SIN ____
EMPLOYER ____ WORK PHONE ____
IS THIS PERSON CURRENTLY A PATIENT IN OUR OFFICE? ☐ YES ☐ NO

INSURANCE INFORMATION

NAME OF INSURED ____ RELATIONSHIP TO PATIENT ____
BIRTHDATE ____ SS#/SIN ____ DATE EMPLOYED ____
NAME OF EMPLOYER ____ UNION OR LOCAL # ____ WORK PHONE ____
EMPLOYER ADDRESS ____ CITY ____ STATE/PROV. ____ ZIP/P.C. ____
INSURANCE CO. ____ TEL. # ____ GRP # ____ POLICY / I.D. # ____
INS. CO. ADDRESS ____ CITY ____ STATE/PROV. ____ ZIP/P.C. ____
HOW MUCH IS YOUR DEDUCTIBLE? ____ HOW MUCH HAVE YOU USED? ____ MAX ANNUAL BENEFIT? ____

DO YOU HAVE ANY ADDITIONAL INSURANCE? ☐ YES ☐ NO IF YES, COMPLETE THE FOLLOWING:

NAME OF INSURED ____ RELATIONSHIP TO PATIENT ____
BIRTHDATE ____ SS#/SIN ____ DATE EMPLOYED ____
NAME OF EMPLOYER ____ UNION OR LOCAL # ____ WORK PHONE ____
EMPLOYER ADDRESS ____ CITY ____ STATE/PROV. ____ ZIP/P.C. ____
INSURANCE CO. ____ TEL. # ____ GRP # ____ POLICY / I.D. # ____
INS. CO. ADDRESS ____ CITY ____ STATE/PROV. ____ ZIP/P.C. ____
HOW MUCH IS YOUR DEDUCTIBLE? ____ HOW MUCH HAVE YOU USED? ____ MAX ANNUAL BENEFIT? ____

X ____
SIGNATURE OF PATIENT OR PARENT/GUARDIAN IF MINOR
PATIENT NUMBER

REGISTRATION

B

Figure 7-11 A, Front of an alternative patient registration form. (Courtesy Patterson Office Supplies, Champaign, IL.) **B,** Common registration form. (Courtesy Patterson Office Supplies, Champaign, IL.)

PATIENT'S MEDICAL HISTORY

PATIENT'S NAME _____ DATE OF BIRTH _____

ALTHOUGH DENTAL PERSONNEL PRIMARILY TREAT THE AREA IN AND AROUND YOUR MOUTH, YOUR MOUTH IS A PART OF YOUR ENTIRE BODY. HEALTH PROBLEMS THAT YOU MAY HAVE, OR MEDICATION THAT YOU MAY BE TAKING, COULD HAVE AN IMPORTANT INTERRELATIONSHIP WITH THE DENTISTRY THAT YOU WILL BE RECEIVING. THANK YOU FOR ANSWERING THE FOLLOWING QUESTIONS.

	YES	NO
1. ARE YOU IN GOOD HEALTH.		
2. HAVE THERE BEEN ANY CHANGES IN YOUR GENERAL HEALTH WITHIN THE PAST YEAR.		
3. DATE OF YOUR LAST PHYSICAL EXAM: _____		
4. PHYSICIAN'S NAME _____ PHONE NO. _____		
5. ARE YOU NOW UNDER THE CARE OF A PHYSICIAN.		
6. HAVE YOU EVER BEEN HOSPITALIZED FOR ANY SURGICAL OPERATION OR SERIOUS ILLNESS PLEASE EXPLAIN.		
7. ARE YOU TAKING ANY MEDICINE(S) INCLUDING NON-PRESCRIPTION MEDICINE. IF YES, WHAT MEDICINE(S) ARE YOU TAKING.		
8. HAVE YOU HAD ANY ABNORMAL BLEEDING.		
9. DO YOU BRUISE EASILY.		
10. HAVE YOU EVER REQUIRED A BLOOD TRANSFUSION.		
11. HAVE YOU HAD A RECENT WEIGHT LOSS.		

	YES	NO
12. HAVE YOU EVER TAKEN FEN-PHEN/REDUX.		
13. HAVE YOU EVER TAKEN FOSAMAX, BONIVA, ACTONEL OR ANY CANCER MEDICATIONS CONTAINING BISPHOSPHONATES.		
14. HAVE YOU TAKEN VIAGRA, REVATIO, CIALIS OR LEVITRA IN THE LAST 24 HOURS.		
15. DO YOU USE TOBACCO.		
16. DO YOU OR HAVE YOU USED CONTROLLED SUBSTANCES.		
17. ARE YOU WEARING CONTACT LENSES.		
18. DO YOU HAVE A PERSISTENT COUGH OR THROAT CLEARING NOT ASSOCIATED WITH A KNOWN ILLNESS (LASTING MORE THAN 3 WEEKS).		
19. DO YOU HAVE ANY DISEASE, CONDITION OR PROBLEM NOT LISTED ABOVE THAT YOU THINK I SHOULD KNOW ABOUT.		

WOMEN ONLY:

	YES	NO
ARE YOU PREGNANT OR THINK YOU MAY BE PREGNANT.		
ARE YOU NURSING.		
ARE YOU TAKING BIRTH CONTROL PILLS.		

ARE YOU ALLERGIC TO OR HAVE YOU HAD REACTIONS TO:	YES	NO
LOCAL ANESTHETICS LIKE NOVOCAINE.		
PENICILLIN OR OTHER ANTIBIOTICS.		
SULFA DRUGS.		
BARBITURATES, SEDATIVES OR SLEEPING PILLS.		
ASPIRIN.		
IODINE.		
ANY METALS (E.G., NICKEL, MERCURY, ETC.).		
LATEX / RUBBER.		
OTHER (PLEASE LIST).		

DO YOU HAVE OR HAVE YOU EVER HAD THE FOLLOWING:

	YES	NO
RHEUMATIC HEART DISEASE OR RHEUMATIC FEVER.		
SCARLET FEVER.		
HEART DEFECT OR HEART MURMUR.		
HEART TROUBLE, HEART ATTACK OR ANGINA.		
CHEST PAIN.		
SHORTNESS OF BREATH.		
PACEMAKER.		
HEART SURGERY.		
HIGH/LOW BLOOD PRESSURE.		
CONGENITAL HEART PROBLEM.		
SWELLING OF FEET, ANKLES, HANDS.		
HEPATITIS, JAUNDICE OR LIVER DISEASE.		
STROKE.		
SINUS TROUBLE.		
LUNG OR BREATHING PROBLEMS.		
ASTHMA OR HAY FEVER.		

	YES	NO
HIVES OR SKIN RASH.		
FAINTING OR DIZZY SPELLS.		
DIABETES.		
AIDS OR HIV INFECTION.		
THYROID PROBLEMS.		
ALLERGIES.		
ARTHRITIS OR RHEUMATISM.		
JOINT REPLACEMENT OR IMPLANT.		
STOMACH ULCER.		
KIDNEY TROUBLE.		
TUBERCULOSIS.		
PERSISTENT COUGH.		
COUGH THAT PRODUCES BLOOD.		
CHEMOTHERAPY (CANCER, LEUKEMIA).		
SEXUALLY TRANSMITTED DISEASE.		
EPILEPSY OR SEIZURES.		
ANEMIA.		
GLAUCOMA.		
NERVOUSNESS.		
TONSILLITIS.		
TUMORS.		
MENTAL HEALTH CARE.		
BACK PROBLEMS.		
CHEMICAL DEPENDENCY.		
MITRAL VALVE PROLAPSE.		
CORTISONE TREATMENT.		
COLD SORES/FEVER BLISTERS.		
HYPOGLYCEMIA.		
EATING DISORDERS.		

PATIENT'S NUMBER _____

HEALTH HISTORY

PATIENT'S DENTAL HISTORY

PATIENT'S NAME _____ DATE OF BIRTH _____

REASON FOR THIS VISIT _____

WHEN WAS YOUR LAST DENTAL VISIT _____ WHAT WAS DONE THEN _____

HOW OFTEN DID YOU VISIT THE DENTIST BEFORE THEN _____

PREVIOUS DENTIST (NAME AND LOCATION) _____

HAVE YOU HAD A COMPLETE SERIES OF DENTAL FILMS (X-RAYS) TAKEN WHEN/WHERE _____

HOW OFTEN DO YOU BRUSH YOUR TEETH _____ HOW OFTEN DO YOU FLOSS YOUR TEETH _____

IS YOUR DRINKING WATER FLUORIDATED _____

	YES	NO
DO YOUR GUMS BLEED WHILE BRUSHING OR FLOSSING.		
ARE YOUR TEETH SENSITIVE TO HOT OR COLD LIQUIDS/FOODS.		
ARE YOUR TEETH SENSITIVE TO SWEET OR SOUR LIQUIDS/FOODS.		
DO YOU FEEL PAIN TO ANY OF YOUR TEETH.		
DO YOU HAVE ANY SORES OR LUMPS IN OR NEAR YOUR MOUTH.		
HAVE YOU HAD ANY HEAD, NECK OR JAW INJURIES.		
HAVE YOU EVER EXPERIENCED ANY OF THE FOLLOWING PROBLEMS IN YOUR JAW? CLICKING.		
PAIN (JOINT, EAR, SIDE OF FACE).		
DIFFICULTY IN OPENING OR CLOSING.		
DIFFICULTY IN CHEWING.		
DO YOU HAVE FREQUENT HEADACHES.		
DO YOU CLENCH OR GRIND YOUR TEETH.		

	YES	NO
DO YOU BITE YOUR LIPS OR CHEEKS FREQUENTLY.		
HAVE YOU NOTICED ANY LOOSENING OF YOUR TEETH.		
DOES FOOD TEND TO BECOME CAUGHT BETWEEN YOUR TEETH.		
HAVE YOU EVER HAD PERIODONTAL TREATMENT (GUMS).		
EVER WORN A BITE PLATE OR OTHER APPLIANCE.		
HAVE YOU EVER HAD ANY DIFFICULT EXTRACTIONS IN THE PAST.		
HAVE YOU EVER HAD ANY PROLONGED BLEEDING FOLLOWING EXTRACTIONS.		
DO YOU WEAR DENTURES OR PARTIALS. IF YES, DATE OF PLACEMENT.		
HAVE YOU EVER RECEIVED ORAL HYGIENE INSTRUCTIONS REGARDING THE CARE OF YOUR TEETH AND GUMS.		

IF YOU COULD CHANGE ANYTHING ABOUT YOUR SMILE, WHAT WOULD YOU CHANGE? _____

AUTHORIZATION AND RELEASE

I CERTIFY THAT I HAVE READ AND UNDERSTAND THE ABOVE INFORMATION TO THE BEST OF MY KNOWLEDGE. THE ABOVE QUESTIONS HAVE BEEN ACCURATELY ANSWERED. I UNDERSTAND THAT PROVIDING INCORRECT INFORMATION CAN BE DANGEROUS TO MY HEALTH. I AUTHORIZE THE DENTIST TO RELEASE ANY INFORMATION INCLUDING THE DIAGNOSIS AND THE RECORDS OF ANY TREATMENT OR EXAMINATION RENDERED TO ME OR MY CHILD DURING THE PERIOD OF SUCH DENTAL CARE TO THIRD PARTY PAYORS AND/OR HEALTH PRACTITIONERS. I AUTHORIZE AND REQUEST MY INSURANCE COMPANY TO PAY DIRECTLY TO THE DENTIST OR DENTAL GROUP INSURANCE BENEFITS OTHERWISE PAYABLE TO ME. I UNDERSTAND THAT MY DENTAL INSURANCE CARRIER MAY PAY LESS THAN THE ACTUAL BILL FOR SERVICES. I AGREE TO BE RESPONSIBLE FOR PAYMENT OF ALL SERVICES RENDERED ON MY BEHALF OR MY DEPENDENTS.

X _____ DATE _____
SIGNATURE OF PATIENT OR PARENT/GUARDIAN IF MINOR

DOCTOR'S COMMENTS _____

_____ _____
SIGNATURE DATE

ITEM 07-0615776/7011 Patterson Office Supplies 800-637-1140

PATIENT'S NUMBER _____

HEALTH HISTORY

Figure 7-12 Adult patient health history form. (Courtesy Patterson Office Supplies, Champaign, IL.)

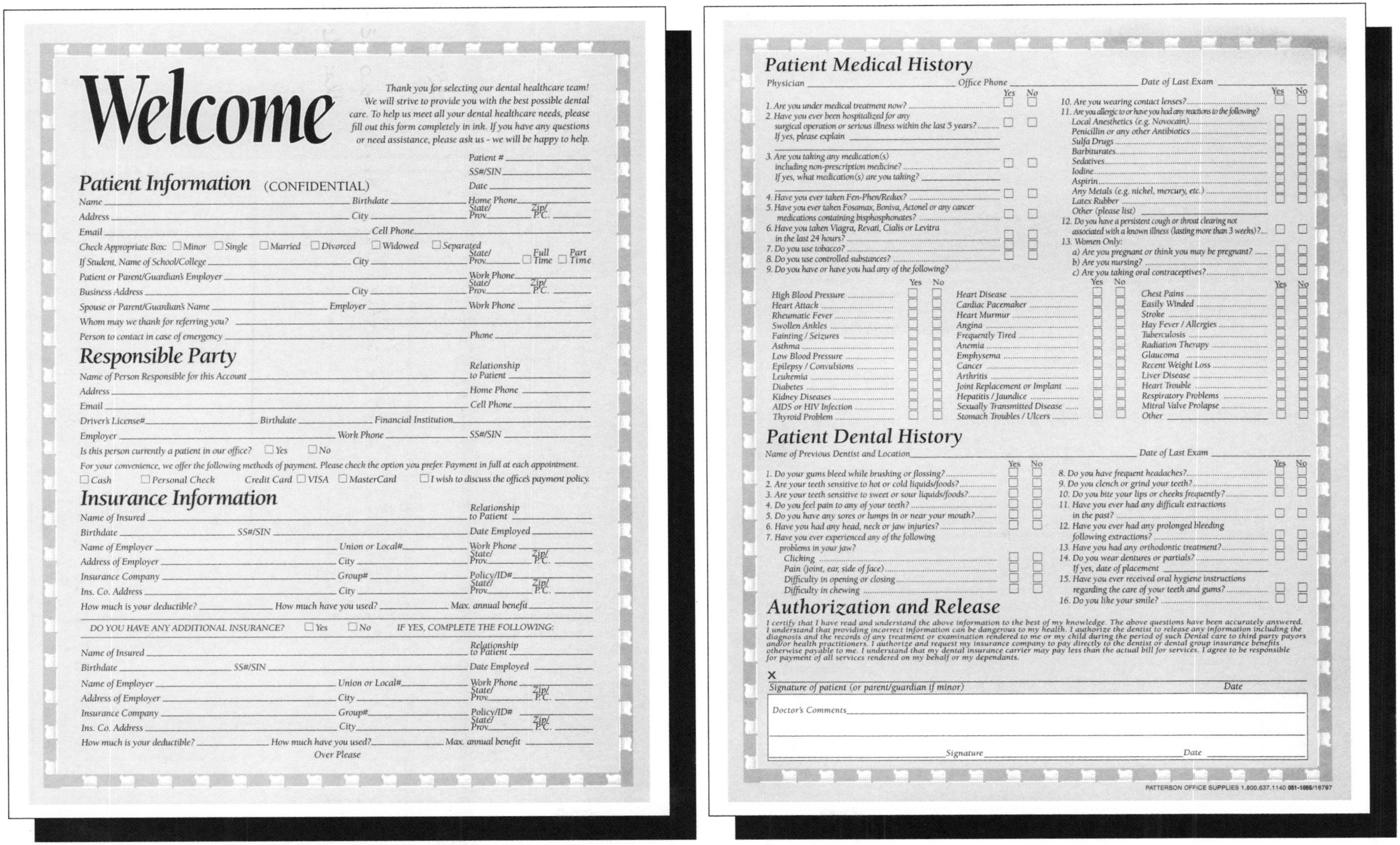

Figure 7-13 Combination history and registration form. (Courtesy Patterson Office Supplies, Champaign, IL.)

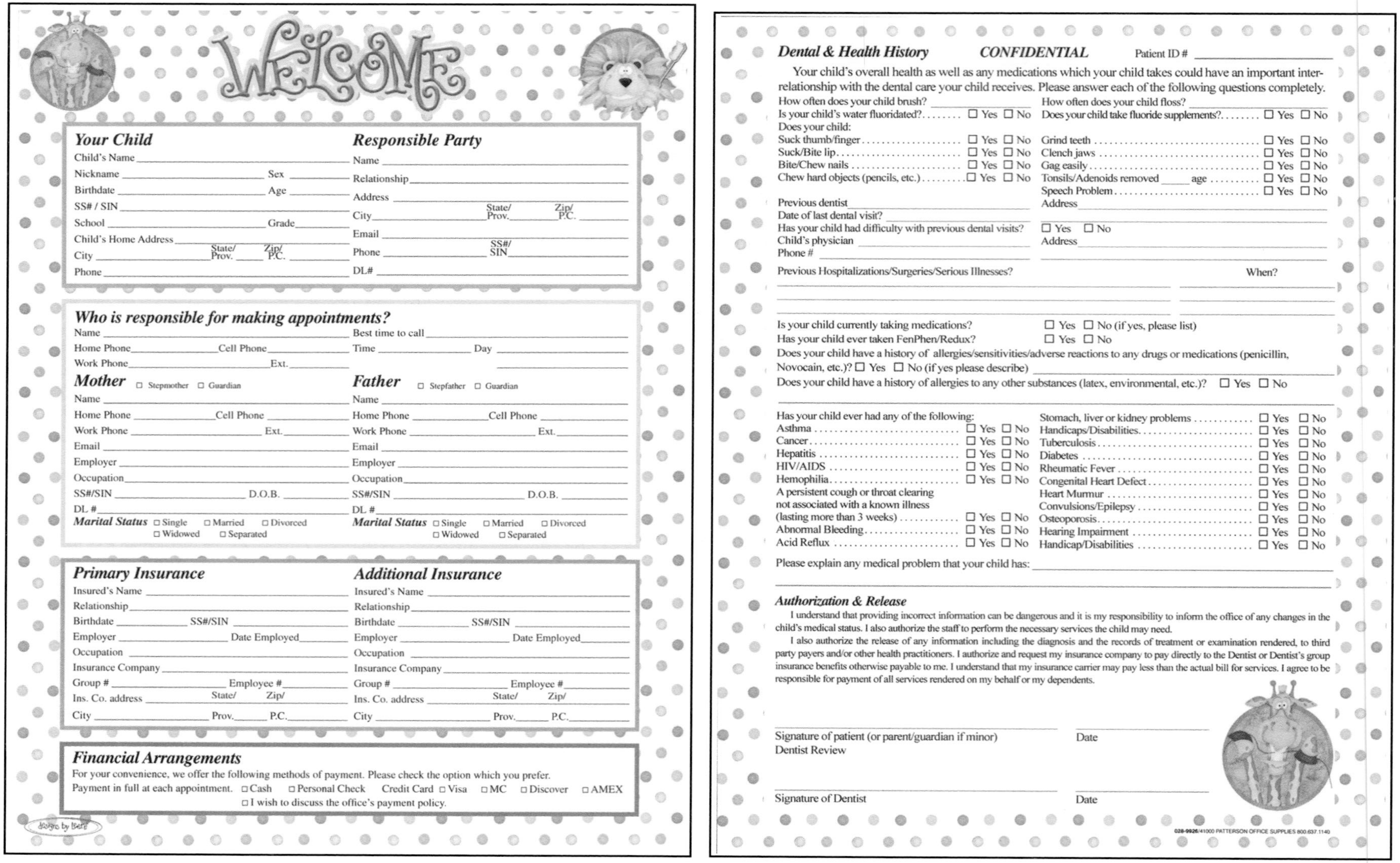

WELCOME

Your Child
Child's Name
Nickname Sex
Birthdate Age
SS# / SIN
School Grade
Child's Home Address
City State/Prov. Zip/P.C.
Phone

Responsible Party
Name
Relationship
Address
City State/Prov. Zip/P.C.
Email
Phone SS#/SIN
DL#

Who is responsible for making appointments?
Name
Home Phone Cell Phone
Work Phone Ext.
Best time to call
Time Day

Mother □ Stepmother □ Guardian
Name
Home Phone Cell Phone
Work Phone Ext.
Email
Employer
Occupation
SS#/SIN D.O.B.
DL #
Marital Status □ Single □ Married □ Divorced □ Widowed □ Separated

Father □ Stepfather □ Guardian
Name
Home Phone Cell Phone
Work Phone Ext.
Email
Employer
Occupation
SS#/SIN D.O.B.
DL #
Marital Status □ Single □ Married □ Divorced □ Widowed □ Separated

Primary Insurance
Insured's Name
Relationship
Birthdate SS#/SIN
Employer Date Employed
Occupation
Insurance Company
Group # Employee #
Ins. Co. address State/ Zip/
City Prov. P.C.

Additional Insurance
Insured's Name
Relationship
Birthdate SS#/SIN
Employer Date Employed
Occupation
Insurance Company
Group # Employee #
Ins. Co. address State/ Zip/
City Prov. P.C.

Financial Arrangements
For your convenience, we offer the following methods of payment. Please check the option which you prefer.
Payment in full at each appointment. □ Cash □ Personal Check Credit Card □ Visa □ MC □ Discover □ AMEX
□ I wish to discuss the office's payment policy.

Dental & Health History **CONFIDENTIAL** Patient ID #

Your child's overall health as well as any medications which your child takes could have an important interrelationship with the dental care your child receives. Please answer each of the following questions completely.

How often does your child brush?
How often does your child floss?
Is your child's water fluoridated? □ Yes □ No
Does your child take fluoride supplements? □ Yes □ No
Does your child:
Suck thumb/finger □ Yes □ No
Suck/Bite lip □ Yes □ No
Bite/Chew nails □ Yes □ No
Chew hard objects (pencils, etc.) □ Yes □ No
Grind teeth □ Yes □ No
Clench jaws □ Yes □ No
Gag easily □ Yes □ No
Tonsils/Adenoids removed ____ age □ Yes □ No
Speech Problem □ Yes □ No

Previous dentist Address
Date of last dental visit?
Has your child had difficulty with previous dental visits? □ Yes □ No
Child's physician Address
Phone #
Previous Hospitalizations/Surgeries/Serious Illnesses? When?

Is your child currently taking medications? □ Yes □ No (if yes, please list)
Has your child ever taken FenPhen/Redux? □ Yes □ No
Does your child have a history of allergies/sensitivities/adverse reactions to any drugs or medications (penicillin, Novocain, etc.)? □ Yes □ No (if yes please describe)
Does your child have a history of allergies to any other substances (latex, environmental, etc.)? □ Yes □ No

Has your child ever had any of the following:
Asthma □ Yes □ No
Cancer □ Yes □ No
Hepatitis □ Yes □ No
HIV/AIDS □ Yes □ No
Hemophilia □ Yes □ No
A persistent cough or throat clearing not associated with a known illness (lasting more than 3 weeks) □ Yes □ No
Abnormal Bleeding □ Yes □ No
Acid Reflux □ Yes □ No
Stomach, liver or kidney problems □ Yes □ No
Handicaps/Disabilities □ Yes □ No
Tuberculosis □ Yes □ No
Diabetes □ Yes □ No
Rheumatic Fever □ Yes □ No
Congenital Heart Defect □ Yes □ No
Heart Murmur □ Yes □ No
Convulsions/Epilepsy □ Yes □ No
Osteoporosis □ Yes □ No
Hearing Impairment □ Yes □ No
Handicap/Disabilities □ Yes □ No

Please explain any medical problem that your child has:

Authorization & Release
I understand that providing incorrect information can be dangerous and it is my responsibility to inform the office of any changes in the child's medical status. I also authorize the staff to perform the necessary services the child may need.
I also authorize the release of any information including the diagnosis and the records of treatment or examination rendered, to third party payers and/or other health practitioners. I authorize and request my insurance company to pay directly to the Dentist or Dentist's group insurance benefits otherwise payable to me. I understand that my insurance carrier may pay less than the actual bill for services. I agree to be responsible for payment of all services rendered on my behalf or my dependents.

Signature of patient (or parent/guardian if minor) Date
Dentist Review
Signature of Dentist Date

Figure 7-14 Registration and health history form for children. (Courtesy Patterson Office Supplies, Champaign, IL.)

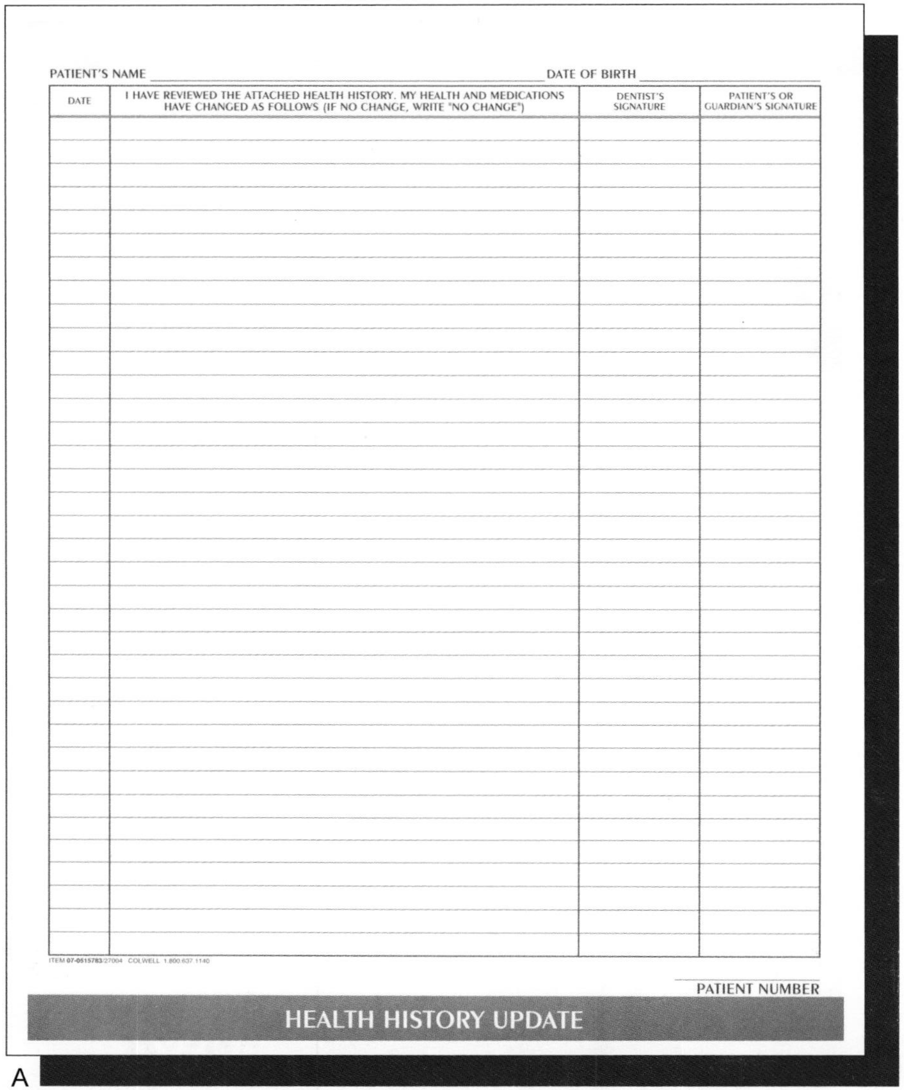
PATIENT'S NAME ______ DATE OF BIRTH ______

DATE	I HAVE REVIEWED THE ATTACHED HEALTH HISTORY. MY HEALTH AND MEDICATIONS HAVE CHANGED AS FOLLOWS (IF NO CHANGE, WRITE "NO CHANGE")	DENTIST'S SIGNATURE	PATIENT'S OR GUARDIAN'S SIGNATURE

PATIENT NUMBER

HEALTH HISTORY UPDATE

A

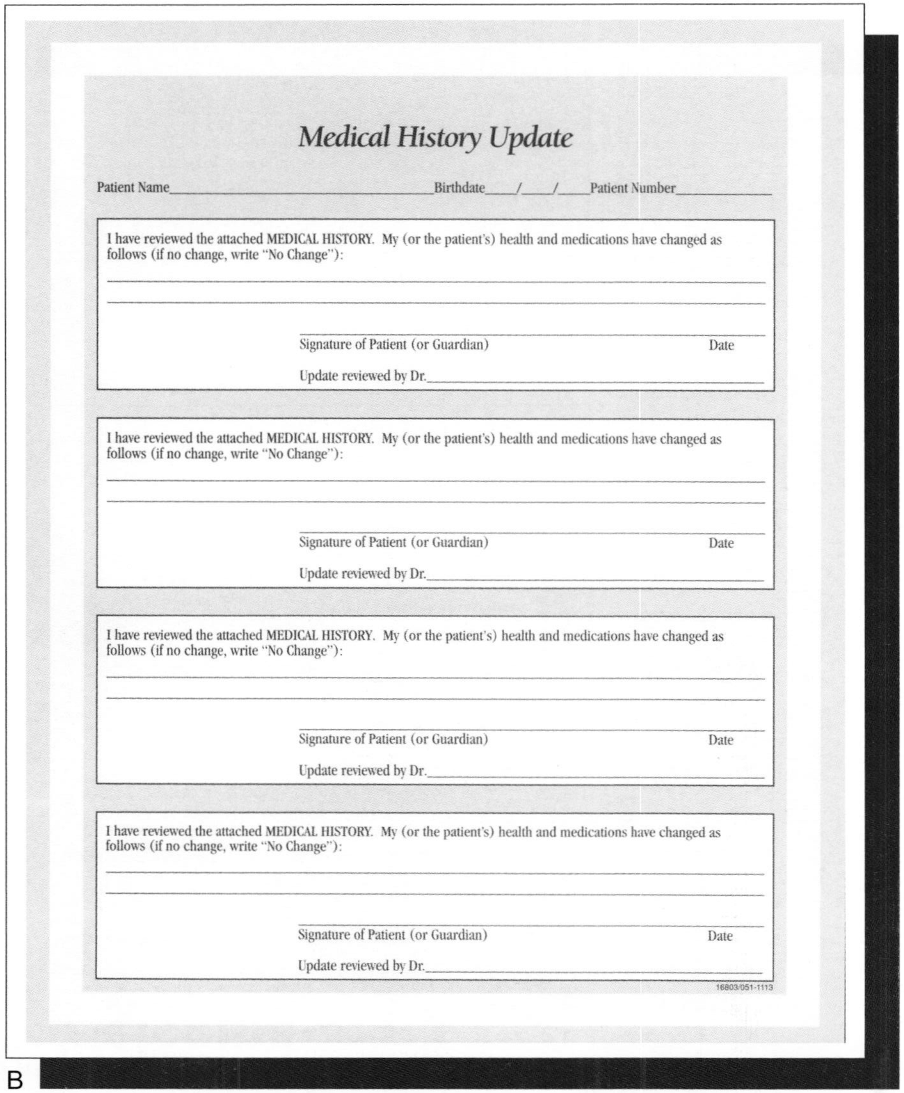
Medical History Update

Patient Name______ Birthdate___/___/___ Patient Number______

I have reviewed the attached MEDICAL HISTORY. My (or the patient's) health and medications have changed as follows (if no change, write "No Change"):

Signature of Patient (or Guardian) Date

Update reviewed by Dr.______

I have reviewed the attached MEDICAL HISTORY. My (or the patient's) health and medications have changed as follows (if no change, write "No Change"):

Signature of Patient (or Guardian) Date

Update reviewed by Dr.______

I have reviewed the attached MEDICAL HISTORY. My (or the patient's) health and medications have changed as follows (if no change, write "No Change"):

Signature of Patient (or Guardian) Date

Update reviewed by Dr.______

I have reviewed the attached MEDICAL HISTORY. My (or the patient's) health and medications have changed as follows (if no change, write "No Change"):

Signature of Patient (or Guardian) Date

Update reviewed by Dr.______

16803/051-1113

B

Figure 7-15 Common (**A**) and alternative (**B**) health history update forms. (Courtesy Patterson Office Supplies, Champaign, IL.)

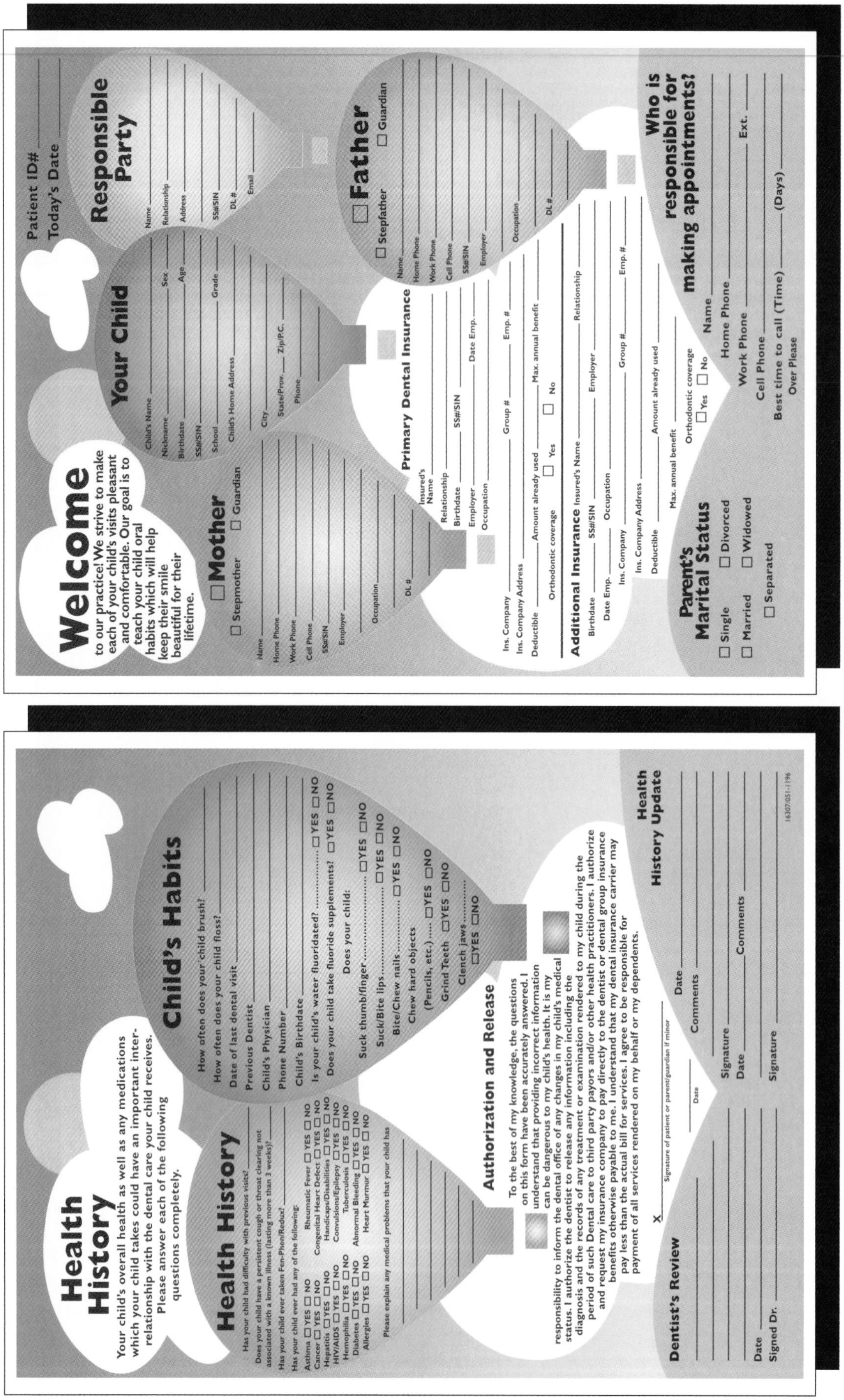
Patient ID#
Today's Date

Welcome
to our practice! We strive to make each of your child's visits pleasant and comfortable. Our goal is to teach your child oral habits which will help keep their smile beautiful for their lifetime.

Your Child
Child's Name
Nickname
Sex
Birthdate
Age
SS#/SIN
School
Grade
Child's Home Address
City
State/Prov.
Zip/P.C.
Phone

Responsible Party
Name
Relationship
Address
SS#/SIN
DL #
Email

☐ Mother
☐ Stepmother ☐ Guardian
Name
Home Phone
Work Phone
Cell Phone
SS#/SIN
Employer
Occupation
DL #

☐ Father
☐ Stepfather ☐ Guardian
Name
Home Phone
Work Phone
Cell Phone
SS#/SIN
Employer
Occupation
DL #

Primary Dental Insurance
Insured's Name
Relationship
Birthdate
SS#/SIN
Employer
Date Emp.
Occupation
Group #
Emp. #
Ins. Company
Ins. Company Address
Deductible
Amount already used
Max. annual benefit
Orthodontic coverage ☐ Yes ☐ No

Additional Insurance
Insured's Name
Relationship
Birthdate
SS#/SIN
Employer
Date Emp.
Occupation
Ins. Company
Group #
Emp. #
Ins. Company Address
Deductible
Amount already used
Max. annual benefit
Orthodontic coverage ☐ Yes ☐ No

Parent's Marital Status
☐ Single ☐ Divorced
☐ Married ☐ Widowed
☐ Separated

Who is responsible for making appointments?
Name
Home Phone
Work Phone
Ext.
Cell Phone
Best time to call (Time) (Days)
Over Please

Health History
Your child's overall health as well as any medications which your child takes could have an important interrelationship with the dental care your child receives. Please answer each of the following questions completely.

Health History
Has your child had difficulty with previous visits?
Does your child have a persistent cough or throat clearing not associated with a known illness (lasting more than 3 weeks)?
Has your child ever taken Fen-Phen/Redux?
Has your child ever had any of the following:
Asthma ☐ YES ☐ NO
Cancer ☐ YES ☐ NO
Hepatitis ☐ YES ☐ NO
HIV/AIDS ☐ YES ☐ NO
Hemophilia ☐ YES ☐ NO
Diabetes ☐ YES ☐ NO
Allergies ☐ YES ☐ NO
Rheumatic Fever ☐ YES ☐ NO
Congenital Heart Defect ☐ YES ☐ NO
Handicaps/Disabilities ☐ YES ☐ NO
Convulsions/Epilepsy ☐ YES ☐ NO
Tuberculosis ☐ YES ☐ NO
Abnormal Bleeding ☐ YES ☐ NO
Heart Murmur ☐ YES ☐ NO
Please explain any medical problems that your child has

Child's Habits
How often does your child brush?
How often does your child floss?
Date of last dental visit
Previous Dentist
Child's Physician
Phone Number
Child's Birthdate
Is your child's water fluoridated? ☐ YES ☐ NO
Does your child take fluoride supplements? ☐ YES ☐ NO
Does your child:
Suck thumb/finger ☐ YES ☐ NO
Suck/Bite lips ☐ YES ☐ NO
Bite/Chew nails ☐ YES ☐ NO
Chew hard objects (Pencils, etc.) ☐ YES ☐ NO
Grind Teeth ☐ YES ☐ NO
Clench jaws ☐ YES ☐ NO

Authorization and Release
To the best of my knowledge, the questions on this form have been accurately answered. I understand that providing incorrect information can be dangerous to my child's health. It is my responsibility to inform the dental office of any changes in my child's medical status. I authorize the dentist to release any information including the diagnosis and the records of any treatment or examination rendered to my child during the period of such Dental care to third party payors and/or other health practitioners. I authorize and request my insurance company to pay directly to the dentist or dental group insurance benefits otherwise payable to me. I understand that my dental insurance carrier may pay less than the actual bill for services. I agree to be responsible for payment of all services rendered on my behalf or my dependents.

X
Signature of patient or parent/guardian if minor
Date

Dentist's Review
Date
Signed Dr.

Health History Update
Date
Comments
Signature
Date
Comments
Signature

16307/051-1196

Figure 7-16 Alternative registration and health history form for children. (Courtesy Patterson Office Supplies, Champaign, IL.)

REGISTRATION SLIP

PLEASE PRINT   Date _____

Name _____

Address _____

City _____ Zip/P.C. _____

Telephone _____ Birth Date _____ Sex _____

Cell Phone _____ E-Mail _____

☐ Single   ☐ Married   ☐ Widowed   ☐ Divorced

Occupation _____ Phone _____

Employed by _____

Employer's address _____

Insurance Co. _____ Policy No. _____

Name of Spouse/Parent/Guardian _____

Occupation _____ Phone _____

Employed by _____

Employer's address _____

Referred by _____

Physician _____ SS#/SIN _____

HEALTH QUESTIONS: Yes   No

Is your general health good? .... ☐   ☐

Are you under a physician's care now? .... ☐   ☐

Have you ever had heart trouble, rheumatic fever,
  diabetes, infectious hepatitis, tuberculosis or AIDS? ..... ☐   ☐

Have you ever had trouble with bleeding after surgery? ... ☐   ☐

Have you ever had an unusual reaction to any
  drug or local anesthetic? .... ☐   ☐

Have you ever taken Fen-Phen/Redux? .... ☐   ☐

Do you have a persistent cough or throat clearing not
  associated with a known illness (lasting more
  than 3 weeks)? .... ☐   ☐

Is there any other information about your health
  which should be known? .... ☐   ☐

ITEM **07-0567008**/3370

Figure 7-17 Short-form registration and health history form. (Courtesy Patterson Office Supplies, Champaign, IL.)

available for each type of practice. The dentist may purchase a standard form or may design one specifically suited for the needs of the practice. Most supply companies offer a special service for dentists who want to design their own charts.

Most charts are 8½ × 11 inches, made of heavy paper stock, and printed on both sides. Many of these charts are die-punched to fit into a file folder. One side of the record contains a dental chart, a review of the patient's health history, and general patient information. The reverse side provides space for entering the treatment plan and recording services rendered. Some charts have space for entering the fee, but this should not become the patient's financial ledger card, and it need not include a record of payments and balances.

A review of Figures 7-18 to 7-20 will help familiarize the assistant with some of the different types of dental charts. Figures 7-18 and 7-19 show general practice charts that provide similar basic information. Figure 7-20 on p. 115 is a periodontal specialty chart. Figure 7-21 on p. 116 is a separate form that is added to the chart as a progress sheet for treatment entries.

Figure 7-22 on p. 116, 117 and 118 is a pediatric clinical chart that emphasizes clinical conditions unique to pediatric patients. A smaller form may be used as an oral surgery chart (see Figure 7-23 on p. 119). Re-examination charts (see Figure 7-24 on p. 120 and 121) may be used at the time of the periodic examination; these forms may be supplied individually or in pads of 50 or more. Many companies also provide self-adhesive anatomical labels to make charting and communication easier (see Figure 7-25 on p. 122).

Dental Diagnosis Estimate Form

This form includes the dentist's diagnosis and the treatment plan recommended for the patient (see Figure 7-26 on p. 123). In many cases the patient can select options in the treatment plan. After the consultation has been completed and treatment has been accepted by the patient, the form is signed by the person responsible for the account. Often a clause is included explaining that the fee quoted is an estimate and that unforeseen circumstances may affect the final fee for the service.

Consultation and Referral Report

In some cases, the dentist refers a patient to another dentist for examination, evaluation, and diagnosis. The form shown in Figure 7-27 on p. 124 includes information about the patient, the reason for the referral, and an anticipated treatment plan. This form is sent to the referring dentist with a copy to the patient. The consultant enters an evaluation and recommendation on the form and returns it to the dentist.

Medications History Form

As in a medical practice, medications are prescribed for a dental patient on a prescription form (see Figure 7-28, *A* on p. 125). Some states require specific formats for prescription forms and as of April 2009, a special form is required for Medicare patients. Having a history of a patient's medications helps prevent the prescription of drugs that could lead to unsafe interactions. The form in Figure 7-28, *B* is used to record a patient's medication history.

Prescription or Laboratory Requisitions form

Many states require that a prescription or laboratory requisition form (see Figure 7-29 on p. 126) accompany each case a dentist sends to a dental laboratory. This blueprint improves communication between the dentist and the laboratory technician and helps eliminate illegal dental practices, thereby protecting the patient.

Consent Form

A consent form (see Figure 7-30 on p. 127 and 128) is commonly used in dentistry as a preventive measure against malpractice suits. The form, which is signed by the patient or the parent or guardian of a pediatric patient, grants permission for administration of an anesthetic and other specified procedures. It is impossible to have a consent form for every phase of treatment, and it is unrealistic to believe that a general consent form covering every possible procedure would be upheld in court. Therefore a written summary of the treatment plan, as agreed upon by the patient and dentist, dated and signed by both parties, is a more acceptable format for such consent. Chapter 4 reviews the use of various types of consent forms in the dental office.

Refusal of Treatment

There may be a time in the dental practice when a patient refuses to have recommended treatment for a condition that presents potential risks. To ensure that litigation does not ensue, the dentist should have the patient sign a refusal of treatment form Figure 7-31 on p. 129 that includes the nature of the treatment, alternative treatment, treatment risks and risks if *no* treatment is rendered.

Letters

Copies of all written communications sent to or concerning a patient should become part of the patient's clinical record. The fact that these documents may become evidence in a malpractice suit warrants caution in writing and retaining them.

Postal Receipts

Radiographs or other records transferred to another dentist should be sent by certified mail with return receipt requested. The receipt verifies that the films were mailed and by whom the package was received.

Radiographic Films

The radiographic films stored in a patient's record should be labeled with the patient's full name, the date of exposure, the number and type of films, and the dentist's name. If radiographs are copied and transferred to another practitioner, the name and date of transfer should be noted on the clinical chart. In addition, a signed request from the patient and a letter of transmittal must be retained in the file envelope.

Patient Sign-in Sheets

The sign-in sheet is not a direct part of a patient's record but is often used for patients upon arrival in the office. In a busy
(Text continued on p. 115)

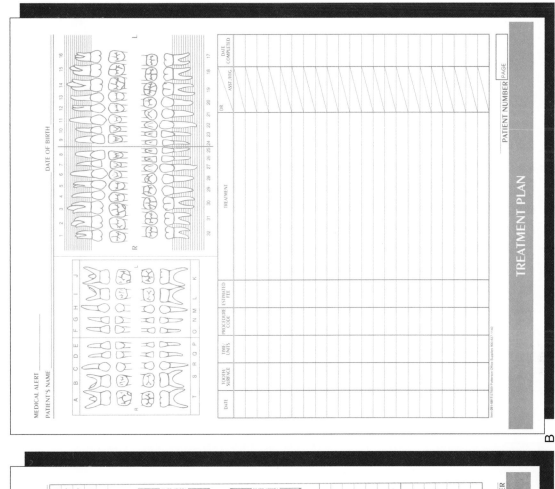

Figure 7-18 A, Adult clinical chart (general practice). **B,** Treatment plan that may accompany a clinical chart. (Courtesy Patterson Office Supplies, Champaign, IL.)

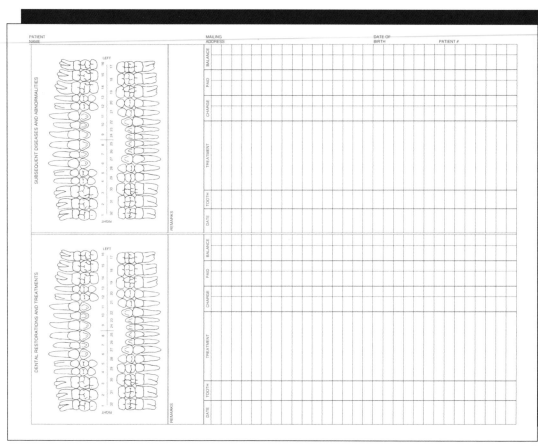

Figure 7-19 Alternative adult clinical chart (general practice) combining the clinical charting and treatment plan information. (Courtesy Patterson Office Supplies, Champaign, IL.)

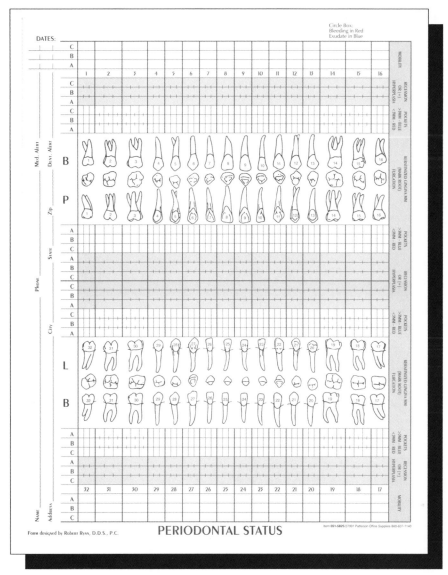

Figure 7-20 Periodontal specialty clinical chart, front. (Courtesy Patterson Office Supplies, Champaign, IL.)

office, the patient is asked to sign in on a sheet located on the receptionist's desk. Caution should be taken that this patient name is not available to the public. Tear-off labels such as shown in Figure 7-32 on p. 130 should be used, so that as soon as the patient has signed in, the label can be removed so that the name is not available for others to see. Crossing off the name on some forms often does not obliterate the name completely.

Entering Data on a Clinical Chart

Several types of data are entered in the various components of a patient's record, such as charting of existing conditions, which is done with a variety of symbols and codes; recording of treatment procedures on progress notes, written in clear, concise detail using codes; treatment plans; and discussions

with the patient about recommended treatment. Some clinical charts provide space for data entry on the back of the form. As entries are made and the form becomes complete, or as a separate form, many dentists opt to use a progress sheet to enter clinical data. All data entered in a patient's clinical chart or progress note should be dated, accurate and complete, and initialed by the treating dentist and assistant (see Figure 7-33 on p. 131). One of the major concerns in legal action is the incompleteness of data on a patient record. All action should be recorded in the clinical record. If a patient declines treatment, this notation should be entered on the record, dated, and signed. Failure to document any activity completely and accurately may prove costly in a lawsuit. Box 7-3 (see Figure 7-34 on p. 131) lists several rules for entering data, beginning with creation of the record.

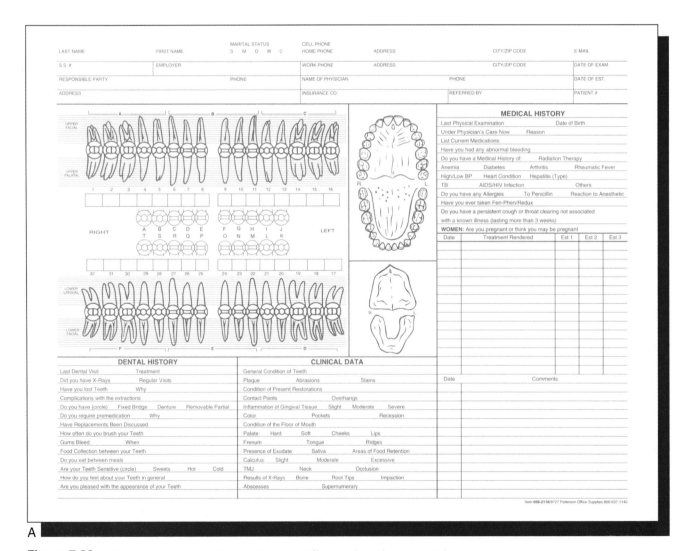

Figure 7-21 Progress sheet added to a clinical chart to record treatment data. (Courtesy Patterson Office Supplies, Champaign, IL.)

A

Figure 7-22 A, Pediatric chart, front. (Courtesy Patterson Office Supplies, Champaign, IL.)

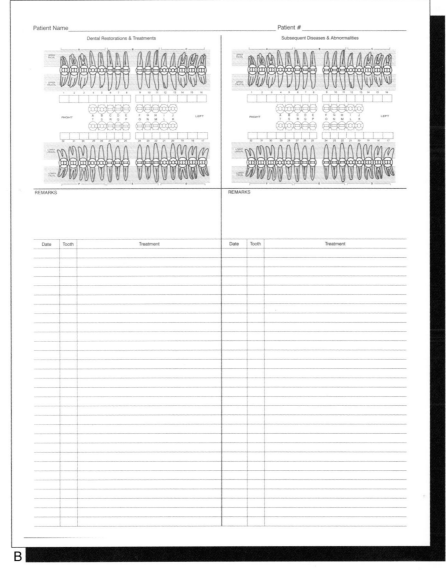

Figure 7-22, cont'd **B,** Pediatric chart, back. (Courtesy Patterson Office Supplies, Champaign, IL.)

(Continued)

Types of Clinical Data Entries

Entering information on the patient's clinical chart or progress notes involves the use of tooth numbering systems and an assortment of abbreviations and symbols. The administrative assistant must understand each of these systems, as well as the basic descriptions of the oral cavity. For example, there are two arches, the maxilla, or maxillary arch (upper jaw), and the mandible, or mandibular arch (lower jaw). There are four quadrants, maxillary right and left and mandibular right and left. There are six segments: the maxillary and mandibular right and left segments, which include the molars and premolars, and the two anterior segments, which include all anterior teeth on the right and left in both arches from canine to canine.

 PRACTICE NOTE
Failure to document any activity completely and accurately may prove costly in a lawsuit.

Tooth Nomenclature

To begin with, the administrative assistant should be able to identify the names and numbers of teeth in both the primary and permanent dentition (see Box 7-4 on p. 132). Mixed dentition (a combination of primary and permanent teeth) usually exists from approximately 6 to 12 years of age. Mixed dentition occurs when the permanent teeth begin to erupt while some of the primary teeth are still present. This is a common condition in a child of about 7 years of age. For example, the child may have lost the primary central incisors, and the first permanent molars may have erupted. Mixed dentition occasionally occurs in an adult when a primary tooth is retained and is not replaced by a permanent tooth.

Teeth present a good appearance and provide support for other structures. They also aid in swallowing, mastication, digestion, and the production of speech and phonetics. The primary dentition creates the framework for eruption of a healthy permanent dentition. Premature loss of the primary teeth can be directly related to future dental disease or other dental anomalies. Likewise the loss of a single permanent tooth, if not replaced, can be the start of serious dental impairment. The administrative assistant plays an important role in patient education and must take advantage of seminars promoting dental health, gaining knowledge that will make the assistant an ambassador for maintaining teeth for a lifetime.

It is important to understand the correct identification of a tooth in the oral cavity and the sequence of terms used to identify it. Confusion in the order of identification can cause many communication problems. The correct sequence of identification is: the dentition, the arch, the quadrant, and the specific tooth (see Box 7-5 on p. 132).

For example, in describing a patient's complaint, define the problem tooth as the permanent maxillary right first molar. This sequence of identification is commonly used in dental offices.

Tooth Numbering Systems

Every dental office has a specific numbering system that is used in charting a patient's oral cavity or referring to dental treatment to be performed. There are several numbering systems, and the dentist and staff choose which will be used in the office. The objective of a numbering system is to name and code each tooth

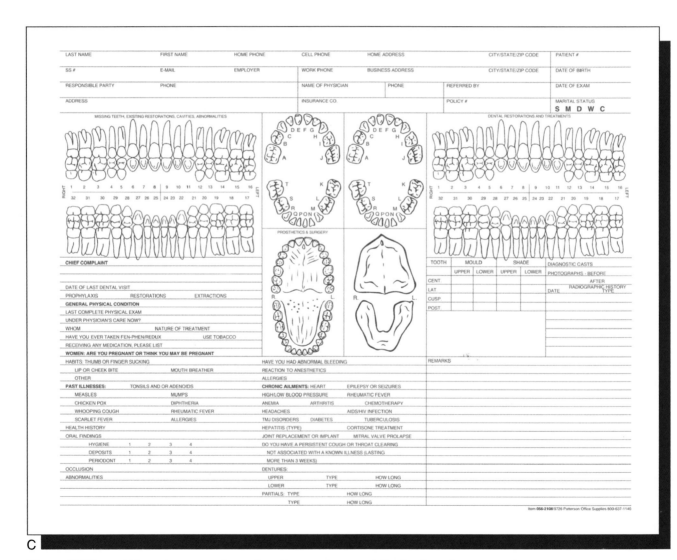

Figure 7-22, cont'd C, Alternative pediatric chart. (Courtesy Patterson Office Supplies, Champaign, IL.)

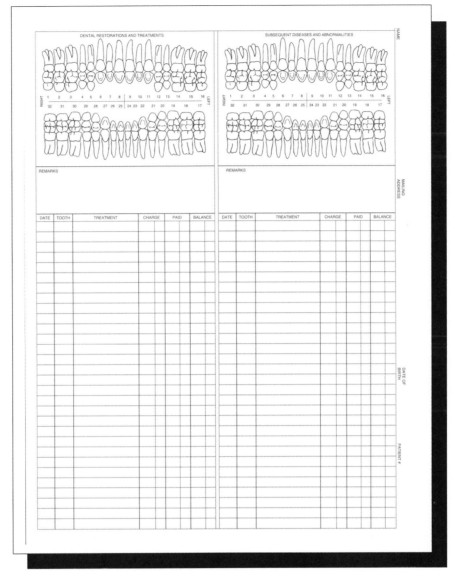

Figure 7-22, cont'd **C,** Alternative pediatric chart. (Courtesy Patterson Office Supplies, Champaign, IL.)

numerically or alphabetically. This number or letter provides an abbreviated form of tooth reference and aids in consistency in records management. The three most common numbering systems are the **universal numbering system**, the **Palmer notation system**, and the **Federal Dentaire International (FDI) system**.

Universal Numbering System. The most popular numbering system is the universal numbering system. It uses the Arabic numerals from 1 to 32 for the permanent dentition and the letters *A* to *T* for the primary dentition.

The universal system begins numbering the teeth with the most posterior tooth on the patient's maxillary right quadrant, the third molar (i.e., tooth #1), or the permanent maxillary right third molar. If the numbering is for the primary dentition, the tooth is labeled in an alpha code beginning with *A* for the primary maxillary right second molar. The numbering continues toward the anterior midline to the central incisor, or tooth #8 of the permanent dentition (tooth #*E* of the primary dentition). The numbering continues to the maxillary

left quadrant, from the midline to the most posterior tooth, either #16 of the permanent dentition or #*J* of the primary dentition. The numbering then drops to the mandibular left quadrant to permanent tooth #17 (primary tooth #*K*) across the arch to the mandibular right most posterior tooth, #32 (or #*T*) (see Figure 7-35 on p. 132).

Palmer Notation System. The Palmer notation system assigns each of the four quadrants a bracket to designate the area of the mouth where the tooth is found. In Figure 7-36, *A* on p. 133, the left side of the chart represents the patient's right side, and the right side of the chart represents the patient's left side. It might be depicted as follows:

Maxillary right	Maxillary left
Mandibular right	Mandibular left

PRE-OP EVALUATION

PATIENT NAME: DATE:

CHIEF COMPLAINT

PAST MEDICAL HISTORY

Current meds:

Previous general anesthetic:

Family history:

Allergic to:

Sensitive to:

TREATMENT TODAY

DIAGNOSIS

☐ Impacted teeth #'s: _____

☐ Infected teeth #'s: _____

☐ Nonfunctional teeth #'s: _____

☐ Other:

TREATMENT PLAN

☐ Extract teeth #'s: _____

☐ Expose crown #: _____

☐ Other:

X-RAY FINDINGS

☐ panorex   ☐ periapical   ☐ occlusal

CLINICAL FINDINGS

SURGICAL RISKS DISCUSSED

☐ Inferior alveolar/lingual nerve paresthesia

☐ Sinus perforation

☐ Possible damage to adjacent crown or large restoration

☐ Possible incomplete bone fill or exposed cementum

☐ Other:

ANESTHESIA PLAN

☐ Local Anesthesia

☐ Nitrous Oxide/Oxygen

☐ I.V. Sedation

RETURN VISIT

Figure 7-23 Chart that might be used in an oral surgery office. (Courtesy Patterson Office Supplies, Champaign, IL.)

Each permanent tooth in any quadrant is assigned the same number with #1 beginning at the midline and increasing to #8 distally. For instance:

Maxillary right central incisor 1
Maxillary left central incisor 1
Mandibular left central incisor 1
Mandibular right central incisor 1

The direction of the bracket determines the arch, and the number within the bracket determines the tooth, as follows:

Maxillary right third molar 8
Maxillary left second molar 7
Mandibular right first premolar 4
Mandibular left lateral incisor 2

For the primary dentition, brackets are used to assign a quadrant, but the teeth are designated by the letters *A* to *E*. *A* specifies the central incisors, and *E* specifies the second molars (see Figure 7-36, *B* on p. 133).

Federal Dentaire International System. The Federal Dentaire International (FDI) system (see Figure 7-37 on p. 134) assigns a two-digit number to each tooth in any quadrant. The first number indicates the quadrant in which the tooth is positioned, and the second number identifies the specific tooth. The numbers 1 to 4 are assigned to the permanent dentition, and 5 to 8 are assigned to the quadrants of the primary dentition. Therefore, the first number would be designated as follows:

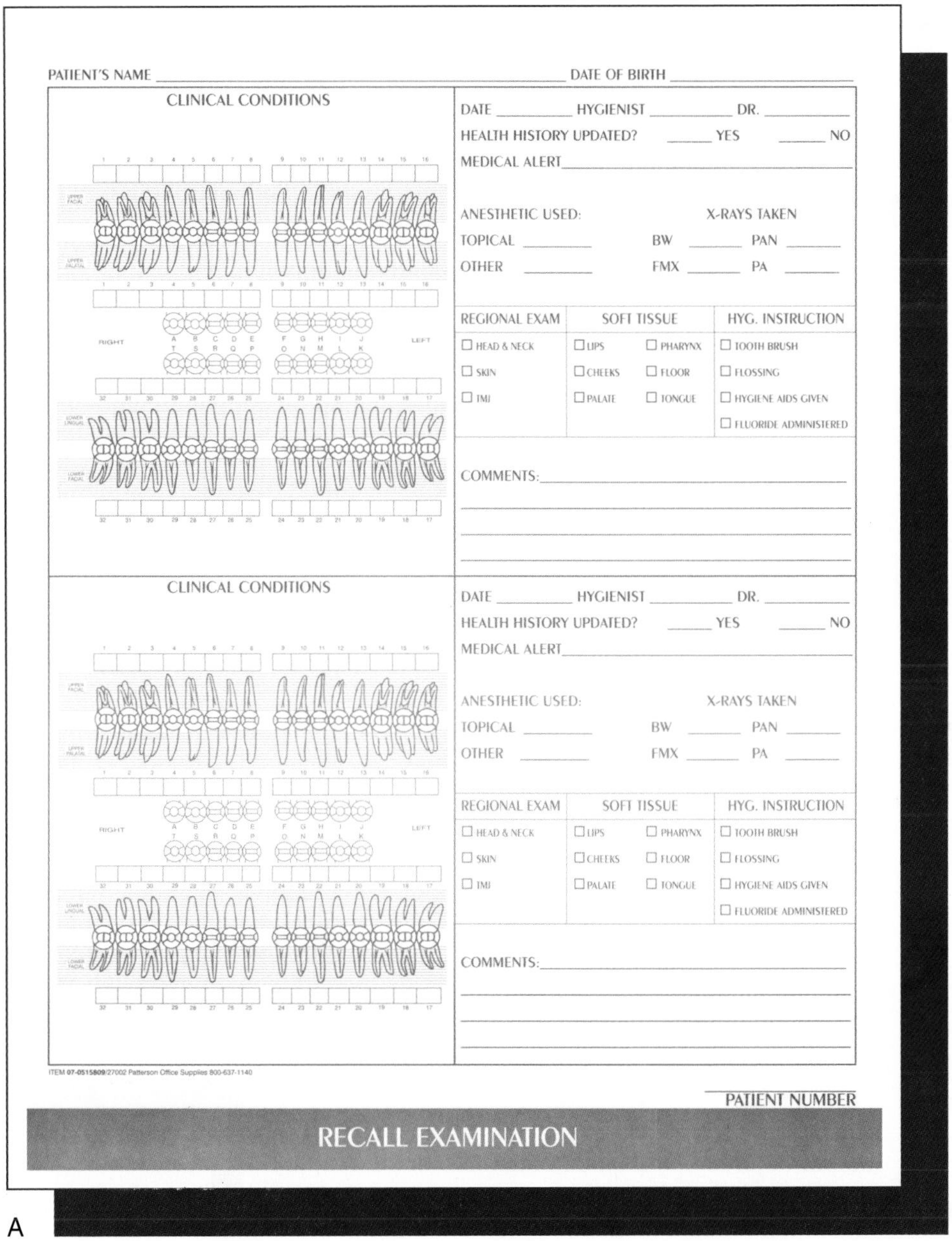

Figure 7-24 A, Recall examination form. (Courtesy Patterson Office Supplies, Champaign, IL.)

(Continued)

Number	Quadrant
1	Permanent maxillary right
2	Permanent maxillary left
3	Permanent mandibular left
4	Permanent mandibular right
5	Primary maxillary right
6	Primary maxillary left
7	Primary mandibular left
8	Primary mandibular right

The second number identifies the specific tooth in the arch. The numbers 1 to 8 are assigned to the permanent dentition and 1 to 5 to the primary dentition. The #1 in both instances begins with the central incisors, and the numbering of the teeth proceeds posteriorly so that the last tooth in the quadrant is the highest number in the sequence. Some examples are as follows:

Permanent maxillary right central incisor: #11 (which is read, "number one one")

Permanent maxillary left central incisor: #21 (number two one)

Permanent mandibular left central incisor: #31 (number three one)

Permanent mandibular right central incisor: #41 (number four one)

The primary dentition is handled in the same manner, but because there are only five teeth per quadrant, the numbers would range from 1 to 5 for each tooth and 5 to 8 for the quadrants. Therefore the primary maxillary right first molar is #54 (number five four) and the primary mandibular left lateral incisor is #72 (number seven two).

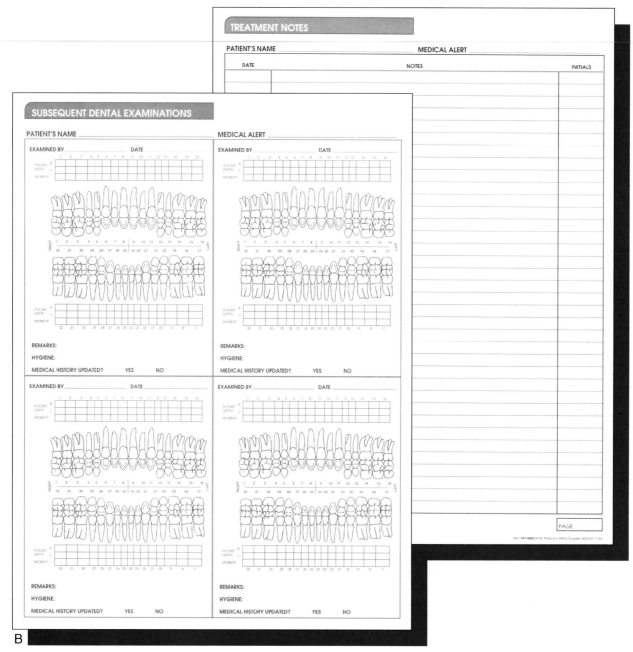

Figure 7-24, cont'd **B,** Alternative re-examination record. (Courtesy Patterson Office Supplies, Champaign, IL.)

Tooth Surfaces

During routine charting procedures, the chairside assistant uses various alpha codes for tooth surface annotation. Using tooth nomenclature and surface annotation makes it easy to identify a specific location on a tooth in which there may be dental decay, a fracture, or a restoration. The administrative assistant must be familiar with this terminology to complete insurance forms and to consult with other dentists about patient treatment.

All crowns of the teeth are divided into surfaces, which are identified by their position in relation to the oral cavity. For example, the surfaces nearest the lips are referred to as the labial, or facial, surfaces. The posterior teeth (the premolars and molars) have five surfaces. The anterior teeth (the incisors and canines) have four surfaces with a ridge. Both anterior and posterior teeth have four axial surfaces. The **axial surface** runs vertically from the biting surface to the apex of a tooth. The posterior teeth have one additional surface, the **occlusal surface**, which is the horizontal surface that runs perpendicular to the other axial surfaces.

The surfaces of the teeth not only have names but are also identified by letters or numbers. This surface annotation is used to simplify charting notations and for all insurance reports.

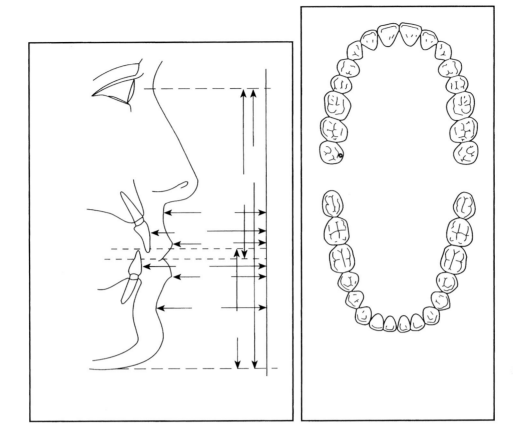

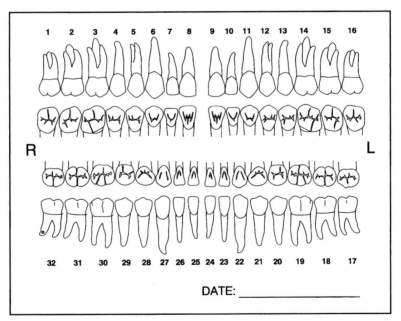

Figure 7-25 Examples of custom self-adhesive anatomical labels can be used to make special notations on a clinical chart. (Courtesy Patterson Office Supplies, Champaign, IL.)

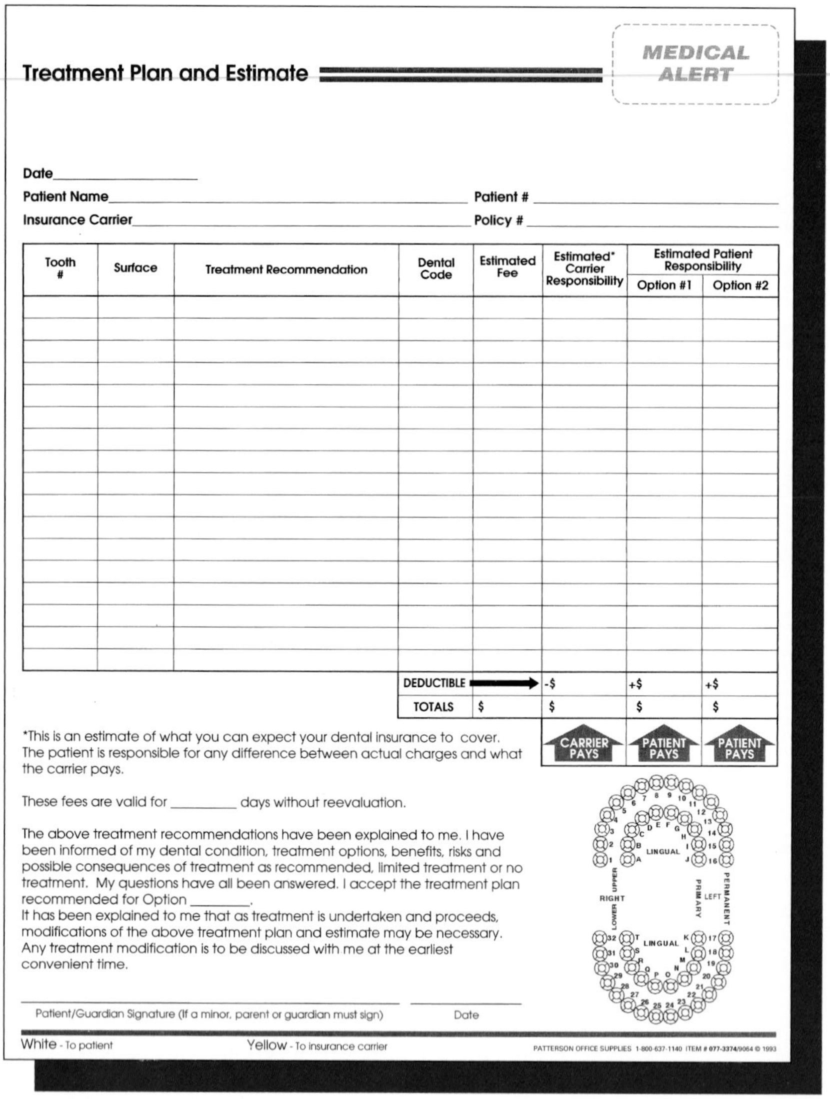

Treatment Plan and Estimate

MEDICAL ALERT

Date________________

Patient Name________________ Patient # ________________

Insurance Carrier________________ Policy # ________________

Tooth #	Surface	Treatment Recommendation	Dental Code	Estimated Fee	Estimated* Carrier Responsibility	Estimated Patient Responsibility	
						Option #1	Option #2
			DEDUCTIBLE	→	-$	+$	+$
			TOTALS	$	$	$	$
					CARRIER PAYS	PATIENT PAYS	PATIENT PAYS

*This is an estimate of what you can expect your dental insurance to cover. The patient is responsible for any difference between actual charges and what the carrier pays.

These fees are valid for ________ days without reevaluation.

The above treatment recommendations have been explained to me. I have been informed of my dental condition, treatment options, benefits, risks and possible consequences of treatment as recommended, limited treatment or no treatment. My questions have all been answered. I accept the treatment plan recommended for Option ________.
It has been explained to me that as treatment is undertaken and proceeds, modifications of the above treatment plan and estimate may be necessary. Any treatment modification is to be discussed with me at the earliest convenient time.

Patient/Guardian Signature (If a minor, parent or guardian must sign) Date

White - To patient Yellow - To insurance carrier PATTERSON OFFICE SUPPLIES 1-800-637-1140 ITEM # 077-3374/9064 © 1993

Figure 7-26 Dental treatment plan and estimate form. (Courtesy Patterson Office Supplies, Champaign, IL.)

The letter or number is commonly placed as a superscript (above the print line) next to the tooth number. For example, using the Universal numbering system to describe a procedure involving the mesial surface of the permanent maxillary left first molar, the assistant would write: $\#14^{M}$ or $\#14^{1}$. The surfaces of the teeth are as follows (see Figure 7-38 on p. 134):

- The *mesial surface* (M or 1) is the axial surface closest to the midline of the mouth.
- The *distal surface* (D or 2) lies directly opposite the mesial surface and is the axial surface farthest from the midline.
- The *facial surface* (F or 3) faces the cheek and lips, or the exterior of the mouth.
- The *labial surface* (LA or 3) is the same as the facial surface but is found facing only the lips on the anterior teeth. This letter combination is not used frequently because it requires an extra space in data entry; the designation *facial* (F) is used more often.
- The *buccal surface* (B or 3) is the same as the facial surface but is found on posterior teeth only, facing the cheeks.
- The *lingual surface* (L or 4) is the surface closest to the tongue.
- The *occlusal surface* (O or 5) is found only on posterior teeth on a vertical plane, or the biting surface of the teeth.
- The *incisal ridge* (or *edge* or *surface*) (I or 5) is found only on anterior teeth that have a biting edge.
- The *proximal* areas or surfaces are the areas or surfaces where two teeth abut or face each other. Most teeth have two proximal surfaces, the mesial and the distal proximal surfaces. In the third molars, however, only the mesial surface may be considered a proximal surface.

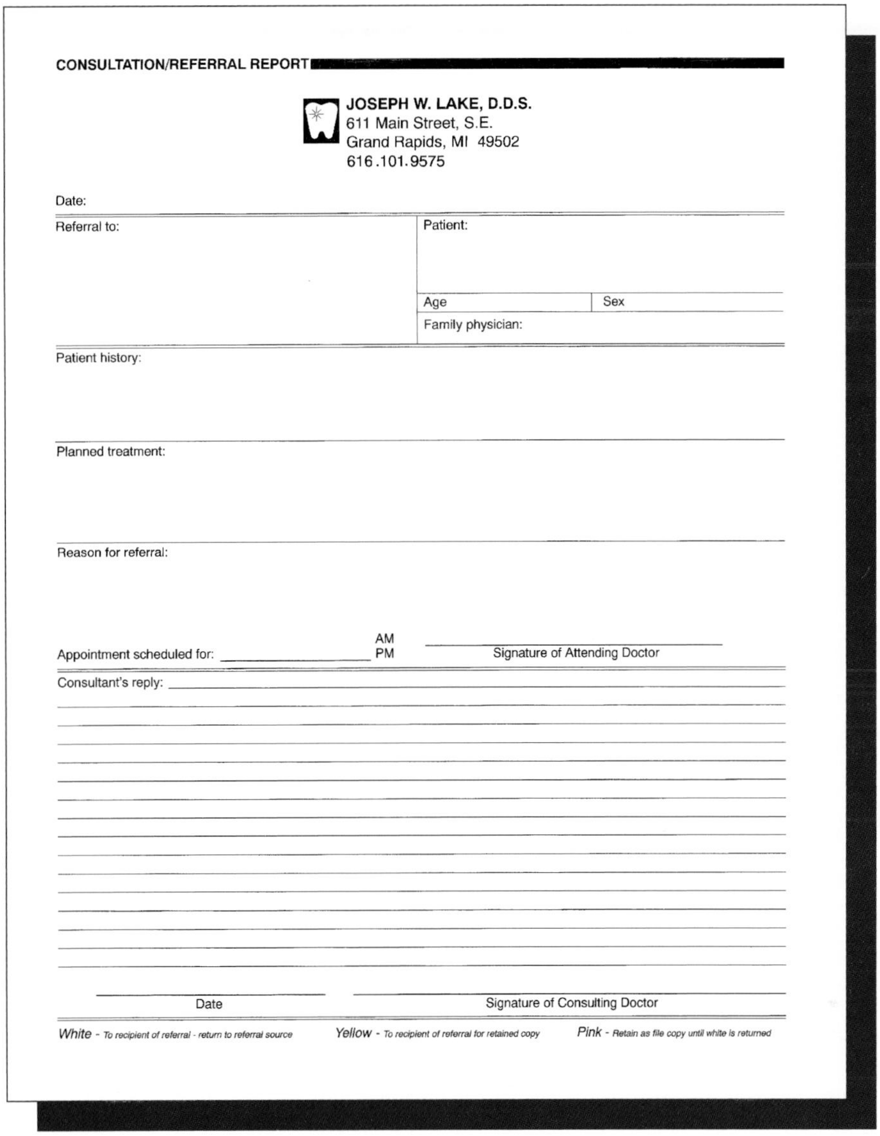

CONSULTATION/REFERRAL REPORT

JOSEPH W. LAKE, D.D.S.
611 Main Street, S.E.
Grand Rapids, MI 49502
616.101.9575

Date:

Referral to:

Patient:

Age | Sex

Family physician:

Patient history:

Planned treatment:

Reason for referral:

Appointment scheduled for: ______ AM PM ______ Signature of Attending Doctor

Consultant's reply:

Date ______ Signature of Consulting Doctor

White - To recipient of referral - return to referral source Yellow - To recipient of referral for retained copy Pink - Retain as file copy until white is returned

Figure 7-27 Examples of custom consultation and referral report form. (Courtesy Patterson Office Supplies, Champaign, IL.)

When more than one surface is involved (e.g., mesial, occlusal, and distal), the surface annotations are placed in order from mesial to distal: for example, $\#19^{MOD}$ instead of $\#19^{DOM}$ or $\#19^{ODM}$. This standardization provides for uniform communication between dental professionals.

Charting Symbols and Abbreviations

Charting symbols are a form of shorthand in the dental office. They allow the clinical assistant to quickly outline a condition on a graphic chart. The dentist later can use this information for the diagnosis, or the administrative assistant can quickly identify conditions in the patient's mouth without reading through a lengthy description. Figure 7-39 on p. 135 presents a variety of symbols commonly used in a dental office. **Clinical abbreviations** are short versions of or initials for common clinical terminology. Table 7-1 on p. 136 and 137 is a detailed list of abbreviations commonly used for data entry on dental records.

Records Retention

The question often is asked, "How long should a patient's records be retained?" The answer seems awkward: The record should be retained for the period of time consistent with the statute

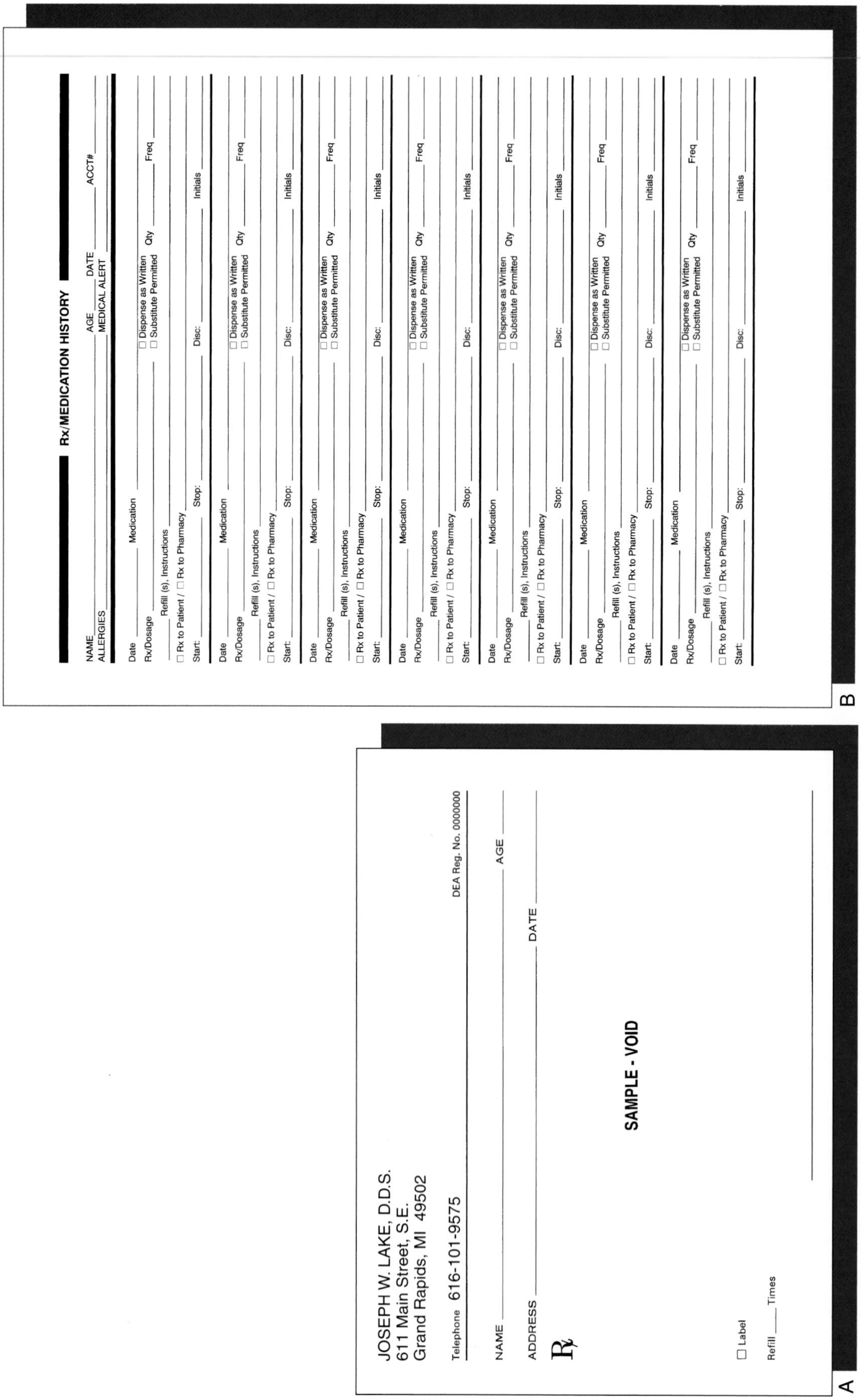

Figure 7-28 A, Prescription form. **B,** Custom medication history form. (Courtesy Patterson Office Supplies, Champaign, IL.)

WARD | a dti company

1068 Charles H. Orndorf Drive • Brighton, MI • 48116 • P 810 534 9273 • F 810 534 9278

Crown and Bridge Rx

RX DATE _____

CASE # _____

| DATE WANTED | TIME |

DOCTOR INFORMATION
Name _____
Address _____
_____
Telephone _____

PATIENT INFORMATION
Name _____
Sex _____ Age _____
○ Diagnostic wax up ○ Pearltemps™ (provisionals)
○ Call me (before proceeding with case)

Rx _____
_____
_____
_____
_____
_____
_____
_____
_____
_____
_____
_____

HAVE YOU INCLUDED THE FOLLOWING?
○ Impression
○ Bite
○ Opposing
○ Shade
○ Pre-op model
○ Photos
○ Model of temps
○ Bite stick
○ Face bow

PLEASE SEND
○ Prescription forms
○ Plastic bags
○ Case boxes

RETURN FOR
○ Die Trim
○ Metal try-in
○ Finish
○ Evaluation
○ Wax check
○ Bisque bake try-in

IF INSUFFICIENT ROOM
○ Reduce and mark
○ Metal occlusion
○ Reduction coping
○ Please call

IF CASE WILL NOT DRAW
○ Make reduction copings
○ Please call

○ Surgical Stent

SHADE _____ STUMP _____

AMOUNT OF TRANSLUCENCY
○ Light ○ Medium ○ Heavy

VALUE
○ Bright ○ Medium ○ Low

MIDLINE SHIFT
R _____ MM L _____ MM
_____ MM
Length of centrals from cervical margin
○ Close Diastema

CIRCLE TEETH NUMBERS
1 2 3 4 5 6 7 8 9 10 11 12 13 14 15 16
32 31 30 29 28 27 26 25 24 23 22 21 20 19 18 17

METAL
○ High noble ○ Noble

OCCLUSION
○ Metal ○ Porcelain

LATERAL EXCURSION
○ Cuspid guidance ○ Group function

LABIAL MARGIN
○ Fine metal collar on tooth # _____ ○ Show no metal standard on # _____
○ Show no metal 360° on tooth # _____ ○ Porcelain Butt Margin on tooth # _____

CONTACTS
○ Broad ○ Normal ○ Point

OCCLUSAL CLEARANCE
○ Positive Contact ○ Cusp Fossa ○ Out of Occlusion ○ Foil Relief

OCCLUSAL STAINING
○ None
○ Light
○ Medium
○ Dark
○ Hypo-calcification
○ Shade tab enclosed

MOLD OF CROWN DESIRED
○ Follow study model
○ Match existing
○ Make ideal

SURFACE ANATOMY
○ Smooth
○ Textured
○ Mamelon development
○ Match existing

PONTIC DESIGN
Harmony Ovate Ridge Lap
Cone Hygienic

PONTIC TISSUE RELIEF
○ Yes mm deep _____ ○ No _____

Doctor's Signature _____ License # _____

White - Lab Copy Yellow - Lab Copy Blue - Doctor's Copy

Figure 7-29 A, Example of a laboratory prescription/requisition form for a crown and bridge. (Courtesy Ward Dental Laboratory, Brighton, MI.)

(Continued)

of limitations within the state. The **statute of limitations,** the period within which a civil suit for alleged wrongdoing may be legally filed, varies from state to state. The average minimum for retention of a patient's records is approximately 6 years after performance of the last treatment, but it is better to retain the records longer than that. Chapter 8 offers suggestions for longer-term storage.

Records Transfer

Requests for transfer of records are made for many reasons such as: (1) the patient wants to change dentists; (2) the patient is moving out of the area; (3) the dentist wants to consult with another dentist; and (4) the patient has been referred to another dentist.

Care must be taken in completing a request for transfer of a patient's records. By law, any information regarding a patient's care and treatment is confidential and privileged. This privilege belongs to the patient, not to the dentist. Therefore, for the dentist's protection, it is prudent to obtain a written consent signed by the patient or the patient's legal representative before transferring records to anyone other than the patient. Certain exceptions exist to this privilege prohibiting disclosure, such as legal action or court orders involving the dentist. In general if the following suggestions are followed, record transfer can be handled efficiently and confidentially.

PRACTICE NOTE
By law, any information regarding a patient's care and treatment is confidential and privileged.

Figure 7-29 cont'd B, Laboratory prescription form with provisions for dentures, crowns, and bridges. (Courtesy Patterson Office Supplies, Champaign, IL.)

- Provide accurate and complete dental records.
- Never change dental records without maintaining the readability of the original entry; date any changes, and record the reason for the change.
- Obtain a signed consent form from the patient or the advice of legal counsel before providing copies of or allowing access to a patient's dental records to anyone other than the patient.
- Retain records in accordance with the state statute.
- Keep original records.
- Charge a reasonable clerical fee for furnishing records in accordance with local standards.
- Charge a reasonable professional fee for preparing and furnishing a narrative report for the patient.
- Require advance payment for clerical and preparation service in accordance with local standards.
- If records are mailed, send them certified mail with return receipt requested. The receipt will verify that the materials were received.

Records Maintenance

Financial records are as important as clinical records but must be maintained separately. A financial record protects the patient and the dentist, provides information for tax purposes, and verifies data for a business analysis. Inadequate or incomplete financial records can result in poor public relations and can create unnecessary legal problems with state and federal governments and third-party payers. Chapter 15 details the step-by-step procedure for creating and managing various financial records. At this point, suffice it to say that financial records differ from clinical records in that a ledger card can be used for a family unit or

PATIENT'S NAME: ____________________ DATE: __________

TIME: __________ (A.M.) (P.M.)

I HEREBY AUTHORIZE DR. ____________________ AND HIS/HER ASSOCIATES AT ____________________ TO PERFORM UPON ME OR THE NAMED PATIENT THE FOLLOWING PROCEDURE(S): ____________________ (EXPLAIN IN PLAIN ENGLISH).

DR. ______________ HAS FULLY EXPLAINED TO ME THE PURPOSE OF THE PROCEDURE(S) AND HAS ALSO INFORMED ME OF EXPECTED BENEFITS AND COMPLICATIONS (FROM KNOWN AND UNKNOWN CAUSES), ATTENDANT DISCOMFORTS AND RISKS THAT MAY ARISE, AS WELL AS POSSIBLE ALTERNATIVES TO THE PROPOSED TREATMENT, INCLUDING NO TREATMENT. THE ATTENDANT RISKS OF NO TREATMENT HAVE ALSO BEEN DISCUSSED. I HAVE BEEN GIVEN AN OPPORTUNITY TO ASK QUESTIONS, AND ALL MY QUESTIONS HAVE BEEN ANSWERED FULLY AND SATISFACTORILY. I ACKNOWLEDGE THAT NO GUARANTEES OR ASSURANCES HAVE BEEN MADE TO ME CONCERNING THE RESULTS INTENDED FROM THE PROCEDURE(S).

I UNDERSTAND THAT DURING THE COURSE OF THE PROCEDURE(S), UNFORESEEN CONDITIONS MAY ARISE WHICH NECESSITATE PROCEDURES DIFFERENT FROM THOSE CONTEMPLATED. I, THEREFORE, CONSENT TO THE PERFORMANCE OF ADDITIONAL PROCEDURE(S) WHICH THE ABOVE-NAMED DENTIST OR HIS/HER ASSOCIATES MAY CONSIDER NECESSARY.

I ALSO UNDERSTAND THE FINANCIAL OBLIGATION ATTACHED TO THIS PROCEDURE AND AGREE TO COMPLY AS LISTED BELOW: AMOUNT DUE __________ TO BE PAID IN __________ MONTHLY PAYMENTS OF $__________ STARTING __________. BALANCE TO BE PAID IN FULL BY __________.

I UNDERSTAND THAT I AM RESPONSIBLE FOR ALL FEES REGARDLESS OF INSURANCE COVERAGE. I ALSO UNDERSTAND THAT AS TREATMENT PROGRESSES THE ABOVE FEES MAY HAVE TO BE ADJUSTED, BUT THAT I WILL BE INFORMED OF THESE ADJUSTMENTS AND HOW THEY WILL AFFECT MY PAYMENT PLAN. IN THE EVENT THAT MY PAYMENTS ARE NOT RECEIVED WITHIN 30 DAYS OF THEIR DUE DATE, I AGREE TO PAY ALL COSTS OF COLLECTIONS, INCLUDING, BUT NOT LIMITED TO, REASONABLE ATTORNEY'S FEES.

I CONFIRM THAT I HAVE READ AND FULLY UNDERSTAND THE ABOVE AND THAT ALL BLANK SPACES HAVE BEEN COMPLETED PRIOR TO MY SIGNING.

I HEREBY CONSENT TO THE PROPOSED DENTAL TREATMENT.

SIGNATURE OF PATIENT OR PARENT/GUARDIAN IF MINOR — DATE

INTERPRETER (IF USED) — DATE

SIGNATURE OF WITNESS — DATE

DENTIST CERTIFICATION:

I HEREBY CERTIFY THAT I HAVE EXPLAINED THE NATURE, PURPOSE, BENEFITS, RISKS OF, AND ALTERNATIVES (INCLUDING NO TREATMENT AND ATTENDANT RISKS), TO THE PROPOSED PROCEDURE(S). I HAVE OFFERED ANSWERS TO ANY QUESTIONS AND HAVE FULLY ANSWERED ALL SUCH QUESTIONS. I BELIEVE THAT THE PATIENT/PARENT/GUARDIAN FULLY UNDERSTANDS WHAT I HAVE EXPLAINED AND ANSWERED.

DENTIST'S SIGNATURE ____________________

PRINT NAME ____________________ DATE __________

Item 051-5742/27005 Patterson Office Supplies 800-637-1140

PATIENT NUMBER

CONSENT TO DENTAL TREATMENT

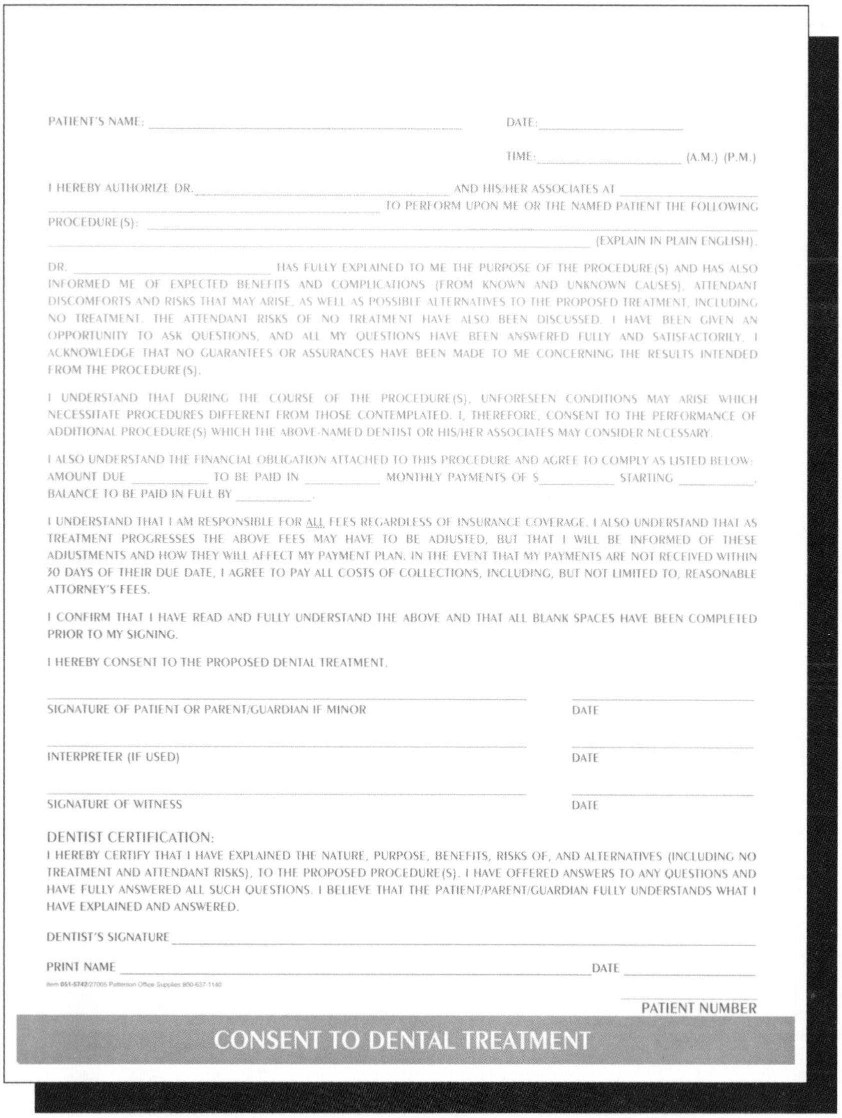

Figure 7-30 Consent form. (Courtesy Patterson Office Supplies, Champaign, IL.)

a responsible party, whereas clinical records are created for each individual. Therefore if one person is responsible for payment for several dependents, all entries can be made on one ledger card.

Occupational Safety and Health Administration Records

Chapter 17 details the responsibility of the administrative assistant in disease prevention. Specific records must be maintained for OSHA. The *Regulatory Compliance Manual* (see Figure 17-2, *B*), developed by the American Dental Association, is an important source of samples and suggestions for developing the documents required by federal regulations.

Several employee records must be maintained in the office. These must be accurate and must be maintained with strict confidentiality. The administrative assistant is responsible for periodically updating these records. Many of the records relate to payroll, and these are discussed in Chapter 16.

Employee records are classified into various categories, such as:

Employment Forms
- Applications for employment (see Chapter 18)
- Employment agreements (see Chapter 18)
- Merit evaluation forms (see Chapter 18)
- Health forms and medical records (see Figure 7-40 on p. 138)
- Federal Employment Eligibility Verification forms (Form I-9; see Figure 2-8)

Employment Tax Information Forms (see Chapter 16)
- Employer identification number
- Amounts and dates of all wage, annuity, and pension payments
- Names, addresses, Social Security numbers, and documents of employees and recipients

REFUSAL OF PERIODONTAL TREATMENT

I have been advised and understand on this date that I have periodontal disease that may cause gum and bone inflammation or loss, and that it can lead to loss of my teeth. The severity of my condition today is slight/moderate/advanced. I have been informed that I have pocket depths as follows:

Depth	Tooth Number(s)
3-5 mm	_____
6-7 mm	_____
8+ mm	_____

Various treatment options for this condition have been explained to me, including gum surgery, replacement, extraction, as well as my right to refuse treatment. I have had the opportunity to read this form and ask questions, and my questions have been answered to my satisfaction. I am electing to refuse treatment and agree to release and hold harmless this office and the undersigned dentist from any liability for any adverse effects of my decision.

Signature of Patient/
Parent or Guardian _____

Print Name _____ Date _____

Interpreter (if used) Signature _____

Print Name _____ Date _____

Witness Signature _____

Print Name _____ Date _____

Dentist Certification:

I hereby certify that I have explained the nature, purpose, benefits, risks of, and alternatives (including no treatment and attendant risks), to the proposed procedures. I have offered answers to any questions and have fully answered all such questions. I believe that the patient/parent/guardian fully understands what I have explained and answered.

Dentist's Signature _____

Print Name _____ Date _____

REFUSAL OF PERIODONTAL TREATMENT

Item 051-3713/9085 Patterson Office Supplies 800-637-1140

Figure 7-31 Refusal of treatment form for periodontics. (Courtesy Patterson Office Supplies, Champaign, IL.)

- Periods for which employees and recipients are paid while absent due to sickness or injury, and the amount and weekly rate of payments made by the dentist or third-party payers
- Copies of employees' and recipients' income tax withholding allowance certificates
- Any employee copies of federal form W-2 that were returned as undeliverable
- Dates and copies of tax deposits made
- Copies of returns filed

- Record of fringe benefits provided including substantiation under the Internal Revenue Service (IRS) Code Section 274 and related regulations

OSHA Records Relating to Each Employee
- Medical records
- Copies of employee hepatitis B vaccination records
- Hepatitis B declination forms
- Exposure incident forms
- Follow-up documents for exposure incidents
- OSHA training records

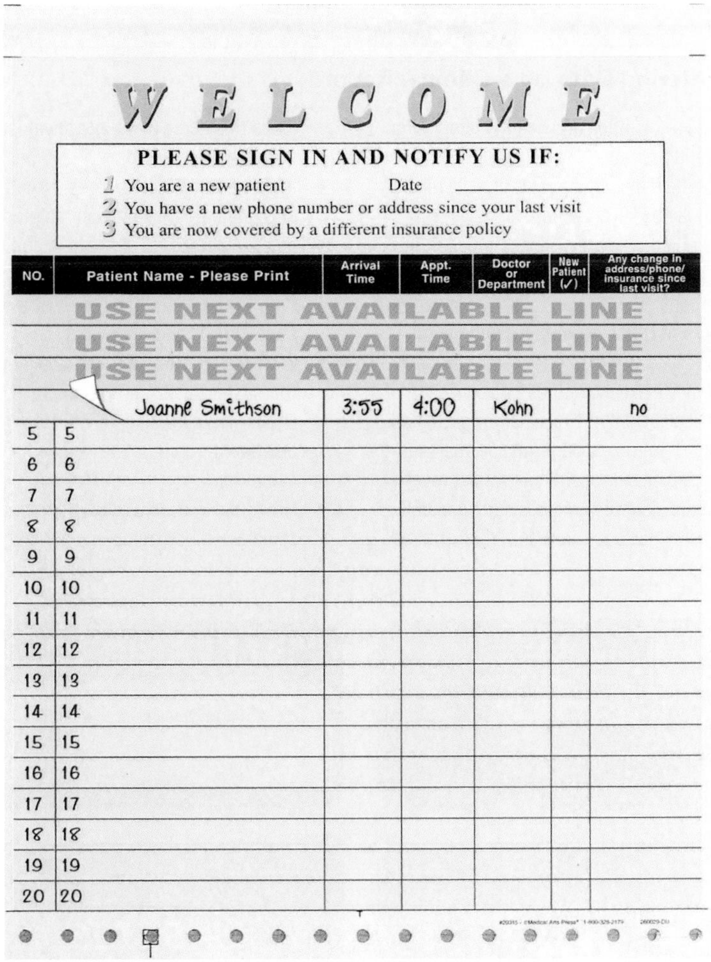

WELCOME

PLEASE SIGN IN AND NOTIFY US IF:

1. You are a new patient Date ____________
2. You have a new phone number or address since your last visit
3. You are now covered by a different insurance policy

NO.	Patient Name - Please Print	Arrival Time	Appt. Time	Doctor or Department	New Patient (✓)	Any change in address/phone/insurance since last visit?
USE NEXT AVAILABLE LINE						
USE NEXT AVAILABLE LINE						
USE NEXT AVAILABLE LINE						
	Joanne Smithson	3:55	4:00	Kohn		no
5	5					
6	6					
7	7					
8	8					
9	9					
10	10					
11	11					
12	12					
13	13					
14	14					
15	15					
16	16					
17	17					
18	18					
19	19					
20	20					

Figure 7-32 Sign-in form with removable lines. (Courtesy Medical Arts Press, Brooklyn Park, MN.)

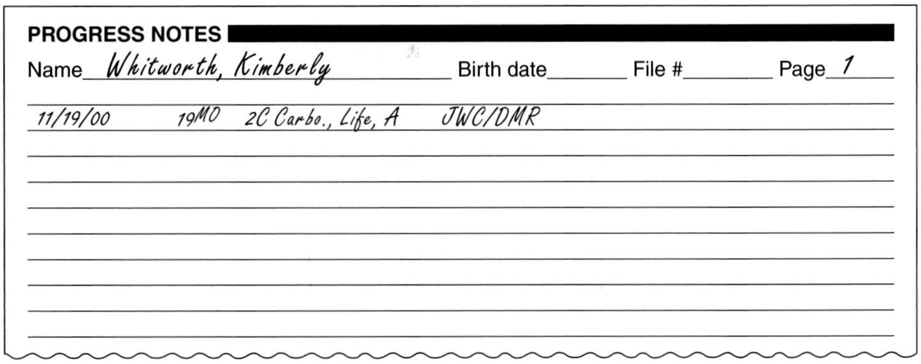

PROGRESS NOTES

Name *Whitworth, Kimberly* Birth date______ File #______ Page *1*

11/19/00 19MO 2C Carbo., Life, A JWC/DMR

Figure 7-33 Data entry on a clinical chart, initialed by the treating dentist and dental assistant.

BOX 7-3 — Rules for Entering Data on a Clinical Record

- Transfer the information from the registration and health history form to the dental chart completely and accurately.
- Enter general information about the patient neatly (the clinical record must be completed in ink, or it may be keyboarded).
- Underline in red any notation about a serious illness or allergies. Small, brightly colored labels (see Figure 7-34) also may be used to draw attention to special notations. These labels must be inserted inside the patient chart to adhere to HIPAA regulations and maintain patient confidentiality.
- The clinical assistant or dentist may make the entries for services rendered in the clinical record. Data can be entered on a barrier-protected keyboard in the treatment room or on a keyboard outside the treatment room. Both methods provide a neater record and, when properly implemented, can improve infection control in records management.
- Check information to ensure that it has been transferred or entered correctly.

- Place the record in the file envelope or folder with the patient's name visible on the record.
- After each patient has been treated, check each record carefully to determine if it has been completed for the day.
- Verify that the record has been initialed by the dentist and the clinical assistant who performed the treatment (see Figure 7-33). In offices with a large staff, this serves as a reference for follow-up and may be needed in case of a lawsuit.
- Ensure that all codes and charting techniques are consistent with the system used in the office. A list of these codes and symbols should be available to all staff members and be posted in each treatment room or be available in a drop down screen on the computer.
- Never make a derogatory remark about a patient in the record that could prove damaging in a lawsuit.

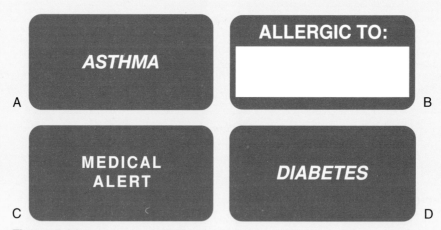

Figure 7-34 Colored chart labels draw attention to special medical conditions. (Courtesy Patterson Office Supplies, Champaign, IL.)

BOX 7-4 — Primary and Permanent Dentition

Primary Dentition

2	Central incisors
2	Lateral incisors
2	Cuspids (canines)
2	First molars
2	Second molars
TOTAL:	10 in each arch

Permanent Dentition

2	Central incisors
2	Lateral incisors
2	Cuspids (canines)
2	First premolars
2	Second premolars
2	First molars
2	Second molars
2	Third molars (may not develop)
TOTAL:	16 in each arch (including third molars)

BOX 7-5 — Categories of Tooth Identification

Dentition
Primary
Permanent

Arch
Maxillary
Mandibular

Quadrant
Right
Left

Specific Tooth
(e.g., first premolar, central incisor)

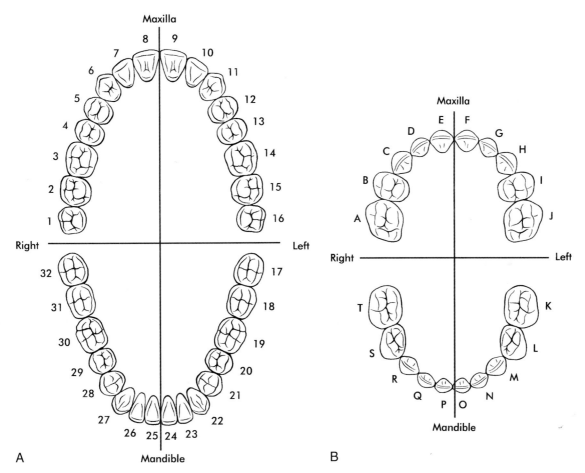

Figure 7-35 Universal numbering system. **A,** Permanent dentition. **B,** Primary dentition.

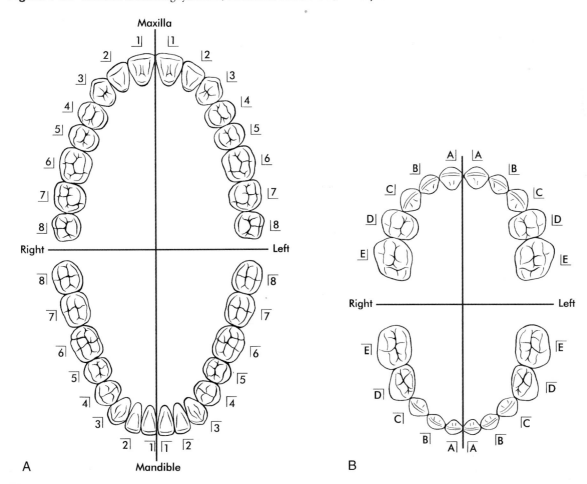

Figure 7-36 Palmer notation numbering system. **A,** Permanent dentition. **B,** Primary dentition.

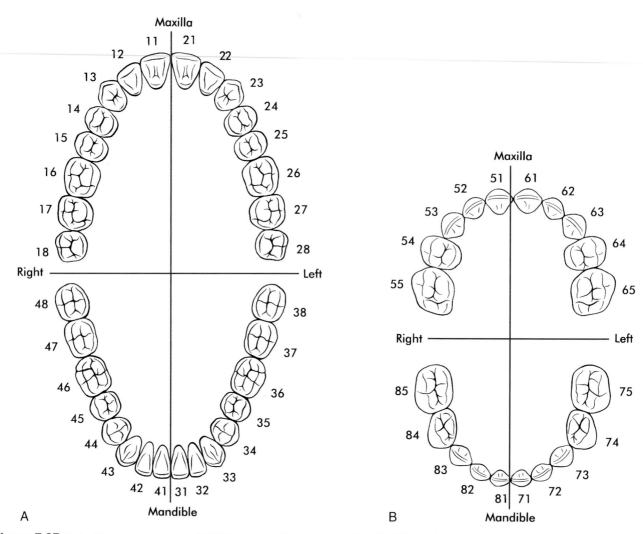

Figure 7-37 Federal Dentaire International (FDI) system. **A,** Permanent dentition. **B,** Primary dentition.

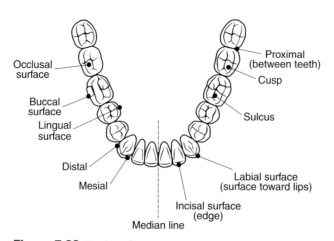

Figure 7-38 Tooth surface annotation.

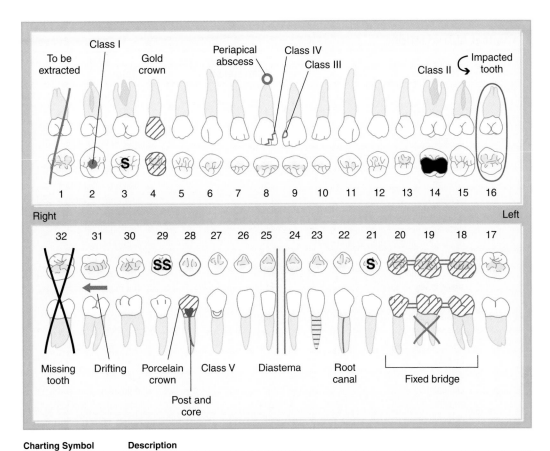

Charting Symbol	Description
Amalgam	Outline the surfaces that are involved (refer to teeth 2 and 14).
Composite	Outline the surfaces involved (refer to teeth 9 and 27).
Porcelain fused to metal (PFM)	Outline the tooth and draw diagonal lines on the occlusal or lingual surface where metal appears (refer to tooth 28).
Gold	Outline the crown of the tooth and place diagonal lines (refer to tooth 4).
Sealant	Place an "S" on the occlusal surface (refer to teeth 3 and 21).
Stainless steel crown	Outline crown of tooth and place "SS" on occlusal surface (refer to tooth 29).
To be extracted	Draw a red diagonal line through the tooth. An alternative method is to draw two red parallel lines through the tooth (refer to tooth 1).
Missing tooth	Draw a black or blue "X" through the tooth. It does not matter if the tooth was extracted or it never erupted, just as long as the tooth is not visible in the mouth. If a quadrant, or arch, is edentulous, make one "X" over all teeth (refer to tooth 32).
Impacted or unerupted	Draw a red circle around the whole tooth, including the root (refer to tooth 16).
Decay	Depending on the caries classification, outline and color the area for amalgam (refer to tooth 2), or outline the area for composite (refer to tooth 9).
Recurrent decay	Outline the existing restoration in red to indicate decay in the area (refer to tooth 14).
Root canal	Draw a line through the center of each root involved (refer to tooth 22).
Periapical abscess	Draw a red circle at the apex of the root to indicate infection (refer to tooth 8).
Post and core	Draw a line through the root that requires a post; then continue the line into the gingival one third of the crown, making a triangle shape (refer to tooth 6).
Rotated tooth	If a tooth has rotated in its position, indicate the direction the tooth has turned by placing a red arrow to the side of the tooth (refer to tooth 15).
Diastema	When there is more space than normal between two teeth, draw two red vertical lines between the areas (refer to teeth 24 and 25).
Fixed bridge	Draw an "X" through the roots of the missing tooth or teeth involved. Then draw a line to connect each of the teeth that make up the bridge. The type of material used to make the bridge will determine whether you outline the crown for porcelain, use diagonal lines for gold, or use a combination of the two (refer to teeth 18-20).
Full crown	Outline the complete crown if it is to be a porcelain crown, or outline and place diagonal lines if it will be a gold crown (refer to tooth 4).
Drifting	Place a red arrow pointing in the direction a tooth is drifting (refer to tooth 31).
Implant	In red, draw horizontal lines through the root or roots of a tooth (refer to tooth 23).
Bonded veneer	Veneers cover only the facial aspect of a tooth. Outline the facial portion only (refer to tooth 26).
Fractured tooth or root	If a tooth or a root is fractured, draw a red zigzag line where the fracture occurred (refer to tooth 8).

Figure 7-39 Example of an anatomic diagram for charting conditions of the mouth. (From Bird DL, Robinson DS: *Torres and Ehrlich modern dental assisting*, ed 9, St Louis, 2009, Saunders.)

TABLE 7-1 Clinical Abbreviations

Abbreviation	Term	Abbreviation	Term
@	at	est	estimate, estimation
ac	before meals	et	and
ad	to, up to	et al	and others
a, ag, am	amalgam	etc	and so on, and so forth
AIDS	acquired immune deficiency syndrome	evac	evacuate, evacuation
amp	ampule	eval	evaluate, evaluation
amt	amount	ext	extract, external
anat	anatomy	F	Fahrenheit, female, field, formula
anes	anesthesia	FB	foreign body
ant	anterior	FBS	fasting blood sugar
appl	applicable, application, appliance	FH	family history
approx	approximate	FLD	full lower denture
BF	bone fragment	FMS	full mouth series
bid	twice a day	FMX	full mouth x-ray
bio, boil	biological, biology	FR or frac	fracture
BP	blood pressure	frag	fragment
Br	bridge	freq	frequent, frequency
BW	bitewing radiograph	FUD	full upper denture
Bx	biopsy	G	gold
c–	with	GF	gold foil
C	composite	GI	gold inlay
caps	capsules	ging	gingiva, gingivectomy
carbo	carbocaine	GP	general practitioner
cav	cavity	HBP	high blood pressure
CC	chief complaint	Hdpc	handpiece
CDA	Certified Dental Assistant	hosp	hospital
cm	centimeter	hr	hour
CM	cast metal	hs	hour of sleep
comp	compound, composite	ht	height
conc	concentrate	Hx	history
cond	condition	I&D	incision and drainage
CSX	complete series x-rays	IA	incurred accidentally
cur	curettage	IH	infectious hepatitis
CV	cardiovascular	IM	intramuscular
CVA	cerebrovascular accident	IMP	impacted
D	distal	inc	incisal, incisive, incise
DV	devital	inf	infected, inferior, infusion
dbl	double	imp	impression
DDS	Doctor of Dental Surgery/Science	inj	injection, injury
DEF	defective	inop	inoperable, inoperative
Dg or Dx	diagnosis	IV	intravenous
DM	diagnostic models	L	lingual
DMD	Doctor of Dental Medicine	LA	labial
DMF	decayed, missing, and filled	lab	laboratory
DO	distoocclusal	lac	laceration
DOB	date of birth	lat	lateral
DR	doctor	lig	ligament
dwt	pennyweight	ling	lingual
EDDA	Expanded duties dental assistant	liq	liquid
emerg	emergency	LLQ	lower left quadrant
EMT	emergency medical treatment	LN	lymph node
ENT	ears, nose, and throat	LRQ	lower right quadrant
epith	epithelial	lt	left

TABLE 7-1	Clinical Abbreviations—cont'd		
Abbreviation	**Term**	**Abbreviation**	**Term**
M, mes	mesial	qid	4 times a day
mand	mandibular	qn	every night
max	maximum, maxillary	R	respiration
MDR	minimum daily requirement	Rx, RX	prescribed
med	medicine, medical	rad	radiograph
mg, mg, m	milligram	RC	root canal
micro	microscopic	RDA	Registered Dental Assistant
ML	midline	RDH	Registered Dental Hygienist
MM	mucous membrane	reg	regular
mm	millimeter	req	requisition
MO	mesiocclusal	resp	respiration
mo	month	RHD	rheumatic heart disease
MOD	mesiocclusodistal	ROA	received on account
MS	multiple sclerosis	SBE	subacute bacterial endocarditis
narc	narcotic	Sig	write on label
nc	no change, no charge	sol	solution
NCP	not clinically present	stat	immediately
neg	negative	stim	stimulate, stimulator
nonrep	nonrepetitive	strep	*Streptococcus pyogenes*
norm	normal	surg	surgery, surgeon
NPO	nothing by mouth	Sx	symptom
occ, occl	occlusal	T	temperature
OH	oral hygiene	tab	tablet
OHI	oral hygiene instructions	TAT	tetanus antitoxin
opp	opposite	TB	tuberculosis
P	pulse	TBI	toothbrush instructions
PA	periapical	temp	temperature
Pan	panoramic oral examination	tid	three times a day
path	pathology	TLC	tender loving care
PDR	*Physicians' Desk Reference*	TMJ	temporomandibular joint
Ped	pediatrics	TPR	temperature, pulse, respiration
PLD	partial lower denture	Tr.P	treatment plan
PO, postop	postoperative	U, u	unit
preop	preoperative	unk	unknown
prep	preparation, prepare for treatment	ULQ	upper left quadrant
prn	as needed	URI	upper respiratory infection
prog	prognosis	URQ	upper right quadrant
pt	patient	VD	venereal disease
Px, Pro, Proph	prophylaxis	wh	white
q	every	wnd	wound
qd	every day	x	times (e.g., 4×); x-ray
qh	every hour	YOB	year of birth
q2h	every 2 hours	yr	year

Confidential employee medical record

Employee medical record

Employee name ____________________

Employee address ____________________

Employee social security number ____________________

Employee starting date ____________________

Employee termination date (if any) ____________________

History of HBV vaccination ____________________

(date received, or, if not received, a brief explanation of why not)

History of other immunizations ____________________

History of exposure incident(s) (dates, brief explanation, attachments) ____________________

Results of medical exams and follow-up procedures regarding exposure incident or hepatitis B immunity, including written opinion of healthcare professional (dates, brief explanation, attachments)

Information provided to the health care professional regarding hepatitis B vaccination and/or exposure incident(s) (dates, brief explanation, attachments)

Attach pre-employment health records to this document.
Note: maintain the record for duration of employment plus 30 years

Figure 7-40 Custom employee health and medical records form. (Courtesy Patterson Office Supplies, Champaign, IL.)

KEY TERMS

Axial surface—The tooth surface that runs vertically from the biting surface to the apex of a tooth.

Charting symbols—A type of shorthand in the dental office that is used to enter clinical data on tooth symbols on a patient's chart.

Clinical abbreviations—Initials or short terms used to explain a clinical condition in a patient's oral cavity.

Clinical record—A collection of all information about a patient's dental treatment.

Consent form—A form that is signed by the patient or by the parent or guardian of a pediatric patient, which grants permission for administration of an anesthetic and other specified procedures.

Federal Dentaire International (FDI)—A tooth numbering system that assigns a two-digit number to each tooth in any quadrant. The first number indicates the quadrant in which the tooth is positioned, and the second number identifies the specific tooth.

Health history form—A form that provides the patient's complete health history and is signed by the patient.

Health history update form—This form should be completed periodically to keep both the health history and the personal information current. The patient should sign and date this form.

Health Portability and Accountability Act (HIPAA)—Federal act that requires dental offices that transmit certain health information electronically to protect patient health information.

Important records—Records for the office operation that are extremely valuable but not vital. They include accounts payable and receivable, invoices, canceled checks, inventory and payroll records, and other federal regulatory records.

Information management—See *records management.*

Laboratory prescription/requisition—A form that accompanies each case a dentist sends to a dental laboratory and includes information about the case.

Nonessential records—Documents that lie around, have little importance, and take up space. They include such items as notes to you, reminders of meetings, outdated announcements, and pamphlets.

Occlusal surface—Biting surface

Palmer notation system—A tooth numbering system that assigns each of the four quadrants a bracket to designate the area of the mouth where the tooth is found.

Patient registration form—A form containing general information such as addresses and phone numbers, as well as employment and insurance information. It may also be combined with a health history form.

Record—Data in forms such as text, numbers, images, or voice that is kept for future reference.

Records management—The process of establishing a logical, functional system for storing and retrieving information. Also called *information management.*

Statute of limitations—Period within which a civil suit for alleged wrongdoing may be legally filed.

Universal numbering system—The most popular numbering system. It uses Arabic numerals 1 to 32 for the permanent dentition, and the letters *A* to *T* for the primary dentition.

Useful records—Records that include employment applications, expired insurance policies, petty cash vouchers, bank reconciliations, and general correspondence.

Vital records—Essential documents that cannot be replaced, including patient clinical and financial records and the office's corporate charter and deed, mortgage, or bill of sale.

LEARNING ACTIVITIES

1. Describe the impact of HIPAA on a dental practice. Why is this important to a patient and healthcare professional?
2. List the various categories of records, and give examples of dental office documents that fit each category.
3. Explain why the clinical record is a vital record in the dental office.
4. Describe the parts of a clinical record.
5. Describe the retention and transfer of clinical records in the dental office.

Please refer to the student workbook for additional learning activities.

BIBLIOGRAPHY

Fulton-Calkins PJ: *The administrative professional*, ed 13, Mason, OH, 2007, Thomson South-Western.

Furlong A: *Electronic claims filing made easy: new ADA tool shows dental community how [online]*, Chicago, 2005, American Dental Association. Available at www.ada.org. Accessed April 28, 2009.

Michigan Dental Association: *Disposal of dental records [member's only]*, Lansing, MI, 2008, Author. Available at www.smilemichigan.com. Accessed November 10, 2008.

Michigan Dental Association: *Dental records access and release [member's-only]*, Lansing, MI, 2008, Author. Available at www.smilemichigan.com Accessed November 10, 2008.

Schulte D: The latest changes in Michigan's dental records law, *J Mich Dent Assoc* 89(5):30, 2007.

Schulte D: Your most-asked questions about dental records, *J Mich Dent Assoc* 89(5):36, 2007.

RECOMMENDED WEB SITES

www.ada.org/prof/resources/topics/hipaa/index.asp
www.hhs.gov/ocr/hipaa
www.hipaacomply.com/hipaafaq.htm
www.hipaadvisory.com
http://answers.hhs.gov/cgi-bin/hhs.cfg/php/enduser/std_alp.php
www.marygovoni.com
www.smilemichigan.com

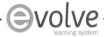

Please visit http://evolve.elsevier.com/Finkibeiner/practice for additional practice activities.

8

Storage of Business Records

CHAPTER OUTLINE

Preparing Records for Filing
    Basic Steps
    Records Retention
Classification of Filing Systems
    Five Basic Systems
    Selecting the Appropriate Filing System
Electronic Files
    Storage
    Care of Recordable Media
Electronic Media
Storage Supplies
Managing Workstation Records Effectively

LEARNING OUTCOMES

- Define key terms.
- Identify and distinguish among the different storage systems.
- Apply basic alphabetical indexing rules.
- Determine the most efficient storage methods for various documents in a dental office.
- Select supplies for the storage of records.

Vast amounts of information are generated in the dental office each day. The idea of a paperless office sounds exciting, but it has proved to be a myth. Reality dictates that traditional methods of record storage will be used for some time. In Chapter 7, disposition is identified as the final stage of a dental record—either destruction or storage. The administrative assistant is responsible for managing and maintaining records, both paper and electronic files. This chapter discusses records storage. A sound understanding of records management and the indexing rules associated with records storage will continue to be an essential skill for the administrative assistant.

A dental office produces many kinds of information, including clinical and financial records, radiographs, and diagnostic models. Inability to find a document quickly is frustrating and can often delay a decision, diagnosis, or payment. Such delays can be costly and stressful.

A record is stored information on any media created or received by the office that is evidence of its operations or that has value requiring its retention for a period of time. For example, information may be:

- Written and recorded on paper as in a patient's clinical or financial record
- Written forms such as an employee records
- Completed and written federal forms for Occupational Safety and Health Administration (OSHA) records, tax and insurance records, and accounts receivable and payable
- Any written and recorded information on some type of electronic form or microform

- An oral record that captures the human voice and is stored on DVD or other electronic storage media.
- E-mail, spreadsheets, databases, word processing document, or other computer software systems stored in an electronic folder
- Radiographs, video, digital photographs, stored on DVDs or other media
- Models or other replicas of patient's oral cavity

Records are assets to the dental practice. They provide legal value by providing evidence of treatment and business transactions. Records may provide information of articles of incorporation, real estate, and contracts. Records provide information on day-to-day operation of the practice and historical evidence of treatment, employee data, and financial activity. Thus the maintenance of these records becomes a major responsibility of the administrative assistant—to ensure a smooth flow of the practice as well as a safe and secure practice.

To many administrative assistants, filing is one of those dreaded, procrastinated, routine jobs done when the administrative assistant can "get around to it" or "has the time."

Anyone with office experience knows that records must be readily available. Wise planning can save a tremendous amount of time and effort. The heart of any professional office is its filing system. Business office files should not be a place to *put* materials, but rather a place to *find* materials. A systematic plan for storage, retrieval, transferring, protection, and retention must be established. When planning for the office files, consider ease in retrieval, confidentiality, and safety. The needs of the office, the size of the dental practice, and the space available for equipment are determining factors in establishing an efficient filing system.

PRACTICE NOTE
The heart of any professional office is its filing system.

PREPARING RECORDS FOR FILING

Basic Steps

Certain routines should be followed in preparing materials for filing: (1) set aside some time each day or every few days for filing paper records; (2) keep papers or records to be filed in a basket marked *to be filed;* (3) file electronic records immediately in the appropriate electronic folder. Make backup copies of all electronic files as they are completed.

Before mastering the different filing systems, it is necessary to learn and understand some basic steps, which are generally done in the order of inspecting, indexing, coding, sorting, and storing:

- *Inspecting:* Review each record to determine if it is something that must be filed. If it can be disposed of (check the retention schedule or the originator of the form), dispose of it. If it is to be retained, continue to the next step.
- *Indexing:* Determine under which caption or name an item is to be filed. Indexing is a mental process that requires making a decision. For instance, if the record is a receipt for

a payment that was just made from the dentist's checking account, the administrative assistant must decide into which file to place the receipt. If files are organized by subject, file the receipt under the subject to which it pertains (e.g., a receipt for an electric bill might be filed under "utilities" or "electricity"). For a patient's clinical record, use an alphabetical system and break down the name into first, second, and third units to consider for filing.

Electronic records are indexed by determining in what directory the file should be located and by following a uniform procedure for naming the files. Do not name electronic files with characters or words that do not identify the subject of the record.

- *Coding:* Once the caption or title of the record has been determined, assign a code by highlighting, typing, or writing a caption on a paper record or by giving the electronic file a name. On an electronic record, this is done by creating a descriptive file name and including it on the document under the initials of the creator. If an electronic file also exists in paper form, the file name on the document allows for quick, easy retrieval. Examples of coding are shown in Figure 8-1. The clinical record is coded with the patient's name, and the electronic document is coded with the name of the originator and other important information about the document.
- *Sorting:* The records are arranged in the order in which they are to be placed in the file (e.g., if the file is alphabetical, put the records in alphabetical order). Electronic files are sorted

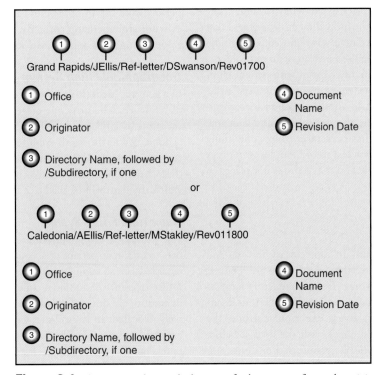

Figure 8-1 Electronic coding at the bottom of a document refers to the originator of the document, the directory name, the subdirectory (if used), and the document name.

as the files are saved in the correct directory or on the correct disk. The system then sorts the files either alphabetically by file name, date, or by any other designation made.

- *Storing:* Put documents in folders and bulkier records in file drawers. Check and double-check that documents are being filed correctly. Also be sure to put CDs, DVDs, or other media, such as microfilm, in the correct place.

> **PRACTICE NOTE**
> Check and double-check that you are filing a document correctly.

Two other aspects of document storage, cross-referencing and retrieval, deserve special consideration, as follows:

1. **Cross-referencing** alerts staff members that a record normally kept in a specific location has been stored elsewhere. A cross-reference can be provided by making a copy of the record and filing it in the referenced file with a note that it is a copy, or a cross-reference sheet can be put in the file. A cross-reference sheet contains the name of the document, the date it was filed, a brief description of the subject of the record, and the places where the record could be found. This type of cross-referencing is often found in a library card catalog.

> **PRACTICE NOTE**
> Cross-referencing alerts staff members that a record normally kept in a specific location has been stored elsewhere.

2. **Retrieval** is the removal of records from files using proper "charge-out" methods. When an entire file folder is removed, an out-folder is put in the place of the removed folder. The out-folder has the name of the individual or department that removed the folder and the date it was removed. Out-guides or substitution cards may be used instead of an out-folder.

Although it does not commonly happen with patient clinical charts during routine treatment, a record may need to be removed from a file and used in another location for consultation or study. In such cases, the out-folder should denote the area to which the record has been taken. Electronic filing appears to lessen the chance for a lost record, but loss can occur when coding is done incorrectly and the record is not placed in the correct file.

Records Retention

It is not cost-effective to maintain unnecessary records and filing cabinets. Many records in the dental office are retained in accordance with state statutes. If the practice is large, a retention schedule may have been developed for various documents. If the office does not have a retention schedule, the administrative assistant should check with the dentist before deciding how documents should be transferred or destroyed. The National Archives and Records Service, a federal agency, has produced a helpful reference, *Guide to Record Retention Requirements.* It is available from the Superintendent of Documents, U.S. Government Printing Office, Washington, DC 20402.

Retention and destruction of files have taken on additional importance since the federal Revised Rule 26 of the Rules of Civil Procedure was approved in December 1993. This rule requires organizations to make available all relevant records that must be kept in compliance with prevailing statutes and regulations. Delay or failure to find information makes an office vulnerable to financial loss and adverse legal judgments.

CLASSIFICATION OF FILING SYSTEMS

Five Basic Systems

The five basic classification systems of filing are the alphabetical system, the geographical system, the numerical system, the subject system, and the chronological system. All these methods except the chronological system basically apply alphabetical procedures. The method used in a dental office depends on the type of practice, but it is not uncommon to use several of these methods for various types of filing.

> **PRACTICE NOTE**
> Delay or failure to find information makes an office vulnerable to financial loss and adverse legal judgments.

Selecting the Appropriate Filing System

Alphabetical System
In an **alphabetical filing system** the arrangement of names appears in sequence from A to Z. The alphabetical filing system accounts for about 90 percent of the filing a person is likely to perform and can be applied to various captions. Standard rules exist for alphabetizing correctly. Box 8-1 illustrates alphabetical indexing rules applied to a variety of situations.

Geographical Filing System
In a **geographical filing system** location is the important factor of reference. The principle of geographical filing is essentially the same as alphabetical filing, except that geographical filing is done by a territorial division (e.g., state, city, or street) rather than by name. Coding should be done in a manner similar to that of the alphabetical system by marking the caption under which the item will be filed (see Figure 8-1).

Numerical Filing System
The **numerical filing system** uses a method of assigning numbers to each new patient or account. Numbers assigned are then recorded on an alphabetical card index or computer file for future reference. Additional papers relating to the same patient or account are subsequently filed according to the number originally allocated. In large clinics with access to computer centers, a numerical system can be used to great advantage because computers handle numerical data faster than alphabetical characters.

Subject Filing System
The **subject filing system** is the alphabetical arrangement of papers according to the subject or topic of the papers. This system is used when it is more desirable to assemble information

BOX 8-1 Indexing Rules for the Alphabetical System

Names of individuals are indexed by units. The last name (surname) is the key unit, followed by the first name (given name), which is the second unit, and then by the middle name or initial, the third unit. Alphabetize names by comparing the first units of the names, letter by letter. Consider second units only when the first units are identical. Consider third units only if the first and second units are identical, and so on.

Name	1	2	3
Alice J. Gooding	Gooding	Alice	J.
Alice Marie Goodman	Goodman	Alice	Marie
William Grafton	Grafton	William	

If the last names are the same, consider the second indexing unit.

Name	1	2	3
Frank Martin	Martin	Frank	
George Martin	Martin	George	
George C. Martin	Martin	George	C.

If the last names are the same but vary in spelling, consider each letter.

Name	1	2	3
Joy Read	Read	Joy	
Janice Reed	Reed	Janice	
Phyllis J. Reid	Reid	Phyllis	J.

Initials are considered the same as a whole word and are filed before names beginning with the same initial. Names with no initial are filed before those with an initial ("nothing before something").

Name	1	2	3
Arthur Stone	Stone	Arthur	
C. Stone	Stone	C.	
Charles Stone	Stone	Charles	

If two people have the same name, they are indexed according to the alphabetical order of the city of residence, then by state. If two people have the same name and live in the same city, they are indexed according to street name.

Name	1	2	3
Richard Murphey (Grand Rapids)	Murphey	Richard	Grand Rapids
Richard Murphey (Grandville)	Murphey	Richard	Grandville

Surname prefixes are considered part of the last name, not separate words. A hyphenated surname (e.g., Meyer-Schafer) is considered a single indexing unit. A compound personal name that is not hyphenated (e.g., Catherine Myers Schafer) is treated as separate indexing units.

Name	1	2	3
Connie MacDonald	MacDonald	Connie	
Connie McDonald	McDonald	Connie	
Alice Meyer-Schafer	Meyer-Schafer	Alice	
Martin O'Connor	O'Connor	Martin	
Frank M. O'Dell	O'Dell	Frank	M.
Catherine Myers Schafer	Schafer	Myers	Catherine

If the first word in a compound surname is one of the standard prefixes (St. in St. James), the surname is indexed as a single unit.

Name	1	2	3
Edward St. James	Saint James	Edward	
William St. Johns	Saint Johns	William	
James E. Sutton	Sutton	James	E.

Titles and degrees are disregarded but may be placed in parentheses after the names.

Name	1	2	3
Professor Joseph C. Kline	Kline	Joseph	C. (Prof.)
Father Patrick O'Reilly	O'Reilly	Patrick (Fr.)	
Capt. C. J. Walters	Walters	C.	J. (Capt.)

A seniority designation is not considered an indexing unit but is used as an identifying element to distinguish between identical names.

Name	1	2	3
Charles D. Flynn Jr.	Flynn	Charles	D. (Junior)
Charles D. Flynn Sr.	Flynn	Charles	D. (Senior)

Titles used without a complete name should be considered as the key indexing unit.

Name	1	2	3
Father Patrick	Father	Patrick	
Sister Mary Martha	Sister	Mary	Martha

Articles, conjunctions, and prepositions are disregarded in indexing.

Name	1	2	3
The Litton Dental Clinic	Litton	Dental	Clinic (The)

A firm or business name is indexed in the order written unless it contains an individual's name.

Name	1	2	3	4	5
The Harvey F. Andrew Dental Laboratory	Harvey	F.	Andrew	Dental	Laboratory (The)
Grand Rapids Dental Laboratory	Grand	Rapids	Dental	Laboratory	
Horton Dental Ceramics	Horton	Dental	Ceramics		

(Continued)

Indexing Rules for the Alphabetical System—cont'd

Agencies of the federal government are indexed under United States Government and then according to department, division, subdivision, and location for adequate differentiation.

Name	1	2	3	4	5	6
Federal Bureau of Investigation	United	States	Govt. Justice	Federal Investigation	(Dept. of) (Bur. of)	
Bureau of Labor	United	States	Govt. Labor	Labor	Statistics	(Dept. of) (Bur. of)

State, county, and city governments are indexed according to location and then by department, division, or subdivision.

Name	1	2	3
Park Department, Kent County	Kent	County	Park (Dept.)
Michigan State Department of Education	Michigan	State	Education (Dept. of)
Grandville Department of Health	Grandville	City	Health (Dept.)

Numbers spelled as words in business names are filed alphabetically. Numbers written in digit form are filed before letters or words.

Name	1	2	3	4
5-Cent Copy Center	10	Cent	Copy	Center
Four Seasons Health Spa	Four	Seasons	Health	Spa
Seventh Street Photo Center	Seventh	Street	Photo	Center

- Names of schools are first indexed by the name of the city in which the school is located and then by the name of the school.
- Local banking or other institutions with branch offices are indexed as the name is written; however, if banks from several cities are involved, the first indexing unit is the city where the bank is located, and the name of the bank follows.
- Numbers, including Roman numerals, are filed before alphabetical information. However, all Arabic numerals come before Roman numerals.
- Acronyms, abbreviations, and television and radio call letters are treated as one unit, and company names are filed as you see them.

by topic than by name. For example, a subject file may be preferred if the dentist is involved in research or writing for publications. If a subject area is very broad, it can be broken down into smaller divisions by the use of secondary guides. This system is effective only if the administrative assistant is totally aware of the dentist's involvement in the relevant subject areas, or it may be used for filing receipts for the accounts payable.

Chronological Filing System

Basic System. The **chronological filing system** is a method of filing by date. It can be used within an alphabetical, geographical, subject, or numerical system by filing the most recent correspondence in the front of the file folder. This system can also be used for treatment records in a patient's clinical chart. The most current treatment data sheet would appear first, followed by past treatment records.

Tickler File. Another type of chronological classification system is a **tickler file**, or follow-up file. The most common type of tickler file contains the days of the month and the months of the year. Manually the tickler file is a card file that contains the days of each month, from 1 to 31. Items to be completed are filed in the slot of the day planned to complete the task. Take time each day to review the tickler file. Perform the task to be done on that day, or move the notation to the appropriate day

if the activity has been rescheduled. Electronically this can be done in software that provides a calendar. Simply insert the task to be done on the day to be reminded, and the calendar comes up on that day with the various tasks listed. A separate task card can even be created for each task with information entered specific to that task, as shown in Figure 8-2. Care should be taken to ensure that an activity is not placed on a weekend day or holiday on which the office will be closed. The files for these days should be carefully checked in advance to ensure that the task is done before the weekend or holiday or that the task is placed in the slot of a later day.

ELECTRONIC FILES

Storage

Storage of electronic records requires a knowledge of computer systems and the storage of word processing, database, or spreadsheet files, as well as knowledge of tasks required to sort, search, retrieve, and print reports. As mentioned, a dental office will probably most often use a manual filing system, but may also use at least one type of electronic storage system: CD or DVD, hard disk, zip disk, tape cartridge, and jump drive. (These forms of storage are discussed in Chapter 5.)

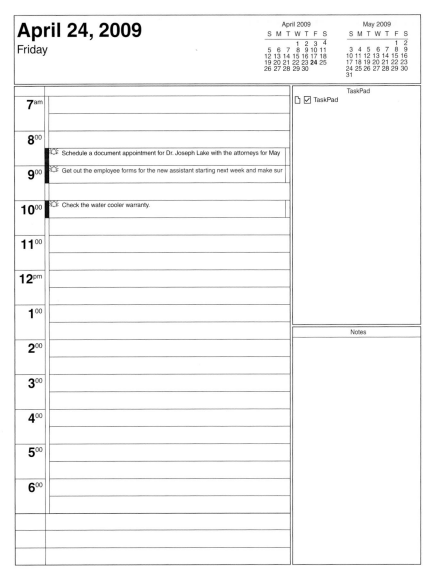

Figure 8-2 An electronic calendar used as a tickler file easily reminds the administrative assistant of tasks to be done on a specific day.

In most dental offices where microcomputers are used, all files are stored from the hard drive on a removable disk or tape. One way to keep track of which files are on each storage unit is to label each storage unit with its own identifying number or code. A separate index stored in a database can list all the file names and the numbers or codes of the storage units on which they may be found. To retrieve a file, search the index for the file by file name; the index will show in what storage unit or directory the file is located.

Care of Recordable Media

Recordable media includes magnetic disks, optical disks (CDs and DVDs), tape, PC cards, Smart cards, and flash drives.

Special attention must be paid to the storage of recordable media to prevent damage and loss of data. Each manufacturer may recommend specific care for its products, but in general, disks should be protected from dust, magnetic fields, extreme temperatures, liquids, and vapors. Box 8-2 (Figure 8-3) presents several suggestions for ensuring safe storage of data.

ELECTRONIC MEDIA

Once an appropriate filing system has been chosen, the administrative assistant must determine what types of supplies and equipment are necessary to maintain the system. The equipment should be practical for day-to-day use and storage.

The term *filing equipment* refers to the actual structures that store files or records. Most manufacturers supply a variety of models in different colors with assorted features. Many practices still use vertical files, but open-shelf or lateral filing has become very popular, especially if space is limited. A **vertical file** stores records in drawers; file folders are placed

BOX 8-2 Recordable Media Care

- Never touch the internal disk; handle disks only by the protective outer cover (Figure 8-3).
- Do not expose disks to magnetic fields, such as those produced by telephones, radio speakers, or computer screens.
- Keep media at temperatures of 50 to 140° F (10–60° C); avoid extreme temperatures.
- Protect media from dust and foreign particles.
- Do not expose media to water or other liquids.
- If media contains permanent information, use the *write-protect* system to prevent data loss. (Write-protect is a feature on a CD or DVD or tape that prevents writing over existing data.)

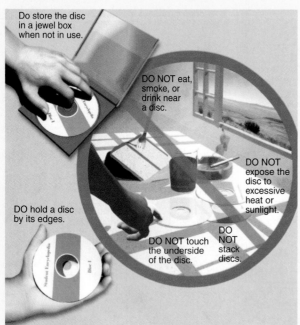

Figure 8-3 Some guidelines for the proper care of optical discs. (Image from Shelly GB, Cashman TJ, Vermaat ME: *Discovering Computers 2008: Complete,* Stanford, CT, 2008, Course Technology, a part of Cengage Learning.)

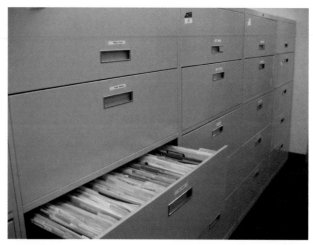

Figure 8-4 Lateral file.

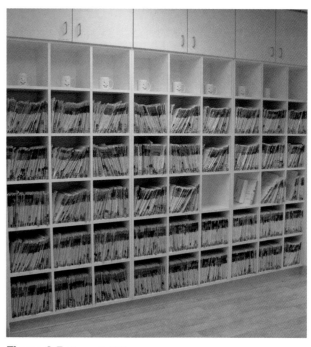

Figure 8-5 Open-shelf file.

on the folder's edge and arranged according to the filing method selected. Vertical files are available in cabinets with one to five or more drawers and may accommodate either an 8½ × 11-inch (letter size) or 8½ × 14-inch (legal size) file. These are not the best file cabinets to use for saving space. Allow room for the cabinet as well as the pull-out drawer space. This means that approximately double the space of the vertical cabinet is needed.

A **lateral file** (Figure 8-4) is similar to a vertical file, except that the longest side opens and the files are stored as if they were placed on a bookshelf. Lateral files have the added advantage of providing a countertop for reviewing files removed from the cabinet or for displaying books and other materials. Like vertical files, lateral files also are designed to accommodate letter- or legal-size files. Less actual floor space is needed because these cabinets can store more files and require less floor and pullout drawer space.

Open-shelf filing is the most popular filing system among modern dental practices. This arrangement saves space and speeds filing and retrieval. The visibility and accessibility of open-shelf filing have proved to be two of the many advantages of this arrangement (Figure 8-5). Compared to a closed drawer filing system, open-shelf units hold twice as many files on half the floor space. The files give a visible sense of location and allow users to take full advantage of index guides and color-coding techniques. Misfiled information becomes less of a problem. However, because the files are open, dirt and dust may accumulate if covers are not used.

A **card file** can be used to store small cards (3 × 5-inch, 4 × 6-inch, or larger) that are used for specialized systems. An example of the use of the rotary or Rolodex file (Figure 8-6) is for addresses, e-mail addresses, telephone and fax numbers of dental suppliers, laboratories, and dental associates commonly contacted.

When selecting filing equipment for a dental office, the administrative assistant should also consider a fire-protection file. As a precaution against fire destruction, the patients' ledger cards, the appointment book, CDs or DVD copies, and other vital records should be placed in the file at the end of each work day. Many dentists buy an additional file for storing valuable records away from the office.

STORAGE SUPPLIES

Filing supplies for paper storage include file guides, file folders, folder labels (in a variety of colors for color-coding), cross-reference sheets, and out-guides.

File guides, usually heavy cardboard, divide the file drawer into separate sections. The division is indicated by a tab that extends above the guide. The guides divide the alphabet into sections, or they may show a division in a numerical sequence. The file drawer is marked on the outside to correspond with the division of the filing arrangement.

File folders are usually made of Manila paper or another heavy type of material. Folders may be obtained in a variety of cuts. Using a variety of cuts allows the tabs to be arranged in a staggered fashion. The tabs may be on the far-left side, or they may be center-cut, one-third cut, or one-fifth cut.

Most dental practices prefer to use patient file folders or envelopes with labels that come in a variety of colors. This type of file and label guards against misplaced records (e.g., x-ray films) and provides space for the patient's name, address, and telephone number. Most file folders can be labeled with gummed labels, available in a variety of styles (rolls of labels, peel-off labels, and continuous folded strips) and colors that will make the folders easier to locate and re-file (Figure 8-7). In a group practice, a different color may be used to designate the patients of each dentist. Color-codes may also be used for other pertinent patient information.

Points to remember when making the labels are: (1) the labels should be keyed, not handwritten; (2) the keying should begin two or three spaces from the left edge of the label and at a uniform distance (usually one line space) from the top edge of the label; (3) the name may be keyed in all capital letters, or the first letter of each important word may be capitalized; and (4) the established format should be followed consistently.

Color-coding of file folders aids in fast retrieval and re-filing. Figure 8-8 shows a typical open-shelf, end-tab filing

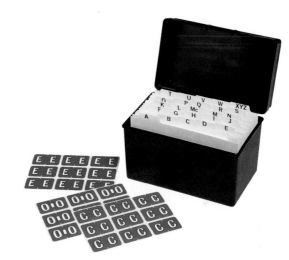

Figure 8-7 Label kit with assorted colored labels. (Courtesy Patterson Office Supplies, Champaign, IL.)

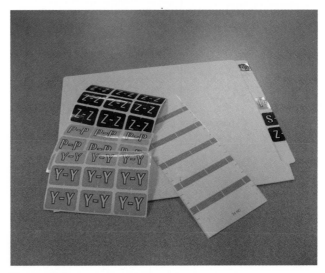

Figure 8-8 Patient file folders using colored filing labels.

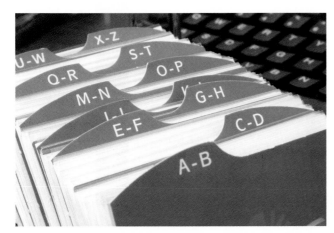

Figure 8-6 Rolodex file. (Copyright 2009 JupiterImages Corporation.)

system that uses colored filing labels on each file folder to translate the alphabetical rules discussed earlier into a color "code." The assignment of color to each alphabetical character has long been recognized by efficiency experts as a time and energy saver. When patient charts are filed alphabetically and when each letter in the alphabet has a different file label color, color block patterns begin to form in the open-shelf system "block" patterns that immediately direct the eye toward the proper filing areas. This virtually eliminates the misfiling common in non–color-coded systems. By assigning a different color to each number, large filing systems that use the numerical system can also benefit from the added efficiency of color-coding.

Sometimes cross-referencing is necessary within the filing system. Cross-referencing helps the administrative assistant to locate or file the information in its proper location. For example, if a letter is to be filed by the dental clinic name rather than by the name of the individual who has written the letter, the administrative assistant may look under the individual's name and find the cross-reference sheet, which will indicate the name of the clinic (Figure 8-9).

The electronic supplies necessary for records management include specially designed storage units for disks or tapes. These may be small plastic or fabric units that hold one to five CDs or DVDs, plastic or wooden desktop boxes, rotary files, or ring binders with vinyl pages that have pockets. A digital tape backup system is necessary when large amounts of data stored on hard disks must be recorded. Some of these systems store the entire contents of a hard disk on a single minicassette. Consideration might be given to an online back up system that is done each day at an office down time. Such an online system should be thoroughly investigated for security before enrollment. At the end of this chapter is a recommended web site.

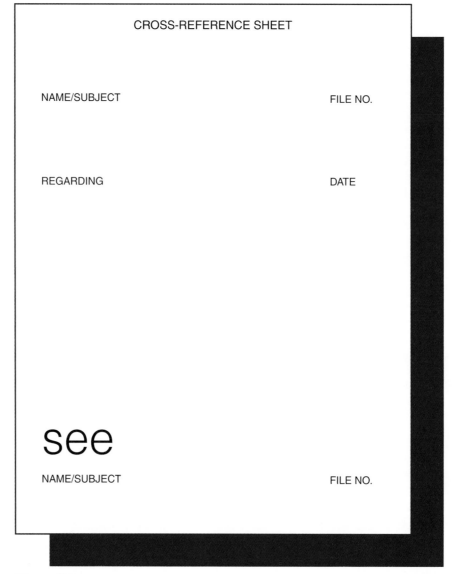

Figure 8-9 Cross-reference sheet.

MANAGING WORKSTATION RECORDS EFFECTIVELY

Regardless of the types of records or systems used in a dental office, organization of the workstation is an absolute necessity for successful records management. Almost all assistants spend some of their work day filing records of some type. Even if filing duties are limited to organizing individual files

develop and follow a simple system. The goal should be to establish a system that allows for easy retrieval. Successful retrieval means being able to find a record or document when needed in a minimal amount of time. As stated earlier, this type of efficiency eliminates time and motion and ultimately financial loss. Box 8-3 presents tips for successful records management.

BOX 8-3 **Tips for Successful Records Management**

Paper Records
- Organize incoming and outgoing papers in an In/Out box. Use a stackable style that has two or three trays. Label each tray In, Out, or Hold. The Hold tray is for papers that do not have to be acted upon immediately.
- Use desk drawer files for personal records, forms, stationery, procedural handbooks, and other routinely used items.
- Use logbooks to record recurring events or data, such as long distance telephone calls, petty cash, and appointment call lists.
- Keep correspondence in a loose-leaf binder called a *correspondence* or *chronological file,* and date each folder for the year. This will provide a fingertip reference of all correspondence pertaining to any patient or given activity. Of course, a copy of the correspondence must also go into the patient's record.
- File copies of insurance claims in a loose-leaf binder in chronological or numerical order. Include a log sheet with an up-to-date reference on the status of each claim form. As forms are completed and paid, re-file them in the patient record.
- Plan a work schedule that includes filing as a daily routine.
- When placing records in a folder, remove the folder from the file far enough so that the material can be placed completely in the folder and does not extend over the top edge of the folder or tab.
- Be careful to place materials *in* a folder, not behind or in front of another folder.

- Do not use paper clips on filed material. It is easy for other materials to attach themselves to the clips. Staples are better if materials must be held together, but remove the first staple before adding another.
- To avoid filing errors, designate as few people as possible to file and retrieve records.
- When searching for lost records, check transposition and alternate spellings of names.
- Replace folders as they become worn out.
- Avoid overuse of the *Miscellaneous* file. Be ready to begin a separate file for a patient or an associate.

Electronic Records
- Store recordable media in a file box specifically designed for the media style.
- Label each media with a general classification.
- Print an index of the documents currently on the media each time a new document is added. The index can be folded and placed in the jacket or kept in a reference notebook.
- When the media source becomes full and the same label is wanted for a new disk, number the disks in consecutive order (e.g., "Letters 1," "Letters 2"). Mark each new media with the date it was first used.
- Store documents in electronic folders named to represent the activity (e.g., "correspondence," "recall," "patient charts").

KEY TERMS

Alphabetical filing system—Method of filing in which the arrangement of names appears in sequence from A to Z.

Card file—A file that can be used to store small cards (3 × 5-inch, 4 × 6-inch, or larger) that are used for specialized systems.

Chronological filing system—Method of filing by date. This system can be used within an alphabetical, geographical, subject, or numerical system by filing the most recent correspondence in front of the file folder.

Cross-referencing—This system alerts staff members that a record normally kept in a specific location has been stored elsewhere.

Geographical filing system—Method of filing in which location is the important factor of reference. The principle is essentially the same as alphabetical filing, except that it is done by territorial division (e.g., state, city, or street) rather than by name.

Lateral file—A file that is similar to a vertical file, except that the longest side opens and the files are stored as if they were placed on a bookshelf.

Numerical filing system—Method of filing that assigns a number to each new patient or account.

Open-shelf filing—Method of filing that is similar to lateral filing but with no doors to close.

Retrieval—Removal of records from files using proper "charge-out" methods.

Subject filing system—Method of filing that uses an alphabetical arrangement of papers according to the subject or topic of the papers.

Tickler file—A chronological method of filing that serves as a follow-up file and contains the days of the month and the months of the year to alert the administrative assistant to perform a task.

Vertical file—A file that stores records in drawers. File folders are placed on the folder's edge and arranged according to the filing method selected.

LEARNING ACTIVITIES

1. List four steps for preparing materials to be filed.
2. Define the five basic methods of filing.
3. Describe the use of the following filing equipment:
   a. Vertical file
   b. Open-shelf file
   c. Card file
   d. Rolodex file
   e. Tickler file
   f. Electronic file
4. Explain how color-coding can be used in dental office files.
5. List six helpful hints for more efficient filing.

Please refer to the student workbook for additional learning activities.

BIBLIOGRAPHY

Fulton-Calkins PJ: *The administrative professional*, ed 13, Mason, OH, 2007, Thomson South-Western.

Mosley DC, et al: *Supervisory management*, ed 6, Cincinnati, 2004, South-Western.

Oliverio ME, Pasewark WR, White BR: *The office: procedures and technology*, ed 5, Mason, OH, 2007, Thomson South-Western.

Shelly GB, Vermaat ME: *Discovering computers 2009*, Boston, 2008, Course Technology.

RECOMMENDED WEB SITE

www.drbackup.net.

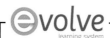

Please visit http://evolve.elsevier.com/Finkibeiner/practice for additional practice activities.

9

Written Communications

CHAPTER OUTLINE

LEARNING OUTCOMES

- Define glossary terms
- Describe the various types of written communication in a dental office.
- Select stationery supplies.
- Identify the characteristics of effective correspondence.
- Identify the parts of a letter.
- Review rules of punctuation and capitalization.
- Describe the basic steps for preparing written communication.
- Apply various formatting styles to written communication.
- Describe standard procedures for preparing outgoing mail.
- Observe ethical and legal obligations in written communication.
- Explain the use of e-mail in the dental office.
- Apply common business etiquette to the use of e-mail.
- Identify the classifications of mail.
- Identify special mail services.
- Explain the function of a postage meter.
- Discuss the process for packaging laboratory cases.
- Explain the procedure for sorting incoming mail.

Today one may ask if written communication is as important in the dental office as it has been in the past. The answer is a resounding *yes*. Because e-mail is such a widely used vehicle for communicating today, the administrative assistant will probably write more than in the past. Many professionals find themselves writing more than telephoning their colleagues.

Written communication in all of its forms remains extremely important. In addition to e-mail, the administrative assistant will use instant messaging via the Internet and write memorandums, letters, and reports. Effective written correspondence promotes good will for the office, whereas ineffectively written correspondence can cost the dental office greatly in unhappy patients and good will. The cost can include, but not limited to, loss of patients, profit, patient satisfaction, and good will.

Good business and professional writing should sound like a person talking to another person. Using an easy-to-read style makes the reader respond more positively to stated ideas. Make writing easier to read in two ways. First, make individual sentences and paragraphs easy to read so the reader can easily skim the first paragraph or read the entire document in as short a time as possible. Second, make the document visually pleasant and structure signposts that lead the reader through the document.

Good business and professional writing is closer to a conversation and less formal than the style of writing that has traditionally earned high marks on college essays and term papers. However, many dental professionals also use professional papers that are easy to read and use good visual impact.

Most people have several styles of talking, which they vary instinctively, depending on the audience. So it will be with writing in the dental office. A letter to a dentist regarding a professional technique or a letter to a dental supplier demanding better service may be formal, whereas an e-mail to a colleague will be informal and perhaps even chatty.

Chapter 7 examined the various types of documents generated in the dental office. Now it is time to review the importance of other types of written communication in a dental practice, specifically the use of letters, forms, and newsletters. These documents are all created by the administrative assistant for a variety of reasons. This chapter discusses the creation and production of written communication, how it is distributed, and how incoming written communication is processed, both in the manual and electronic form.

LETTERS

A variety of written documents are generated in the dental office, but none are as important as the letters that seek to enhance public relations with patients and professional colleagues. These letters should be original and create a professional image. Most important, these letters should be one that the administrative assistant is proud to mail from the office.

With the use of word processing in the dental office, the dreaded task of creating an original letter each time one is needed is eliminated. Today's administrative assistant can have a supply of sample letters stored as templates in an electronic file. When necessary, the assistant can transform the sample into an original letter that is professional and can be personalized within minutes.

The types of written communication most commonly sent from a dental office include thank you notes for referral of patients, letters of appreciation, birthday or holiday greetings, congratulatory letters, sympathy messages, patient transfer letters or letters of consultation, recall notices, collection letters, order letters, and newsletters.

Thank You for Referral Letter

The dentist should be appreciative of the confidence expressed by a patient who refers a new patient to the office and should acknowledge such a referral with a personally signed letter. Although this letter should mention the name of the referred patient, it should never divulge any confidential information about the treatment. However, if this letter is to be sent to a physician or another dentist, a reference statement may be made about the patient's diagnosis and/or prognosis, if this was discussed with the patient and the patient has signed the appropriate disclosure forms. Several examples of this type of thank you letter are shown in Figure 9-1. Note that the differences in content vary according to the situation.

Letter of Appreciation to a Cooperative Patient

A cooperative patient is often overlooked and taken for granted. Often one thinks only of the patient who creates frustration. A dentist should acknowledge a patient who is prompt for appointments, maintains a regular payment plan, and cooperates with prescribed home care plans. This is an opportunity to give sincere compliments. When the opportunity presents itself, try writing a letter as in Figure 9-2 on p. 155 and see how appreciative the patients are. A letter of appreciation should be sincere, state the purpose briefly, and be written as though conversing with the patient in person.

Birthday Letter and Holiday Greetings

Patients, especially children and older adults, like to be recognized on their birthdays. These letters should be cheerful and friendly. Figure 9-3 on p. 156 shows a letter that could be sent to an older adult on a special birthday. Another method of handling this form of public relations is to send a birthday card. Many professional stationers provide appropriate greeting cards for all occasions and dental specialties (see Figure 9-4 on p. 156).

Congratulatory Letter

Through conversations with patients and via the daily newspaper, the administrative assistant may learn the outstanding achievements of patients. Such accomplishments should not go unnoticed by the dental office staff. A letter sent to congratulate a patient must be sent promptly. Include how the event was learned of and include a sincere expression of congratulations

Dental Associates, PC
Joseph W. Lake, DDS - Ashley M. Lake, DDS

September 15, 20—

Mr. Carl Ladley
3567 Wines Drive
Wyoming, MI 49507

Dear Carl:

It was good of you to refer one of your employees, Raymone Hunchez, to me for treatment. My staff and I are always glad to be of assistance to you and your employees whenever possible.

You and your family have been valuable members of my dental practice. We hope that we will be able to provide Mr. Hunchez the same quality service that we have provided your family in the past.

Give my best regards to Mary and the boys.

Sincerely,

Ashley M. Lake, DDS

je

611 Main Street, SE – Grand Rapids, MI 49502   Phone: 616.101.9575 Fax: 616.101.9999
E-mail: office@dapc.com or Visit us at: www.Lakedental.com

B

Dental Associates, PC
Joseph W. Lake, DDS - Ashley M. Lake, DDS

April 17, 20—

Mr. Edward Aprill
347 North Wixom
Frankfort, MI 48223

Dear Mr. Aprill:

Your expression of confidence in referring Mr. Robert Smith to my office for treatment is greatly appreciated. It is always a pleasure to welcome new patients to our practice, especially when they are referred by another satisfied patient.

It gives my staff and me a sense of satisfaction that you have been pleased with the treatment we have rendered. We will make every effort to provide Mr. Smith with the same complete and thorough dentistry we have provided you during these past five years.

Thank you again for your confidence.

Sincerely,

Joseph W. Lake, DDS

je

611 Main Street, SE – Grand Rapids, MI 49502   Phone: 616.101.9575 Fax: 616.101.9999
E-mail: office@dapc.com or Visit us at: www.Lakedental.com

A

Figure 9-1 A, Thank you for referral letter. **B,** Informal thank you for referral letter to a patient who is a personal friend of the dentist.

(Continued)

Dental Associates, PC
Joseph W. Lake, DDS – Ashley M. Lake, DDS

December 19, 20—

Robert W. Wells, DDS, MS
2146 Rochester Avenue
Grand Rapids, MI 49502

Dear Dr. Wells:

Mrs. Roger (Amy) Browne was in my office today for an examination. I confirmed your diagnosis of advanced periodontitis. We have set up a series of appointments for x-rays and beginning periodonatal curettage.

The prognosis is favorable and Mrs. Browne was eager to begin treatment. Thank you for this referral and the kind remarks you made to her.

Sincerely,

Joseph W. Lake, DDS

je

611 Main Street, SE – Grand Rapids, MI 49502   Phone: 616.101.9575   Fax: 616.101.9999
E-mail: office@dapc.com or Visit us at: www.Lakedental.com

D

Dental Associates, PC
Joseph W. Lake, DDS – Ashley M. Lake, DDS

September 19, 20—

Ms. Angela Gualandi
2492 Plymouth Road
Comstock, MI 49829

Dear Ms. Gualandi:

I would like to take this opportunity to thank you for your confidence in referring your friend, Judy McKay, and her children, Debbie and Rick, to our office for treatment.

My staff and I are pleased to learn of your satisfaction. We will make every effort to justify the confidence you have shown in us during the treatment of Ms. McKay and her children.

Thank you again for your expression of confidence.

Sincerely,

Ashley M. Lake, DDS

je

611 Main Street, SE – Grand Rapids, MI 49502   Phone: 616.101.9575   Fax: 616.101.9999
E-mail: office@dapc.com or Visit us at: www.Lakedental.com

C

Figure 9-1, cont'd C, General thank you for referral letter. **D,** Thank you for referral letter to a colleague.

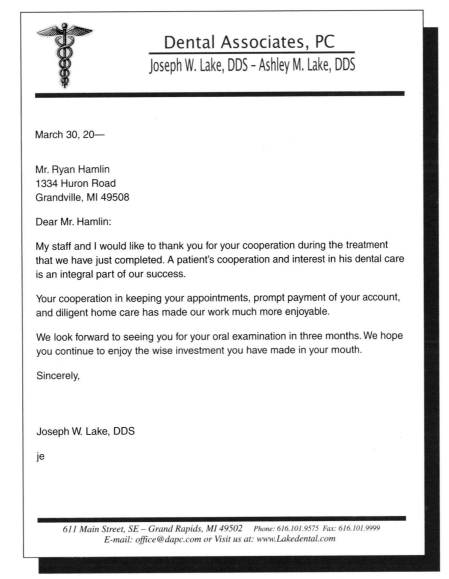

Dental Associates, PC

Joseph W. Lake, DDS – Ashley M. Lake, DDS

March 30, 20—

Mr. Ryan Hamlin
1334 Huron Road
Grandville, MI 49508

Dear Mr. Hamlin:

My staff and I would like to thank you for your cooperation during the treatment that we have just completed. A patient's cooperation and interest in his dental care is an integral part of our success.

Your cooperation in keeping your appointments, prompt payment of your account, and diligent home care has made our work much more enjoyable.

We look forward to seeing you for your oral examination in three months. We hope you continue to enjoy the wise investment you have made in your mouth.

Sincerely,

Joseph W. Lake, DDS

je

611 Main Street, SE – Grand Rapids, MI 49502   Phone: 616.101.9575 Fax: 616.101.9999
E-mail: office@dapc.com or Visit us at: www.Lakedental.com

Figure 9-2 Letter of appreciation to a cooperative patient.

(see Figure 9-5 on p. 157). Congratulations can also be sent for the birth of a child, a wedding, or a graduation. A greeting card or brief letter is appropriate.

Referral for Consultation or Treatment

During the treatment of a patient, it is often necessary to call upon the services of a specialist. A series of letters may be sent between the two dental offices concerning the patient's treatment. A good example of such an experience is the transfer of a patient to an orthodontist for treatment (see Figure 9-6 on p. 158). Figure 9-7 on p. 159–161 shows examples of several forms of communication that might be used during a patient's treatment. Note that the specialist's office has used a basic format that provides information about the patient's treatment. This letter can be stored electronically, or a pre-prepared form can be used in a specialty office, such as an orthodontics office, because there is a large patient volume and a similarity of basic

treatment. Regardless of the type of form used, note that in each case the patient's name is referenced, the message is brief, and each tooth or condition is diagrammed or written out completely to avoid error in interpretation.

Sympathy Message

Many people find it difficult to express sympathy in a letter. Therefore one of the best ways to handle this difficult situation is to send a sympathy card. It is the unexpected message that often means a great deal to family members in their time of grief.

Miscellaneous Letters

Many letters are not public relations letters and are not included in this chapter. Specific examples of recall, broken appointment, and collection letters are discussed in the chapters that specifically address each of these topics.

Dental Associates, PC
Joseph W. Lake, DDS – Ashley M. Lake, DDS

May 17, 20—

Mr. Michael Russo
1145 Collins Drive
Grand Rapids, MI 49502

Dear Mr. Russo:

My staff and I wish to send our best wishes for a happy birthday tomorrow. We hope you will enjoy your ninety-fifth birthday and reflect on your many accomplishments.

Your longevity may be attributed to your good health and heritage, but your continued personal contributions to the community are evidence of your unselfishness. We hope your example of good citizenship will impact the youth of this city.

Again, best wishes for a happy birthday and continued good health in the future.

Sincerely,

Ashley M. Lake, DDS

je

611 Main Street, SE – Grand Rapids, MI 49502   Phone: 616.101.9575 Fax: 616.101.9999
E-mail: office@dapc.com or Visit us at: www.Lakedental.com

Figure 9-3 Birthday letter to an older adult.

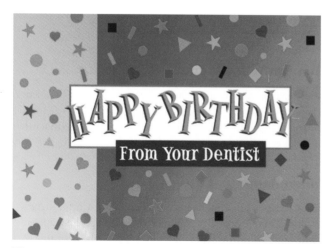

Figure 9-4 Birthday card. (Courtesy Patterson Office Supplies Champaign, IL.)

SELECTING STATIONERY SUPPLIES

If the administrative assistant begins working in an established dental practice, the stationery supplies will already be available. However, he or she may have to choose business supplies if asked to order them. Many of these supplies are listed in Chapter 6.

The office stationery (letterhead) is usually selected on the basis of simplicity, neatness, and quality. Bond paper, because of its quality, is often used. It can be made from all-cotton fiber (sometimes called rag), all-sulfite (a wood pulp), or any proportion of the two. High-cotton fiber bond indicates quality and prestige, and it ages without deterioration or chemical breakdown.

The following information may be used as a guide for future stationery needs:

Dental Associates, PC
Joseph W. Lake, DDS – Ashley M. Lake, DDS

September 28, 20—

Mr. Jason Henkle
1135 Hollyhock Lane
Grand Rapids, MI 49503

Dear Mr. Henkle:

Last night the staff and I read in the *Grand Rapids News* about your promotion to Vice President of the Michigan Trust Company. We want to send our congratulations to you on this promotion.

It is a pleasure to learn of your advancement and I send my best wishes for success in this new position. I am certain this will be a challenging experience.

Again, my sincerest best wishes on your fine achievement.

Sincerely,

Ashley M. Lake, DDS

je

611 Main Street, SE – Grand Rapids, MI 49502   Phone: 616.101.9575 Fax: 616.101.9999
E-mail: office@dapc.com or Visit us at: www.Lakedental.com

Figure 9-5 Congratulatory letter.

- A color theme for stationery items, such as letterheads, envelopes, appointment cards, prescription pads, medicine envelopes, and notepads, may be used. Color coordinates such as light and dark brown or blue, or contrasting tones of gray with black print are attractive combinations. Most dental stationery supply or chain office supply houses have samples of stationery stock and logo designs from which to select.
- A popular alternative to purchasing stationery is to create the letterhead using appropriate computer software. A fine bond paper can be purchased. When a new letter is to be keyboarded, the letterhead is removed from the file where it is stored, the letter is prepared, and then it is printed on bond paper. This becomes less expensive and allows for more frequent changes and creativity. Clip art is available that makes it easy to create a professional letterhead that provides the office staff many options. Labels with the same clip art and office information can also be created in this manner. It is important that the labels selected are compatible with the office printer.

Letterheads
Standard office use:
Business size 8½ × 11 in.

Usually 16# or 20# bond,
25% cotton fiber (rag)
Executive use:
Standard and Monarch size

(Monarch size: 7¼ × 10 in.)
Usually 24# bond, 100%
cotton-fiber

Matching Envelopes
No. 10 ($4^1/_8$ × 9½ in.)
Same weight and fiber content as
letterhead

No. 10 and No. 7 ($3^7/_8$ × 7½ in.)
Same weight and fiber content as
letterhead

CHARACTERISTICS OF AN EFFECTIVE LETTER

Effective letters that generate good public relations have certain common elements. Keep in mind that direct, simple writing is easier to read. The best word depends on context: the situation,

Dental Associates, PC
Joseph W. Lake, DDS – Ashley M. Lake, DDS

September 25, 20—

Daniel R. Jacobsen, DDS, MS
2495 Packard Road SE
Grand Rapids, MI 49506

Dear Dr. Jacobsen:

I am referring Michael Moran, age 12, to you for an orthodontic evaluation. Mrs. Moran will be calling your office for an appointment. Michael appears to have a Class II malocclusion with crowding of the mandibular anterior teeth.

Enclosed you will find a complete series of radiographs that were taken on September 11, 20-- .

I will look forward to your diagnosis and assistance with this case.

Sincerely,

Joseph W. Lake, DDS

je

Enclosure: Full mouth series radiographs

611 Main Street, SE – Grand Rapids, MI 49502   Phone: 616.101.9575 Fax: 616.101.9999
E-mail: office@dapc.com or Visit us at: www.Lakedental.com

Figure 9-6 Referral of a patient to an orthodontist.

the purpose, the audience, and the words used. Following are some general guidelines:

- *Use words that are accurate, appropriate, and familiar.* Accurate words mean what is wanted to say. Appropriate words convey the attitudes wanted to create and fit well with the other words in the document. Familiar words are easy to read and understand.
- *Use technical terminology sparingly.* The exception to this rule is if the administrative assistant is communicating with another professional and needs to describe a condition or treatment in technical terms. However, when communicating with patients or laypersons, it is wise to use a "plain English" equivalent instead of a technical term.
- *Use active verbs most of the time.* This is common in writing for a job application or referring a patient to a specialist. If the verb describes something that the subject is doing, the verb is active. If the verb describes something that is being done to the grammatical subject, the verb is passive.

Active: I recommend that the patient's third molar be removed.
Passive: It was recommended by me for the patient to have the third molar removed.
Active: I can expose digital radiographs.
Passive: Digital radiography is something I could do.

- *Tighten the writing.* Eliminate words that say nothing. Combine sentences to eliminate unnecessary words. Put the meaning of the sentence into the subject and verb. Cut words if the idea is already clear from other words in the sentence. Substitute single words for wordy phrases.

Wordy: Keep this information in the patient's file for future reference.
Tighter: Keep this information for reference.
or: File this information.

Phrases beginning with *of, which,* and *that* can often be shortened.

John G. Clinthorne, D.D.S., M.S.
H. Ludia Kim, D.M.D., M.S.
Professional Corporation
Specialists in Orthodontics
1303 Packard
Ann Arbor, Michigan 48104
(734) 761-3116

«Todays_date_in_words»

«Responsible_party_name»
«Responsible_party_address»
«Responsible_party_city_state_zip»

Dear «Responsible_party_greeting»:

Welcome to our practice! My staff and I look forward to meeting you and «Patient_first_name» on «Next_appoint-ment_date» at «Next_appointment_time». Be assured that «Patient_first_name possessive» first visit with us will be a pleasant and rewarding experience.

Please bring with you the enclosed information sheet as well as any insurance forms and information we may need to file with your insurance carrier.

At «Patient_first_name possessive» first visit to our office, we will proceed with an oral examination and discuss the findings with you. If a more thorough diagnosis is advisable, the following materials may be requested at an addi-tional charge:

• Models of Teeth
• Panoramic X-ray
• Profile X-ray
• Diagnostic Photographs

After the above materials have been studied and the best course of therapy determined, the overall treatment plan will be discussed with you at a consultation appointment.

Sincerely,

John G. Clinthorne, D.D.S., M.S.
H. Ludia Kim, D.M.D., M.S.

Members American Association of **Orthodontists**

A

John G. Clinthorne, D.D.S., M.S.
H. Ludia Kim, D.M.D., M.S.
Professional Corporation
Specialists in Orthodontics
1303 Packard
Ann Arbor, Michigan 48104
(734) 761-3116

«Todays_date_in_words»

«Referring_party_name»
«Referring_party_address—line 1»
«Referring_party_address—line 2»«Referring_party_city_state_zip»

RE: «Patient_full_name»   «Age: Patients_age»

Dear «Referring_party_greeting»:

DISPOSITION: ( ) Orthodontic treatment is indicated at this time and:
                    ( ) They intend to proceed with treatment.
                         Records and consultation appointments have been made.
                    ( ) They are to notify us if and when they wish to proceed.
                    ( ) They do not intend to proceed with treatment.

               ( ) «Patient_first_name» has been referred to your office for:
                    ( ) Dental examination and prophylaxis.
                    ( ) _____

               ( ) Orthodontic treatment may be indicated in the future and
                    «Patient_first_name» has been placed on recall _____
                    ( ) They prefer to call our office at a later date.

               ( ) Orthodontic treatment is not indicated.

REMARKS:

Members American Association of **Orthodontists**

B

Figure 9-7 **A,** Basic form letter from an orthodontist to welcome a new patient. Diagnosis text from the patient's record may be inserted. **B,** Basic form letter from an orthodontist to a refer-ring dentist upon examination of a patient. (Courtesy JG Clinthorne, D.D.S., and HL Kim, D.M.D., Ann Arbor, MI.)

(Continued)

D

C

Figure 9-7, cont'd **C,** Letter to a patient confirming consultation appointment and explaining the process. **D,** Final letter from an orthodontist to a referring dentist informing of completed treatment. (Courtesy JG Clinthorne, D.D.S., and HL Kim, D.M.D., Ann Arbor, MI.)

JOHN G. CLINTHORNE, D.D.S., M.S.
H. LUDIA KIM, D.M.D., M.S.

ORTHODONTICS   1303 PACKARD, ANN ARBOR, MI. 48104   **734-761-3116**

DR. _____ PHONE _____

NAME _____ PHONE _____

_____

_____

_____

_____

_____

_____

_____

_____

DATE _____   _____ D.D.S.

Extract Teeth Encircled

PERMANENT TEETH

UPPER

1 2 3 4 5 6 7 8 │ 9 10 11 12 13 14 15 16

PATIENT'S RIGHT   PATIENT'S LEFT

32 31 30 29 28 27 26 25 │ 24 23 22 21 20 19 18 17

LOWER

DECIDUOUS TEETH

UPPER

A B C D E │ F G H I J

PATIENT'S RIGHT   PATIENT'S LEFT

T S R Q P │ O N M L K

LOWER

☐ Enclosure - X-Rays
☐ Return Requested
☐ Please Keep For Your Records

If any questions ...... Please Telephone

E

Figure 9-7, cont'd E, Requisition used by an orthodontist to refer a patient for extraction. (Courtesy JG Clinthorne, D.D.S., and HL Kim, D.M.D., Ann Arbor, MI.)

Wordy: The issue of most importance
Tighter: The most important issue.
Wordy: The estimate that is enclosed
Tighter: The enclosed estimate
Wordy: It is the case that Registered Dental Assistants are more qualified clinicians in the office.
Tighter: Registered Dental Assistants are more qualified clinicians in the office.

Combine sentences to eliminate unnecessary words. In addition to saying words, combining sentences focuses the reader's attention on key points, makes your writing sound more sophisticated, and sharpens the relationship between ideas, thus making your writing more coherent.

Wordy: I conducted a survey by telephone on Monday April 17th. I questioned 18 dental assistants, some Registered Dental Assistants, and some Certified Dental Assistants, who according to the state directory were all currently working. The purpose of this survey was to find out how many of them were performing advanced functions that were delegated by the state. I also wanted to find out if there were any differences between their salaries.

Tighter: On Monday April 17th, I phoned Registered and Certified working dental assistants to determine (1) if they were performing the state delegated advanced functions, and (2) whether there was a distinction between salaries for these two credentials.

- *Vary sentence length and sentence structure:* A readable letter mixes sentence lengths and varies sentence structure. A really short sentence is under 10 words and can add punch to your letter. Really long sentences of 30 to 40 words can raise a danger flag.

A simple sentence has one main clause:

We will open a new office this month.

A compound sentence has two main clauses joined with and, but, or, or another conjunction. Compound sentences are used best when the ideas in the two clauses are closely related.

[Clause 1]We have hired three new dental assistants, and [Clause 2]they will complete their orientation next week.
[Clause 1]We hired a new intern, but [Clause 2]she will be unable to begin work until the end of the month.

Complex sentences have one main and one subordinate clause; they are good for showing logical relationships.

[Subordinate clause] When the new office opens, [Main clause] we will have an open house for local dentists and offer refreshments and door prizes.
[Subordinate clause] Because we already have a strong patient base in Livingston County, [Main clause] we expect the new office will be as successful as the Ann Arbor office.

- *Use parallel structure:* Parallel structure puts words, phrases, or clauses in the same grammatical and logical form. Clarity eliminates long, meaningless words and uses language that the reader will understand. Thus it is certain that each statement will not be misinterpreted.

  Nonparallel: The position is prestigious, challenging, and also offers good money.
  Parallel: The position offers prestige, challenge, and good money.
  Nonparallel: The steps in the planning process include:
  Determining the objectives
  An idea of who the reader is
  A list of the facts
  Parallel: Determine the objective
  Consider the reader
  Gather the facts

- *Put your readers in your sentences:* Use second person pronouns (you) rather than third person (he, she, one) or first person (I) to give your writing a greater team approach. The "you" approach to letter writing requires the writer to place the reader at the center of the message. When writing the letter, put yourself in place of the reader.

  Third person: References for patients in this office are made by our office manager, and the patient will be contacted as soon as the appointment has been confirmed with the specialist.
  Second person: Once you are referred to a specialist, you will receive a confirmation of your appointment from our office manager.

PRACTICE NOTE
The "you" approach to letter writing requires the writer to place the reader at the center of the message.

In addition to the ideas presented in the preceding, the administrative assistant should review the basic characteristics of effective correspondence. These factors should be used in a review of the letter before it is sent. Remember that the letter sent from the dental office is representative of the quality of work or treatment produced in that practice and should contain the following characteristics:

- *Completeness:* Include all necessary data the reader needs to make a decision or take action.
- *Conciseness:* State the information briefly.
- *Confidentiality:* Release information only about the case that is relative to the contents of the letter and only after the patient has given consent to release specific information.
- *Courtesy:* Use good manners for good public relations. Don't make derogatory statements.
- *Accuracy:* Make sure all of the data are correct. Check details carefully. Use correct spelling and grammar.
- *Neatness:* Avoid smudges, tears, or wrinkles.
- *Positive language:* Use positive words that indicate helpfulness and caring (Box 9-1).
- *Orientation to reader:* Use "you-oriented" pronouns.

PARTS OF A BUSINESS LETTER

A review of the parts of a business letter and the proper placement and purpose for each part is appropriate before selecting a letter style creating the letter. Most business letters contain the following parts:

- Date line
- Inside address (letter address)
- Salutation
- Body
- Complimentary close
- Keyboarded signature
- Reference initials
- Special notations such as attention line, subject line, or enclosures

When using most word processing software, many preformatted letter styles are available. Dates are automatic, and in most systems alignment and letter parts are already defined.

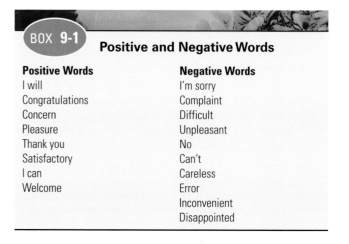
BOX 9-1 **Positive and Negative Words**

Positive Words	Negative Words
I will	I'm sorry
Congratulations	Complaint
Concern	Difficult
Pleasure	Unpleasant
Thank you	No
Satisfactory	Can't
I can	Careless
Welcome	Error
	Inconvenient
	Disappointed

Date Line

The date line contains the date the letter is keyboarded. When using printed letterhead stationery, the date usually begins a double space below the lowest line of the letterhead. (The letterhead usually takes up about 2 inches, but this may vary depending on the style and design of the letterhead.) Many times the length of the letter determines whether the heading should be started lower on the paper; good judgment is needed. When keyboarding a personal business letter, the individual's return address is placed as the first two lines directly above the date line. The date line can be affected by the length of the letter. When using the computer, you may go to "Print Preview" to check the appearance of the letter. Necessary changes can be made before printing. General guidelines that relate to letter length are shown in Box 9-2.

Inside Address

The inside address provides all of the information for mailing the letter. The letter address should match the envelope address. When using word processing, the envelope often is addressed from the letter address by a minor key function on the computer. The information to be included is the recipient's name, the name of company (if appropriate), street number and name, city, and zip code. Three lines of space are left between the date and the first line of the letter address.

Use titles preceding the individual's name (Mr., Mrs., Ms., or Dr.). Do not use a double title, such as Dr. L. B. Crown, D.D.S.; this is redundant. An official title, such as President, may follow the name, for example, Ms. M. P. Coleman, President. The person's official title is often placed on the second line if it helps to balance the inside address lines. The city, state, and zip code are placed on the last line. The appropriate two-letter state abbreviation should be set in capital letters without a period. Leave two spaces after the abbreviation before entering the Zip code.

Salutation

The salutation formally greets the reader. If the writer wishes the letter to be directed to an individual within a firm, it is acceptable to use an attention line. The salutation line should begin one double space below the letter address and should be even with the left margin. If you are writing to an individual, the most appropriate salutation is the individual's name. For example, if the letter is addressed to Mr. Ted Monroe, the salutation would be Dear Mr. Monroe. The salutation can be altered to be Dear Ted if the dentist is a close friend of the recipient. This

change in formality should be recognized before keyboarding the letter. Special situations occur when the letter is to be sent to unknown individuals or more than one person. Suggestions for salutations to be used in common situations are shown in Box 9-3, *A*. Addresses and salutations used for governmental and academic officials are shown in Box 9-3, *B*.

Body of the Letter

The body of the letter contains the message. It begins a double space after the salutation. The paragraphs within the body are single spaced with double spacing between paragraphs. Paragraphs may or may not be indented, depending on the format selected. Refer to Figures 9-2 to 9-7 for selection of the format. Many illustrations in this chapter demonstrate variations in format styles.

Complimentary Close

The complimentary close provides a courteous ending to the letter. It is keyboarded a double space after the last line of the body of the letter. The complimentary close is entered at the same point as the date line position if using the modified block style, or aligned with the left margin if using the block style. Only the first word of the complimentary close should be capitalized. The most common complimentary closes are "Very truly yours" and "Sincerely." Other acceptable closures are "Yours very truly" and "Sincerely yours."

Keyboarded Signature

The keyboarded signature appears four line spaces below the complimentary close. If the name and title of the individual are short, they may be placed on the same line and separated by a comma. If, however, the name and title are relatively long, the name is keyboarded on the first line and the title is placed on the second line. The comma is not placed after the name. You should attempt to make the lines as even as possible.

Reference Initials

Reference initials are the initials of the person who keyboards the letter and should appear in lowercase one double space after the keyboarded signature, even with the left margin. If it is policy to enter the dentist's initials in capital letters before the keyer's in lowercase, it appears as JWL:db or JWL/db.

Attention Line

You may wish to direct a letter to a particular individual or department within an organization. This can be done by using an attention line. The following example illustrates how an attention line is used if the letter has been addressed to a firm:

Apex Dental Laboratories
Attention Mr. W. W. Thomas, President
1616 W. Riverfront Street
Grand Rapids, MI 49502

BOX 9-2 Placement of a Date Line		
Letter Length	**Side Margins**	**Top/Bottom Margins**
Short (Less than 100 words)	2 in.	3 in.
Average (101-200 words)	1½ in.	2 in.
Long (201-300 words)	1 in.	1 in.

BOX 9-3,A   Appropriate Salutations for Various Situations

- *One person, gender unknown:* Dear M.R. Rieger
- *One person, name unknown, title known:* Dear Director of Surgical Technology
- *One woman, title unknown:* Dear Ms. Hartwig
- *Two or more women, titles known:* Dear Ms. Martin, Mrs. Leverett, and Ms. Grey
- *If all women are married:* Dear Mrs. Franks, Mrs. Johnson, and Mrs. Sullens, or Dear Mesdames Franks, Johnson, and Sullens
- *If all women are unmarried:* Dear Miss Franks, Miss Johnson, and Miss Sullens, or Dear Misses Franks, Johnson, and Sullens

- *If all recipients are women:* Dear Ms. Franks, Johnson, and Sullens, or Dear Mses. or Mss. Franks, Johnson, and Sullens
- *A woman and a man:* Dear Ms. Johnson and Mr. Ladley
- *A group or organization composed entirely of women:* Ladies or Mesdames
- *A group or organization composed entirely of men:* Gentlemen
- *A group composed of women and men:* Ladies and Gentlemen

BOX 9-3,B   Addresses and Salutations for Government and Academic Officials

The following addresses and salutations are recommended in correspondence with governmental or academic officials. In each case, the proper ways to address letters are illustrated. On the left are addresses, and on the right, salutations. When one or more examples are given, they are arranged in order of decreasing formality.

Correspondence with Government Officials

The President

The President	Dear Sir, Madam
The White House	Dear Mr. (Mrs. or Ms.) President
Washington, DC 20500	Dear Mr. President; Dear Madam
or	President
The President of the United States	
The White House	
Washington, DC 20500	

Chief Justice of the Supreme Court

The Chief Justice of the	Dear Sir, Madam
United States	Dear Mr. or Madam Chief Justice
Washington, DC 20543	
or	
The Honorable (full name)	
United States Supreme Court	
Washington, DC 20543	

Associate Justice of the Supreme Court

The Honorable (full name)	Dear Sir, Madam
Associate Justice of the Supreme Court	Dear Mr. or Madam Justice
Washington, DC 20543	My dear Justice (surname)
	Dear Justice (surname)

Cabinet Member

The Honorable (full name)	Dear Sir, Madam
Secretary of State	My dear Mr. or Madam Secretary
Washington, DC 20520	

or	
The Secretary of State	Dear Mr. or Madam Secretary
Washington, DC 20520	

Senator

The Honorable (full name)	Dear Sir, Madam
The United States Senate	My dear Mr. or Madam Senator
Washington, DC 20510	My dear Senator (surname)
or	Dear Senator (surname)
Senator (full name)	
The United States Senate	
Washington, DC 20510	

Representative

The Honorable (full name)	Dear Sir, Madam
The House of Representatives	My dear Representative (surname)
Washington, DC 20515	Dear Representative (surname)
or	
Representative (full name)	
The House of Representatives	
Washington, DC 20515	

Chief, Director, or Commissioner of a Government Bureau

Mr., Ms., Mrs., or Miss (full name)	Dear Sir, Madam
Director of Public Information	My dear Mr., Ms., Mrs., or Miss
Department of Justice	(surname)
Washington, DC 20530	Dear Mr., Ms., Mrs., or Miss
or	
Director of Public Information	
Department of Justice	
Washington, DC 20530	

BOX 9-3 Addresses and Salutations for Government and Academic Officials—cont'd

Governor

The Honorable (full name)
Governor of Ohio
Columbus, OH 43215
or
The Governor of Ohio
Columbus, OH 43215

Dear Sir, Madam
My dear Governor (surname)
Dear Governor (surname)
Dear Governor

State Senator

The Honorable (full name)
The State Senate
Columbus, OH 43215
or
Senator (full name)
The State Senate
Columbus, OH 43215

Dear Sir, Madam
My dear Senator
My dear Senator (surname)
Dear Senator (surname)
My dear Mr., Ms., Mrs., or Miss
   (surname)
Dear Mr., Ms., Mrs., or Miss

State Representative

The Honorable (full name)
House of Representatives
Columbus, OH 43215
or
Representative (full name)
House of Representatives
Columbus, OH 43215

Dear Sir, Madam
My dear Representative (surname)
Dear Representative (surname)
My dear Mr., Ms., Mrs., or Miss
   (surname)
Dear Mr., Ms., Mrs., or Miss
   (surname)

Mayor of a City

The Honorable (full name)
Mayor of the City of Ann Arbor
City Hall
Ann Arbor, MI 48105

My dear Sir or Madam
Dear Sir or Madam
Dear Mr. or Madam Mayor
My dear Mayor (surname)
Dear Mayor (surname)

Correspondence with Educators

President (College or University)

Dr. (full name)
or
(full name), Ph.D.
President
Ohio University
Athens, OH 45701

My dear Sir, Madam
Dear Sir, Madam
My dear President (surname)
Dear President (surname)

Dean of a College

Dean (full name)
College of Business Administration
University of Cincinnati
Cincinnati, OH 45221
or
Dr. (full name)
Dean of the College of Business Administration
University of Cincinnati
Cincinnati, OH 45221
(If the individual has a doctorate degree, the salutation may be Dear
Dr. Wilson instead of Dear Dean Wilson.)

My dear Sir, Madam
Dear Sir, Madam
My dear Dean (surname)
Dear Dean (surname)

Professor (College or University)

(full name), Ph.D.
Dr. (full name)
Vanderbilt University
Nashville, TN 37203
Dear Mrs. Mr. Ms., or Miss (surname)

My dear Sir, Madam
Dear Sir, Madam
My dear Professor (surname)
Dear Dr. (surname)

Note: Window envelopes require the date line to be placed on a line 2 inches below the top of the page.

The attention line indicates that the letter writer prefers that the letter be directed to a particular individual. The salutation should agree with the inside address, not the attention line.

Subject Line

The **subject line** clearly states what the letter is about. For example, if writing to a patient regarding the office policy on broken appointments, the subject line is written as follows— Subject: Broken Appointments. The subject line is entered a double space after the salutation and is followed by a double space before continuing with the body of the letter. The subject line may be centered, begun at paragraph point, or aligned with the left margin when using block style. The style of letter will often determine the best position for the subject line. The word *subject* or abbreviation RE may be entered in all capital letters or in capitals and lowercase, or it may be underlined.

Acceptable methods using the subject line are illustrated as follows:

Dear Mrs. Calloway:
SUBJECT: Broken Appointments
or
Dear Mrs. Calloway:
RE: BROKEN APPOINTMENTS
or
Dear Mrs. Calloway:
RE: Broken Appointments

In place of a subject line, a reference number may be used. For example, in a clinical situation, the patient's registration number will appear in the same position as the subject line and is preceded by "Reference" or "Re":

Dear Dr. Wilcox:
Reference: No. 06920

Enclosures

It is common to transfer radiographs with a letter to another dentist when requesting a consultation. When the letter has mentioned that an item is enclosed or attached, an enclosure notation should be made. This notation is keyboarded after double spacing below the reference initials, even with the left margin. Two acceptable methods are as follows:

> je
> Enclosure

or

> je
> Enclosures 2

Copy Notation

When additional copies of the letter are made for distribution to various persons, reference to each recipient is commonly made in the **copy notation.** This informs the recipient to whom copies were sent. Several types of notations are possible, including mail, computer copy, blind copy, postscript, as well as second-page headings.

Special Mailing Notations

Notations such as registered mail, special delivery, or certified are keyboarded in all capital letters between the date and inside address, aligned with the left margin. Other special notations, such as confidential or personal, are entered in the same location.

Types of Copy Notations

With the use of word processing in the office today, copies of correspondence are stored electronically; however, paper copies of all business correspondence should be available in the office. When additional copies are made for distribution, it is necessary for the addressee to know this. A notation is keyboarded a double space below the enclosure, if used, or below the reference initials if there is no enclosure. When more than one person is to receive a copy, list each person on a succeeding line, indenting three spaces from the left margin. Because not all copies are photocopies or com-

puter copies, variations may be used as they apply to the various copy styles. The notation may be keyboarded as follows:

> Copy to O.J. Fox, D.D.S.
> *or*
> c O.J. Fox, D.D.S. (copy)
> *or*
> cc O.J. Fox, D.D.S. (courtesy copy)
> *or*
> cc O.J. Fox, D.D.S. (courtesy copies to multiple parties)
> R.C. Campbell, D.D.S.
> M.A. Reynolds, RDA

Blind Copy

If the person who receives the original letter does not need to know that a copy is being sent to a particular person, then a blind copy notation can be made. To do this, the original copy is removed from the computer or machine, and the notation is keyboarded on the copy one inch from the top at the left margin, as in the following example:

> bc Barbara Rice

Postscript

A postscript is often used to highlight a particular point. It is not necessarily an item that has been omitted in the body of the letter. If a postscript is used, it is the last line entered. It is not necessary to precede the postscript with P.S.; however, the postscript paragraph should be blocked or indented, depending on the style of letter used (Figure 9-8).

Second-Page Heading

When writing a patient referral letter, it is sometimes necessary to send a lengthy letter to provide adequate information about the patient. If a second page is necessary, the continuation is made on plain paper that is the same size, color, and quality as the letterhead. Leave a one-inch bottom margin on the first page. Include at least two lines of a paragraph at the bottom of the first

You were right, Daniel. The experience of working alongside my father in his practice has been invaluable. I only hope it has been as rewarding for him as it has been for me. Again, thank you for your continued interest in my success.

Very truly yours,

Ashley M Lake, DDS

je

Please make a note to join us for the Martinique Open on December 29th.

Figure 9-8 Letter with a postscript.

page, and continue with at least two lines of the same paragraph on the succeeding page. A heading consisting of the addressee, page number, and date is single-spaced, 1 inch (line six) from the top of the sheet. The following are two acceptable arrangements for beginning the second page.

Block form (used when the letter is in block style):
Ms. Margaret Thompson
Page 2
October 27, 2009
Horizontal form (used when the letter is in modified block style):
Ms. Margaret Thompson 2 October 27, 2009
(triple space)

PUNCTUATION STYLES IN BUSINESS LETTERS

Two common styles of punctuation are used in business letters: open punctuation and mixed or standard punctuation. **Open punctuation** omits all punctuation (except periods after abbreviations) in the salutation and complimentary close lines. **Mixed** or standard **punctuation** requires a colon after the salutation and a comma after the complimentary close. Either style of punctuation may be used with any of the basic letter styles.

The administrative assistant will frequently use titles and academic degrees in writing. The traditional rule is to never omit the period after the element of an academic degree or religious order and never include internal spaces: B.S., Ph.D., LL.B., D.M.D., C.D.A., R.D.A., R.D.H., or Ed.D. This rule may need to be altered, however, in contemporary use when addressing envelopes or completing specialized federal, state, or insurance forms that limit space for computerization or scanning. Addressing envelopes is discussed in greater detail later in this chapter.

Correct punctuation is based on certain accepted rules and principles rather than on the whim of the writer. Punctuation is also important so that the reader can correctly interpret the writer's thoughts. The summary of rules given in this chapter will be helpful in using correct punctuation. The common use of periods, commas, colons, and other types of punctuation is reviewed in the following sections.*

The Period

- The period indicates a full stop and is used at the end of a complete declarative or imperative sentence.
- It is also used following an abbreviation, and after a single or double initial that represents a word (does not apply to addressing envelopes).

acct. etc. Ph.D.
U.S. viz. P.M.
N.E. i.e. pp.

*Descriptions and examples of punctuations from Fulton PJ: *General office procedures for colleges*, ed 8, Cincinnati, 1983, South-Western, a part of Cengage Learning, Inc.

- Some abbreviations that are made up of several initial letters do not require periods.

FDIC (Federal Deposit Insurance Corporation)
ADA (American Dental Association)
AAA (American Automobile Association)
YWCA (Young Women's Christian Association)

- Insert a period between dollars and cents (period and cipher are not required when an amount in even dollars is expressed in numerals).

$42.65 $1.47 $25

- Insert a period to indicate a decimal.

3.5 bushels   12.65%   6.25 feet

The Comma

The comma indicates a partial stop and is used in the following instances:
- To separate coordinate clauses that are connected by conjunctions, such as *and, but, or, for, neither,* or *nor,* unless the clauses are short and closely connected

We have a supply on hand, but I think we should order an additional quantity.
She had to work late, because the auditors were examining the books.

- To set off a subordinate clause that precedes the main clause

Assuming that there will be no changes, I suggest that you proceed with your instructions.

- After an introductory phrase containing a verb form

To finish his work, he remained at the office after hours.
After planning the program, she proceeded to put it into effect.

If an introductory phrase does not contain a verb, it usually is not followed by a comma.

After much deliberation the plan was revoked. Because of the vacation period we have been extremely busy.

- To set off a nonrestrictive clause

Our group, which had never lost a debate, won the grand prize.

- To set off a nonrestrictive phrase

The beacon, rising proudly toward the sky, guided the pilots safely home.

- To separate from the rest of the sentence a word or a group of words that breaks the continuity of a sentence

  The business manager, even though his work was completed, was always willing to help others.

- To separate parenthetical expressions from the rest of the sentence

  We have, as you know, two persons who can handle the reorganization.

- To set off names used in direct address or to set off explanatory phrases or clauses

  I think you, Mr. Bennett, will agree with the statement. Ms. Linda Tom, our vice-president, will be in your city soon.

- To separate from the rest of the sentence expressions that might be interpreted incorrectly without punctuation

  Misleading: Ever since we have filed our reports monthly.
  Better: Ever since, we have filed our reports monthly.

- To separate words or groups of words when they are used in a series of three or more

  Most executives agree that dependability, trustworthiness, ambition, and judgment are required of their office workers.
  Again I emphasize that factory organization, correlation of sales and production, and good office organization are all necessary for maximum results.

- To set off short quotations from the rest of the sentence

  He said, "I shall be there." "The committees have agreed," he said, "to work together on the project."

- To separate the name of a city from the name of a state

  Our southern branch is located in Atlanta, Georgia.

- To separate abbreviations of titles from the name

  William R. Warner, Jr.
  Ramona Sanchez, Ph.D.

The Semicolon

The semicolon is used in the following instances:
- Between independent groups or clauses that are long or that contain parts that are separated by commas

  He was outstanding in his knowledge of word processing, database, spreadsheets, and related software applications; however, he was lacking in many desirable personal qualities.

- Between the members of a compound sentence when the conjunction is omitted

  Many executives would rather dictate to a machine than to a secretary; the machine won't talk back.

- To precede expressions used to introduce a clause, such as namely, viz., e.g., and i.e.

  We selected the machine for two reasons; namely, because it is as reasonable in price as any other and because it does better work than others.
  There are several reasons for changing the routine of handling mail; i.e., to reduce postage, to conserve time, and to place responsibility.

- In a series of well-defined units when special emphasis is desired

  Emphatic: The prudent secretary considers the future; he or she ensures that all requirements are obtained, and he or she uses his or her talents to attain the desired goal successfully.
  Less emphatic: The prudent secretary considers the future, ensures that all requirements are obtained, and uses his or her talents to attain the desired goal successfully.

The Colon

The colon is used in the following instances:
- After the salutation in a business letter, except when open punctuation is used

  Ladies and Gentlemen:
  Dear Ms. Carroll:

- Following introductory expressions, such as *the following, thus, as follows,* and other expressions that precede enumerations

  Please send the following by parcel post:
  Officers were elected as follows: president, vice-president, and secretary-treasurer.

- To separate hours and minutes when indicating time

  2:10 PM 4:45 PM 12:15 AM

- To introduce a long quotation

  The agreement read: "We the undersigned hereby agree…"

- To separate two independent groups having no connecting words between them and in which the second group explains or expands the statement in the first group

  We selected the machine for one reason: in competitive tests it surpassed all other machines.

The Question Mark

The question mark (interrogation point) is used in the following instances:
- After each direct question

  When do you expect to arrive in Philadelphia?

  An exception to the foregoing rule is a sentence that is phrased in the form of a question, merely as a matter of courtesy, when it is actually a request.

  Will you please send us an up-to-date statement of our account.

- After each question in a series of questions within one sentence

  What is your opinion of the IBM word processor? the Xerox? the CPT?

The Exclamation Point

The exclamation point is used ordinarily after words or groups of words that express command, strong feeling, emotion, or an exclamation.

  Don't waste office supplies!
  It can't be done!
  Stop!

The Dash

The dash is used in the following instances:
- To indicate an omission of letters or figures

  Dear Mr.—   Date the letter July 16, 20—

- Sometimes in letters, especially sales letters, to cause a definite stop in reading the letter

  This book is not a revision of an old book—it is a brand new book.

  Usually the dash is used in such cases for increased emphasis. One must be careful, however, not to overdo the use of the dash.
- To separate parenthetical expressions when unusual emphasis is desired on the parenthetical expression

  These sales arguments—and every one of them is important—should result in getting the order.

The Apostrophe

The apostrophe should be used in the following instances:
- To indicate possession

  the patient's record
  the dentist's coat
  the assistants' responsibilities
  the dentists' records

- To form the possessive singular, add 's to the noun

  man's work
  bird's wing
  hostess's plans

- An exception to this rule is made when the word after the possessive begins with an *s* sound.

  for goodness' sake
  for conscience' sake

- To form the possessive of a plural noun ending in an *s* or *z* sound, add only the apostrophe to the plural noun.

  workers' rights
  hostesses' duties

- If the plural noun does not end in an *s* or *z* sound, add 's to the plural noun.

  women's clothes
  alumni's donations

- Proper names that end in an *s* sound form the possessive singular by adding 's.

  Williams's house
  Fox's automobile

- Proper names ending in *s* form the possessive plural by adding the apostrophe only.

  The Walters' property faces the Jones' swimming pool.

- To indicate the omission of a letter or letters in a contraction

  it's (it is)
  you're (you are)
  we'll (we shall)

- To indicate the plurals of letters, figures, words, and abbreviations

  Don't forget to dot your i's and cross your t's.
  I can add easily by 2's and 4's, but I have difficulty with 6's and 8's.
  More direct letters can be written by using shorter sentences and by omitting and's and but's.
  Two of the speakers were Ph.D.'s.

Quotation Marks

The following basic rules should be followed when using quotation marks:
- When a quotation mark is used with a comma or a period, the comma or period should be placed inside the quotation mark.

She said, "I plan to complete my program in college before seeking a position."

- When a quotation mark is used with a semicolon or a colon, the semicolon or colon should be placed outside the quotation mark.

The treasurer said, "I plan to go by train"; others in the group stated that they would go by plane.

- When more than one paragraph of quoted material is used, quotation marks should appear at the beginning of each paragraph and at the end of the last paragraph.

"_____
_____
_____
_____
_____.

"_____
_____
_____
_____ "

Quotation marks are used in the following instances:
- Before and after direct quotations

The author states, "Too frequent use of certain words weakens the appeal."

- To indicate a quotation within a quotation, use single quotation marks

The author states, "Too frequent use of 'very' and 'most' weakens the appeal."

- To indicate the title of a published article

Have you read the article, "Automation in the Office?"
He asked, "Have you read 'Automation in the Office'?"

Omission Marks or Ellipses

Ellipses marks (… or ***) are frequently used to denote the omission of letters or words in quoted material. If the material omitted ends in a period, four omission marks are used (….?). If the material omitted is elsewhere in the quoted material, three omission marks are used (…).

He quoted the proverb, "A soft answer turneth away wrath: but. …"
She quoted Plato, "Nothing is more unworthy of a wise man … than to have allowed more time for trifling and useless things than they deserved."

Parentheses

Although parentheses are frequently used as a catchall in writing, they are correctly used in the following instances:
- When amounts expressed in words are followed by figures

He agreed to pay twenty-five dollars ($25) as soon as possible.

- Around words that are used as parenthetical expressions

Our letter costs (excluding paper and postage) are much too high for this type of business.

- To indicate technical references

Sodium chloride (NaCl) is the chemical name for common table salt.

- When enumerations are included in narrative form

The reasons for his resignation were three: (1) advanced age, (2) failing health, and (3) a desire to travel.

CAPITALIZATION*

In addition to understanding the rules for punctuation, it is necessary to review the rules for capitalizing various initials and words. A summary of the rules for capitalization is convenient for reference purposes and is provided as follows.

Common Usage

The following are examples of the most common usage of capitalization:
- The first word of every sentence should be capitalized.
- The first word of a complete direct quotation should be capitalized.
- The first word of a salutation and all nouns used in the salutation should be capitalized.
- The first word in a complimentary close should be capitalized.

Outline Form

Capitalize the first word in each section of an outline form.

First Word After a Colon

Capitalize the first word after a colon only when the colon introduces a complete passage or sentence having independent meaning. In conclusion I wish to say: "The survey shows that…" If the material following a colon is dependent on the preceding clause, the first word after the colon is not capitalized.

I present the following three reasons for changing: the volume of business does not justify the expense; we are short of people; and the product is decreasing in popularity.

---

*This section from Fulton PJ: *General office procedures for colleges*, ed 8, Cincinnati, 1983, South-Western, a part of Cengage Learning, Inc.

Names

- Capitalize the names of associations, buildings, churches, hotels, streets, organizations, and clubs.

  The American Dental Association, Merchandise Mart, Central District Dental Society, Peabody Hotel, Seventh Avenue, Administrative Management Society, Chicago Chamber of Commerce

- Capitalize all proper names.

  Great Britain, John G. Hammitt, Mexico

- Capitalize names that are derived from proper names.

  American, Chinese

- Do not, however, capitalize words that are derived from proper nouns and that have developed a special meaning.

  pasteurized milk, china dishes, moroccan leather

- Capitalize special names for regions and localities.

  North Central states, the Far East, the East Side, the Hoosier State

- Do not, however, capitalize adjectives derived from such names or localities that are used as directional parts of states and countries.

  far eastern lands, the southern United States, southern Illinois

- Capitalize names of government boards, agencies, bureaus, departments, and commissions.

  Civil Service Commission, Social Security Board, Bureau of Navigation

- Capitalize names of the deity (deities), the Bible, holy days, and religious denominations.

  God, Easter, Yom Kippur, Genesis, Church of Christ

- Capitalize the names of holidays.

  Memorial Day, Labor Day

- Capitalize words used before numbers and numerals, with the exception of the common word, such as *page, line,* and *verse.*

  The reservation is Lower 6, Car 27.
  He found the material in Part 3 of Chapter X.

Titles Used in Business and Professions

The following are rules for capitalizing titles in business and professions.

- Any title that signifies rank, honor, and respect, and that immediately precedes an individual's name should be capitalized.

  She asked President Harry G. Sanders to preside.
  He was attended by Dr. Howard Richards.

- Academic degrees should be capitalized when they precede or follow an individual name.

  Constance R. Collins, Ph.D., was invited to direct the program.
  Fred R. Bowling, Master of Arts

- Capitalize titles of high-ranking government officers when the title is used in place of the proper name in referring to a specific person.

  Our Senator invited us to visit him in Washington.
  The President will return to Washington soon.

- Capitalize military titles signifying rank.

  Captain Meyers, Lieutenant White, Lieutenant Commander Murphy

TELEPHONE NUMBERS

There are several ways of entering telephone numbers in a letter. The parentheses method (734) 956-9800 is frequently used, but does not work well in text material when the telephone number as a whole has to be enclosed in parentheses. One reason it is suggested not to use the parentheses is because of the growing use of the mandatory area code where there is a shortage of numbers. In these areas, the use of the parentheses with the telephone number might suggest you would not need to use the area code. Three other methods of entering telephone numbers are 707-555-3998, 707 555 3998, and 707.555.3998. The latter system seems to be gaining popularity as it uses periods or dots to separate the elements. This is because these periods resemble the dots in e-mail addresses.

PREPARING AN EFFECTIVE LETTER

To prepare an effective letter, it is necessary to follow several basic steps:

- Collect the information.
- Make an outline.
- Develop the letter.
- Select a format style.
- Review and revise the letter.
- Produce the letter.
- Proofread the letter.

- Distribute the letter.
- Store the document.

Before beginning each step of letter writing, it is necessary to determine who will receive the letter and what the person knows about the subject. If a letter is to be written to another dentist about a patient, it will require using technical language. On the other hand, if a patient is to receive a letter about an unknown subject, the educational level of the person needs to be determined so the letter can be written in understandable language.

Collecting Information

Before beginning to write the letter, gather the important facts to be included in the letter. In general gather the following information: to whom the letter is being sent, by whom the letter is being written, and the subject of the letter. If it is a letter of referral, the name of the patient and any necessary personal information for which consent has been given, the nature of the problem, any possible symptoms or diagnosis, enclosures if any, anticipated response, deadline dates, and how the patient will contact the office. If it is a letter of inquiry, the nature of the inquiry, product names if available, quantity or specifications of the product, and date of needed reply.

Making an Outline

One may ask, "Why is it necessary to make an outline if I know what I want to say?" After writing several letters, it may be natural to be organized. However, if a beginner or someone who dislikes letter writing, making an outline will provide organization and a framework that forces a person to get his or her thoughts on paper, and in the process it may be discovered that all the needed facts have not been gathered. An outline helps clarify relationships between topics and determine if the letter is written in a logical sequence.

Developing the Letter

It is often said that once the outline is completed, the letter is nearly finished. This is partially true, but give special attention to how each part of the letter is developed and determine its format. A variety of format styles are illustrated in this chapter.

PRACTICE NOTE

 An outline helps you to see relationships between topics and determine if your letter is written in a logical sequence.

As the letter begins to develop, remember that the first paragraph is the most important one of any letter. It should get the reader's attention and set the tone for the letter. This paragraph places the emphasis on the reader and uses the "you" approach. Review each paragraph in the letter to determine if it gets the reader's attention first and clearly states the purpose

---

BOX 9-4 **Special Considerations for Letter Content**

Order Letter
- Indicate the quantity.
- Provide description of the material or product.
- List the price.
- Define the method of payment.
- Indicate the shipping preference.

Referral Letter
- Provide the complete and proper name of patient.
- State the condition and expected type of consultation or examination.
- Always write out tooth names or provide an illustration; avoid using tooth numbers only.
- Refer to enclosures.
- Indicate timeliness if necessary.
- Maintain confidentiality and provide only information for which consent is given.
- Extend courteous expression of appreciation.

Inquiry Letter
- State the objective.
- Give all the necessary facts.
- Close with good will.

Thank-You Letter
- State the purpose.
- Explain your appreciation.
- Maintain confidentiality.
- Close with a sincere expression of good will.

---

of the letter. Make a natural transition from one paragraph to the next. Special consideration should be given to factors such as data and confidentiality that are included in various types of letters. Box 9-4 includes several suggestions for writing various types of letters.

Selecting the Format

The administrative assistant may select a template from the word processing software in the office, but the letter will still require decisions about punctuation styles. Letter style is a personal choice that relates to a particular practice and complements the office stationery most effectively.

Most word processing software provides several templates for a variety of letter styles, which can be modified to meet the dentist's preference and saved in the letter file as a specialized template. Several basic styles are shown in Figure 9-9, including the block style with mixed punctuation, block style with open punctuation, modified block style with mixed punctuation, block style with attention line and enclosure, and the Administrative Management Society (AMS) simplified style. The first styles are self-explanatory.

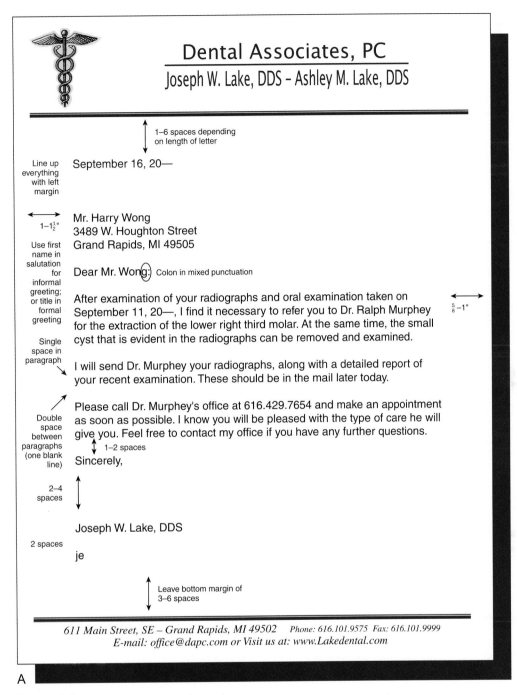

Figure 9-9 A, Block-style letter with mixed punctuation.

(Continued)

The AMS simplified style can be put to good use when informing all patients about a policy change or announcing that an associate will be joining the practice. The style has two basic rules, as follows:

1. The letter must have a subject line. The word *subject* is omitted, and the subject line is keyboarded in all capital letters with a triple space before and after the subject line.

2. The writer's name and title are keyboarded in all capital letters at least four lines below the last line of the letter.

Reviewing the Letter

Once the letter has been written, determine if the letter meets all of the criteria of an effective letter, as described in Box 9-1. If the letter does not meet most of these criteria, take time to

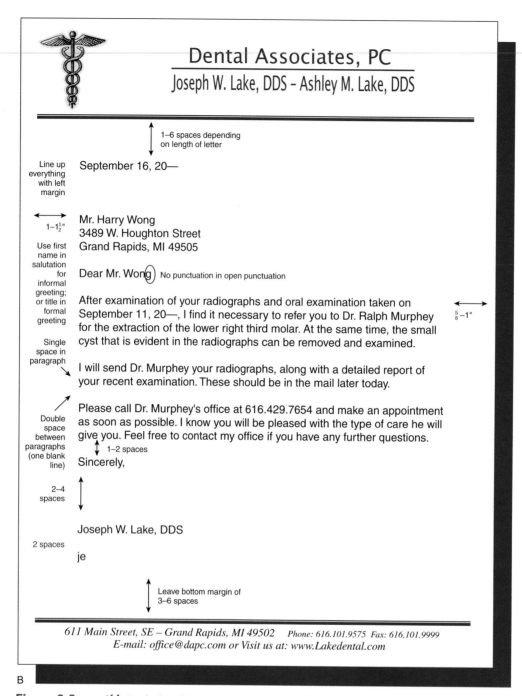

1–6 spaces depending on length of letter

Line up everything with left margin

September 16, 20—

1–1½"

Mr. Harry Wong
3489 W. Houghton Street
Grand Rapids, MI 49505

Use first name in salutation for informal greeting; or title in formal greeting

Dear Mr. Wong No punctuation in open punctuation

After examination of your radiographs and oral examination taken on September 11, 20—, I find it necessary to refer you to Dr. Ralph Murphey for the extraction of the lower right third molar. At the same time, the small cyst that is evident in the radiographs can be removed and examined.

⅝–1"

Single space in paragraph

I will send Dr. Murphey your radiographs, along with a detailed report of your recent examination. These should be in the mail later today.

Double space between paragraphs (one blank line)

Please call Dr. Murphey's office at 616.429.7654 and make an appointment as soon as possible. I know you will be pleased with the type of care he will give you. Feel free to contact my office if you have any further questions.

1–2 spaces

Sincerely,

2–4 spaces

Joseph W. Lake, DDS

2 spaces

je

Leave bottom margin of 3–6 spaces

611 Main Street, SE – Grand Rapids, MI 49502   Phone: 616.101.9575 Fax: 616.101.9999
E-mail: office@dapc.com or Visit us at: www.Lakedental.com

B

Figure 9-9, cont'd B, Block-style letter with open punctuation.

modify it. If unsure about a letter, ask another person to review and evaluate it. Make the necessary changes until all criteria are met.

Producing the Final Letter

Before the final printing of the letter, use spell-check and grammar-check, if available. Whether the letter is created on a typewriter or electronically using word processing software, the letter needs to be produced on quality stationery that creates a professional image of the office.

Proofreading the Letter

Do not rely completely on an electronic system to proofread a letter. Although software packages provide spell-check, many

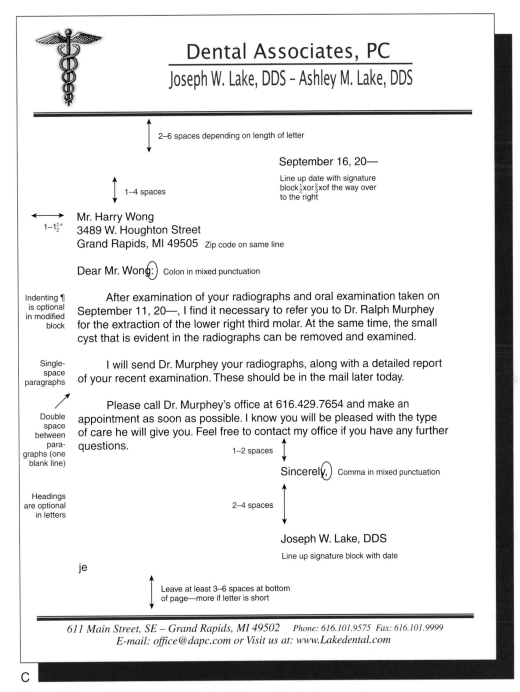

Dental Associates, PC

Joseph W. Lake, DDS – Ashley M. Lake, DDS

2–6 spaces depending on length of letter

September 16, 20—

Line up date with signature block $\frac{1}{2}$x or $\frac{2}{3}$x of the way over to the right

1–4 spaces

1–1$\frac{1}{2}$"

Mr. Harry Wong
3489 W. Houghton Street
Grand Rapids, MI 49505   Zip code on same line

Dear Mr. Wong: Colon in mixed punctuation

Indenting ¶ is optional in modified block

After examination of your radiographs and oral examination taken on September 11, 20—, I find it necessary to refer you to Dr. Ralph Murphey for the extraction of the lower right third molar. At the same time, the small cyst that is evident in the radiographs can be removed and examined.

Single-space paragraphs

I will send Dr. Murphey your radiographs, along with a detailed report of your recent examination. These should be in the mail later today.

Double space between paragraphs (one blank line)

Please call Dr. Murphey's office at 616.429.7654 and make an appointment as soon as possible. I know you will be pleased with the type of care he will give you. Feel free to contact my office if you have any further questions.

1–2 spaces

Sincerely,   Comma in mixed punctuation

Headings are optional in letters

2–4 spaces

Joseph W. Lake, DDS

Line up signature block with date

je

Leave at least 3–6 spaces at bottom of page—more if letter is short

611 Main Street, SE – Grand Rapids, MI 49502   Phone: 616.101.9575 Fax: 616.101.9999
E-mail: office@dapc.com or Visit us at: www.Lakedental.com

C

Figure 9-9, cont'd C, Modified-block-style letter with mixed punctuation.

(Continued)

dental terms are not in the dictionary, unless they have been inserted. Likewise, English words are often misused, such as *there* or *their.* Both of these words will come up as correct, but may have been misused. Not all word processing systems can be relied on for complete grammar accuracy. Therefore, make a final review of the letter to be certain the grammar, spelling, and punctuation are correct. Proofreading a letter is much like the final check of the margins on an amalgam restoration. It is an individual creation, and it should be perfect.

 PRACTICE NOTE
Do not rely completely on an electronic system to proofread letters.

Distributing the Letter

There are several methods of distributing the letter: E-mail, traditional postal services, fax, or some form of specialized mail service. Each of these is explained in detail later in this chapter.

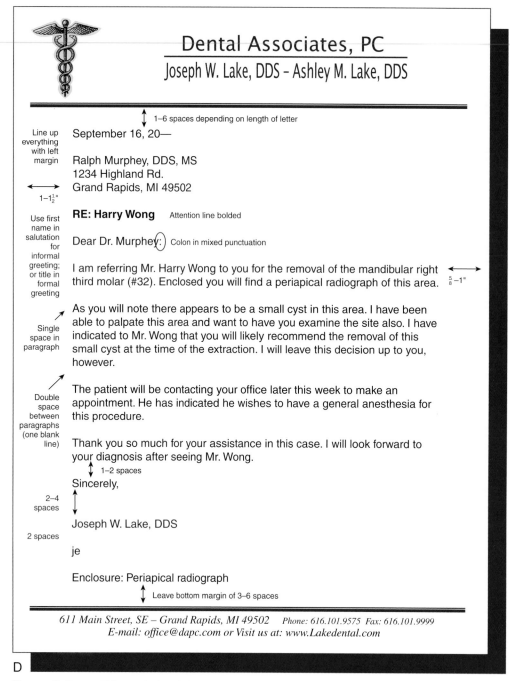

Figure 9-9, cont'd D, Block-style letter with attention line and enclosure.

Before creating the letter, be aware of the method of distribution to determine the type of envelope or mailing label necessary for production.

is appropriate for the document. Remember, if striving for the paperless office, maximize the use of the electronic filing system.

Storing the Document

If the letter is to be stored electronically, the procedure discussed in Chapter 8 should be followed. If not, a hard copy should be made and filed in the patient record or other location that

PREPARING THE ENVELOPE

It is possible to prepare the envelope as part of the word processing procedure, or the envelope may be keyboarded on a typewriter. Larger mailing envelopes may require special

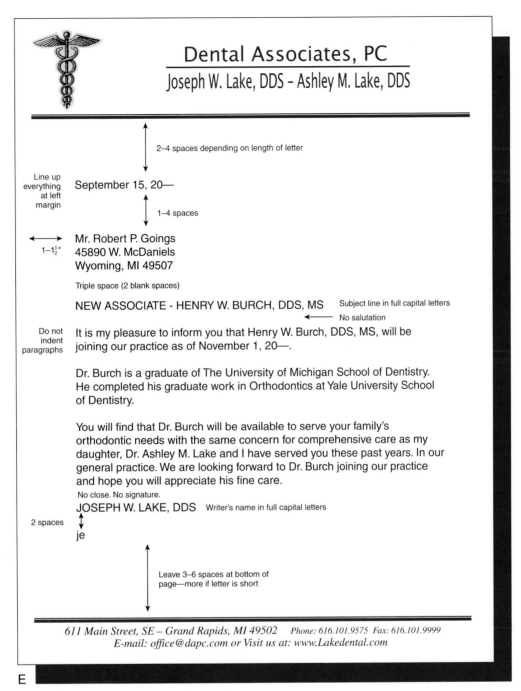

Figure 9-9, cont'd E, Administrative Management Society (AMS) simplified style.

labeling. In either case, it is necessary to prepare the envelope or package with a standardized delivery address. Most postal services use automatic sorting equipment, which begins an automatic sorting process with an optical character reader (OCR). A standardized address, readable by an OCR, contains the correct city name, state, and zip+4 code. To obtain Zip codes for any address, visit the U.S. Postal Service web site at www.usps.com, and select the Zip code navigation bar. The address on the envelope should agree with the inside address of the letter, although the inside address may contain punctuation not recommended by the postal service for the envelope.

The address should be single-spaced, even if the address is only two lines. In this case, the name of the individual or firm is on the first line, and the city, state, and Zip code are on the second line. The two-letter state abbreviations, approved and recommended by the U.S. Postal Service, should be used. These abbreviations appear in Box 9-5. For further information,

BOX 9-5

Two-Letter Abbreviations for States

Alabama	AL	Montana	MT
Alaska	AK	Nebraska	NE
Arizona	AZ	Nevada	NV
Arkansas	AR	New Hampshire	NH
California	CA	New Jersey	NJ
Colorado	CO	New Mexico	NM
Connecticut	CT	New York	NY
Delaware	DE	North Carolina	NC
District of Columbia	DC	North Dakota	ND
Florida	FL	Ohio	OH
Georgia	GA	Oklahoma	OK
Hawaii	HI	Oregon	OR
Idaho	ID	Pennsylvania	PA
Illinois	IL	Rhode Island	RI
Indiana	IN	South Carolina	SC
Iowa	IA	South Dakota	SD
Kansas	KS	Tennessee	TN
Kentucky	KY	Texas	TX
Louisiana	LA	Utah	UT
Maine	ME	Vermont	VT
Maryland	MD	Virginia	VA
Massachusetts	MA	Washington	WA
Michigan	MI	West Virginia	WV
Minnesota	MN	Wisconsin	WI
Mississippi	MS	Wyoming	WY
Missouri	MO		

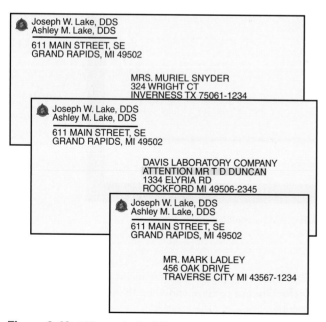

Figure 9-10 Address styles for different size envelopes. Note placement of attention line.

request Publication 28, Postal Addressing Standards, from the local Postal Business Center or online at www.usps.gov. Figure 9-10 illustrates how an address should be keyboarded on various business envelopes.

Other important elements of the address are suffixes, directionals, apartment or suite numbers, post office box numbers, and complete rural/highway contract route addresses with box numbers. All of these elements must be spelled correctly and clearly written. If the address is not electronically readable, the letter or package will be delayed for manual handling. If the Zip+4 code is not known, it can be obtained at www.usps.gov.

Address Format

Using the universal format for addresses expedites the processing capability of automated equipment at the post office. The format requires that the use of a uniform left margin. Type the address in uppercase letters as follows:

MS MARY BALL
3347 MAPLE RD
ROCKFORD MI 48167-2345

A secondary address unit, such as an apartment (APT) or suite (STE) number, should be printed as part of the address. Always use APT or STE rather than the # (pound) sign. Common designations are APT, BLDG FLOOR (FL), STE, UNIT, ROOM (RM), and DEPARTMENT (DEPT). Using this format, the address line might appear as follows:

1334 RIVERSIDE APT 201
or
3745 KINSEY DR STE 301
or
845 KELSAY BLVD BLDG 5
or
1234 KELLOGG PL RM 136

If the letter or package is sent to the attention of an individual, that information precedes the line of the name of the firm or building. The attention line varies from the traditional format that many people have used. For example:

ATTN: MS MARY CLINE
ACME DENTAL COMPANY
134 FLETCHER
CUTLERVILLE MI 49504-2345

Avoid using dual addresses, even though both a box number and street address may be available. Place the delivery address on the line immediately above the city, state, and zip+4 code.

Punctuation on Address Labels

The U.S. Postal Service prefers that punctuation, special characters, or multiple blanks in the address are not used, with the exception of a hyphen in the zip+4 code or a hyphen that appears in the primary number of the delivery address, such as 51-234 HANCOCK ST. Spell out city names completely. If an abbreviation must be used because of labeling/space constraints, use existing abbreviations first for suffix or directional words. For instance:

EAST MARKET becomes E MARKET
JEFFERSON MOUNTAIN becomes JEFFERSON MT

The eight standard directionals can be abbreviated to one or two characters. For instance:

255 NW WASHINGTON ST
133 CHERRY DR S

If the first word in a street name is a directional word and no other directional is to the left of it, abbreviate it. For example:

NORTH CHERRY ST becomes N CHERRY ST
or
LAKE DRIVE WEST becomes LAKE DRIVE W

When two directional words appear before the street name, the first one is abbreviated:

NORTH EAST SUGAR ST becomes N EAST SUGAR ST

Folding and Inserting the Letter

After all enclosures have been checked to be certain they correspond to the letter and the items are correct, the letters must be signed and it must be ensured that the right letter gets into the right envelope. (Letters get into the wrong envelopes surprisingly often.) The letter is placed into the envelope so that the date and inside address are visible upon opening the letter. The reader should not be forced to turn the paper around to begin reading the letter. Figure 9-11 illustrates a step-by-step procedure for folding and inserting the letter in the proper size envelope.

ELECTRONIC MAIL (E-MAIL)

Basic Considerations

With the wide use of computers today, electronic mail (e-mail) has opened the doors to sending mail between computers within networked locations. E-mail within a large clinic or dental school has become the choice for sending memoranda to the staff. With more patients having e-mail, this becomes another source of communication between the office and patient. As mentioned in Chapter 7, attention should be given to including a patient's e-mail address on the personal questionnaire on admission and asking the patient if this is a mode of communication he or she would prefer to use. Some patients may even indicate that text messaging is also an option for them to receive messages. The patient's e-mail can be integrated into various software programs and may even be used to confirm appointments or act as a reminder for routine recalls. E-mail has many advantages as a communication tool, as follows:

- E-mail reaches its destination in a matter of seconds after it is sent, even if its destination is across the world.
- Multiple individuals may be sent the same message quickly, with all the recipients receiving the message instantly.
- Paper is saved. It is not necessary to make a hard copy of e-mail.
- E-mail may be filed electronically for later reference.
- E-mail may be forwarded to another party.
- E-mail may be destroyed immediately after it is read.
- E-mail takes less time to write than a paper letter. Only the receiver's name, the sender's name, and the body of the letter need to be entered. The date and time is entered automatically, and the letter or envelope does not need to be printed.
- Other documents and graphic images may be transferred as attachments through e-mail.
- The recipient is notified of the arrival of an e-mail by a message that appears at the bottom of the computer screen or an audio signal that is emitted through the computer.
- A hard copy of the e-mail may be printed if necessary for retention in a manual file.
- Notations such as "confidential" and "urgent" can be made on the e-mail message.

As with any new system, a person often overlooks the need to follow basic protocol. E-mail should not become a quick system for communication with no concern given to punctuation or formatting.

 PRACTICE NOTE
E-mail should not become a quick system for communication with no concern given to punctuation or formatting.

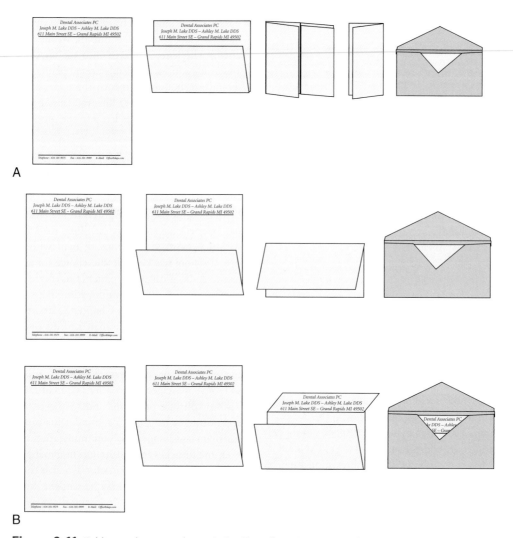

A

B

Figure 9-11 Folding and inserting letter. **A,** Small envelope. **B,** Large envelope.

Consider the following guidelines when using e-mail:
- Be certain to think about the purpose of the e-mail before beginning to write; in other words, know what is wanted to achieve with the e-mail message.
- Be succinct. Before sending an e-mail, reread it. Delete unnecessary phrases, words, or sentences.
- Be polite. Think of an e-mail as a short letter, and follow etiquette rules. Use *please* and *thank you.*
- Be suitably formal when writing e-mail. The rule of thumb is to be almost as formal in e-mail as in standard memorandums to an employer, coworkers, or patients.
- Always capitalize the appropriate words, be specific about needs, and use proper closing.
- Use the subject line that is provided on the e-mail form. This line should be concise yet convey the purpose of the message to the reader.
- If replying to a message but changing the subject of conversation, change the subject also.

- Edit and proofread carefully. Do not send an e-mail that contains inaccuracies or incorrect grammar.
- Use complete sentences.
- Capitalize and punctuate properly.
- Do not run sentences together; it is difficult to read e-mail constructed in this manner.
- Insert the nature of the message on the subject line.
- Include a salutation.
- Use a colon after the salutation. A comma can be used in a nonbusiness application.
- Use complete sentences and paragraph structure.
- Check the letter for spelling and grammatical errors.
- Insert a blank line after each paragraph.
- Always include the sender's name and title (if appropriate) when replying to an e-mail.
- Assume that any message sent is permanent. The message can be sitting in someone's private file or in a tape archive.

E-mail Ethics and Etiquette

There is a growing body of ethical issues in regard to e-mail. Some organizations have developed a code of ethics for using e-mail. This form of communication should follow the same ethical guidelines used in any form of written communication in the dental office. Box 9-6 provides a checklist of items to help guide users in the ethical use of e-mail.

The contents of an e-mail can be retained as a permanent record, so anything that you do not wish to be documented in writing should not be entered into an e-mail message. Users should be mindful of the following:

- Confidentiality must be maintained.
- Rules of courtesy should be followed.
- An appropriate closing should be included.

In addition, e-mail and e-mail attachments can be used as an alternative to dictation equipment, discussed later in this chapter. A dentist may wish to keyboard a document and not dictate it. This is often easier than handwriting. This could be done in word processing and sent to the administrative assistant via e-mail. The administrative assistant can download the document, print it, and store it in the appropriate file.

OTHER TYPES OF WRITTEN COMMUNICATION

Other types of written communication routinely prepared by the administrative assistant include postal cards, interoffice memorandums, and manuscripts. For many of these documents, there are templates available that aid in formatting and eliminate the steps of setting up the document.

Postal Cards

There will be times in a dental office when it is more practical to send a patient a postal card (e.g., for recall or confirmation of an appointment) rather than to write a letter. Figure 9-12 illustrates how a postal card should be addressed and the placement for the message.

Interoffice Memoranda

Although most office correspondence is keyboarded on office letterhead, the interoffice memorandum is a timesaving form and is entered on plain paper (Figure 9-13). This type of communication is often used within a clinic or group practice or within a professional building where several dental offices are located. The form provides space for the name of the department or individual(s) to whom the memorandum is being sent, the date, subject or reference line, and space for the sender's name. The memorandum should be brief, clearly stated, well-organized, and easy to read. A copy of the memorandum should be made for the office files. If several people are to receive the memorandum, their names are inserted in the space provided, or additional copies are made and the individual names entered on each memorandum.

Manuscripts

In the first part of this chapter, emphasis was placed on general correspondence. In both the academic and health environments, the administrative assistant may be asked to write a report or research paper for the employer. Such reports could range from a business proposal to a research paper. Whether writing a business report or an academic report, follow standard style when preparing it.

BOX 9-6 Guidelines to Promote Ethics and Etiquette with E-mail

- Do not send personal e-mail from an office computer.
- When people send inappropriate e-mail, let them know politely that it cannot be received.
- Do not use e-mail to berate or reprimand an employee or patient.
- Do not use e-mail to send information that involves any type of legal action; third parties who should have no knowledge of the action may obtain the information.
- Do not forward junk mail or chain letters.
- Do not forward an e-mail unless it is known to be true.
- Do not include credit card numbers.
- Do not forward confidential patient information.
- Do not criticize or insult third parties.
- Do not use e-mail to send information that might involve legal action.

- Be cautious about using different types of fonts, colors, clip art, and other graphics in e-mail. It clutters the message and may be difficult for the reader to view.
- Do not write in all CAPITALS.
- Avoid sending messages when angry.
- Observe the Golden Rule in cyberspace; treat others as you would like to be treated.
- Act responsibly when sending e-mail or posting messages to a discussion group.
- Use a style and tone that are appropriate to the intended recipient(s).
- Before replying to an e-mail, ask if a reply is really necessary.
- Read the e-mail before sending it.
- Use a meaningful subject.
- Answer e-mail promptly.

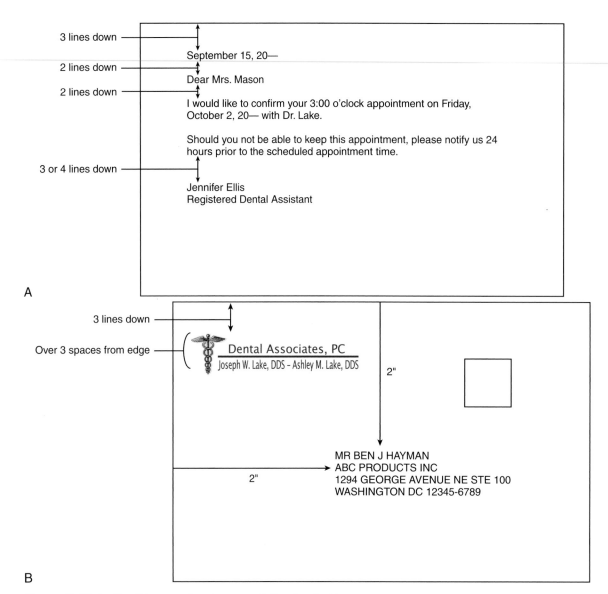

3 lines down

September 15, 20—

2 lines down

Dear Mrs. Mason

2 lines down

I would like to confirm your 3:00 o'clock appointment on Friday, October 2, 20— with Dr. Lake.

Should you not be able to keep this appointment, please notify us 24 hours prior to the scheduled appointment time.

3 or 4 lines down

Jennifer Ellis
Registered Dental Assistant

A

3 lines down

Over 3 spaces from edge

Dental Associates, PC
Joseph W. Lake, DDS – Ashley M. Lake, DDS

2"

MR BEN J HAYMAN
ABC PRODUCTS INC
1294 GEORGE AVENUE NE STE 100
WASHINGTON DC 12345-6789

2"

B

Figure 9-12 **A,** 5½ × 3½-in. postal card message. **B,** Postal card address.

Many styles exist for manuscript preparation, depending on the nature of the report. Each style requires the same basic information. For example, one style may use the term *bibliography,* whereas another uses *references,* and a third prefers *works cited.* Although a publisher may provide the author with a format for a manuscript, a popular documentation style used today for research papers is presented by the Modern Language Association (MLA), as shown in Figure 9-14. When preparing a paper, adhere to some form of documentation style. Therefore, if none are given it is wise to select the MLA style, which is summarized in Box 9-7.

Dictation and Transcription

Some dentists prefer to use dictation and transcription equipment as part of a written communication system. The use of dictation and transcription equipment (Figure 9-15) has become a vital link between the dentist and the administrative assistant. Studies show that machine dictation is six times faster than longhand and almost three times faster than shorthand. After considering the many advantages of dictation equipment, its importance in the word processing system can be easily recognized in the increase of both input and output.

INTEROFFICE MEMORANDUM

TO: Jennifer Ellis, RDA

FROM: Dr. Ashley Lake

SUBJECT: Reassignment to business manager position

DATE: October 19, 20--

For some time I have been thinking that we should promote you to the position of office manager. After our discussion last Friday, I would like to confirm this reassignment. Both my father and I feel that you have considerable expertise in patient management and have excelled in the recent courses in small business management in which you have been enrolled. Both of us would like to discuss this transition with you.

Let's meet on Friday, October 25, at 2 P.M. to discuss this matter. If this date is inconvenient for you, please let me know.

Figure 9-13 Interoffice memorandum. (Note that image is not to size; this memo would be placed on a letter-size piece of paper.)

At the conclusion of the workday or between patients, the dentist may use the dictation equipment for referral letters or for recording information to be transferred to clinical records, etc.

Effective dictation requires following a few guidelines:

- Indicate the message disposition to the transcriber before beginning to dictate the message: the number of copies to be made and to whom the copies are to be sent. If the material has priority over other dictation, this too should be indicated at the beginning. State what is being dictated (e.g., letter, memo, report). Also indicate whether the item is a rough draft or finished product, as well as spacing and margins.
- Spell out any words that might not be easily understood, as well as names, streets, and cities.
- Organize correspondence materials before beginning to dictate.
- Dictate clearly, at an easy pace, and in a conversational tone. Most dictation equipment provides for control of speed and volume, but the fewer adjustments that have to be made, the faster the material will be transcribed.

The administrative assistant can schedule the daily work to include transcription periods to complete correspondence and reports on a priority basis. The following are some guidelines for effective transcription:

- Assemble all materials and necessary equipment.
- Use reference sources such as a dictionary, written communication reference book, spelling and grammar checker and thesaurus, and a name and address file.
- Listen to special instructions on the dictated material to determine priority. Some systems have audible indexing that gives a single tone signal to indicate the end of each document and double tones for special instructions. Determine whether other materials are needed for enclosures or if there are special mailing procedures.
- If the dictation does not make sense or there is a question regarding the information, ask the dentist rather than transcribing incorrect information.
- Proofread the entire transcription before printing the document.

MANAGING OFFICE MAIL

With the increase in written communications in today's dental office, more demands for efficient processing and distribution of both incoming and outgoing mail must be met by the administrative assistant. Because of the constant flow of incoming and outgoing mail, the administrative assistant must know proper techniques for handling the mail.

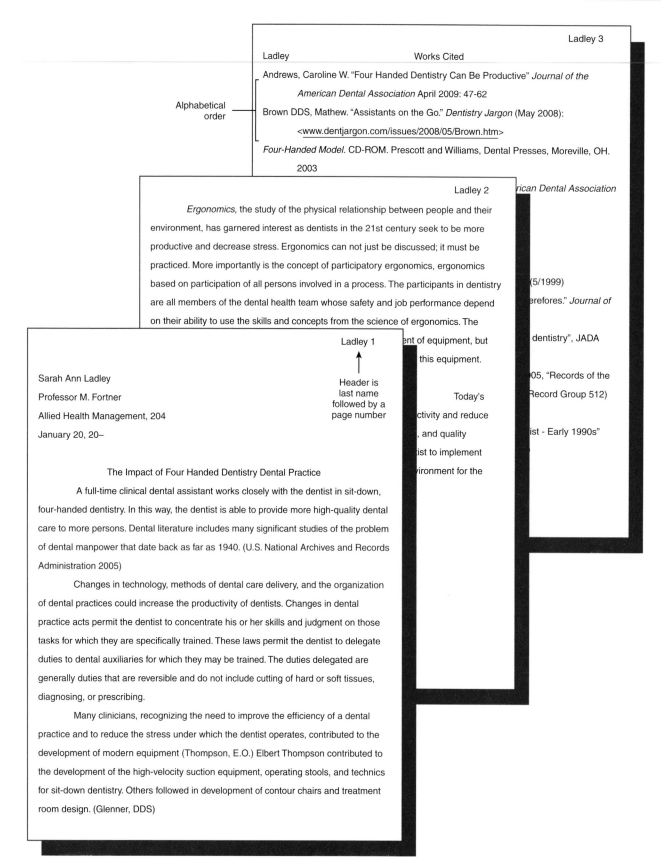

Ladley 3

Ladley   Works Cited

Andrews, Caroline W. "Four Handed Dentistry Can Be Productive" *Journal of the*
American Dental Association April 2009: 47-62

Alphabetical order — Brown DDS, Mathew. "Assistants on the Go." *Dentistry Jargon* (May 2008):
<www.dentjargon.com/issues/2008/05/Brown.htm>

Four-Handed Model. CD-ROM. Prescott and Williams, Dental Presses, Moreville, OH.
2003

Ladley 2

Ergonomics, the study of the physical relationship between people and their
environment, has garnered interest as dentists in the 21st century seek to be more
productive and decrease stress. Ergonomics can not just be discussed; it must be
practiced. More importantly is the concept of participatory ergonomics, ergonomics
based on participation of all persons involved in a process. The participants in dentistry
are all members of the dental health team whose safety and job performance depend
on their ability to use the skills and concepts from the science of ergonomics. The

Ladley 1

Sarah Ann Ladley

Professor M. Fortner

Allied Health Management, 204

January 20, 20–

Header is
last name
followed by a
page number

The Impact of Four Handed Dentistry Dental Practice

A full-time clinical dental assistant works closely with the dentist in sit-down,
four-handed dentistry. In this way, the dentist is able to provide more high-quality dental
care to more persons. Dental literature includes many significant studies of the problem
of dental manpower that date back as far as 1940. (U.S. National Archives and Records
Administration 2005)

Changes in technology, methods of dental care delivery, and the organization
of dental practices could increase the productivity of dentists. Changes in dental
practice acts permit the dentist to concentrate his or her skills and judgment on those
tasks for which they are specifically trained. These laws permit the dentist to delegate
duties to dental auxiliaries for which they may be trained. The duties delegated are
generally duties that are reversible and do not include cutting of hard or soft tissues,
diagnosing, or prescribing.

Many clinicians, recognizing the need to improve the efficiency of a dental
practice and to reduce the stress under which the dentist operates, contributed to the
development of modern equipment (Thompson, E.O.) Elbert Thompson contributed to
the development of the high-velocity suction equipment, operating stools, and technics
for sit-down dentistry. Others followed in development of contour chairs and treatment
room design. (Glenner, DDS)

Figure 9-14 MLA manuscript format. Notice setup for first page, footnotes, and works cited page.

BOX 9-7 Modern Language Association (MLA) Writing Style

- Use 8½ × 11-in. paper.
- Double-space all pages of the paper with 1-in. top, bottom, left, and right margins.
- Indent the first word of each paragraph ½ in. from the left margin.
- At the right margin of each page, place a page number ½ in. from the top margin and 1 in. from the right margin. Double-space between the header and the body. Only use Arabic numbers; do not use pp, p, or the # sign.
- On each page, precede the page number with the author's last name.
- When a quote contains fewer than six lines, set it off with quotation marks and keep it within the normal text, followed by the reference. When a quote contains six or more lines, set it off by indenting it 1 in. from the right and left margins. Check MLA sources for other requirements regarding longer quotes, special circumstances, and quotes within quotes.
- Each figure and table needs to be labeled and numbered. Place the words *figure* or *table* (and the number) a double space before the actual figure or table. Other materials, such as charts, photographs, and drawings, also need to be labeled and numbered, and should include a caption.
- No title page is required. Instead, on the first page only place the author's name on the first line and double space each successive line followed by the instructor's name, the course name and number,

and the date. This should be in a block at the left margin beginning 1 in. from the top of the page.

- Center the title two double spaces below the date and other related information (e.g., the course number). The title's first, last, and principal words should be capitalized. Do not underline, italicize, or use all caps in the title. Do not end with a period. A question or exclamation mark may be used if appropriate.
- Place author references in the body of the paper in parentheses with the page number(s) where the referenced information is located. These parenthetical citations are used instead of footnoting each source at the bottom of the page. Footnotes are used only for explanatory notes. In the body of the paper, use superscripts (raised numbers) to signal that an explanatory note exists. Explanatory notes are optional. If used, the note is placed either at the bottom of the page as a footnote or at the end of the paper as an endnote.
- MLA style uses the term *works cited* for bibliographic references. These are placed on a separate numbered page. Center the title (Works Cited) one inch from the top margin. List references in alphabetic order by each author's last name. Double-space all lines. Works cited from books, journals, magazines, newspapers, letters, online sites, and compact disks each have their own MLA reference style that should be followed.

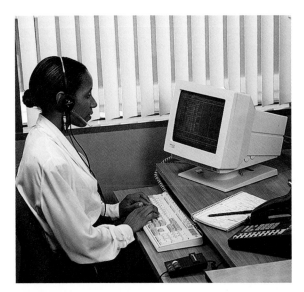

Figure 9-15 Dictation and transcription equipment. (From Young AP: *Kinn's the administrative medical assistant*, ed 6, St. Louis, 2007, WB Saunders.)

Processing Outgoing Mail

Outgoing correspondence may be prepared earlier in the day, but is often organized for mailing at the end of the day, as part of the daily routine.

Classification of Mail

Some of the outgoing mail will be sent as first-class mail, some as fourth class, some insured, and some special handling using the address guidelines in Figure 9-16. The administrative assistant must be aware of these various classes of mail and services available to select the best classification for the type of item being mailed.

Certified Mail

Certified Mail provides a receipt stamped with the date of mailing. A unique article number allows verification of delivery online. As an additional security feature, the recipient's signature is obtained at the time of delivery and a record is maintained by the post office. Certified mail does not include insurance, and is not available for international mail. For valuables and irreplaceable items, it's better to use services such as express mail, insured mail, or registered mail.

Collect on Delivery

Although items may not be shipped from the dental office often, items may be shipped to the office for which the post office must be paid. With Collect on Delivery (COD), the Post Office delivery person will collect payment by cash or check and postage from the addressee for the items being delivered.

Follow these simple guidelines to help mail get where it's going faster.

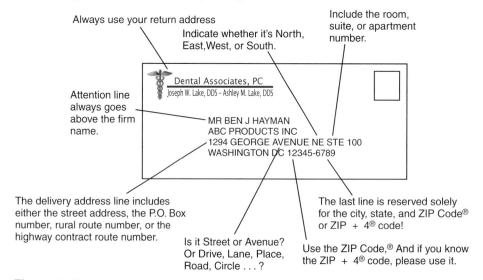

Figure 9-16 Guidelines recommended by the U.S. Postal Service for addressing mail correctly.

Delivery Confirmation

Delivery Confirmation is a special service that provides the date of delivery or attempted delivery for Priority Mail and Standard Mail parcels, Bound Printed Matter and Library Mail. Delivery Confirmation is available at a retail fee and an electronic fee. The retail fee can be purchased at the local post office and uses the fluorescent green Delivery Confirmation label, PS Form 152. Delivery information is available online and by phone (for retail fee customers only).

Express Mail

Express Mail is the postal service's premium delivery service, providing guaranteed overnight delivery for documents and packages weighing up to 70 pounds. Both domestic and international services are offered. This form of mail is automatically insured for $100.

First-Class Mail

First-class is a class of mail including letters, postcards, and all matter sealed or otherwise closed against inspection. This service is required for personal correspondence, handwritten or typewritten letters, and bills or statements of account.

Periodicals

Periodicals describes a class of mail formerly called *second-class mail,* which consists of magazines, newspapers, and other publications.

Insured Mail

This type of mail insures against loss or damage to the articles being mailed. Security is key when sending valuable documents or materials from the office.

Priority Mail

Priority Mail is a 1- to 3-day nonguaranteed delivery service.

Registered Mail

Items sent with Registered Mail are placed under tight security from the point of mailing to the point of delivery, and insured up to $25,000 against loss or damage. The date and time of delivery as well as delivery attempts can be verified online.

Return Receipt

A return receipt is available with Certified or Registered mail when proof of delivery (information about the recipient's signature and actual delivery address) is wanted. A return receipt may be purchased before or after the mailing. A mailer purchasing return receipt service at the time of mailing may choose to receive the return receipt by mail or e-mail. (The e-mail option is available at most post offices. Contact the local post office for availability.)

Signature Confirmation

If mailing something important, the administrative assistant may want to be sure that it reaches not just the right address, but the right hands as well. Signature Confirmation provides confirmation of delivery—including date, time and location. The sender can request to have a letter faxed or mailed to him or her with a copy of the recipient's signature.

Standard Mail

Standard Mail is a mailing service offered for any item, including advertisements and merchandise weighing less than 16 ounces, that is not required to be sent using First-Class Mail. Standard Mail is typically used for multiple delivery addresses and bulk advertising.

Other questions that arise regarding outgoing mail can be answered by checking with the U.S. Postal Service. Manuals are available from the Superintendent of Documents, Government Printing Office, Washington, DC 20402\MDomestic Mail Manual, 19 and International Mail Manual, 14 or by visiting the web site at www.usps.gov.

Mailing Accessories and Methods

Postage Scale

A postage scale, to determine the weight of outgoing mail, is an asset in the dental business office. Mail sent with insufficient postage might be returned to the sender. This causes a delay in delivery of statements to patients and insurance forms to the carrier, thus delaying the return of money to the practice.

Postage Meter

A postage meter can be a timesaving device for the administrative assistant. Although various sizes of postage meters are available, a desk model is practical for a private practice. Group practices and clinics may need a larger meter that feeds envelopes through the machine automatically, both stamping and sealing them. The meters are purchased outright, but the meter mechanism is leased. A meter license is obtained from the U.S. Postal Service. With new electronic models, meter resetting is done by means of a telephone call. All that is needed is an active account with the Postage-by-Phone System and the appropriate meter. No special telephone hookups, computers, or software are required. The customer signs up for the system and then writes a check to put funds into an account to draw on as postage is ordered. Monthly reports listing the account activities are sent to the customer. In keeping with this new technology, postage scales are now available that weigh and automatically determine correct postage rates (Figure 9-17). The accuracy of electronic scales helps to eliminate overpayment in postage. The meter can also be set for the amount of postage required for packages. The amount is printed on a tape, which is then affixed to the package.

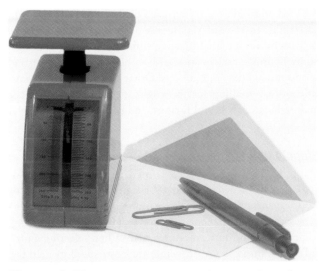

Figure 9-17 Postage scale. (Copyright 2009 JupiterImages Corporation)

Outgoing mail that is addressed correctly, has the proper amount of postage, and is pre-postmarked goes through the post office faster and will arrive at its destination sooner.

E-Mail

Dental practices often make use of e-mail through a computer network system. This is a type of message service (software) that allows users to communicate directly with other users by sending messages electronically over communication channels. E-mail can be used to leave messages for other staff members, and messages are safeguarded because the users must have their own identification code to access the messages. E-mail has gained wide use in processing insurance claim forms. Turnaround time has been greatly reduced, and the result is an increase in cash flow for the office.

Facsimile

Another electronic means of communication is the facsimile (fax) machine. A fax machine is a scanning device that transmits an image of a document over standard telephone lines; it is described in detail in Chapter 10. The dentist may find this method of transmitting written communication very effective when it is necessary to have an immediate response or if the information involves an emergency procedure. The use of such a transmission requires a transmission cover sheet and requires that transmitted information be maintained confidentially.

Mailing Services

Mailing services are service enterprises that specialize in mail communications. A mailing service is an independent postal service that is a complete business center that processes metered and bulk mail, first-class mail, UPS, FedEx, DHL, air freight, and so on. Making use of such a service might be very useful for a dental practice with high-volume mailings. Some mailing services specialize in direct mail advertising, promotional sales, and billings. Other types of services available from a mailing service might include data entry, file maintenance, labels and listings, and personalized letters.

Shipping Providers

Shipping providers, such as United Parcel Service (UPS), FedEx, DHL, Greyhound Package Express, Purolator Courier, and many others, are gaining popularity with businesses that wish letters or packages delivered the next day or need to send fourth-class material. When selecting a provider, it is important to consider the cost, speed of delivery, and convenience. Most providers will require the completion of a special form, and some are even moving toward online generation of this paperwork.

The following list provides information about shipping providers:

- Rates are determined by weight, size of the package, distance to the destination, and required time of delivery.
- Maximum weight varies with carrier.
- Each package will be protected against loss or damage.
- Most general commodities may be shipped.
- Packages to be shipped can be picked up at the dental office or place of business. Deliveries are made to the exact address indicated on the parcel.
- Deliveries are not made to post office boxes.
- Delivery reattempts are typically made at no additional charge.
- The sender is not charged for return of an undeliverable package.
- Shipping providers are available in most areas. Check local listings for providers near you.

Laboratory Services

In areas in which there is no local dental laboratory, cases must be shipped to the laboratory via the U.S. mail or commercial delivery services. The dental laboratory provides a dentist with a sturdy cardboard or plastic, insulated mail carton. All impressions or devices that have been placed in the patient's mouth must be disinfected in compliance with OSHA guidelines before packaging. The contents should be carefully wrapped. The case should be disassembled from articulators and each item wrapped separately to be reassembled when received by the laboratory. The laboratory requisition is enclosed in the box and a mailing label, supplied by the laboratory, is attached to the carton.

Processing Incoming Mail

The location of the dental practice may determine whether the mail is delivered to the office by a regular postal mail carrier or whether a post office box is rented and the mail is picked up at the post office or postal station. For a clinic within an institution, mail may be routed from a central mailroom within the building. Whatever the situation, the administrative assistant is responsible for proper sorting and distribution of the mail.

When the mail is first sorted, distinguish among the various types:

- First-class mail, including priority mail, personal mail, special delivery, registered or certified mail, payments, invoices, and general correspondence
- Printed matter, such as announcements of professional meetings, solicitations for contributions, collegiate newsletters, and other semiprofessional materials
- Magazines and newspapers for the reception room, as well as professional journals and periodicals
- Advertisements
- Samples of dental products and drugs
- Materials from laboratories
- Supplies ordered from a dental supply company

After the initial sorting, distribute the personal mail to the intended receiver and place it so that it will receive prompt attention.

When payments are received, attach the returned portion of the statement, or note on the envelope the amount of money received. Enclosures should be clipped to the letter, invoice, or statement, and all incoming correspondence should be stamped with the date and time received. Many offices find that an automated time-stamp machine, which stamps the date and time received, is practical, especially if a question arises as to the time and date a particular item was received (Figure 9-18). If a time-stamp machine is not

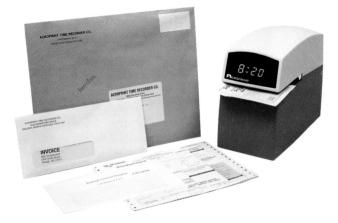

Figure 9-18 Automatic time-stamp machine. (Courtesy Acroprint Time Recorder Co., Raleigh, NC.)

available, then the date and time the correspondence is received have to be written on the correspondence. Also, the administrative assistant may have the responsibility for opening and reading some first-class mail and highlighting the significant portions of the correspondence. When doing so, use a colored pen to make notations. This procedure saves the dentist valuable time when he or she reads through important mail. If the incoming mail item makes reference to previous correspondence, copies of the latter can be attached or clinical records pulled and attached. This will save time when replying and also serves as a reminder of a previous conversation or correspondence. In a group practice or clinic, a routing slip may be used for a piece of correspondence when several people need to be informed of the contents (Figure 9-19). When discarding the envelopes of incoming mail, be sure the entire contents have been removed and all important data, such as company name, individual name, postmark date, and time if significant, have been recorded. The envelope in some situations may even be retained. If an envelope is to be discarded, it should be shredded so that personal information such as return addresses remain confidential.

Some printed material such as meeting notices will be opened by the dentist and should be placed on his or her desk along

with the personal mail. The magazines for the office should be distributed to the reception room and the older issues removed and recycled.

The administrative assistant may be asked to scan the professional magazines and make notes in the margins of special meetings and conferences that may be of interest to the dentist. This saves the dentist's time when reading the magazine.

The dental office receives many advertisements, and many of them are regarded as "junk" mail. It is the administrative assistant's responsibility to sort through the advertisements to determine which material should be examined by the dentist. The dentist will indicate the types of advertisements for review. If the advertisements are of no value, throw them away, always making certain that confidential labels are destroyed properly.

When dental supplies are received in the office through the mail, they need to be processed as soon as possible. This procedure is detailed in the inventory chapter, Chapter 12. Care should be taken, however, to ensure that any MSDSs that accompany the products remain with the products until the materials are checked in, stored, and appropriate labels and data entry are made.

Open any samples received in the mail, and place them on the dentist's desk. Most of these samples accompany literature that should remain with the product.

Extreme care should be taken when opening materials from dental laboratories. Follow appropriate disinfection procedures, inform the dentist of the arrival of a lab case, and then confirm the patient's appointment.

Managing Mail in the Dentist's Absence

When the dentist is away from the office, the administrative assistant is responsible for handling all mail. Decisions will have to be made regarding the following:

- Contacting the dentist regarding any of the correspondence
- Forwarding mail to the dentist
- Answering mail and explaining that the dentist is away from the office
- Determining which correspondence can wait for an answer when the dentist returns

Before the dentist leaves the office for any length of time, a policy regarding handling of mail should be established.

Dental Associates, PC

Joseph W. Lake, DDS - Ashley M. Lake, DDS

INTEROFFICE

ROUTING SLIP

Please read the attached _____
and record the date passed on to the persons indicated.

Refer to:	Date Received	Date Passed on
Dr. Austin	_____	_____
Dr. Baker	_____	_____
Dr. Downing	_____	_____
Dr. Green	_____	_____
Dr. Mann	_____	_____
Dr. Powers	_____	_____
Routed by:	_____	

Figure 9-19 Mail routing slip.

KEY TERMS

Attention line—A line at the beginning of a letter that directs the letter to a particular individual or department within an organization.

Body—The main portion of a letter that include the message.

Complimentary close—A courteous ending to a letter, such as "Sincerely," "Yours truly," or "Sincerely yours."

Copy notation—This informs the recipient to whom copies were sent. Several types of notations are possible, including mail, computer copy, blind copy, postscript, as well as second-page headings.

Date line—The line that contains the date the letter is keyboarded. When using printed letterhead stationery, it usually begins a double space below the lowest line of the letterhead.

E-mail—Electronic mail used to communicate within the office and with external sources.

Inside address—The address that provides all information for mailing the letter and includes the recipient's name, the name of the company (if appropriate), street number and name, city, and zip code.

Interoffice memorandum—Communication within the organization or office.

Keyboarded signature—The name and title of the person sending the letter or communication.

Mixed punctuation—The use of punctuation within a letter; a colon follows the salutation and a comma follows the close.

Open punctuation—The elimination of punctuation after the salutation and the close.

Reference initials—The initials of the person who produced the letter or memo if different than the signature.

Salutation—Formal greeting to the reader.

Subject line—A statement that concisely states what the letter is about.

LEARNING ACTIVITIES

1. List and explain the characteristics of an effective letter.
2. Outline the acceptable format for addressing envelopes.
3. Outline the procedures for sorting incoming mail.
4. List and define the four classifications of mail.
5. Discuss the special mail services that might be used by a dental office.
6. Explain the functions of a postage meter.
7. List the advantages of using a commercial delivery service.
8. Explain a situation that could be handled through a fax process.

Please refer to the student workbook for additional learning activities.

Bibliography

Alred GJ, Brusaw CT, Oliu WE: *The business writer's handbook*, ed 8, New York, 2006, St. Martin's Press.

FedEx service guide, Dallas, 2009, FedEx Corporation.

Fulton-Calkins PJ: *The administrative professional*, ed 13, Mason, OH, 2007, Thomson South-Western.

Gibaldi J: *MLA handbook for writers of research papers*, ed 6, New York, 2003, Modern Language Association of America (for high school and undergraduate students).

Lipson C: *Cite right: a quick guide to citation style-MLA, APA, Chicago, the sciences, professions, and more*, Chicago, 2006, University of Chicago Press.

Locker KO: *Business and administrative communication*, ed 6, New York, 2007, McGraw-Hill/Irwin.

Sabin WA: *The Gregg reference manual*, ed 10, New York, 2004, McGraw-Hill/Irwin.

U.S. Postal Service: *The postal manual*, Washington, DC, 2007, U.S. Government Printing Office.

Recommended Web Sites

www.fedex.com
www.mla.org/style
www.albion.com/netiquette
www.usps.gov

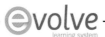

Please visit http://evolve.elsevier.com/Finkibeiner/practice
for additional practice activities.

10 Telecommunications

CHAPTER OUTLINE

Telecommunications in Dentistry
  Telephones
  Pagers
  Personal Digital Assistant
  iPhone
  Instant Messaging System
  Facsimile (FAX) Communication System
  Long Distance Services
  Telephone Directories
Developing Effective Telephone Etiquette
  Speaking Voice
  Creating a Good Image
  Managing Incoming Calls
  Managing Outgoing Calls
  Recording Telephone Messages Carefully
  Personal Telephone Calls
  Cellular Telephone Etiquette
  Telegrams

LEARNING OUTCOMES

- Define key terms.
- Explain the application of telecommunications in a dental office.
- Describe various types of telecommunication systems commonly used by the dental team.
- Practice efficient telephone techniques.
- Receive, transmit, and record telephone messages.
- Plan and place outgoing telephone calls.
- Describe cell phone rules of etiquette.
- Describe the use of text messaging.
- Use the features of special telephone equipment and services.
- Describe the best way to manage telephone calls commonly encountered in the dental office.

A revolution is taking place in the field of telecommunications. Trying to keep up with the latest devices in telecommunications is like trying to keep up with all the new brands of composite restorative materials in clinical dentistry. New telecommunications models are being introduced rapidly. Therefore the materials presented here represent the current concepts, although a newer model may have been introduced only yesterday. It is up to the administrative assistant in a busy dental office to complete the research on the most current models and determine the application of the latest telecommunications technology for the office.

If the patient is the most important person in the dental office, then certainly one can say that telecommunications is the most important equipment system in the office. In the past the telephone alone was the most common communication instrument for society. Modern telecommunications is now the most important communication system in the world because it is perhaps the fastest and easiest way to transmit messages.

Considerable attention is paid to choosing modern equipment for the dental treatment rooms, hiring assistants highly skilled in business concepts or clinical procedures, and using the latest technological advances in diagnosis. Yet the most important instrument in the office, the telephone, is often taken for granted and receives less consideration.

 PRACTICE NOTE
The telephone is the most important piece of equipment in the office.

For more than 90% of the patients in a dental office, the first contact is made by telephone. Like it or not, there is no second chance to make a first impression. Thus telephone management should not be entrusted to an inexperienced staff member. This responsibility should be delegated only to a person who has a broad knowledge of dentistry, possesses a high degree of self-confidence, is alert, is able to make decisions, and shows good verbal communication skills. Speaking with a smile in the voice, being enthusiastic, and having a cordial manner may not solve all problems automatically, but speaking with hostility or disinterest ensures that future communications with patients will be more difficult (Figure 10-1).

 PRACTICE NOTE
For 90% of the patients in a dental office, the first contact is made by telephone.

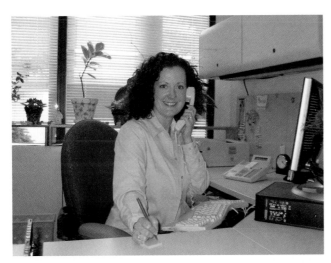

Figure 10-1 A voice that makes the caller feel as though a smile is coming through the receiver is a winning voice.

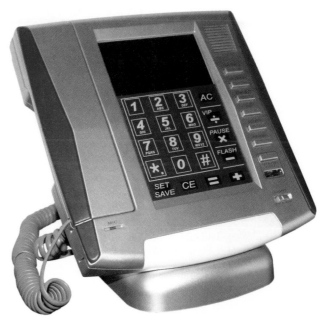

Figure 10-2 A basic, easy-to-use telephone systems for small businesses includes features such as a built-in speakerphone for convenience and the ability to establish three-way conference calls. (Copyright 2009 Beth van Trees. Image from BigStockPhoto.com.)

TELECOMMUNICATIONS IN DENTISTRY

The term **telecommunications** refers to the science and technology of communication by electronic transmission of impulses, as by telegraphy, cable, telephone, radio, or television. In a practical sense, telecommunications in a dental office refers to the different kinds of telephone systems and communication that result from the use of the telephone lines. This chapter discusses the various types of telephone systems, such as key systems, cellular phones, hands-free telephones, conference calls, answering machines, and pagers. It also discusses how to manage communication using these systems.

Telephones

With the array of specialized telephone equipment now available, the dental staff can take advantage of state-of-the-art equipment to become more efficient. For a modest price, dental business owners can buy sophisticated telephone systems that can improve the productivity and profitability of their enterprise. Telephone companies and agencies usually are very accommodating in helping businesses determine their needs for telephone equipment and making recommendations. Various types of equipment also can be explored at product web sites (e.g., www.lucent.com). The equipment and services listed in the following can be useful in the dental office:

- Integrated business communication systems offer features designed for a small business such as a dental practice. A system such as the one shown in Figure 10-2 automatically redials the last outside number dialed at the touch of a button; easily establishes a three-way conference call with the conference button; and, on most system phones, allows dialing and talking without picking up the handset. It includes basic transfer and hold functions, as well as programming of multiple numbers to allow speed dialing of frequently called numbers. Information can be displayed

in multiple languages such as English, French, or Spanish. An alternative version of this system provides most of the same features but includes multiple handsets with only one base charger. A dentist may feel that only a basic, traditional telephone is required; however, a versatile telephone system with the features described allows more efficient handling of the many telephone calls the office receives daily.

Communications can be improved from one area of the office or clinic to another through the paging and intercom features of this system. With single-button access, the person to be contacted can be reached quickly. Often the individual can answer intercom calls without touching the phone or interrupting work.

- PC-linked telecommunications systems let businesses manage incoming and outgoing calls, organize personal information, and store patient information (e.g., telephone numbers) in a database file that can be retrieved for autodialing. It also allows programming of phones from a personal computer (Figure 10-3).

With this type of computer-telephone integration, incoming calling information can be used to provide an automatic pop-up window on a personal computer that displays a caller's database file; this allows the administrative assistant to greet the caller by name and have detailed information readily available for answering questions. This system brings the efficiency and productivity of advanced telecommunications technology to small and medium-size businesses.

- Cordless telephone systems provide an extended mobility range in the office (Figure 10-4). This allows staff members

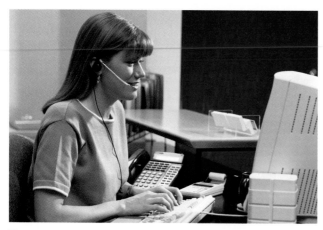

Figure 10-3 A telecommunications system linked to personal computers provides rapid access to patient data.

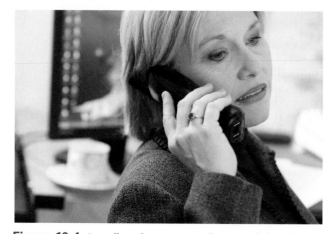

Figure 10-4 A cordless phone systems allow extended mobility in the dental office. (Copyright 2009 JupiterImages Corporation.)

to leave the base station and communicate with other areas without having to use answering machines or voicemail or play telephone tag.

- A mobile or cellular phone (cell phone) is a portable communication device (Figure 10-5). When a dentist or staff member needs to maintain contact with a central location while driving from one place to another, cellular technology makes it possible to use a fully functional telephone. This technology breaks down a large service area into smaller areas, called *cells*. Each cell is served by a low-powered receiver-transmitter. As the mobile caller moves from one cell to another, a switching office automatically moves the call in corresponding fashion. The mobile telephone switching office communicates with a land-based subscriber to complete mobile calls to fixed locations serviced by telephone lines.
- A hands-free telephone allows the administrative assistant to work on the computer, access records, or perform some other task while talking on the telephone. This time-saving device is becoming very popular in clinics and private dental offices. The concept of a hands-free system can be carried into other methods of communication (e.g., pagers and walkie-talkie types of systems), allowing staff members to obtain messages from other areas of the office without using a keyboard or dialing system (Figure 10-6).

Selecting a Telephone System

When a telephone service is selected for an office or when an existing service is changed, consultation with a telecommunications professional from the company responsible for service to the office may be required. Several factors should be considered in the purchase of a telephone system, including cost, flexibility,

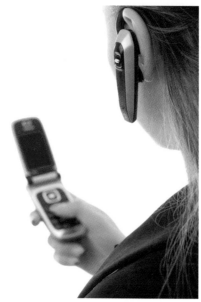

Figure 10-5 Cellular phones allow dentists and staff members to communicate while outside of the dental office. Some advanced cellular models include additional features such as multimedia access or the ability to capture and send or receive digital images. (Copyright 2009 JupiterImages Corporation.)

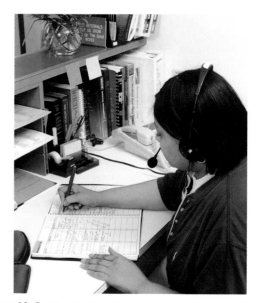

Figure 10-6 A hands-free telephone system allows the administrative assistant to perform other tasks while speaking on the telephone. (From Young AP: *Kinn's the administrative medical assistant*, ed 6, St Louis, 2007, Saunders.)

mobility, and future expansion. Before consulting with a telephone specialist, it is wise to do a task analysis to determine present and future needs.

Cost generally is the primary factor in selecting a telephone system. Today telephones can be purchased at a variety of stores. However, be certain that the system purchased is from a reliable source that will provide support when needed. The telephone market is cost competitive, but costs can vary considerably. Before selecting a system, examine the specifications carefully to determine the cost of the standard features and the cost of each of the optional features. Also, be sure to consider the cost of operating and maintaining the system. A reliable system often saves money in future maintenance. In some areas suppliers provide maintenance contracts as insurance for multiple service calls.

Flexibility should also be a major consideration. Expansion or updating of the telephone system must be possible as the practice grows. The ability to move telephones between systems and facilities is also important.

Voice and data switching capabilities are important considerations. A dental office staff must be sure that a telephone system can meet existing and future needs. For instance, a system equipped with data handling capabilities allows for data transmission and reception between users and equipment, such as computers linked to the system.

Telephone Features

As noted, telephones offer a multitude of features, from the very basic to the highly technical. The following sections describe some of the basic features.

Speakerphone. The dentist may find the hands-free speakerphone feature very convenient. With most systems, with just a push of a button the speaker's voice is picked up by a microphone and is heard anywhere in the office. The handset need not be picked up, and the volume of the loudspeaker is adjustable. The speakerphone function can be canceled, even in the middle of a conversation, by picking up the handset. Speakerphones are particularly valuable for group meetings.

Voicemail Messaging. Voicemail messaging, or phone mail, uses advanced recording and routing functions to combine the features of a telephone, a computer, and a recording device. This feature can be learned quickly and is simple to use. The only equipment needed is a touch-tone telephone.

Users of **voicemail** can dial their voice mailboxes at any time, regardless of the location. A caller may hear previously recorded messages or may leave a message with such options as replaying the message, erasing it, adding to it, sending it by normal or urgent delivery, switching the call to another line, or having it directly recorded to a voice mailbox. Dental office applications include voice-recorded daily updates of office activities and directions to callers on ways to obtain emergency care.

The dentist usually decides which type of message service meets the particular needs of the practice. Alternatives to voicemail could include an answering machine or answering service.

The stand-alone answering machine differs from voicemail in that it does not have the option of sending messages to various locations. However, callers can leave a message and receive information from the office.

An answering service with operator-answered calls can be used when patients call after office hours, on weekends, or on scheduled days off. The answering service operator informs the caller where the dentist can be reached for emergencies or takes the information from the caller and then notifies the dentist. This type of service is frequently used in an oral surgery practice, in which the likelihood of emergencies is greater than in a general practice.

Regardless of whether a voicemail system or a separate automatic answering device is used, some basic courtesies must be observed:

- If an answering machine is used, turn it on before leaving the office.
- In the outgoing message, indicate that the caller has reached an answering system. Give the name of the office, not the telephone number, so the caller knows she or he has reached the correct office.
- Give clear information about office hours or ways to contact the dentist.
- Ensure that the answering message includes specific information about emergency contacts.
- Make sure the caller has adequate time to record a message.
- Arrange to have messages checked periodically by the doctor or a staff member if the administrative assistant is out of the office over a period of time.
- Upon returning to the office, check the calls on the voicemail or recorder.
- Take care of any necessary follow-up to the recorded calls. Most systems allow the user to access the answering machine or voice mailbox to receive messages even when off site.
- Update the outgoing messages regularly.
- Do not leave nonprofessional messages that may distract the caller.

Conference Calls. If the dentist needs to talk to several people in various locations simultaneously, a **conference call** may be placed. Such a call is arranged through a conference call operator, who is given the names and telephone numbers of the individuals included in the call and the time the call should be made. With special equipment, several people can hear and participate in the call at each location.

Caller ID. The **caller ID** feature can help identify a caller before the telephone is answered by displaying the number of the telephone from which the person is calling. A number may be blocked from appearing by pressing a special key.

Call Forwarding. A telephone call can be automatically forwarded to another telephone number with **call forwarding**.

Call Holding. **Call holding** is frequently used in dental offices, which often receive calls in rapid succession. This feature allows answering a second call while the first caller "holds"

BOX 10-1 **Using Call Holding**

- Excuse oneself from the first caller before answering a second call.
- Greet the second caller with the standard office greeting.
- If the second caller requires only a short response, complete the call and return to the first caller.
- If the second caller appears to need more extensive assistance, explain that there is another call, ask the caller if he or she can wait, and place the call on hold. If the caller does not want to wait, ask where the person can be reached and say that the call will be returned. Always return the call promptly.
- In returning to the first caller, always thank the person for waiting before proceeding with the conversation.

---

on the line. Care should be taken to extend maximum courtesy to the caller asked to hold (Box 10-1).

Music on Hold. The music-on-hold system provides the caller with music or a short narrative about treatment in the dental office while the person is on hold. The system can be personalized to address specific types of treatment in the office and then revert to music periodically. This feature tends to ease the caller's impatience and can offer short educational clips that may market certain aspects of the practice.

Automatic Call Back. A caller can give instructions to a busy station to call back as soon as the busy station is free.

Automatic Call Stacking. Calls that arrive at a busy station are automatically answered by a recorded wait message.

Speed Dialing. Commonly called numbers can be stored in the telephone's memory, and the call can be made by keying in a one- or two-digit code. **Speed dialing** cuts down on the time the administrative assistant spends dialing other offices or laboratories that are contacted frequently.

Call Timing. This feature is used in professional offices that charge clients by the time spent handling their business on the telephone. It is common in law and accounting firms and other professional offices that bill for consultation on the telephone.

Call Restriction. Unauthorized long distance telephone calls can be eliminated with this feature. If an individual is authorized to make a long distance call, the call is given an authorization code that must be keyed into the telephone before the call can be processed. The telephone may also be programmed not to accept long distance calls.

Identified Ringing. This feature provides distinctive ringing tones for different categories of calls. For example, internal calls may have one long ring, whereas outside calls may have two short rings.

Liquid Crystal Display. A **liquid crystal display (LCD)** allows the user to see the number dialed, prompts the user with instructions, and displays the number of minutes the individual remains on the telephone. When used for incoming calls, an LCD also displays the number of the caller.

Multiple Lines or Key Telephones. Multiple lines are a standard feature on most telephones in a dental office. Special care must be taken when using them to ensure privacy and avoid interfering with other calls in progress.

If multiple lines are available for receiving or placing calls, one of the lines often is for a number that is not listed in the telephone directory or printed on the business stationery; this line should be used for outgoing calls, leaving the other lines available for incoming calls.

A telephone system with multiple lines can be used for both inside and outside calls. This can be a very efficient system, but the administrative assistant must remember several key points, which are presented in Box 10-2.

Pagers

A **pager** is a telecommunication device that allows a person to receive accurate messages instantly. The pager can receive numeric messages, including phone numbers and special codes that have been devised, or alphanumeric messages. Most pagers, such as the one shown in Figure 10-7, are easy to read, have various alert tones, display the date and time, offer various-size message slots, and retain messages in memory.

BOX 10-2 **Using a Multiple-Line Telephone System**

1. Determine which line is to be answered; this usually is indicated by a ring or buzz, and the button flashes until the line is answered. Depress the key to be answered before lifting the receiver.
2. If placing an outside call, determine which line is available (indicated by an unlighted button). Depress the key for that line and then dial the number. If accidentally selecting a line that has been placed on hold, depress the hold key again to put the call back on hold.
3. If placing an incoming call on hold, indicate to the caller that this is being done. Depress the hold key, which keeps the caller on the line. (The hold key then returns to its normal position.) The line key remains lighted, which indicates that the line is in use. Other calls then can be placed or received on another line.
4. Before transferring a call, be sure to inform the caller that this is being done, because the person may not want the call transferred. Give the caller the extension number to which he or she is being transferred in case the call is disconnected. This allows the caller to call the person back directly.

   To transfer an outside call with the button system, first place the call on hold. Then push the button for local, which lights when in use (the local button is for in-office transfers only). Dial or buzz a number in the office telephone system; the telephone is answered on local in another office. Inform the dentist of a call on a particular line, and the dentist completes the call from that telephone. If returning to the incoming line, remember which line the caller used. "Hold reminder" is a feature on advanced telephone systems that gives a reminder tone at various intervals to indicate that a caller is still waiting. Depress that button, which opens the line once more and allows completion of the call.

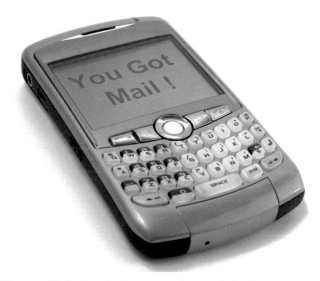

Figure 10-8 The Blackberry provides a mobile telephone plus Internet access as well as a variety of other services. (Copyright 2009 Edcel Mayo. Image from BigStockPhoto.com.)

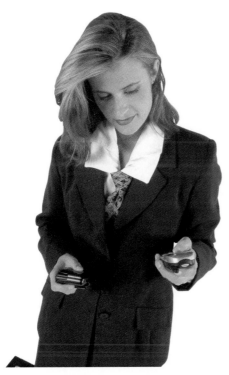

Figure 10-7 A dentist calls the office from a cellular phone after receiving a message from a portable pager. (Copyright 2009 JupiterImages Corporation.)

Personal Digital Assistant

The BlackBerry is a wireless, handheld personal digital assistant (PDA) (Figure 10-8). In 2002, when the SMART phone BlackBerry was released, it supported push e-mail, mobile telephone, text messaging, Internet faxing, web browsing, and other wireless information services as well as a multi-touch interface. Today's BlackBerry models all have color displays. The BlackBerry includes PDA applications (address book, calendar, to-do lists, etc.) as well as telephone capabilities on newer models. The BlackBerry has gained a reputation for its ability to send and receive e-mail wherever it can access a wireless network of certain cellular phone carriers. The BlackBerry has a built-in keyboard, that enables the user to use of only the thumbs to type. System navigation is primarily accomplished by a scroll ball in the middle of the device. Some models also incorporate a Push-to-Talk (PTT) feature, similar to a two-way radio. The latest devices are very popular with some dental practices, in which they are primarily used to provide e-mail access to roaming employees. To fully integrate the BlackBerry into a practice's systems, the installation of BlackBerry Enterprise Server (BES) is required.

iPhone

The iPhone is like having your own personal computer within your hand (Figure 10-9). This device is designed with a touch screen that enables the user to have a cell phone that's also an

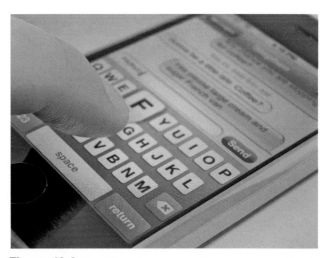

Figure 10-9 The iPhone features a touch screen and provides the user with three technologies in a single device: telephone, Internet, and iPod. (Copyright 2008 Jeff Metzger. Image from BigStockPhoto.com.)

iPod, a video as well as still camera, and a mobile Internet device with email and GPS maps. The technology in this device has been expanded to a level that can provide the user access to a world of information at their fingertips and for the dental professional easy access to all lines of communication. For the latest features of this device visit the web site at www.apple.com/iphone/features/wireless.html

Instant Messaging System

The intercom system is discussed in Chapter 6 as a method of interoffice, nonverbal communication by means of a light system. A more comprehensive messaging system can be established through part of the DataMate family. IMiN Lite is an instant messaging program designed specifically for the small office. It provides secure, instant communication within the dental office. The result is a cost-effective, local area network (LAN) messaging program that delivers the benefits of larger, more expensive messaging systems. This system is easy to use and easy administer and can support networks of up to 50 users.

How Does It Work?

While the dentist is at chairside, an important telephone call comes in. To let the dentist know who is calling, the administrative assistant uses IMiN (Figure 10-10) to type a message, such as "The patient is ready," and sends it to the dentist in the treatment room. The message instantly pops up on the computer screen in the treatment room. To reply, the dentist simply selects the desired response from the customizable message palette with a click of the mouse or by hitting the corresponding function key. The reply, such as "I'll be right there" or "I'll be just another 5 minutes," now appears on the administrative assistant's screen. This system prevents frantic waving, running back and forth, and cryptic hand signals about what to do with the call. The system is clear, crisp, and professional, and the keyboard and mouse can be protected with a barrier to prevent cross-contamination.

Features

The IMiN Lite system has the following features:

- *Instant Messaging:* Unlike e-mail, IMiN Lite is designed to provide secure, instantaneous communication. Messages can be sent to one or more users, one or more groups, or to all online users.
- *Security:* Unlike many Internet-based instant messaging services currently available, IMiN Lite operates in the privacy of the dental office's computer network. The result is secure, private, internal communication among the dental staff without the risk of messages being viewed by outside parties.

- *Fast Responses:* A fully customizable 10-button message palette provides for quick, one-touch responses. Fast Responses can be sent with a single click of the mouse or a push of a button.
- *Visual and Audio Notification:* Pop-up windows and sounds are used to notify users of incoming communications. Both of these features can be turned on or off, depending on the user's preference.
- *AutoReply:* The system can be set to send a response automatically to any incoming message. For example, if the dentist, assistant, or hygienist expects to be involved in a procedure for a period of time and therefore is unable to respond to messages, the AutoReply message "I cannot respond at this time" can be set, and this reply will be sent back for that person's incoming messages.
- *Message History:* The message history allows the user to view, delete, or print stored messages.
- *Customization:* Fast Responses, AutoReplies, sounds, and other features all can be customized to suit the needs of individual users.

Facsimile (FAX) Communication System

Another electronic means of communication is the facsimile (FAX) machine (Figure 10-11). A facsimile transmission machine is a scanning device that transmits an image of a document over standard telephone lines. The machine operates like a photocopy machine that sends an image by wire. At the receiving end, a similar machine receives the transmitted copy. The message may be a handwritten document (in ballpoint pen), a keyboarded page, or a picture. The cost of transmitting a FAX message is the same as a telephone call because the message is transmitted through the telephone lines. Many dental offices prefer to have a dedicated telephone line for the FAX machine rather than using the business telephone number.

Figure 10-10 The IMiN screen indicates a message from the business office to the treatment room. (IMiN screenshot courtesy JustWrks, Inc., www.justwrks.com.)

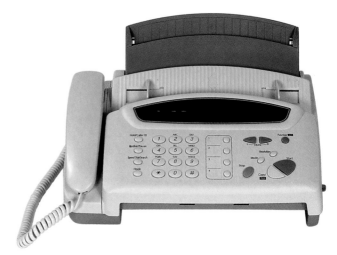

Figure 10-11 A facsimile (FAX) machine uses the telephone line to send copies of documents. (Copyright 2009 JupiterImages Corporation.)

A FAX machine can be a stand-alone unit or may be incorporated into the office computer. The cost of the facsimile machine varies greatly, depending on added features.

In case of an emergency or for consultation purposes, the dentist might find FAX telecommunications very useful for transmitting a patient's clinical dental record either locally or out of town. Documents that require signatures can be transmitted via the FAX system, but most legal transactions require the signing parties eventually to sign the original document.

Long Distance Services

Because many businesses or other resources the dentist uses are more global than in the past, the administrative assistant may be responsible for placing long distance calls. Calls to other areas in the United States and abroad are not uncommon. Several types of services are available for long distance calling, including wide area telephone service (WATS), direct distance dialing (DDD), person-to-person or collect calls, calling cards, and toll-free service.

Wide Area Telephone Service

In offices in which many outgoing long distance calls are made, **wide area telephone service (WATS)** is often used. This service allows the subscriber to make telephone calls from the premises to telephones anywhere within a specified service area at a monthly rate rather than on a per-call basis. The calling area the customer wants determines the monthly charge for the WATS line.

Direct Distance Dialing

With direct distance dialing (DDD), long distance numbers in other parts of the United States or other countries can be dialed on a station-to-station basis. To use the DDD system, dial a 1 plus the area code when charging the call to the number from which the administrative assistant is calling and when she or he is willing to talk to anyone who answers. Therefore, if calling a party in Missouri from Michigan, first check the front pages of the telephone directory to determine the area code and then do the following:

Key: 1 + 314 (or 636) + local number

To access a number in a foreign country, key the international access code (available from the long distance company) plus the country code, city code, and the local number of the company or person.

Person-to-Person or Collect Calls

Person-to-person calls are more costly than direct-dial calls, but in some cases may be necessary. The procedure for making this type of call may vary in certain areas of the country or with various long distance companies. Consult the local telephone directory for specific instructions. In most areas, the call can be made by keying 0, the area code, and the telephone number. If keying is complete, an operator will answer and ask for calling information. Then give the operator the name of the person being called.

A collect call, sometimes referred to as *"reversing the charges,"* can be made from a remote location. Again, when placing such a call, consult the local directory. Usually the same procedure as for placing a person-to-person call is followed. After keying the 0, area code, and the number, the operator will respond. Give the name of the person calling and say that the call is being made collect. The person who answers the call must agree to accept the charges before the conversation can begin.

Calling Card Calls

Many dentists and their administrative assistants now use calling cards. Calling cards allow calls that the person makes while traveling to be charged to the office. The procedure for making a calling card call is similar to that described for the person-to-person call. Key 0, the area code, and then the telephone number. When the operator answers and requests the calling card number, simply key in the number on the card.

Toll-Free Service

A toll-free number beginning 800, 888, 877, or 866 allows callers to reach businesses and/or individuals without being charged for the call. The charge for using a toll-free number is paid by the called party (the toll-free subscriber) instead of the calling party. Toll-free numbers can be dialed directly to a business or personal telephone line.

Toll-free numbers are very common and have proved successful for businesses, particularly in the areas of customer service and telemarketing. Companies that use this service are listed in the telephone directory with an 800/888/877/866 number. If it is known that a company has such a number but it is not available in the local directory, it may be obtained through 800/888/877/866 information by keying 1–800(or other three digit number)-555–1212. As with most information services, a fee may be charged for this service.

Telephone Directories

The telephone directory is a vital tool in the business office. It is important that the administrative assistant look through it and become familiar with the type of information available so that he or she can use the directory as efficiently as possible. Today telephone directories may be received from the telephone service being used as well as private industry, but most of them provide similar information. In some larger cities the yellow pages are separate from the white pages, and areas of the community may be divided into separate directories. The telephone directory provides selected area codes for many cities in North America and foreign countries, as well as **time zones**. In addition, the following information may be found:

1. A community profile
   a. Past and present
   b. Community events
   c. Things to do and see
   d. Parks and recreation
   e. Colleges and universities
   f. Transportation services

2. Maps
   a. Overview of the city
   b. Area maps
   c. Maps of nearby communities
3. Zip codes
4. Senior citizen information

In general, the front pages of the telephone directory provide important information, such as emergency phone numbers, including the police, fire, ambulance, suicide prevention, and poison control numbers. Page 1 of the front pages has a table of contents. Review this page so that other services listed in the directory can be found quickly.

The white pages of the telephone directory generally are divided into three sections: (1) the residence section, which is an alphabetical listing of the names, addresses, and telephone numbers of individuals; (2) the business white pages, which is an alphabetical listing of the names, addresses, and telephone numbers of businesses; and (3) the blue pages, a section that lists the names, addresses, and telephone numbers of local, state, and federal government offices.

The yellow pages list the names of particular businesses according to the type of service the business provides. For example, assume that the administrative assistant is interested in obtaining laundry service for the office, but is not familiar with companies in the area that provide such service. This category could be broken down as follows:

> Laundries
> Laundries—Self-service
> Laundry—Equipment—Commercial

The companies specializing in each area are listed alphabetically. Because this section is used as a sales tool, it has additional advertisements and a variety of print styles.

DEVELOPING EFFECTIVE TELEPHONE ETIQUETTE

Most people take great care to exude a professional business appearance, but few people take as much pride in developing their telephone image. This is unfortunate for an administrative assistant who takes responsibility for telephone calls, because people spend more time listening to than looking at him or her.

People often forget when using the telephone that the person on the other end of the line is a human being. Therefore take time to develop a professional telephone personality. To be effective on the telephone, keep a smile in the voice, answer calls promptly, be attentive and discreet, be cordial and responsive, ask questions tactfully, take messages courteously, speak distinctly, transfer calls carefully, place calls properly, avoid sexism, and be considerate to the caller. The techniques for successful telephone contact, which involves a voice-to-voice relationship, are somewhat different from those of successful personal contact, which involves a face-to-face relationship (Figure 10-12).

 PRACTICE NOTE
To be effective on the telephone, keep a smile in the voice.

Speaking Voice

The speaking voice has four separate but interrelated components: loudness, pitch, rate, and quality.

Loudness refers to the volume of the voice. If the speaker talks too loudly, the listener may be uncomfortable. (Have you ever talked on the telephone with someone who spoke so loudly you had to hold the receiver away from your ear? If you have, then you know how unpleasant excessive volume is to the listener.)

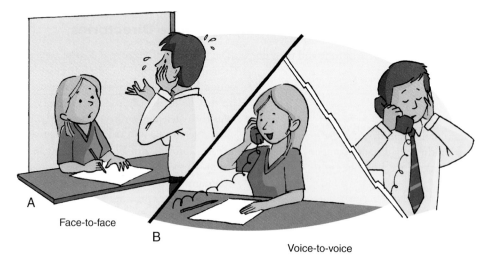

A Face-to-face

B Voice-to-voice

Figure 10-12 A, Face-to-face conversation. Nonverbal cues are apparent; a person smiles or gestures to make a point. Poise, interest, and sincerity provide observable feedback. Facial expressions help indicate the degree of understanding. Discussion is extemporaneous, and notes generally are not used. **B,** Voice-to-voice conversation. The impression of the person is acquired only through hearing. Interpretation comes only from the tone of voice. The degree of understanding is determined by questioning and by rephrasing statements. Notes are advantageous in this situation.

The opposite situation can be equally unpleasant. If lacking confidence, the voice may be so quiet that people will ask for a repetition of what has been said. If this happens, try to increase both confidence and volume.

The *rate* of speaking can determine how well someone is understood. When discussing familiar procedures with a patient, dental assistants may tend to speak rapidly, forgetting that this is new material to the patient. There is no ideal rate, but a general rule is to speak at a rate that does not detract from the clarity of the message and is easy and comfortable to listen to for an extended period.

Pitch is the tone of the voice. This is more difficult to change, because once it has been developed, persistent discipline is required to alter it. A low, gravelly voice or a high, squeaky voice may be unpleasant to listen to and are hard on the throat. Many exercises are available from the local telephone company and reference libraries for improving voice pitch.

The *quality* of a voice is a combination of physical and psychological factors. Changes in each of these alter the effectiveness of the speaking voice. Daily experiences affect this quality, and care should be taken to withhold depression, excitement, and anger from the voice when speaking on the dental office telephone.

To achieve a good telephone personality, develop the qualities of alertness, expressiveness, interest, naturalness, and distinctness.

A patient calling the dental office expects to have the call answered promptly. Answer the phone within the first two rings. Everyone enjoys being recognized, so be attentive to the patient's identity and express this in the voice. When a patient calling the office identifies himself, the alert assistant replies, "Yes, Mr. Jones, how may I help you?"

Furthermore, when the patient presents a problem, don't stammer and stutter and say, "Yeah, well, uh, I don't know." Such a response indicates inexperience to the patient. "I will be glad to check your record" or "Let me check with the dentist and call you back within the next hour" is the type of response that indicates a sincere effort to help and a willingness to seek an answer to the problem. Remember, if a patient is promised a call back, do it at the time promised. Offer to find an answer if information is not known. Don't force the patient to seek the information.

Nothing is more boring than listening to a person who speaks in a monotone. Put expression into what is said. Add enthusiasm to the voice by using natural voice inflections. To create a smile in the voice, place a mirror in front of the telephone. This ensures that a smile on the face before answering the telephone. Try it…it works! Act enthusiastic and one becomes enthusiastic.

> **PRACTICE NOTE**
> Act enthusiastic, and one becomes enthusiastic.

Patients calling the dental office have a definite purpose and expect the assistant to be interested in their problems. Therefore give the patient undivided attention. Don't interrupt or become preoccupied with another matter. Show interest in the patient's problem by asking appropriate questions and not rushing to terminate the conversation.

> **PRACTICE NOTE**
> Give the patient undivided attention.

To be natural, be yourself. Don't be a phony. An unnatural voice is easily detected. Keep the breathy "daaarhling," "sweetie," "honey," and "dear" words out of the vocabulary. Remember, "sugar and syrup" have no place in dentistry, so keep them out of the voice.

> **PRACTICE NOTE**
> To be natural, be yourself.

To speak distinctly, pronounce each syllable of the word completely. When using a handheld telephone, speak directly into the transmitter, which should be ½ to 1 inch from the lips. Don't chew gum, bite on a pencil, or cover the mouth with a hand; these all create mumbled conversation and do not present a good image for the dental office. Avoid slang; it is neither businesslike nor in good taste. Some examples of what to say and what not to say include the following:

Avoid	Say
Bye-bye	Goodbye
Huh?	I do not understand.
	Would you please repeat that?
Uh-huh	Yes
	Of course
Yeah	Yes
	Certainly
	I agree
OK	Yes

Creating a Good Image

In addition to achieving good voice qualities, choose the word or phrase that best communicates the message and makes the best impression. In general, to promote better understanding, use short, simple, descriptive words that are appropriate to the situation. When using technical dental terms, names, numbers, formulas, foreign words, or dictated material, the information should be given slowly and distinctly. Suggestions for identifying letters are presented in Box 10-3 and those for identifying numbers in Table 10-1.

A variety of words and phrases in the dental office can convey an unfavorable image to the patient (Figure 10-13). In Table 10-2 are suggestions for appropriate telephone responses that will create a more positive image. Each time the assistant speaks on the telephone, think about what is being said and ask if that is what is really meant. See things from the patient's point of view to decide whether connotations that should be avoided are being communicated.

BOX 10-3 — Using Words to Identify Letters

The following words might be used to identify letters for a caller:

A as in Alice
B as in Boy
C as in Charles
D as in Dog
E as in Edward
F as in Frank
G as in George
H as in Hat
I as in Ida
J as in Jack
K as in King
L as in Lion
M as in Mary

N as in Nancy
O as in Old
P as in Peter
Q as in Queen
R as in Robert
S as in Susan
T as in Thomas
U as in Union
V as in Victory
W as in William
X as in X-ray
Y as in Young
Z as in Zero

TABLE 10-1 — Pronouncing Numbers Clearly

Number	Sounds Like	Formation of the Sound
0	Zir-o	Well-sounded Z, short I, rolled R, long O
1	Wun	Strong W and N
2	Too	Strong T and OO
3	Th-r-ee	Single roll of the R, long EE
4	Fo-er	Long O, strong R
5	Fi-iv	I changes from long to short; strong V
6	Siks	Strong S and KS
7	Sev-en	Strong S and V, well-sounded EN
8	Ate	Long A, strong T
9	Ni-en	Strong N, well-sounded EN

Managing Incoming Calls

Although each call to and from the dental office presents a unique situation, most calls can be placed in specific categories and certain conditions remain constant in each situation. As a result, the administrative assistant is able to formulate certain questions and answers for each situation. Care should be exercised not to use these statements in a rote manner, but to incorporate the ideas into one's own words and develop a technique that fulfills the philosophy of the dental office. This is especially important when training new personnel who are unfamiliar with the common situations that may arise on the dental office telephone.

The following are examples of typical conversations that illustrate efficient management of the telephone in a dental office. Some suggestions for managing incoming calls are presented in Box 10-4.

> **PRACTICE NOTE**
> Each time the administrative assistant speaks on the telephone, he or she should think about what is being said and ask him or herself if that is what is really meant.

The call: "I would like to make an appointment with the dentist to have my teeth cleaned."

The response: The caller has indicated the nature of the desired treatment, but the administrative assistant must determine whether this is a new patient. Ask, "When was the last time you were seen by Dr. Lake?" This indirectly determines whether this is a former patient (not an "old patient," please). If the patient has never seen Dr. Lake, then further information should be obtained. First, obtain the person's name by asking, "How do I spell your name?" Then ask who referred the patient, the home and business telephone numbers, the home address, and the approximate date of the last dental treatment. Because the person has never been to the office, also ask if the caller knows where the office is located and, if not, give simple, explicit directions. If available, also refer the new patient to the office web site for directions or offer to send an e-mail message with the directions. Conclude the call by saying, "Thank you for calling, Mr. Jones. We look forward to meeting you on Thursday, February 8, at 1:30 PM." Wait for the patient to hang up first.

The call: An unidentified person calls and states, "I would like to speak to the dentist."

The response: This call may be simply to make an appointment, or it may be a personal call that the dentist wishes to receive. It may be someone the dentist does not know, and the person will not state the reason for the call. It is important that a policy be established by the dentist regarding the types of calls he or she will receive personally. Regardless of the form the call takes, follow up the person's initial request to speak to the dentist with, "Dr. Lake is with a patient. How may I help you?" The "how" is important; if simply asked, "May I help you?" the caller may respond, "No, I want to speak to the dentist." Furthermore, if the person refuses to give his or her name, the assistant may say, "The dentist has requested the name of the person calling so that he (or she) may return your call."

> **PRACTICE NOTE**
> Don't hesitate to ask for the spelling of the caller's name.

Fortunately, most people are cooperative at the outset of the conversation, and any message may be recorded on a message form (Figure 10-14) after asking, "May I have your name and phone number?" Don't hesitate to ask for the spelling of the caller's name. Then ask, "Is this call concerning dental treatment?" If so, the assistant should attach the message to the patient's clinical record before giving it to the dentist.

If the call is an emergency that warrants the dentist's immediate attention, a short message may be written and given to him or her in the treatment room. Remember; do not discuss other patients or business in front of the person undergoing treatment.

The call: "Hello, this is Mrs. Harris, and I need to see the dentist today to have him look at a tooth that is bothering me."

The response: This type of call may or may not be an emergency. Therefore it is necessary to ask the patient, "How long has the

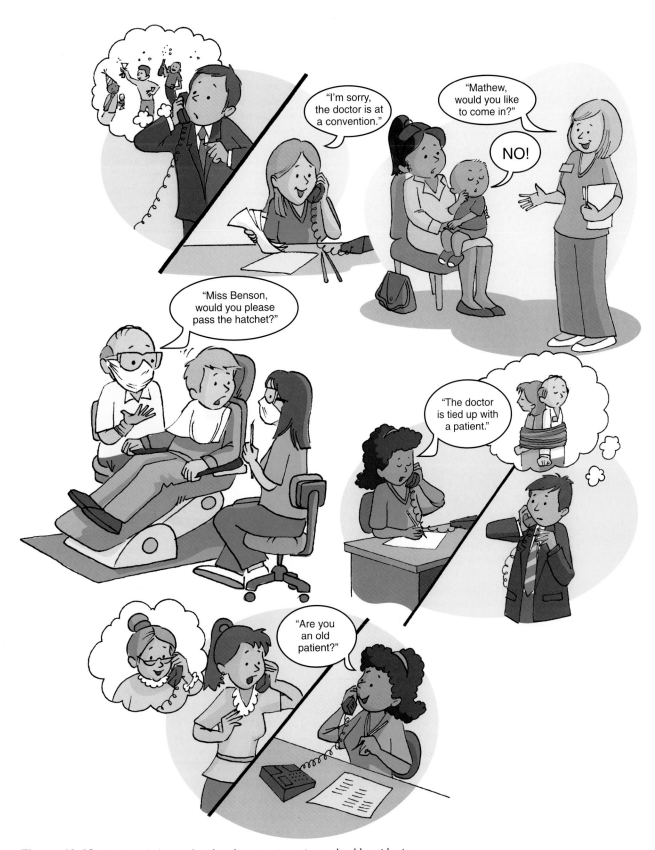

Figure 10-13 Words and phrases that the administrative assistant should avoid using.

TABLE 10-2	Appropriate Words and Phrases to Use in Personal and Telephone Responses

Avoid	Say
Work	Dentistry
Plates	Dentures
Cancellation	Change in the schedule
Waiting room	Reception room
Filling	Restoration
My girl	My assistant or hygienist
Cost	Investment
Pull	Remove or extract
Spit	Empty your mouth
Remind	Confirm
Check-up	Examination
Grind the tooth; drill	Prepare the tooth
Case presentation	Consultation appointment
Rehabilitation	Complete dentistry
Hurt; pain	Uncomfortable
Old patient	Former patient
Operatory	Treatment room
Cost; price; charge	Fee
Bill	Account
Convention	Seminar
Shot	Injection
Joe; Doc; the doctor	Dr. Lake
Doctor is tied up; I'm sorry.	Doctor is with a patient. Doctor is busy.
Would you like to come in now?	Dr. Lake is ready to see you, Mrs. Ward.
Thank you for calling. (without use of name).	Thank you for calling, Mrs. Main.
She is out.	She is not in the office at the present time.
	May I take a message or would you prefer to leave a message on her voice mail?
He is in the men's room.	He has stepped out of the office. Would you like to leave a message?
He hasn't come in yet.	I expect him shortly. Would you like to leave a message?
Doctor is running late.	Doctor has had an interruption in the schedule
When would you like to come in?	Do you prefer mornings or afternoons?

tooth been bothering you?" "How severe is the discomfort?" "Is the tooth sensitive to extreme hot or cold?" These questions help to determine whether an emergency exists. If the situation is an emergency, the patient should be seen immediately, during reserved buffer time. The patient should be informed that this appointment will be given to relieve the immediate discomfort and that if further treatment is necessary, an additional appointment will be scheduled. (If this is not done, the patient may anticipate having all the treatment completed at the emergency appointment.)

If the existing condition is not an emergency, an appointment may be scheduled on another day in the near future.

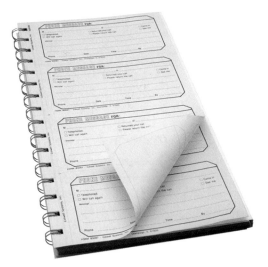

Figure 10-14 Message forms allow the administrative assistant to keep accurate records for other dental team members. (Courtesy Patterson Office Supplies, Champaign, IL.)

The call: "This is Mrs. Alvarez. My daughter, Juanita, just fell off her skateboard and broke her front tooth. It's bleeding. What should I do?" (Caller is frantic.)

The response: Emergencies such as this should be seen immediately. The anxious mother should be told to bring the child into the office immediately. Remain calm and reassure the frantic mother by saying, "Place some cold compresses on the area." Evaluate the situation further and, if the schedule is filled, call some of the later patients and detain them. Don't tell them the office is "running late"; instead, inform them that there has been an unexpected emergency and ask them to come in a half hour later. Patients appreciate consideration of their time.

The call: An unidentified person calls and asks, "How much does Dr. Lake charge for fillings?"

The response: Generally fees should not be quoted on the telephone. However, fees for basic treatment are often quoted. For major treatment the patient should come to the office for an examination to determine the extent of treatment needed, because diagnosis cannot be done on the telephone, nor can the dentist see the conditions in the patient's mouth. It should be remembered that the patient as a consumer has the right to know the basic fees before treatment, and in complex situations the patient should be given an estimate of fees. These factors must be considered when the dentist establishes a policy on quoting fees.

The call: "This is Mr. Huang, and I just received my statement. I think it is awfully high. You must have made a mistake."

The response: Two possibilities exist here: (1) the patient is right, and there is an error on his statement, and (2) there has been a lack of communication with the patient regarding the fee. Regardless of the reason, don't become defensive on the telephone. This always seems to be the first reaction when challenged. Instead, reply, "I'm sorry, Mr. Huang, perhaps I can clarify the statement for you. What is your specific question?" This focuses on the particular problem. Don't make comments until the patient's concern is thoroughly understood. The patient may state, "I sent a check in the mail on the 28th and you didn't deduct it from the statement." To this respond, "Perhaps we didn't receive it before the billing date, Mr. Huang. If you will wait just a moment, I will be glad to get your record and check it for you." Depress the hold button and check the patient's record. In this case, check the patient's record, return to the telephone, thank him for waiting, and inform him whether the check was received. If an error has been made, tell the patient it will be corrected and he will be sent a corrected statement in the mail immediately.

However, if the statement is correct and the patient feels that the fee is too high, return the patient's call rather than keeping him on hold. Such calls are often the result of the dentist's failure to inform the patient of the fee before rendering the service. "Inform before you perform" is a rule that saves many hours on the telephone attempting to explain a patient's statement. Also, the patient may have been informed of the original treatment plan but because of a change in the plan, the fee was higher than originally quoted. It is also possible that the patient still does not understand the treatment plan. In any case, this type of problem is difficult to resolve on the telephone and is best managed by asking the patient to come into the office, where the treatment plan can be reviewed once again in person.

PRACTICE NOTE
Don't become defensive when dealing with callers.

Managing Outgoing Calls

An administrative assistant places many outgoing calls. The following tips are helpful for making such calls:

1. Plan ahead. Be sure to have the telephone numbers written correctly. If calling a patient, list the name with the telephone number; if calling another dentist's office or business, have that number written or easily accessible. Be sure to consult the telephone directory if in doubt about a correct telephone number. Names appear in the telephone directory in alphabetical order; however, some public services or governmental agencies may be listed differently. For example, state offices are listed under the state name first, then alphabetically according to office. County and city offices are also listed by county or city name first, then alphabetically according to the office. Federal offices are listed under United States Government first, then alphabetically according to the office. Parochial and other private schools are listed alphabetically by the name of the school.

   Another source for obtaining the correct telephone number for most businesses is the business white pages or yellow pages directory. If the name of the business is known, check in the business white pages in alphabetical order. If the name of a particular dental laboratory is not known but the location is, find the number by consulting the yellow pages under "Dental Laboratories."

2. If the telephone being used is a lighted push-button system, make sure the line is free before placing the call (the light signals when the line is in use). As the telephone receiver is lifted, make sure the dial tone is heard before starting to dial. When using a rotary telephone, use the index finger to dial the number, and then remove it from the dial opening on the return dial because the return of the dial determines what number is reached. When using a push button phone, press firmly but not too quickly.

3. When the call is answered, the administrative assistant must identify him or herself, as well as the name of the dentist for whom he or she is calling.

4. State the reason for calling. If changing a patient's appointment, have another appointment time available. Indicate why the change is being made, because it may cause a disruption in plans, and the patient may also have to adjust another appointment or work schedule.

5. The person who placed the call should also terminate it. It is discourteous to hang up without an indication that the conversation is finished. End the conversation with a courteous "goodbye" and then replace the receiver gently.

6. If a wrong number is reached, apologize for the inconvenience, verify that the number was dialed correctly, and recheck the number before redialing.

PRACTICE NOTE
The person who placed the call should also terminate it.

Examples of common outgoing calls are provided in the following:

The purpose: Confirmation of a patient's appointment for the following day.

The call: When the patient answers the telephone, identify yourself and state the reason for calling: "Hello, Mrs. Thompson, this is Ms. Benson from Dr. Lake's office." (Do not say, "This is Dr. Lake's office calling." Offices don't make calls-people do!) You may then continue with your message, stating it briefly and completely: "I would like to confirm (not "remind") your appointment for tomorrow at 1:30 PM with Dr. Lake." When the patient acknowledges it affirmatively, you may simply say, "We look forward to seeing you tomorrow at 1:30," and then conclude the call by saying, "Goodbye." Wait for the patient to hang up.

Sometimes patients send up a "trial balloon" and simply state, "I won't be able to keep the appointment tomorrow, and I'll call you later for another one." Although this may be a legitimate statement and the patient does plan to call you at a later date, you should pursue the conversation because it may be a signal that there has been a lack of communication with the patient. Instead of abruptly concluding the conversation, ask the patient, "Would it be possible to reschedule your appointment for a week from today?" If the patient continues to be negative, then asking, "I don't understand, is there something wrong?" will generally bring the patient to the point of explanation.

The purpose: To make plane and hotel reservations for the dentist for a dental meeting out of state.

The call: Many travel reservations can now be made on the computer. However, some doctors prefer working through an agency for more personal service. If this is true, then, before making calls for reservations, obtain information from the dentist about the desired arrival and departure times, type of service, airline preference (if a choice exists), name of the airport (if the city has more than one), name of the hotel, and type of accommodations. Once this preparation is done, contact the travel agency or appropriate airline and ask for "Reservations desk, please." Give the person who answers the necessary information: "I would like to make a reservation for Thursday, January 27, for a flight to Los Angeles, California, from Grand Rapids, Michigan, in the morning, returning on Tuesday, February 1, in the afternoon." Once the clerk has provided the available times, decide which flights will be agreeable to the dentist, then tell the clerk which ones are preferred. For example, "I would like to make a reservation in the business-class section for the flight leaving Grand Rapids at 8:20 AM and arriving at Los Angeles International Airport at 10:57 AM (California time), and returning on the nonstop flight leaving on Tuesday, February 1, at 3:30 PM and arriving at Grand Rapids at 12:35 AM." The reservation is made in the dentist's name. Obtain all flight numbers and details on how the confirmation and boarding passes will be transmitted to the office, and send an interoffice memorandum to the dentist, via e-mail with the information shown in Box 10-5 (which includes the itinerary).

Many hotel reservations can be made through local offices, an 800 number, or online. For instance, because Dr. Lake preferred to stay at an Ocean Inn, his assistant contacted a local Ocean Inn and made the reservation through this office. Specific information should be given to the clerk regarding choice of accommodations, such as preference for a smoking or nonsmoking room or single or double occupancy. Once the reservation has been made and an identification number given, obtain information on the location of the facility. This information is included on the itinerary.

Long distance calls may have to be made when information is needed quickly and there isn't time for an exchange of letters.

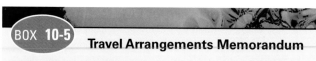

BOX 10-5 **Travel Arrangements Memorandum**

Departure
Leave: Grand Rapids, Thursday, January 27, Spirit Airlines—Flight #846—8:20 AM (nonstop)
Arrive: Los Angeles National Airport—10:57 AM
Hotel: Ocean Front Inn 2100 Wiltshire Boulevard

Return
Leave: Los Angeles National Airport, Tuesday, February 1, Spirit Airlines—Flight #546—3:30 PM (nonstop)
Arrive: Grand Rapids—12:35 AM

The procedure for DDD calls was described previously. However, several factors should be considered when making this type of call. First, when placing a long distance call to different time zones, the time difference must be kept in mind. The United States is divided into four time zones: Eastern, Central, Mountain, and Pacific (Figure 10-15). For example, if it is 2 PM in Grand Rapids, Michigan (Eastern time zone), it is 1 PM in St. Louis, Missouri (Central time zone), 12 PM in Denver (Mountain time zone), and 11 AM in Los Angeles (Pacific time zone). If in doubt about a time zone, check the time at www.time.gov for any area of the country.

If an incorrect number is reached when dialing long distance, obtain the name of the city, the state, and the number reached and immediately notify the operator of the error so that no charge will be made for the call.

Recording Telephone Messages Carefully

Although many offices have voice mail systems to handle messages, be prepared to record messages for the doctor and other staff members. Be prepared for incoming calls by keeping a pencil and message pad handy. Obtaining the correct information on messages is of utmost importance. Repeat the message, spelling of names, and the telephone number if the dentist is to return the call. Take sufficient time to obtain the correct information for the message. Be sure to date the message, indicate the time it was taken, and sign it with your name or initials. The message should always be signed by the person taking it in case questions arise later about the information. If the dentist must first find out who took the message, it takes extra time. Forms similar to the one shown in Figure 10-14 may be ordered from most stationery suppliers.

 PRACTICE NOTE
Be prepared for incoming calls by keeping a pencil and message pad handy.

Personal Telephone Calls

The telephone in the dental office is installed as a service to the dental patients and should be maintained as a business

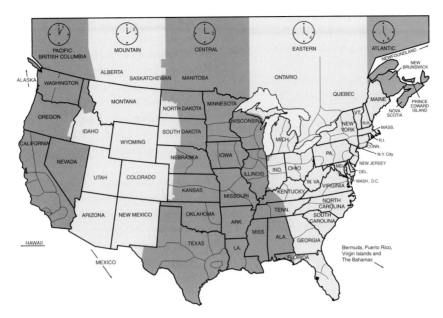

Figure 10-15 Time zones in the United States. (From Young AP: *Kinn's the administrative medical assistant*, ed 6, St Louis, 2007, Saunders.)

telephone. Consequently, staff members should refrain from using the telephone for personal calls, and only emergency calls should be made.

Cellular Telephone Etiquette

Although most of the calls for the dental office will be made on the traditional telephone, a **mobile phone** may be used when out of the office. All of the rules regarding voice and telephone use mentioned in the preceding apply to the cellular phone but since the cellular phone is used when out in public, be aware of special etiquette for its use. Also be aware of how to manage a personal cell phone when at work. Box 10-6 presents a list of suggestions to follow when using a cellular phone.

Telegrams

Although the dentist and staff members use letters and the telephone as the primary means of communication, the need to use a telegram may arise, such as to send an urgent message. Be familiar with telegraph services and know how to prepare a telegram and count chargeable words and characters. One address and one signature are free, and there is no charge for punctuation marks. However, if such words as *stop, period,* or *quote* are used, they are considered chargeable words.

Before calling the Western Union office to relay the telegraph message, compose the message and type a copy of it for the office files. The charge for the telegram is included on the telephone bill. The three basic services are regular telegrams, overnight telegrams, and Mailgrams.

Regular Telegram

A regular telegram can be sent at any time, and the message usually is delivered within 2 hours. The minimum rate is based on

---

BOX 10-6   Cell Phone Etiquette

- Turn off the ringer or set to "vibrate" while at in the office.
- Let family and unimportant calls go to voicemail.
- When using the cell phone, find a private, quiet place to make calls.
- Do not take the cell phone to meetings.
- Never use the cell phone in restrooms.
- Eliminate embarrassing ring tones.
- Maintain a quiet voice during cell phone conversations.
- When possible, use text messages instead of voice calls to maintain professionalism.
- If the phone rings while you are with others, excuse yourself, and move out of listening range to take the call or place on "vibrate."
- If out of the office, do not dial the cell phone while driving.
- Maintain a courteous but succinct introductory message.

---

15 words, exclusive of address and signature. An extra charge is made for each additional word.

Overnight Telegram

Overnight telegrams may be sent at any time up to midnight for delivery the next morning. An overnight telegram is less expensive than a regular telegram. The minimum charge is based on 100 words.

Mailgram

A Mailgram is a combination of night telegram service and postal service. The message (up to 100 words) is wired to the office of the U.S. Postal Service nearest the recipient. The Mailgram is typed from a wired message, placed in a window Mailgram envelope, and delivered in the first mail delivery of the morning.

KEY TERMS

Call forwarding—A telephonic feature that automatically relays a call to another telephone number.

Call holding—A feature of many telephone systems that allows a second call to be answered while the first caller "holds" on the line.

Caller ID—A display that shows the number assigned to the telephone from which the person is calling.

Cellular technology—A mobile telephone system that breaks down a large service area into smaller areas, called cells. Each cell is served by a low-powered receiver-transmitter. As the caller moves from one cell to another, a switching office automatically moves the call in a corresponding fashion.

Conference call—A telephone call in which several people participate, often from a number of different locations. The call is arranged through a conference call operator, who is given the names and telephone numbers of the individuals to be included in the call and the time the call is to be made.

Facsimile (FAX) machine—A facsimile transmission machine, which is a scanning device that transmits an image of a document over standard telephone lines.

Liquid crystal display (LCD)—A device that allows the user to see the number dialed, prompts the user with instructions, and displays the number of minutes the individual remains on the telephone.

Mobile phones—Another term for cellular phone

Pager—A telecommunication device that allows a person to receive accurate messages instantly or that alerts the person to return a call.

Speed dialing—A feature that allows commonly called numbers to be stored in the telephone system's memory and subsequently dialed by keying in a one- or two-digit code.

Telecommunications—The science and technology of communication by electronic transmission of impulses, as by telegraphy, cable, telephone, radio, or television.

Time zones—Geographic regions in which the same standard time is used. The United States is divided into four time zones: Eastern, Central, Mountain, and Pacific.

Voicemail—A telephone system that connects callers directly to an extension or a department and can record messages for that person or department.

Wide area telephone service (WATS)—A telephone service that enables the subscriber to make calls from the premises to telephones anywhere within a specified service area at a monthly rate rather than on a per-call basis.

LEARNING ACTIVITIES

1. List and briefly explain five qualities of a good telephone service.
2. Explain the management of the following calls:
   a. Mr. Sanchez calls the office and says he has broken a tooth and needs to see the dentist right away.
   b. Mrs. Alvarez calls the office and states that she is new in town. She wants to make an appointment for her son, Jim, who needs to have his teeth cleaned.
   c. Mr. Hubbard calls and states that his daughter was just hit in the mouth with a softball bat and has some broken teeth. He asks, "What do I need to do?"
3. Replace the following statements with a statement that would create a better image.
   a. "I'm sorry, the dentist is tied up with a patient."
   b. "Johnny, would you like to come in now?"
   c. "Jennifer, this shot won't hurt much."
   d. "He just went to the men's room. "
   e. "I'm sorry, the dentist is running late."
4. Complete a message form using the following telephone conversation: Mr. Schultz from Pine Mutual Insurance Company calls the office and wants the administrative assistant to tell the dentist he will meet her at the Yacht Club at 4:30 PM today. If this isn't agreeable, Mr. Schultz can be reached at 495.8272.
5. List and briefly define different telephone systems or services available for use in a dental office.

Please refer to the student workbook for additional learning activities.

BIBLIOGRAPHY

Fulton-Calkins PJ: *The Administrative Professional*, ed 13, Mason, OH, 2007, Thomson South-Western.

Oliverio ME, Pasewardk WR, White BR: *The Office, Procedures and Technology*, Mason, OH, 2007, Thomson South-Western.

RECOMMENDED WEB SITES

www.time.gov.
www.cell-phone-etiquette.com.
www.kellyservices.com.

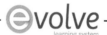

Please visit http://evolve.elsevier.com/Finkibeiner/practice for additional practice activities.

PART III

BUSINESS OFFICE SYSTEMS

Appointment Management Systems

LEARNING OUTCOMES

- Define key terms.
- Describe appointment book styles.
- Describe appointment software options.
- Complete an appointment matrix.
- Identify solutions to common appointment scheduling problems.
- Make an appointment entry.
- Design an appointment schedule list.
- Identify common appointment book symbols.
- Describe the use of a treatment plan.
- Complete an appointment card.
- Complete a daily schedule.
- Describe a call list.
- Explain advanced-function appointment scheduling.

Patients generate revenue, and dentistry is a business. Therefore the administrative assistant must be certain that there is a patient being treated in every chair in the office all day long. If there is an empty chair, then there is no production and no revenue, but the overhead continues. This chapter describes how to manage an appointment system and be aware of common situations that arise frequently in most offices.

Appointment management in today's dental practice most often takes the form of a software system. The traditional **appointment book**, although still available, is used less frequently but is still presented in this chapter, because the concepts of scheduling apply to both the manual and appointment scheduling software systems installed in the office computer. Appointment management on the computer was one of the last holdouts for many dentists. Some thought that electronic appointment scheduling was time consuming and made checking future schedules difficult. This is not true. Box 11-1 lists the advantages of an electronic appointment book.

 PRACTICE NOTE
The practice should be controlled through the appointment system, not by it.

Bill Gates once stated that someday there would be a computer in every household. In the dental practice, you can carry this one step further, as there is likely to be a computer terminal in every treatment room in the near future. For the dental hygienist, this direct access to the appointment scheduler allows more freedom in scheduling appointments and managing the hygiene schedule.

BOX 11-1 **Advantages of an Electronic Appointment System**

- Production goals can aid appointment scheduling.
- Production data are visible daily.
- Data entries are easier to read.
- Auto-scheduling eliminates paging through the book.
- Various screen viewing modes are available.
- Cross-referencing saves time and motion.
- Patient data are more likely to be accurate.
- Searching for appropriate appointment openings is easier.
- Procedures can be posted to several different records from one entry.
- Patient follow-up is easier.
- No manual record filing is necessary.

BOX 11-2 **Tips for Efficient Appointment Management**

1. Put one person in charge of the appointment system.
2. In a traditional appointment book, make accurate, neat entries.
3. Accommodate the patient as much as possible but maintain control of the appointment schedule.
4. Always have a patient being treated in each dental chair.
5. Avoid scheduling repetitive procedures over long periods.
6. Be aware of production goal criteria.
7. Be aware of scheduling in "power blocks."
8. Schedule the workload according to the staff members' body clocks.
9. Assign clinical tasks only to legally qualified personnel.
10. Avoid leaving large blocks of time between appointments.
11. Establish guidelines for problem situations.
12. Make sure the practice is controlled through the appointment system, not by it.

The appointment system, which contains lists of all the scheduled patients and events for the dentist and staff, is the control center of the office and an important factor in the success or failure of a dental practice. The practice should be controlled through the appointment system, not by it. Each dental practice should have a scheduling coordinator who maintains the schedule and keeps patients in the dental chairs. In a dental practice in which there is more than one business assistant with no real defined duties, these individuals are likely to perform the same basic functions in the business office, such as answering the phone, collecting money, opening mail, filing, verifying insurance, and making appointments. When no one person is held responsible for any particular assignment, and as long as the schedule is full, collections are good, and the practice overhead falls within defined goals, inefficiencies in the business office are not noticeable. That doesn't mean there are no inefficiencies, just that these inefficiencies are not glaringly obvious.

An efficient arrangement for the business staff would be to have one person designated as the scheduling coordinator and one person assigned as the financial coordinator. With this arrangement, each staff person can be held accountable for specific assignments, such as scheduling and collections. Job performance, whether good or bad, can then be measured by the amount of downtime (5% or less) and the percentage of collection (a goal of 96% or more).

Whether an appointment book or an electronic system is used, poor management of appointments can result in mounting tension among staff members and can turn the reception room into a waiting room of discontented patients. Basic scheduling concepts (Box 11-2) are the same regardless of the type of system used. Only the process of data entry differs.

The staff of a dental office should analyze the practice and determine an organized system of appointment control that: (1) maximizes productivity, (2) reduces staff tension, and (3) maintains concern for the patients' needs.

Because some dentists still feel strongly about having a hard copy of the appointment book to look at, both the electronic and traditional systems are addressed in this chapter. The concepts presented can be used either in an electronic or a manual system because they are the same for both.

SELECTION OF A TRADITIONAL APPOINTMENT BOOK

When an appointment book is used, the size and design of the book are determined by the needs of the dental practice. The administrative assistant should review the available styles to determine what is best for the office. Time and motion studies have indicated that the most efficient format for an appointment book is the week-at-a-glance style, in which all days of the week can be seen at one time. This allows the assistant to note openings in the schedule quickly (Figure 11-1).

The binding on the appointment book may have three to nine rings or may be spiral. Spiral-bound books appear to withstand a greater amount of use. The books may be printed with or without dates and may have one or more columns.

The individual days are divided into time increments. Some books provide 30-minute increments, others 10- or 15-minute increments. The smallest time increment is referred to as a **unit (u)**. The 15-minute unit has been widely used in dentistry with much success; the 10-minute unit has become generally accepted in advanced-function practices.

OPTIONS FOR THE ELECTRONIC APPOINTMENT BOOK

With the electronic appointment system, appointments can be entered, canceled, rescheduled, and moved easily with one keystroke. The benefits of the electronic system (see Box 11-1) set it apart from the traditional system. Electronic scheduling can be goal oriented, using state-of-the-art technology to set production goals for the practice. With income a consideration, rather than just filling the book, the dentist can begin to maximize

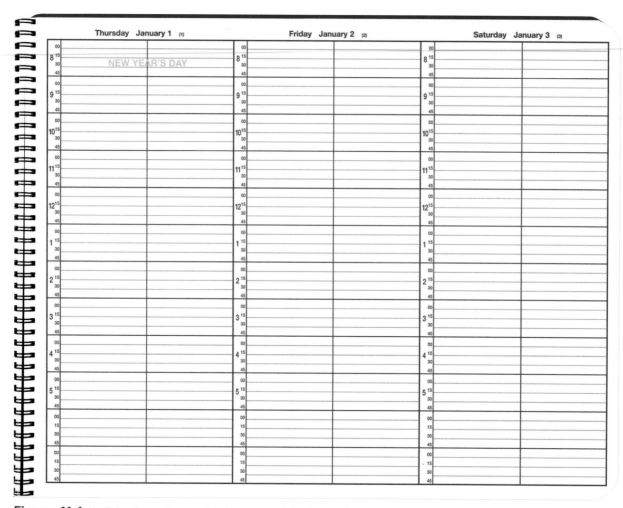

Figure 11-1 Traditional appointment book with spiral binding and multiple columns. (Courtesy Patterson Office Supplies, Champaign, IL.)

profits while controlling where and when certain procedures are performed.

Common electronic software scheduling packages generally have a number of components, as follows:

- *Finding the next available appointment:* This feature allows the staff member to find an open appointment time in a matter of seconds. This feature allows the person scheduling the appointment to search on specific days, during specific hours, and with selected providers and then shows a list of available appointments for the patient to select what works best for him or her.

- *Daily appointment screen:* Most software programs allow for a wide variety of set-up and viewing options for the office schedule. This allows the office staff to select the options that work best for them. Generally these views show the treatment rooms in a column format with the patient's name, treatment information, and resources needed for each time unit (Figure 11-2). An expanded view will show more detail of the appointment book. There is often an easy way to advance from date to date or show the schedule in a weekly format (Figure 11-3).

- *Patient information window:* The patient information screen (Figure 11-4) in most systems shows many types of information, such as demographic, financial, insurance, recall, and appointments. Patient information that can be entered on this record includes the patient's complete name, marital status, gender, age, date of birth, Social Security number, work, cell, and home phone numbers. There is often an easy way to view current balance, pharmacy and medication history, the patient's examination history, the treatment plan, financial information, referrals, medical alerts, treatment completed, and appointment time preferences, each of which are updated on the patient screen when entered in different areas of the program.

- *Locate appointment feature:* Most scheduling software allows searching to see if a patient has an existing appointment. This is very valuable when a patient calls and thinks he or she has an appointment but cannot remember the date (Figure 11-5).

- *Goal tracking:* The dental staff can set monthly goals by provider and enter these goals in the system. The software can then report a summary of the scheduled production, monthly

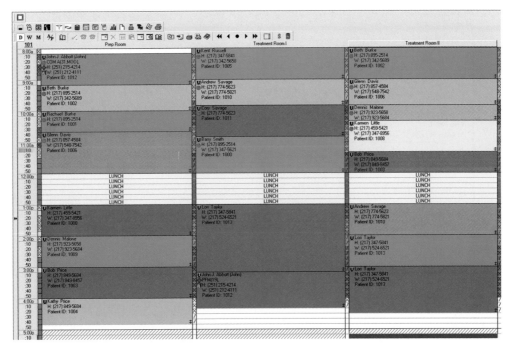

Figure 11-2 Daily appointment screen (expanded view). (Courtesy Patterson Dental, St. Paul, MN.)

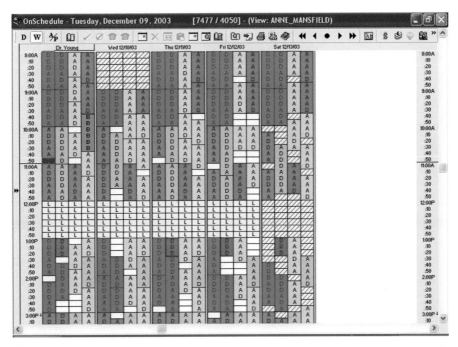

Figure 11-3 Quick-glance screen showing a week at a glance. (Courtesy Patterson Dental, St. Paul, MN.)

goal, percentage of goal, new patients, total appointments, and production totals so the staff can track how they are performing toward goal (Figure 11-6).

- *Short call list:* Electronic appointment books allow for excellent tracking of any appointments that were canceled and not rescheduled—patients who want to come in earlier if something opens up, or who just want to be called when there is a cancellation. Figure 11-7 illustrates a short call list of people who can be contacted quickly to fill an opening in the appointment book.

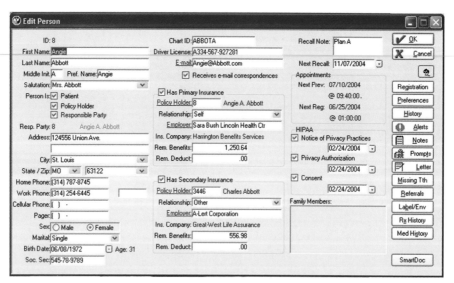

Figure 11-4 Patient information screen. (Courtesy Patterson Dental, St. Paul, MN.)

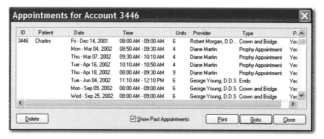

Figure 11-5 Locate appointment screen. (Courtesy Patterson Dental, St. Paul, MN.)

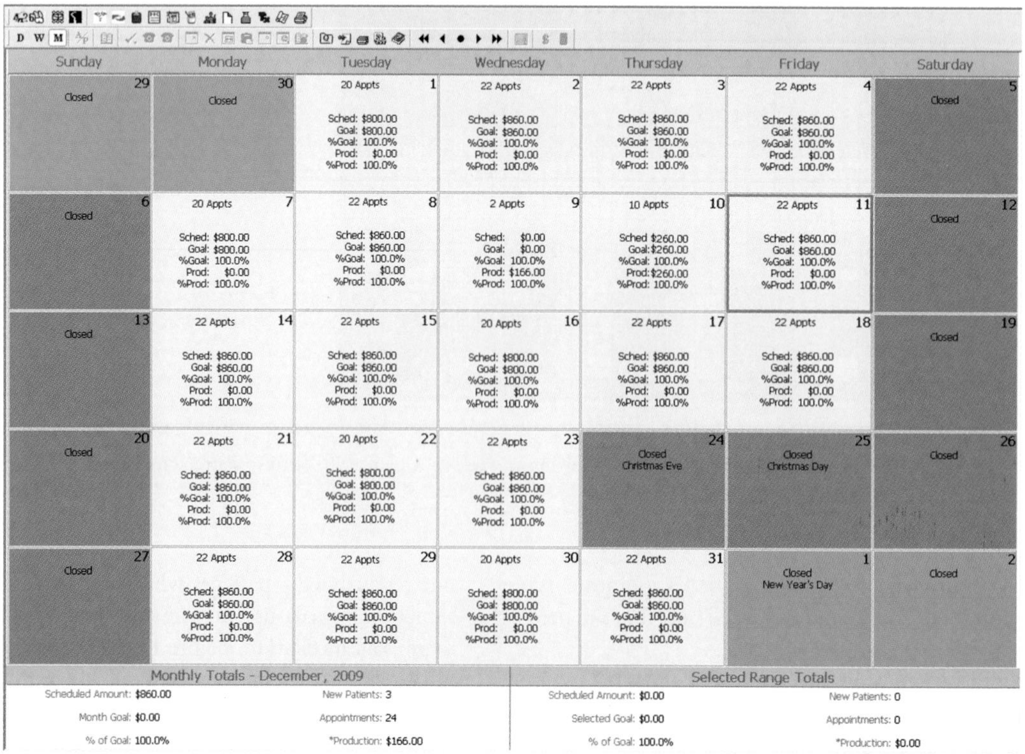

Figure 11-6 Goal tracking screen. (Courtesy Patterson Dental, St. Paul, MN.)

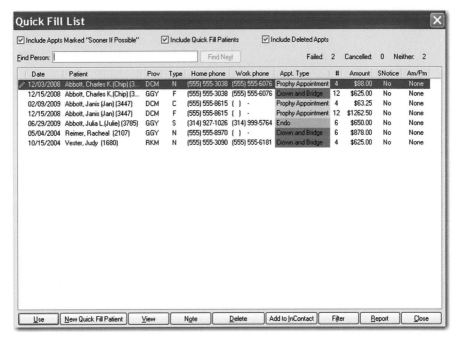

Figure 11-7 Short call list feature. (Courtesy Patterson Dental, St. Paul, MN.)

DESIGNING THE APPOINTMENT BOOK MATRIX

An **appointment book matrix**, or outline of the appointment book, functions like the matrix of a restoration; it provides support. It is the framework around which appointments are made. A matrix should be completed before a new appointment book or electronic system is used. It should include the following elements:
- *Holidays:* In many traditional books and computerized scheduling, holidays are noted by the manufacturer (Figure 11-8, *A*). However, it may be necessary to enter special holidays observed in one's locale or office. This can be done by placing an X across the entire day and marking it with the name of the holiday (Figure 11-8, *B*), or following the software guide to add holidays as necessary to the computerized schedule.
- *Lunch hours:* In traditional appointment books, lines may be used to cross out lunch hours. However, a broad, yellow felt-tip marker accomplishes the same task and can be written over legibly (Figure 11-9, *A*). After becoming experienced with the appointment book it will be unnecessary to mark off these hours. Computerized scheduling will follow a template that the office sets up and will automatically insert lunch hours (Figure 11-9, *B*).
- *Buffer periods:* A **buffer period** is a small amount of time set aside to absorb the hectic workload of the day or to allow for emergencies. A 1-unit increment of time set aside in the morning and again in the afternoon allows time for unexpected emergencies or buffers an already hectic day. If this space is simply colored in with a yellow felt-tip pen, an entry can be made without erasing (Figure 11-10). The buffer period should not be inserted during the busiest periods of the day.

- *School calendar:* In some areas of the country the local dental society provides stick-on labels showing the local scheduled school closings and holidays (Figure 11-11). A school calendar may also be obtained from the local school district. Students and faculty members can then be scheduled for appointments when they are on vacation.
- *Professional meetings:* Some dental societies provide stickers for these dates; otherwise, a notation about the location and nature of the meeting can be made on the appropriate date, with an X blocking out the specified time (Figure 11-12). In the computer schedule the Block feature can be used to notate time that should be blocked.
- *Staff meetings:* Time should be set aside regularly, once or twice a month, for all members of the staff to meet and discuss goals for the office. This time should not be scheduled during the lunch period or after office hours, but should be integrated into regular office hours (see Chapter 2 for suggestions on scheduling staff meetings).
- *Vacation days:* Mark off days that staff will be taking vacations with as much advance notice as possible.

IMPORTANT FACTORS IN SCHEDULING APPOINTMENTS

The administrative assistant must deal with a variety of situations in scheduling appointments. Management of the appointment book requires a well-defined treatment plan, an established appointment sequence, and an ability to maintain strict control over the appointment book while still meeting the needs of patients.

Several of these situations are common to all dental offices. For an assistant with several years of experience, managing such

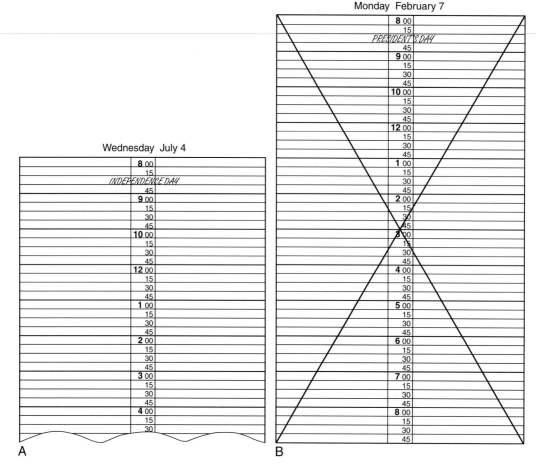

Figure 11-8 A, Holiday page from a traditional appointment book. **B,** An X drawn through a page from an appointment book to indicate a holiday or office closure.

problems is fairly easy, but it may be more difficult for the inexperienced individual. The office staff should identify situations that commonly occur and develop a policy for managing appointments for these situations.

Emergency Patients

Patients who call the office for emergencies should be seen by the dentist during designated buffer periods. When a patient calls and requests an immediate appointment for a toothache, ask the patient the following questions: "How long has the tooth been bothering you?" "Which tooth is it?" "What type of discomfort are you experiencing—a sharp pain or a dull ache?" "Is it sensitive to hot, cold, or pressure?" At this point, determine whether it is a true emergency. It is prudent then to say, "The dentist's schedule is filled for the day, but Dr. Lake could see you to relieve the discomfort at 10:30 this morning. Then, if further treatment is necessary, we can schedule an additional appointment." This eliminates any preconceived idea that the dentist's schedule permits time for extensive treatment that has not been scheduled. If the patient finds it difficult to come in at the suggested time, it may be necessary to schedule the appointment at a later date.

A dentist should always be prepared to see patients of record for emergencies or to make provision for such coverage in his or her absence. Emergency treatment for new patients can become a lifeline for a dental practice. These patients often become excellent patients in the future. They appreciate being seen by the dentist on an emergency basis and often accept treatment plans willingly to avoid future emergencies.

Young Children

Young children should be scheduled at times that will not interfere with their nap periods or regularly scheduled activity times. For these reasons, early morning generally is considered a good time for young children's dental appointments. Have you ever encountered a cross child just before nap time, or have you ever had to call a child in from play to go to the dentist? Ask the mother about the child's daily routine and be considerate in appointment scheduling.

Older Adults

Older patients often require special attention. Some, although they arise early, find rush hour traffic very disconcerting,

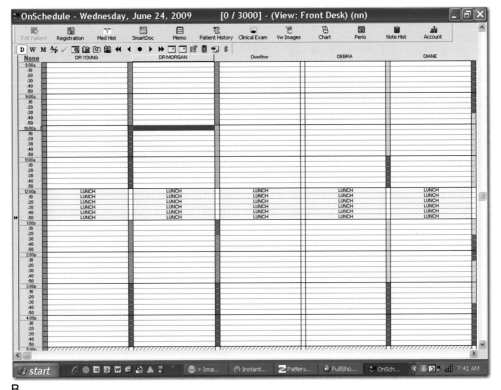

Figure 11-9 A, Lunch hour highlighted in a traditional appointment book with a felt-tip marker. **B,** Computer appointment book with lunch hour indicated. (**B,** Courtesy Patterson Dental, St. Paul, MN.)

whereas others find it difficult to rush about in the morning. Although many older patients need special consideration, remember not to embarrass them by calling attention to their age.

DENTIST'S BIOLOGICAL CLOCK

Difficult cases, such as crown and bridge work, are best scheduled at a time when the dentist is in a peak energy period. Not all people are at their best at all times of the day. Early morning generally has been considered the best time for extensive treatment. However, some dentists do not reach their peak period until 1 or 2 PM, when the early birds who were dynamic at 8 AM have begun to lose energy. This becomes an important factor in determining when certain types of treatment should be scheduled. As a rule, appointments for extensive operative and surgical treatment and management of difficult children should be made at the dentist's peak time.

Scheduling for Productivity

As mentioned earlier in this text, dentistry is a business, and one of the most effective ways to be profitable is to increase productivity. The dentist should focus on procedures that are most profitable while performing the routine tasks or delegating when at all legally possible. Theodore Schumann, a noted CPA (www. dentalbusinesssuccess.com), explains that the typical practitioner produces about $300 to $500 per hour. It is not uncommon to produce even less than this if the scheduling system is not managed effectively. Over the year, if the dentist increases production by just $50 per hour, annual production could increase by $76,000, of which about $60,000 would be additional profit.

This is where the administrative assistant needs to "think outside the box" and modify the old ways of scheduling. To achieve this increased productivity, hourly production must increase. With this concept, considered in conjunction with the dentist's body clock, begin to modify the way scheduling is

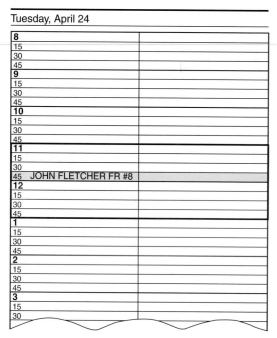

Tuesday, April 24

Figure 11-10 One-unit buffer highlighted in a traditional appointment book with a felt-tip marker.

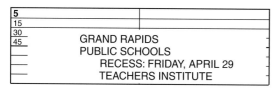

Figure 11-11 Label indicating school closing.

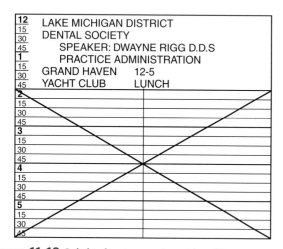

Figure 11-12 Label indicating meeting with an X.

done. If "power blocks" of time are set aside for high productivity/high profit procedures, production will increase. Therefore, if the dentist's body clock is best from 10 AM to 2 PM, all high productivity procedures must be scheduled during that period and *no* other types of treatment. This time must be reserved for productive, profitable procedures, and all attempts to break into the "power blocks" must be forestalled. It takes time to make this system work, and it requires a different mind set at first, but after 6 months this concept will be found to be very effective, and the practice will begin to reap the profits.

Extended Office Hours

Many offices develop a schedule that includes extended office hours, which are hours beyond the traditional work day. These may include early morning, evening time, or weekend days. There is no significant difference in scheduling appointments for this type of practice, but it requires special attention in the selection of an appointment book and designing the matrix. Care should be taken that the days identified for extended hours include times to cover all the hours the office will be open. This situation may require an unmarked appointment book that allows insertion of days and times in accordance with the office schedule Computer scheduling should easily accomplish extended office hours.

Management of Prime Time

Prime time is the time period most often requested by patients; in most offices it generally is the time after 3 PM. Obviously not all who request this time will receive it; therefore, patients must be informed of the need to schedule this time on a rotating basis. Forms are available for students requesting that the patient be excused during class time (Figure 11-13).

Habitually Late Patients

A small number of patients persist in being late for their appointments. Stress the importance of being on time for the appointment by explaining, "Mr. Campbell, the nature of your treatment requires all the time allotted; therefore, we must ask your cooperation in being on time for your appointments." This should be done in a firm but pleasant manner. Another way of handling this situation is to enter an earlier time on the appointment card than is entered in the appointment book. But be careful; this could backfire!

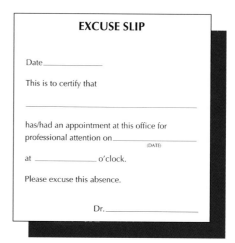

Figure 11-13 School excuse. (Courtesy Patterson Office Supplies, Champaign, IL.)

Series Appointments

Care should be taken not to schedule too many appointments for a patient at one time. The patient who has a long series of appointments is likely to cancel more readily, thinking the appointment can be made up next week, when in reality the appointments may not be of the same length. This disrupts the treatment schedule. Make tentative appointments beyond 2 to 3 weeks, but do not list them on the appointment card until the patient has completed the first series.

Patient Who Arrives on the Wrong Day

No office would be complete without a patient who arrives on the wrong day or at the wrong time. The error may be the patient's, or the assistant may have written the wrong date on the appointment card. Ask to see the appointment card and, if the patient has made the mistake, indicate the actual date and time of the appointment. Of course, if the administrative assistant or another staff member made the error, an apology is necessary and the patient should be seen by the dentist. The scheduled patients may be contacted to explain that an "unexpected change has occurred in the schedule," and delay their arrival. Regardless of who is responsible for the error, the assistant should remain tactful and helpful in correcting the mistake.

Drop-Ins

Nothing is more frustrating than to have a patient drop by the office and say, "I was just in the area, and thought I'd drop in and see if Doc could do something to this tooth that's been bothering me." Seeing a patient on this basis can open Pandora's box and create the concept that a patient can just drop in at any time. Tactfully inform the patient that the dentist sees patients by appointment, and tell the person when the next appointment is available. However, if the drop-in patient is a patient of record and has a legitimate emergency, try to accommodate the person.

This practice does not apply to the many walk-in (convenience) dental clinics established in the past few years. One of the prime objectives of these clinics is to accommodate patients without appointments.

Broken Appointments

At times a patient absolutely must cancel an appointment or is prevented from keeping the appointment by some unforeseen circumstance. Most patients respect the dentist's time, and the dentist should be understanding when a cancellation occurs. Other patients, unfortunately, seem always to find an excuse for breaking an appointment. Although most dentists' initial reaction is to charge for broken appointments, this becomes difficult to accomplish and results in poor public relations. Therefore the patient should be informed of the importance of keeping the appointment; for example, "Mr. Ward, since you failed to keep your 2-hour appointment, the treatment schedule has been delayed." Tactfully explain, "I can only reschedule such a lengthy appointment if we can be assured you will be here." Such cancellations should be noted on the patient's clinical chart (Figure 11-14).

If the patient continues to cancel appointments, he should be told, "Mr. Ward, we are unable to continue to make appointments for you because you have failed to cooperate with us." However, such a policy should be exercised only after it has been approved by the dentist.

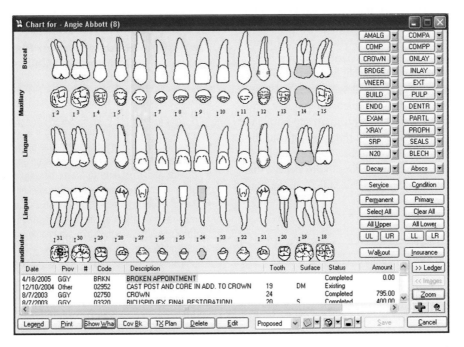

Figure 11-14 Clinical chart showing a broken appointment. (Courtesy Patterson Dental, St. Paul, MN.)

Dovetailing

Minor types of treatment can easily be accomplished in less than 1 unit. **Dovetailing** means working a second patient into the schedule during another scheduled patient's treatment, for example, while the first patient waits for an anesthetic to take effect or an impression to set. The appointment page shown in Figure 11-15 has four places for dovetailing: at 8 AM, while waiting for anesthesia with Hazel Gates; at approximately 8:30 AM, while waiting for the final impression to set; at 8:45 AM, while waiting for anesthesia for John Monroe; and at 9 AM while waiting for John Monroe's final impression to set.

Many types of appointments can be dovetailed, such as denture adjustments, suture removal, healing check, restoration polish, or dressing changes. In an expanded-duties practice, many of these procedures are done by a qualified staff member and must be dovetailed into that person's schedule.

Establishing an Appointment Time

To prevent conflicts with patients over appointment times, the assistant should avoid loaded questions. Don't ask, "What is the most convenient time for you?" "What is your day off?" or "When does Frank get out of school?" It is wiser to ask, "Is morning or afternoon better for you?" and then present two choices for the patient. By leading the patient into making a choice realistically within the office's schedule, the assistant will not be forced to say, "I'm sorry" to each of the patient's suggestions.

Confirming Appointments

To confirm or not to confirm appointments is often a reason for debate. There can be two sides to this discussion. Regardless of the approach the dentist takes for the practice, it is vital to use the term, *confirm* rather than *remind*, as patients do not like to be reminded of an appointment. They will, however, appreciate a confirmation of the appointment.

The issue in "confirming an appointment" is that few other professionals need to call a person to confirm an appointment. Dentistry through the years has adopted the policy of confirming appointments and this practice has been perpetuated over the years. Many practice management consultants believe that when a patient is well educated about the need for complete and

thorough dental care they will respect the appointment time and follow through with all appointment times. Today, with the use of e-mail and answering machines it is easy to make confirmation follow ups if a few basic rules are followed. Before dismissing the patient when a future appointment is needed, ask the patient if he or she needs a courtesy confirmation call or notice. This will allow the retraining of the patient to accept responsibility for the appointment. Box 11-3 lists some suggestions for placing confirmation calls or notices in e-mail.

ENTERING APPOINTMENTS

Overview

As mentioned, one person should be in charge of the appointment system at all times. This does not mean that no one else can make appointments, but this person must routinely check the appointment book and manage it according to the guidelines the staff has determined. The dentist should never encourage friends or relatives to "drop by the office," but rather should direct everyone to contact the administrative assistant for an appointment. Great effort should be made to schedule the next appointment for a patient when the patient is in the office. Never let the patient say, "I will call you," as the person will forget and get distracted by many other activities at home and in his or her personal life.

An entry in the traditional appointment book must be made in pencil. It must be accurate, complete, and legible, and include the information shown in Box 11-4. Appointments entered in a computerized schedule are easily moved from time to time by clicking and dragging the appointment to a new time.

<table>
<tr><td colspan="2">BOX 11-3   **Suggestions for Placing Confirmation Calls or Notices via E-mail**</td></tr>
</table>

- Ask patients if they need a courtesy confirmation call or e-mail.
- If the confirmation is for a preventive recall appointment, do not trivialize that appointment by calling it a "cleaning."
- Avoid leaving confirmation messages on an answering machine for any patient who has a history of broken appointments.
- Do not allow patients to leave messages of cancellation on the office answering machine over the weekend.
- Avoid leaving a message on a patient's answering machine that requires the patient to call back to confirm receipt of the message. This is disruptive to the office's schedule and can be annoying to the dependable patient.
- Use a short succinct message of confirmation.

   "Hello Mrs. Gamez, this is Mary at Dr. Lake's office. I'm calling to confirm your appointment on Wednesday, May 5 at 10 AM. Please call our office within 24 hours of the appointment if there is a change in your schedule. Thank you for your consideration."

- When sending an e-mail confirmation, the message should also be succinct as it is for the telephone.

Friday, April 22	
8 MS. HAZEL GATES (JOHN)	
15 PREP. #7 PVC	
30 H-459-7252	B-454-2100 EXT. 29
45 MR. JOHN MONROE	
9 PREP. #31 F.C.	
15 H-243-6410	B-454-6300
30	
45	

Figure 11-15 Dovetailing on an appointment page in a traditional appointment book.

BOX 11-4 Information to Include in an Appointment Book Entry

- Patient's full name, with cross-reference in case of duplication of names
- Home and business phone numbers to confirm the appointment or to reach the patient in case of an emergency
- Treatment to be done
- Age of patient (if a child)
- Length of the appointment, indicated with an arrow
- Special notations (e.g., new patient, premedication required, case at the laboratory)

Because of the limited amount of space available for each entry, symbols must be used to make special notations about a patient. Table 11-1 lists several symbols commonly used in the appointment book. In the example in Figure 11-16, *A*, note that the two entries in the manual appointment book have been made using these symbols. Each entry was made in pencil and is accurate, complete, and legible. Here the assistant has used the special clinical codes used in Dr. Lake's office to indicate the treatment to be done. Figure 11-16, *B*, shows a description of an appointment using the computer scheduler. It is important to list the complete treatment, because this tells the assistant exactly what is to be done; also, the assistant can easily transfer this information to an appointment list later without referring to the clinical charts, thus saving time.

When appointments are made, the sequence normally followed in a dental office is initial examination and prophylaxis, radiographs, and diagnostic models (Figure 11-17). After the dentist has concluded the diagnosis and treatment plan, the patient returns for a consultation appointment. At this time, the patient accepts the original or modified treatment plan, and the assistant makes the necessary appointments.

Once treatment is complete, the patient is recalled periodically through the preventive recall system outlined in Chapter 12. An appointment sequence must be established, as mentioned, in coordination with the treatment plan. To do this, ask the dentist to establish the sequence and the amount of time needed for each appointment for all types of treatment. In a manual system, this list can be keyed and placed in a celluloid protective cover for easy access. In an electronic system, the information is entered when the system is set up, and the appointment time is entered automatically. If using a manual system, the dentist should identify the number of units needed for a specific treatment, make an appointment schedule list, and have it available for reference during scheduling. After a schedule for the office has been designed, there is no need to guess how much time is needed for each type of appointment. In a computer system, program the amount of time needed according to the type of treatment, and thus eliminate any guessing.

After establishing the appointment sequence, refer to the patient's **treatment plan** to determine the treatment that must be done. The treatment plan is completed at the time of the diagnosis by the dentist and recorded on a treatment plan form (Figure 11-18). The same information is generated in either the manual or electronic treatment plan. The treatment plan in Figure 11-18 indicates that the first need of the patient is a porcelain fused to metal crown on tooth #30. By referring to the appointment list, note that the patient must have two appointments. The first is for preparation (three units); the second, at least 1 week later, is for cementation of the crown and requires two units. This system can be easily followed for all appointment scheduling.

At this point determine the times for the appointments by using the suggestions made previously. Care should be taken to eliminate useless voids in the schedule by: (1) always beginning to schedule appointments at the bottom or top of a large block of time, never in the middle, and (2) not leaving units of time (except for buffers) vacant between appointments.

Appointment Card

An **appointment card** is a written notification of the patient's appointment that the patient takes home. Once the entry has been made in the appointment book, transfer the information to the appointment card. It is entered directly from the appointment book in ink and should be easy to read. Recheck the appointment card before giving it to the patient to make sure the information in the book and on the card is the same.

A traditional appointment card generally is made of medium-weight or lightweight stock and measures about 2 × 3½ inches to fit easily into a wallet. Appointment cards usually are white with black print. However, many offices are now color coding cards, using matching or contrasting ink to carry out a color theme in the office. The information on the card includes the dentist's full name, degrees, address, and phone number and the office policy on broken appointments. Lines are provided for the patient's name and the day, date, and time of the appointment. Figure 11-19 shows a variety of appointment cards that can be used in the dental office.

TABLE 11-1	Symbols for Traditional Appointment Book Entries
Symbol	**Meaning**
N	New patient
*	Patient prefers an earlier appointment.
B	Business phone number
H	Home phone number
L	Case at the laboratory
Ⓛ	Case returned from the laboratory
PM	Premedicate (i.e., medicate before treatment)
÷	In red, denotes confirmed appointment
↓	Length of appointment

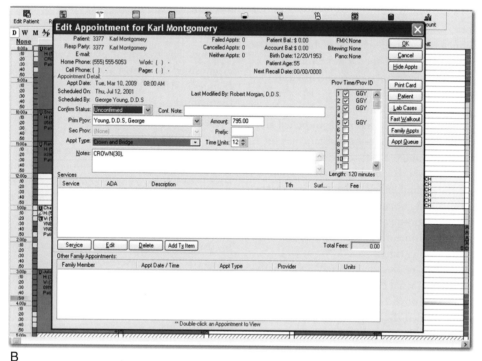

A

B

Figure 11-16 A, Two appointment book entries using symbols in a traditional appointment book. **B,** Appointment entry in a computer appointment book using programmed information. (**B,** Courtesy Patterson Dental, St. Paul, MN.)

The cards shown in *A* and *B* are for only one appointment; the card shown in *C* is a series-type appointment card on which more than one appointment may be listed. The series card saves both the assistant's time and the cost of additional cards. In an electronic system, the appointment often is listed on the exit receipt. It also can be listed on a walkout statement, but many patients like the security of a separate appointment card. If using computerized scheduling, the system should easily print an appointment card for the patient. The electronic system does eliminate the potential for error in writing on the appointment card.

DAILY APPOINTMENT SCHEDULE

Each day the administrative assistant pulls the clinical records for each of the next day's patients and completes a daily schedule. The **daily appointment schedule** is a chronological listing of the day's activities. This schedule is placed in the treatment rooms, laboratory, and dentist's private office. The information transferred from the appointment book may be written or typed onto the daily schedule or entered electronically (Figure 11-20). It should include the patient's name, the treatment to be done, and the time of the appointment. The schedule is placed for easy

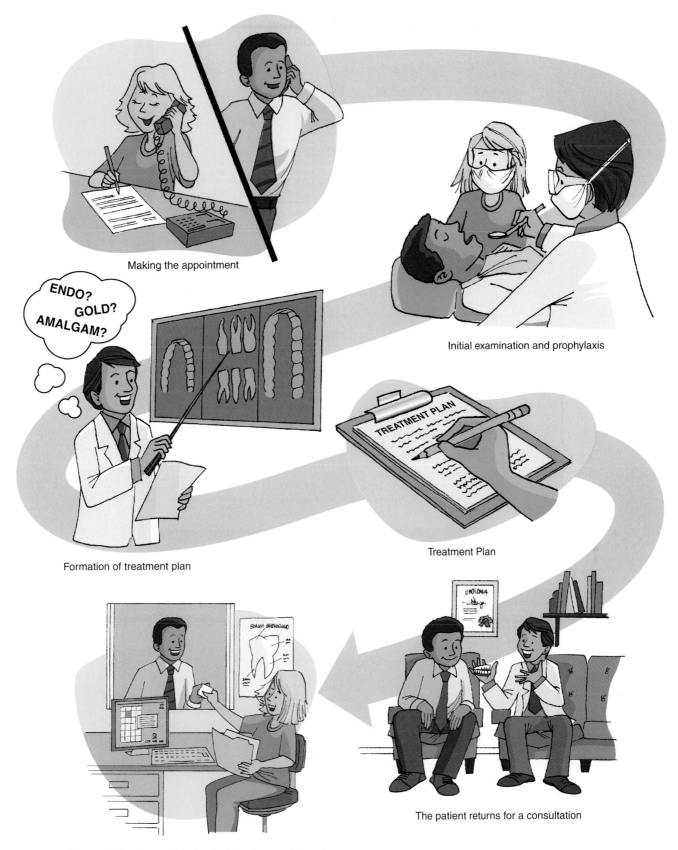

Making the appointment

Initial examination and prophylaxis

Formation of treatment plan

Treatment Plan

The administrative assistant schedules the appointment

The patient returns for a consultation

Figure 11-17 Appointment sequence.

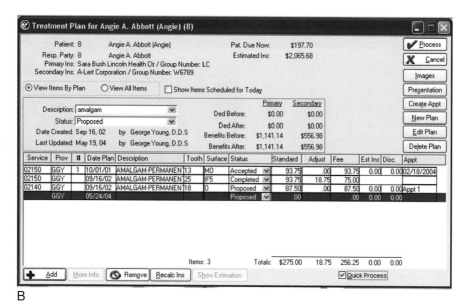

Figure 11-18 A, Traditional treatment plan. **B,** Electronic treatment plan screen. (**B,** Courtesy Patterson Dental, St. Paul, MN.)

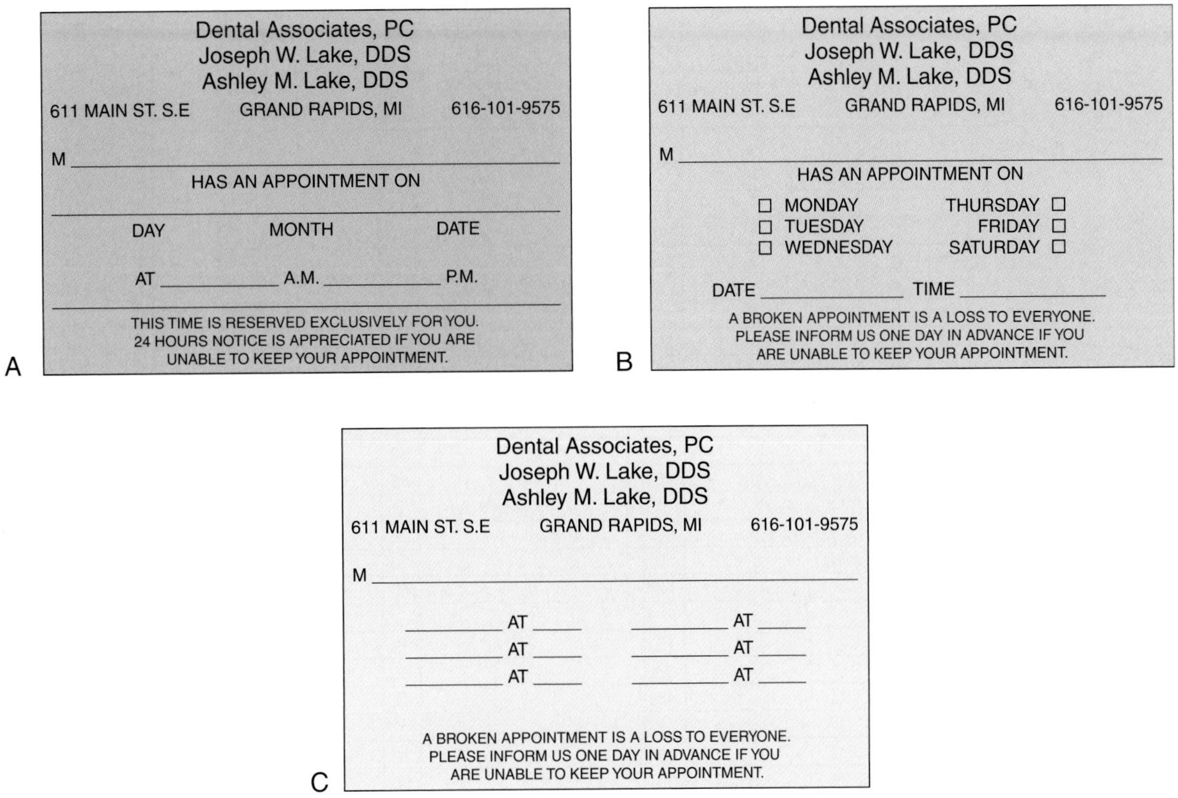

Figure 11-19 Appointment cards. **A** and **B,** Single appointment cards. **C,** Series-style appointment card.

access by the staff; however, to protect confidentiality, it should not be in view to patients or other passersby. The administrative assistant should keep the schedule current if any changes take place during the day. If the office is computerized, the schedule does not need to be printed, as the staff can view the schedule on the computer monitor.

SCHEDULING PATIENTS IN AN ADVANCED-FUNCTION PRACTICE

Scheduling of patients in an office that has an advanced- or expanded-function dental auxiliary requires a different time assignment concept. In such practices the patient does not see the dentist only. Depending on the state dental practice act and the qualifications of the various clinical staff members, time may also be assigned to the advanced-function assistant to perform various clinical tasks without the dentist needing to be assigned to the patient. A variety of tasks that can be assigned to the appropriately qualified assistant may include diagnostic impressions, dental radiographs, periodontal dressing placement or removal, placing or carving of amalgam, or various other specialty tasks.

It is vital that the administrative assistant understand the legal ramifications of assigning an unqualified or noncredentialed person to perform various clinical tasks. The administrative assistant must have a thorough understanding of the state law, and a clinical assistant's qualifications for a task must be verified before the individual is scheduled to treat patients.

Typically the units of time for the operator are modified, but patient chair time remains the same in a specific room, because the advanced functions assistant performs intraoral tasks that might have been performed by the dentist in the past. It takes time on the part of the staff to determine how and by whom the intraoral duties will be performed, but once this is determined, the administrative assistant can plan on such treatment in the scheduling option of the appointment book.

Once familiar with the techniques of appointment book management, it can be a very enjoyable part of the business office. Using time efficiently can make each day in the office more productive and can reduce tension while still meeting the patients' needs. If the rules in Box 11-2 are followed, the dental office can maintain efficiency.

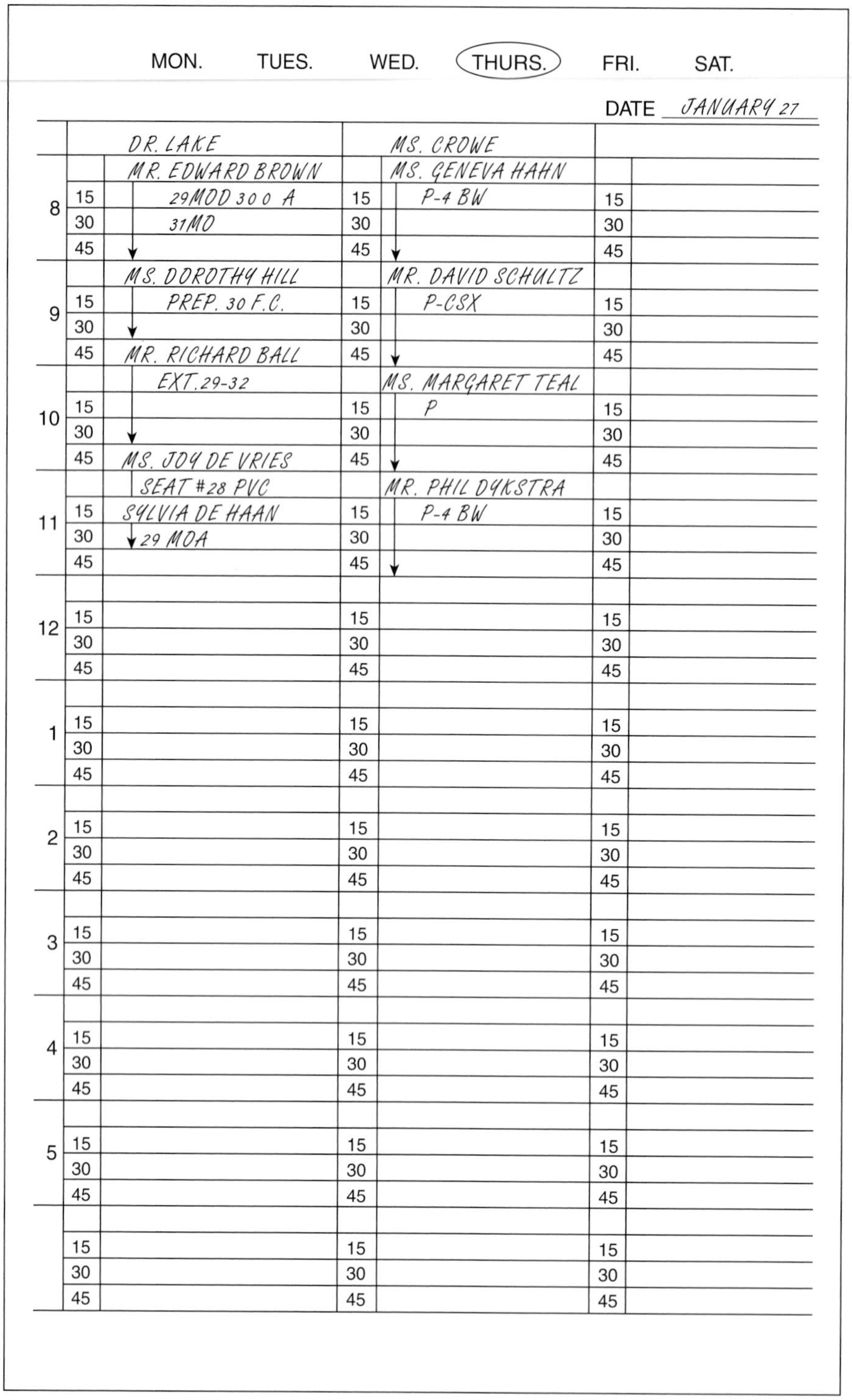

		MON.	TUES.	WED.	THURS.	FRI.	SAT.

DATE _JANUARY 27_

		DR. LAKE		MS. CROWE		
		MR. EDWARD BROWN		MS. GENEVA HAHN		
8	15	29 MOD 300 A	15	P-4 BW	15	
	30	31 MO	30		30	
	45		45		45	
		MS. DOROTHY HILL		MR. DAVID SCHULTZ		
9	15	PREP. 30 F.C.	15	P-CSX	15	
	30		30		30	
	45	MR. RICHARD BALL	45		45	
		EXT. 29-32		MS. MARGARET TEAL		
10	15		15	P	15	
	30		30		30	
	45	MS. JOY DE VRIES	45		45	
		SEAT #28 PVC		MR. PHIL DYKSTRA		
11	15	SYLVIA DE HAAN	15	P-4 BW	15	
	30	29 MOA	30		30	
	45		45		45	
12	15		15		15	
	30		30		30	
	45		45		45	
1	15		15		15	
	30		30		30	
	45		45		45	
2	15		15		15	
	30		30		30	
	45		45		45	
3	15		15		15	
	30		30		30	
	45		45		45	
4	15		15		15	
	30		30		30	
	45		45		45	
5	15		15		15	
	30		30		30	
	45		45		45	
	15		15		15	
	30		30		30	
	45		45		45	

A

Figure 11-20 A, Traditional daily schedule.

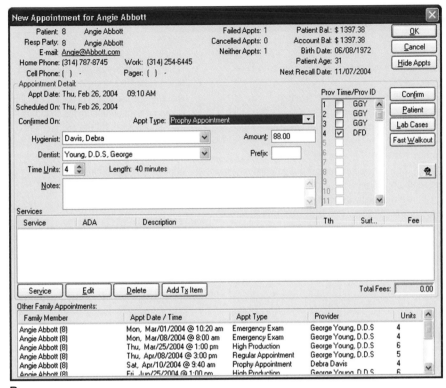

B

Figure 11-20, cont'd B, Electronic daily schedule. (**B,** Courtesy Patterson Dental, St. Paul, MN.)

KEY TERMS

Appointment book—The scheduling software or actual book into which patients and data are entered for appointment times.

Appointment book matrix—An outline of various activities that routinely occur in the dental practice.

Appointment card—The form on which the patient's next appointment is scheduled; it includes the day, date, and time.

Buffer period—A small amount of time set aside to absorb the hectic workload of the day or to allow for emergencies.

Daily appointment schedule—A chronological listing of the day's activities.

Dovetailing—Working a second patient into the schedule during another scheduled patient's treatment.

Prime time—The busiest time in the dental practice.

Treatment plan—A sequential listing of the treatment to be completed for a patient.

Unit (u)—A given amount of time, generally in 10-or 15-minute increments, into which each day of the appointment book is separated.

LEARNING ACTIVITIES

1. Discuss the types of appointment systems available for use in the dental office.
2. Explain the advantages of an electronic appointment system.
3. Explain the components of an appointment matrix.
4. Explain the management of the following appointment scheduling situations:
   a. A mother calls the office, hysterical, because her child, age 8, has just fallen off his bicycle. She states that there is a great deal of bleeding and that his teeth are broken.
   b. A patient who has not been treated by the dentist in more than a year comes into the office about 2:30 PM. He states that he is having some discomfort around a bridge abutment and that he has severe bleeding when he brushes. The schedule for the remaining part of the day is filled.
   c. A patient appears on Monday, January 23, at 10 AM. The assistant greets her, and she says she has a 10 o'clock appointment. On checking the appointment book, her name is not listed for that day.
   d. A patient's appointment was confirmed for 1 PM today. The patient does not show up for the appointment.
5. What information is included on the following forms?
   a. Appointment card
   b. Appointment daily schedule
   c. Call list
   d. Treatment plan

Please refer to the student workbook for additional learning activities.

BIBLIOGRAPHY

DaCosta V: Digital appointment scheduling, *Proofs Magazine,* January 8, 2004.

Miles L: *Dynamic dentistry,* Virginia Beach, VA, 2003, Link Publishing.

Schumann TC: Top five opportunities to improve your profit, *J Mich Dent Assoc,* February 2005 .

RECOMMENDED WEB SITE

www.dentalbusinesssuccess.com

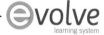

Please visit http://evolve.elsevier.com/Finkibeiner/practice for additional practice activities.

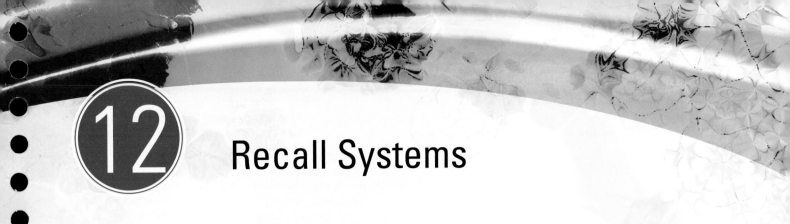

12 Recall Systems

CHAPTER OUTLINE

Keeping Patients Informed
Types of Recall or Recare Systems
    Advanced Appointment System
    Telephone Recall or Recare System
    Mail Recall or Recare System
    Telecommunications (E-mail or Text Messaging) Recall
       or Recare System
Establishing a Recall or Recare System
    Electronic Recall or Recare Files
    Follow-Up
    Purging the System

LEARNING OUTCOMES

- Define key terms.
- Explain the purpose of a recall or recare system.
- Describe motivational techniques to promote a recall or recare system.
- Identify different types of recall or recare systems.
- Develop a recall or recare system.

A **recall or recare system** notifies patients of the timing of routine dental care. Some practitioners have adopted the term *recare* rather than recall, sensing that it has a more caring approach. Whether *recall* or *recare* is used as the term in the office, this system is an integral part of every modern dental practice and is essential to both the patient and the dentist. A recall/recare system is the lifeline of the practice. It helps achieve one of the primary objectives of dentistry—helping patients maintain good oral health for a lifetime. The routine recall appointment generally is assigned to the dental hygienist, but each dental professional in the practice must assume a role in maintaining a successful recall system.

 PRACTICE NOTE
A recall system is the lifeline of the practice. It helps achieve one of the primary objectives of dentistry—helping patients maintain good oral health for a lifetime.

Patients are recalled to the office most often for an oral prophylaxis and examination. However, a recall visit may be scheduled for a variety of other reasons:
- Examination of oral tissues after surgical procedures
- Checking for occlusal relationships
- Examination of prosthetic devices (e.g., full or partial dentures or implants)
- Determination of eruption patterns in children
- Determination of the status of orthodontic treatment
- Follow-up on endodontic treatment
- Follow-up for an implant
- Determination of periodontal tissue status

The success of a recall or recare system depends on three factors: (1) dental health education, (2) motivation, and (3) consistent follow-up. The administrative assistant must help patients develop a sense of responsibility toward their own dental health, even though such a behavioral change is not made quickly. In addition, the patient must be aware of how the practice's recall or recare system operates. As Winston Churchill put it, "People love to learn but hate to be taught."

 PRACTICE NOTE
The success of a recall system depends on three factors: (1) dental health education, (2) motivation, and (3) consistent follow-up.

Education begins when the patient first visits the office. This approach can be delivered in a lifetime and annual format. The dentist or hygienist needs to determine the patient's health goals before beginning treatment. Asking a patient if he or she would like to discuss developing a lifetime approach for their dental health and appearance is vital to determining long-range plans for the patient's dental care. This discussion should take place at the beginning of the appointment when the patient has more energy and is more willing to take the time. By talking about a lifetime strategy toward good dental health and appearance, patients think about lifetime plans rather than simply "fixing a problem" found at a routine prophylaxis. Thus the dentist and hygienist are able to include the routine recall/recare appointment as part of total lifetime care. In fact some dentists have adopted the approach of including the first recall/recare appointment after extensive dental care as part of the total fee.

This lets the patient know how important it is to return to the office for a complete prophylaxis, occlusal adjustment, or other routine care.

Before beginning treatment, the dentist and/or hygienist need to introduce the importance of the annual recall/recare plan. For some patients this may mean returning to the office two or three times for care. This also can rid the patient of thinking solely in a "6-month" mentality and elevates this appointment to higher therapeutic ground. Remember that a successful recall or recare system requires that the administrative assistant use communication skills before clinical skills.

Motivation of patients, which is critical to the effectiveness of the recall/recare system, is the responsibility of the entire dental staff. Once a patient has been educated and motivated to accept a recall/recare system, the administrative assistant is responsible for maintaining the system efficiently. The importance of this step cannot be overemphasized. If an assistant ignores the system even for 1 month, the effect on the patient flow becomes noticeable within a short time, and patients begin to feel ignored.

KEEPING PATIENTS INFORMED

Patients in the dental practice must understand the importance of recall or recare regardless of the reason for the recall appointment. In addition to the initial introduction of the recall or recare program, much can be done through patient education to promote the recall or recare system. Some practical and easy ways to keep patients informed about the dental procedures the office offers and the way the recall or recare system works include the following:

- Updated practice brochures
- Newsletters
- Audiovisual materials in the reception room
- Intraoral cameras
- Before-and-after photographs
- Bulletin boards
- Follow-up e-mails

TYPES OF RECALL OR RECARE SYSTEMS

Any of several types of recall or recare systems can be used. Most dentists find that no one system is perfect; therefore, they often use more than one. The most common systems are the advanced appointment system, the telephone system, the mail system, and more recently telecommunications e-mail or text messaging.

Advanced Appointment System

With the **advanced appointment system**, recall or recare appointments are scheduled before the patient leaves the office. Traditionally, management experts have criticized this system because people cannot predict their schedules 6 months in advance. Chaos can result if the dentist or hygienist is absent

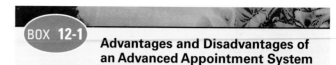

BOX 12-1

Advantages and Disadvantages of an Advanced Appointment System

Advantages
- No cost involved
- No time required of the administrative assistant
- Simple

Disadvantages
- Patients do not know what their future commitments might be.
- Hygienist's appointment book may be filled 6 months in advance, and then staff changes may occur.

from the office and misses a scheduled appointment or if patients constantly cancel their appointments. Advocates of this system contend that most people know their routines and the appointment times that generally are best for them. The office staff should weigh the advantages and disadvantages listed in Box 12-1.

Telephone Recall or Recare System

The **telephone recall or recare system** allows the most immediate response, because the administrative assistant contacts each patient by telephone to schedule a recall/recare appointment. This can be a good practice builder for a new practitioner, but it can be an exhausting and time-consuming task in a large, well-established practice.

When contacting a patient by telephone, use phrases that do not devalue the service. Eliminate such phrases as "for your check-up" or "for your cleaning." Some assistants find it cumbersome to use the words *prophylaxis* and *examination,* because they feel these terms are too technical; also, these words don't accurately convey the importance of the recall or recare visit. This visit includes a complete dental examination, an examination of all oral tissues (to detect oral diseases early), and complete scaling and polishing of teeth. Take the time to inform patients that this is an important preventive service or try using the phrase, *preventive recall* or *recare appointment.*

Because many people have answering machines or voicemail, which allow messages, the telephone system can be an effective technique that provides personal contact with the patient. Care should be taken to avoid personal messages on the telephone unless the patient has indicated in a signed permission form that personal messages may be left on the answering machine or voice mail. Box 12-2 lists a few suggestions for successfully using the telephone in a recall/recare system. The advantages and disadvantages of the telephone system are listed in Box 12-3.

Mail Recall or Recare System

With the **mail recall or recare system**, the patient is responsible for making the appointment. Patients receive a card that: (1) asks them to contact the office to schedule a preventive appointment or (2) gives them an appointment time and asks them to confirm it (Figure 12-1). The card should emphasize the importance of the prophylaxis and should not use words such as *cleaning* or *check-up*. The office manager addresses the card or the patient addresses the card at the previous visit. The latter arrangement can be especially effective, because patients recognize their own handwriting when they receive the card, and this may confirm their interest in the recall/recare system. Despite some drawbacks (Box 12-4), the mail system can be advantageous in a large practice.

Telecommunications (E-mail or Text Messaging) Recall or Recare System

The **e-mail or text messaging system** is becoming more widely used in dental offices today. As patients become accustomed to using e-mail and text messaging for appointment management they will welcome the use of this format from the dental office. Busy patients who often rely on their e-mail and text messaging systems to obtain their daily schedules and messages are often closely linked to these systems and would rather rely on this method of communication than the telephone or U.S. mail. The advantages and disadvantages of an e-mail or text messaging system are shown in Box 12-5.

Several types of recall or recare messages can be used (Figure 12-2). Take care not to underestimate a child's maturity when deciding which type of message to send to pediatric patients.

ESTABLISHING A RECALL OR RECARE SYSTEM

Once the type of system has been determined, the administrative assistant should set up a recall file that is simple, efficient, and accurate. The most efficient recall system is managed electronically. In today's dental practice, this is simply too important a management tool to rely on a manual system.

Electronic Recall or Recare Files

The computer is a valuable component of recall/recare management. With an electronic file, the software system generates a list of patients who need to be contacted (Figure 12-3). The computer also can produce the actual letter or card or create mailing labels for pre-prepared cards. If the office uses a telephone system, generate a master list of patients and their telephone numbers.

Follow-Up

As mentioned, it is critical that patients be recalled routinely. Patients need to be informed of how the recall/recare system works and how they will be notified before they leave the office. The administrative assistant must maintain flawless records and manage the system so as to ensure that the patient returns to the office in a timely manner.

BOX 12-2 **Suggestions for Using the Telephone Recall or Recare System**

- Don't call too early in the morning.
- Make sure your voice conveys a positive attitude; don't make calls if you're tired or grumpy.
- Make the calls in private, out of hearing of other patients.
- Don't pester patients. If they say they will call back, record it on the recall file cards and wait 2 to 3 weeks before contacting them again. If they do not respond after three calls, ask them if they wish to remain on the active recall program.
- Have the patient's recall record in front of you so that you will be well informed.
- Try calling on inclement days; patients are likely to be indoors on such days.
- If an answering machine is reached, speak clearly and leave a complete message, including the reason for the call, the times the office will be open, the telephone number, and a cordial "Thank you."

BOX 12-3 **Advantages and Disadvantages of a Telephone Recall or Recare System**

Advantages
- Immediate response from the patient
- Practice builder

Disadvantages
- May get no answer
- May be unable to reach patient
- May disturb the person called
- Time-consuming in a large practice
- Administrative assistant responsible for most of this system

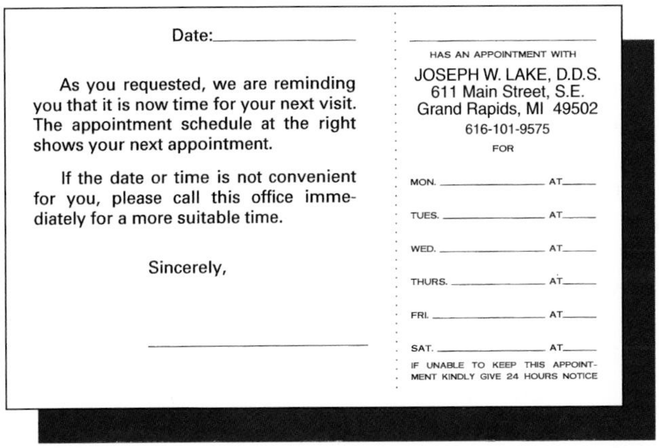

Date:_____

As you requested, we are reminding you that it is now time for your next visit. The appointment schedule at the right shows your next appointment.

If the date or time is not convenient for you, please call this office immediately for a more suitable time.

Sincerely,

_____

HAS AN APPOINTMENT WITH
JOSEPH W. LAKE, D.D.S.
611 Main Street, S.E.
Grand Rapids, MI 49502
616-101-9575

FOR

MON. _____ AT_____
TUES. _____ AT_____
WED. _____ AT_____
THURS. _____ AT_____
FRI. _____ AT_____
SAT. _____ AT_____

IF UNABLE TO KEEP THIS APPOINTMENT KINDLY GIVE 24 HOURS NOTICE

Figure 12-1 Recall card sent to patient to confirm a previously made appointment. (Courtesy Patterson Office Supplies, Champaign, IL.)

Advantages and Disadvantages of a Mail Recall or Recare System

Advantages
- Places responsibility on the patient
- Visible reminder

Disadvantages
- Possible to ignore notice
- Cost of postage
- Lack of immediate response

Advantages and Disadvantages of an E-mail and Text Messaging System

Advantages
- E-mail reaches its destination in a matter of seconds after it is sent, even if its destination is across the world.
- Places the responsibility on the patient to contact the office for an appointment
- Visible reminder
- Good communication tool for those who routinely use this
- Paper is saved. It is not necessary to make a hard copy of e-mail.
- E-mail may be filed electronically for later reference

Disadvantages
- Time consuming for the administrative assistant
- Not all patients prefer this technology
- Patient may quickly delete the message

Purging the System

Periodically, as with any records management system, the recall records must be purged. This can be done electronically for patients who have not been in the practice recall system for a period of years. To avoid the possibility of litigation for negligence, the dental office should inform the patient that the record is being removed from the system. A letter should be sent to the patient (and included in the patient's record) informing the person that he or she is being removed from the recall system. This protects the practice and reminds the patient one last time of the importance of a preventive recall or follow-up appointment.

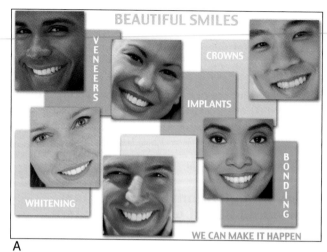

A

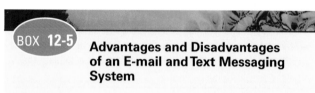

B

DENTAL ASSOCIATES, PC
Joseph W. Lake, DDS – Ashley M. Lake, DDS
611 Main Street, SE
Grand Rapids, MI 49502

PLACE STAMP HERE

Good dental health is important. Please call our office to schedule an appointment for your dental exam and preventive treatment.

C

Figure 12-2 A and **B,** Two styles of recall/recare cards. **C,** The back of a recall card has a message for the patient. (**A** and **B,** Courtesy Patterson Office Supplies, Champaign, IL.)

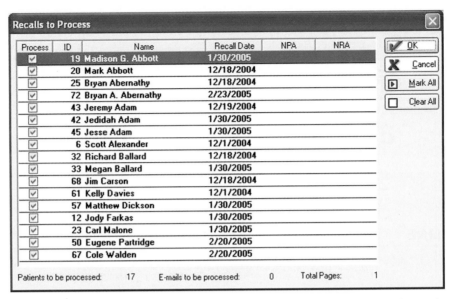

Figure 12-3 An electronic file generates a list of all patients due for recall in a specific month. (Courtesy Patterson Dental, St. Paul, MN.)

KEY TERMS

Advanced appointment system—A recall or recare system in which appointments are scheduled at the time the patient leaves the office.

E-mail or text messaging system—A recall or recare system that electronically notifies the patient that it is time to make an appointment for recall or recare.

Mail recall or recare system—A recall system in which the patient receives a card that: (1) asks the person to contact the office to make an appointment for a preventive recall visit, or (2) gives the patient an appointment time and asks the individual to confirm the appointment.

Recall or recare system—A system by which patients are notified of the timing of routine dental care.

Telephone recall or recare system—A system in which the patient is contacted by telephone for a recall appointment.

LEARNING ACTIVITIES

1. Explain the value of a recall or recare system to (a) a patient and (b) the dentist.
2. Describe the concept of recare versus recall.
3. What are the components to a successful recall/recare system?
4. Explain the advantages and disadvantages of each of the three basic recall/recare systems.

5. What effect would a computer have on a recall/recare system in a dental office?

Please refer to the student workbook for additional learning activities.

BIBLIOGRAPHY

Homoly P: Creating perfect recall, *Dental Economics*, Vol. 90, 4:28, 2001.

Salem G: The periodic exam: a vital key to practice success, *Dental Economics*, Vol. 94, 5:90–96, 2004.

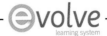

Please visit http://evolve.elsevier.com/Finkibeiner/practice for additional practice activities.

13

Inventory Systems and Supply Ordering

LEARNING OUTCOMES

- Define key terms.
- Identify three types of dental supplies.
- Explain various types of inventory systems.
- Establish an inventory system.
- Explain factors determining supply quantity.
- Describe a technique for receiving supplies.
- Describe a computerized ordering system.
- Identify common supply forms.
- Explain the storage of hazardous materials.

The day-to-day activity of the busy dental office is stressful enough without worrying about supplies. Stress increases when a necessary item is out of stock. Whether it is the dental hygienist who reaches for a fluoride rinse and there is none available, or if the clinical assistant suddenly realizes that there is no more of a specific dental cement, it is a factor that diminishes productivity and profitability. An effective inventory control system in invaluable, and it doesn't have to be complicated. A simple list taped to the inside of the supply cabinet can be just as effective as an inventory control on a computer or an Internet system. An important issue in inventory control is organization. There must be a plan, and each member of the team must understand how it works, and each person must assume responsibility to carry through with their part of the system. In this chapter the reader will learn about a variety of factors that can make the dental office become more organized in inventory control and will have the opportunity to review several systems.

Although one person may be assigned to ordering and maintaining supplies, the actual inventory control is the responsibility of the entire staff. In some dental offices the dental hygienist is responsible for ordering supplies related to the preventive area of practice. Those individuals responsible for the clinical areas of the office must note how much product is left when restocking the treatment rooms. When the product is low, there must be a communication system to indicate it is time to reorder the product. Most systems enable the administrative assistant to keep a record of order dates and product costs. This helps track when a supply is received and how much of a product is being used. In most situations, the person using the last item is required to add the product to the purchasing list or be certain an automated system has logged it into an order.

One person should be in charge of ordering, receiving, and storing supplies; managing hazardous waste; and maintaining **Material Safety Data Sheets (MSDSs)** (p. 244). Because the practice has both a business side and a clinical side, a business staff member may order all the business supplies, and a clinical staff member may be responsible for managing clinical supplies and hazardous materials. However, as mentioned, all staff members are responsible for noting whether supplies are low or exhausted as they perform their daily tasks.

PRACTICE NOTE

Whether at chairside, in the laboratory, or in the business office, dental professionals find it frustrating to reach for an item and find only an empty box.

TYPES OF SUPPLIES

Basic Categories

Supplies can be divided into three basic categories: expendable supplies, nonexpendable supplies, and capital supplies. Expendable supplies are single-use items such as dental cements, stationery, local anesthetics, and gypsum products. Nonexpendable supplies are reusable items that do not constitute a major expense; this category includes most dental instruments. Capital supplies are large, costly items that are seldom replaced, such as computers, sterilizers, and dental units.

Selecting Supplies

Not all materials can be purchased from one supplier, and buying from several suppliers may be more economical. Shopping locally promotes good relations and stimulates the local economy, but for economic reasons a dentist may order supplies from a larger catalog or discount house.

PRACTICE NOTE

Much of the efficiency of a dental office depends on a systematic and economical approach to ordering supplies.

A dental supply house can provide all the basic dental supplies, both brand name and generic. Purchasing from the dealers in a local area is convenient, but many large wholesale supply houses provide quick service and special rates. Making use of toll-free telephone numbers or online ordering also can speed up service. Make sure the vendor is reliable; the materials must be quality products and, where applicable, must meet American Dental Association (ADA) specifications.

Many dealers send a representative to the office routinely to obtain an order. The administrative assistant should have the order prepared or information available as listed in one of the inventory management systems. A manufacturer's representative who wants to see the dentist about a new product may accompany the supply person. If the dentist's schedule does not allow time to meet with the representative, obtain information about new products and relay the information to the dentist later.

Medicaments, which are not specifically dental items, can be purchased from a local pharmacy. Surgical supply companies sell materials such as thermometers, surgical scissors, and hemostats.

Business materials are available from local business office supply stores or by online ordering. Some supplies, such as cleaning materials, must be purchased at local businesses or specialty companies.

For convenience, use an address file on the computer or create a list on the Rolodex of the business addresses and telephone numbers of all the companies patronized routinely (see Chapter 8).

DESIGNING AN INVENTORY SYSTEM

The first step in inventory control organization is to streamline inventory management. An *inventory system* is a list of the stock and assets in the dental office. This list is divided into two parts, capital equipment and expendable and nonexpendable supplies. Become familiar with the types and quantities of products and materials used in the office. Also become quickly familiar with the monetary value of the current inventory and what the minimum and maximum quantities of the products are for the office.

Capital Equipment Inventory Control

A spreadsheet can be used to maintain an inventory of capital equipment. For a spreadsheet, software such as Excel or Access can be used. The administrative assistant can track all the major categories of capital supplies and have vital purchase and warranty information at the fingertips. Figure 13-1, *A*, illustrates the headings on a spread sheet for each capital item and details important information about the item, including date of purchase, serial numbers, and any comments about the product including warranty dates. The system shown in Access in Figure 13-1, *B*, allows the development of a cardlike system within the software for each room or category wished. In both Excel and Access software, templates are available that can be adapted to the individual office needs. A spreadsheet system can save much time and guesswork about the servicing of equipment and can be helpful to the accountant in determining depreciation. This information should be reviewed frequently for necessary preventive maintenance service. Such service is best scheduled when the dentist is out of the office.

Expendable and Nonexpendable Supplies Inventory Control

Dental offices generally do not keep a large stock of nonexpendable supplies on hand; however, a list may be included in an inventory system if the dentist wishes. Because the expendable supplies require more attention, an inventory of these items is important. The inventory can be automated on a computer or maintained manually.

Automated Inventory Systems

An automated inventory system can be created through a special software package or database created individually. The system can be simple or complex. An automated inventory system set up in a centralized database allows the staff simply to enter the shipment data into the system and print new inventory reports. The system enters the inventory numbers in the accounts

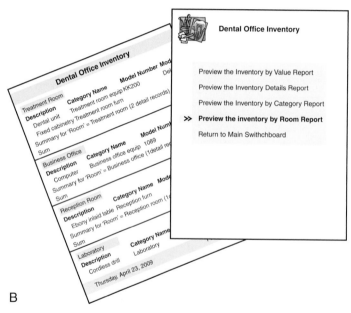

Dental Office Contents
Inventory List

Name	Ashley Lake
Address	611 main St. S.E.
Phone	616.101.9575
Insurance policy number	000-9789-1234
Insurance agent	Michael D. Jones
Insurance agent phone	616.101.4321
Insurance company	Rice and Brinkley
Insurance company phone	616.239.5678
Total estimated value on all items	$587,900.00

Room/area	Item/description	Make/model	Serial number/ ID number	Date purchased	Where purchased	Purchase price	Estimated current value	Notes	Photo?
Laboratory	Tracer Sterilizer	T-78	9325	5/17--	Henry Schein, Inc.				
Treatment Room A	Patient Chair	2001 Integra	743-0122	1/09/20--	HSP	$7,999.00	$6,500.00		
Treatment Room B	Patient Chair	2001 Integra	758-9811	11/09/20--	HSP	$7,999.00	$7,000.00		
Treatment Room A	Dental Unit	Dentassist	432-0321	1/09/20--	HSP	$7,000.00	$6,500.00		
Treatment Room B	Dental Unit	Dentassist	432-0322	11/09/20--	HSP	$7,000.00	$6,500.00		
Treatment Room A	Custom Fixed Cabinetry	HSP - Grande	6450-1	1/09/20--	HSP	$14,800.00	$8,990.00		
Treatment Room B	Custom Fixed Cabinetry	HSP - Grande	6450-1	1/09/20--	HSP	$8,990.00	$8,990.00		
Treatment Room A	Video/MicroEndoscope	CareScope 60	2391	2/12/20--	HSP	$14,800.00	$14,800.00	Warranty expires 48 months from date of purchase	
Treatment Room B	Video/MicroEndoscope	CareScope 60	2499	32/12/20--	HSP	$14,800.00	$14,800.00	Warranty expires 48 months from date of	

A

B

Figure 13-1 **A,** Capital equipment inventory spreadsheet produced in Microsoft Excel. **B,** Two components of a category type system generated using computer software.

automatically, as long as the information is entered correctly. A simple system like this, done in the office, can work as effectively in some offices as a dealer inventory management system.

Most dental supply dealers provide inventory management systems for their customers. The type of system may vary, but some are tag systems in which products are placed in bins or containers with tags that identify the product, quantity to order, and reorder point for the product. When a product needs to be reordered, the tag is removed from the container and placed in a location where the dealer representative can access it and order the product. Other dealers provide systems that reference bar codes on the products or their storage containers/bins (Figure 13-2). When products need to be

Figure 13-2 Bar code used with a scanner for computerized inventory.

ordered, the representative uses a bar code reader to upload the product information and then download it into the dealer's ordering system. Through these automated systems, the dental suppliers can provide customers with reports that summarize expenditures for products and supplies throughout the year, a useful tool in budgeting.

Such an inventory system provides an organized approach that utilizes the capable services of dental supply representatives as an extension of the dental team. This type of system combines inventory management and ordering into simple steps. However, many dealer inventory systems may be limited by the products and supplies that the company carries. Because many dental practices order items from several sources, this may require more than one inventory management system.

An example of an inventory management option is the Cubex system (Figure 13-3). At the end of this chapter is a list of several other inventory management systems. The Cubex system enables users to efficiently manage the ordering, tracking, and costs associated with inventory. The system can be configured to meet the specific needs of dental practices. Cubex can track operative, hygiene, prosthodontic, endodontic, implant, and other similar supplies.

The Cubex modular system enables shelves and drawers to be intermixed within a single cabinet to accommodate supplies of various sizes. Each cabinet can also be combined with auxiliary cabinets to increase storage capacity. The cabinets house more than 400 items and work much like an ATM machine

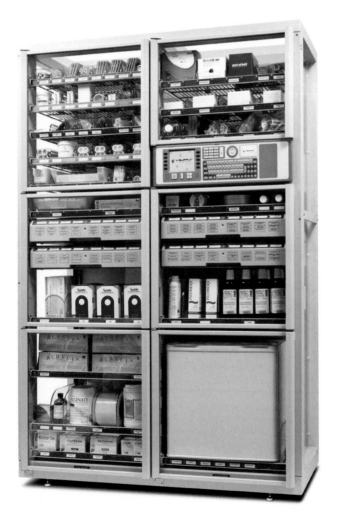

Figure 13-3 Cubex inventory system. (Courtesy VSupply, Scottsdale, AZ.)

that dispenses dental supplies. This system is user friendly and the assistant gains access through manual or badge input. Once access is granted, the user simply presses a button to indicate the removal of an item. Inventory levels are automatically updated.

eMagine is one of the automated supply management software systems used in dentistry. It is a free service for Patterson Supply customers. With eMagine merchandise orders are placed electronically. All special pricing and free goods are included, and many items have pictures and detailed descriptions. eMagine combines the benefits of a mail order catalog with the ease of ordering electronically. Figure 13-4 shows an example of the screen image for this order technique.

Many systems like this are Internet based and the company will provide bar coding or other techniques that staff members can use when taking items out of inventory. When the reorder point is reached, the product information is scanned with the reader and stored until it can be uploaded from the office computer, via the Internet, to the appropriate dealer site. Many programs will give a cost comparison for purchasing products from the company, and can complete an order with just a few extra steps. Users can always order from the dealer of their choice.

When all products have been entered into the system, a total value of the inventory can be provided, which is helpful for tax returns and financial management and budgeting. The system can also track money spent for supplies by category on an ongoing basis. Some systems provide reports in a list or graph/chart format, which is helpful for making monthly or yearly comparisons. When analyzed, these comparisons can provide valuable data for the practice in terms of the amount of money invested in certain types of products and supplies, and help identify where changes might be necessary to increase profitability.

Just as ordering supplies on a timely basis can save shipping costs, maintaining an accurate inventory of products can also save money by avoiding the purchase of too many items with a short shelf-life. If too much of a product is ordered at one time, such as some dental impression materials, not all of that item may be used by the expiration date. Using outdated impression material may result in a poor impression that will need to be discarded and retaken. Inventory management helps to determine the rate of use of items and identify items that are seldom used any more. This is a good predictor of appropriate quantities to have on hand to avoid wasting materials that exceed their expiration date.

Once employed in an office, become familiar with the inventory and work toward better organization to aid the dentist in becoming more efficient and productive. The decision about whether to use any of these types of automated systems depends on the size and needs of the office. Regardless of the system selected, the inventory manager must decide the desired minimum and maximum stock levels ahead of time.

Manual Inventory Systems

Some dentists still find it difficult to hand over the supply ordering system to automation and may find that a manual system is sufficient. If so, either a card system or an alphabetical list may suffice for an inventory system in some offices.

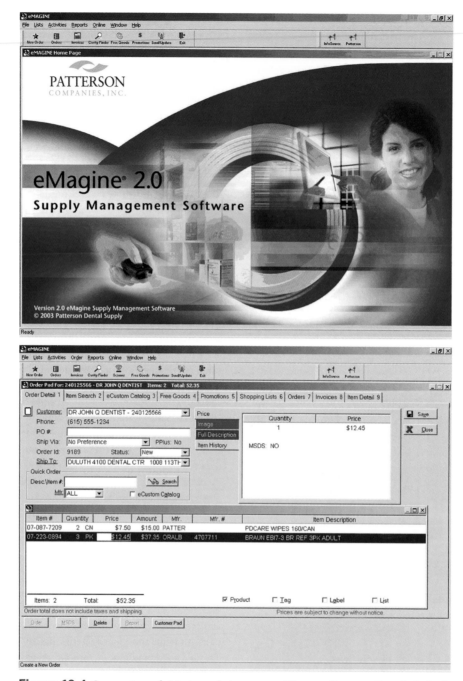

Figure 13-4 Screen views of eMagine ordering system. (Courtesy Patterson Dental, St. Paul, MN.)

Card System

The card system requires a separate card for each product. The cards list complete information about each product and its supplier and are placed in alphabetical order according to the product name. They are kept in a file drawer or notebook. As it becomes necessary to order an item, the card is placed in a section of the file marked *To be ordered*. Once the item has been ordered, the card is moved to the *On order* section of the file. When the item arrives from the supplier, the card is replaced in its original alphabetical position in the file. If the item is currently out of stock and has been placed on back-order by the supplier, the card is placed in the *On back-order* section of the file.

A modification of this system leaves all the cards in the alphabetical section at all times, and the status of the item is indicated with a colored tag (Figure 13-5). A red label might indicate *To be ordered*; blue, *On order*; and yellow, *On back-order*.

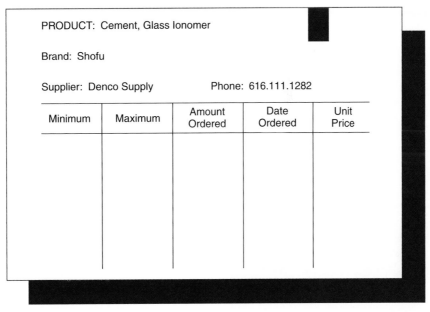

PRODUCT: Cement, Glass Ionomer

Brand: Shofu

Supplier: Denco Supply   Phone: 616.111.1282

Minimum	Maximum	Amount Ordered	Date Ordered	Unit Price

Figure 13-5 Colored tag on an inventory card.

TABLE 13-1   Example of a Master Supply List

Supplier Number	Product Name	Manufacturer	Maximum	Minimum Reorder Point
120	Aerosol spray	Regency	12 btls	3 btls
130	Alcohol, Misopropyl	Stock	2 gal	1 gal
110	Alginate, Jeltrate	Dentsply	250 pkgs	100 pkgs
110	Alloy, TYTIN 400 mg	Kerr	6 cans (500 caps)	10 cans (500 caps)
100	Alloy, TYTIN 800 mg	Kerr	6 cans (500 caps)	10 cans (500 caps)
100	Anesthetic, topical ointment	Schein	12 jars	4 jars
110	Anesthetic, mepivacaine 2% with	Surgimax	50 cans (50)	10 cans (50)
110	Anesthetic, mepivacaine 2% without	Surgimax	20 cans (50)	5 cans (50)
110	Bite blocks—foam	Strident	500	150
110	Cotton rolls #2	Richmond	1000	250
111	Gloves, Reflection, pdw. free fitted	Smart Practice	4 boxes	10 boxes

This system eliminates moving of the cards and the chance of misfiling, and also indicates at a glance the status of the items.

Alphabetical List

Table 13-1 shows an example of an alphabetical list of materials for inventory. This master list includes a code number for each supplier, the name of each product, and columns for the maximum on-hand level and the minimum reorder point. This list is kept in a protective celluloid cover, and when the reorder point is reached, the assistant simply places a red check mark in the appropriate space with a waxed pencil. When visiting the office, the supply representative can review the list, find all the items checked off with the supplier's number, and complete the order. When the items are ordered, the red check marks are erased with a tissue.

MAINTAINING THE INVENTORY SYSTEM

Identifying Reorder Points

In an automated dealer system, the rate of use will aid in determining the reorder point. If using an in-office data system or manual system, some form of identifying the reorder point must be selected. An automated system will have some form of reorder point built into the program. For a manual system, colored tape may be used to indicate the reorder point on small items (Figure 13-6), or a tag can be placed on the item (Figure 13-7). For stationery supplies, a paper tab can be inserted into the stack of materials to indicate the reorder point (Figure 13-8).

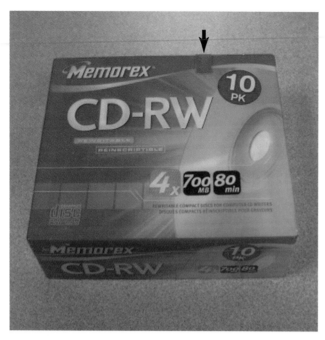

Figure 13-6 Colored tape on small items.

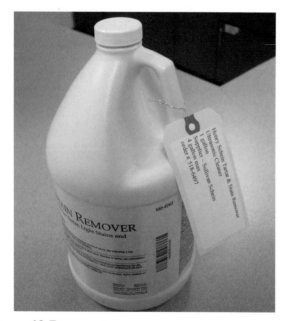

Figure 13-7 Tag on a bottle.

```
RED FLAG
REORDER POINT

PRODUCT IDENTIFICATION
```

Figure 13-8 Paper tab.

- *Shelf-life:* Certain materials, such as x-ray film and some impression materials, begin to deteriorate after a certain period. Some manufacturers indicate an expiration date on the box. Do not purchase a large quantity of items that cannot be used before their expiration date.
- *Amount of capital outlay:* In addition to prices, the amount of cash available often determines whether an item is purchased in bulk amounts.
- *Length of delivery time:* This factor affects the minimum quantity desired to have in stock. If several days are required to receive an order for a frequently used item, increase the minimum amount on hand.
- *Amount of storage space:* In some offices, storage space is a crucial factor, and lack of it prohibits the purchase of large supplies. Consequently, a large storage space is a benefit economically and increases efficiency.
- *Manufacturer's special offers:* Manufacturers routinely offer special rates on various materials. However, a special price is not cost efficient if the item stays on the shelf and collects dust.

Receiving Supplies

All incoming materials should be handled and stored safely. Current regulations require that all manufacturers provide an MSDS with each hazardous material.

Every order that arrives in the office should have an **invoice** or packing slip, or both. A **packing slip** is simply an enumeration of the enclosed items. An invoice (Figure 13-9) is a list of the contents of the package, the price of each item enclosed, and the total charge. Some companies use the invoice as a statement and indicate on the form that this is the statement from which the account is to be paid.

Determining Supply Quantity

Several factors aid in determining the minimum and maximum amounts of an item to be in stock:
- *Rate of use:* Buying large quantities of infrequently used items is not cost efficient. However, buying bulk quantities of supplies used frequently is economical. For example, buying paper products for the dental treatment room in large quantities is a good idea if storage space is available.

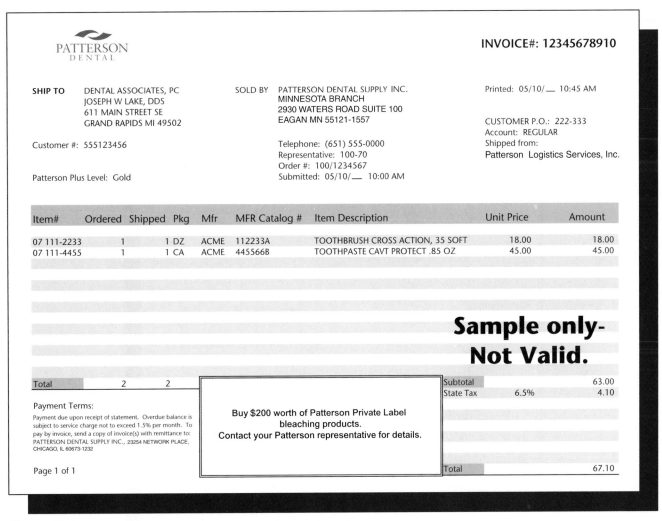

Figure 13-9 Sample invoice. (Courtesy Patterson Dental, St. Paul, MN.)

Make sure that each item listed coincides with the original order, each item on the invoice is in the package, and the total amount listed on the invoice is accurate. Then put the invoice in the *To be paid* file.

At the end of the month, a **statement** or request for payment, will be received from the supplier (Figure 13-10). Each invoice should be checked against the entries on the statement to ensure accuracy before payment is sent.

The check is made payable to the supplier (Chapter 16). The check number is indicated on the retained portion of the statement, the invoices are attached, and these documents are filed in the appropriate subject file.

Receiving Credit

Sometimes supplies must be returned for credit. In such cases the dental supplier sends a **credit memo** (Figure 13-11), which indicates that the dentist's account has been credited for the cost

of the returned item. This amount appears as a credit on the statement at the end of the month.

Back-Ordered Supplies

Sometimes an item ordered is not in stock at the supply house, and a **back-order memo** is received. The supplier sends notification that the article is back-ordered, or this may be noted directly on the invoice. If the product is needed immediately, attempt to obtain it from another supplier or make an alternative selection.

Purchase Orders

In large institutions supplies are ordered through a purchasing agent. All items are listed on a requisition, and the order is keyed into a **purchase order**, a standardized order form for supplies. Each purchase order is given a number and sent to

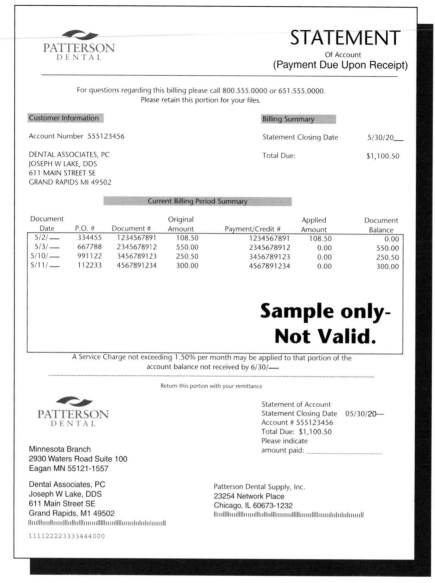

Figure 13-10 Sample statement from a supplier. (Courtesy, Patterson Dental, St. Paul, MN.)

the appropriate supplier, who in turn enters this number on all invoices when shipping the supplies.

Storage of Supplies

All supplies should be stored in an organized manner that allows quick and easy retrieval. Certain materials require a cool, dry, or dark location. In addition, when new materials are received, they should be stocked behind older supplies so that the older supplies are used first.

The administrative assistant must be aware of the federal Occupational Safety and Health Administration (OSHA) guidelines regarding the use and storage of materials in the dental office. MSDSs provided by OSHA should be maintained on hazardous materials. The information on these sheets (Figure 13-12) includes the manufacturer's name, address, and emergency telephone numbers, as well as specific information about the ingredients of the product. Additional information should include storage instructions, health hazard data, spill or leak procedures, and special safety precautions (e.g., storage in a ventilated area). The dentist must make sure that such forms are made available to staff members. If hazardous materials are stored in the office, appropriate labeling must follow the guidelines given in Chapter 17.

When stationery supplies or large boxes are stored, a label describing the contents should be placed on the outside of each box.

Inventory Evaluation

Box 13-1 presents some useful questions to aid the evaluation of an inventory system in a dental office.

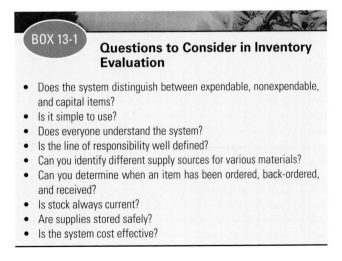

CREDIT MEMO#: 987654321

SHIP TO DENTAL ASSOCIATES, PC
JOSEPH W LAKE, DDS
611 MAIN STREET SE
GRAND RAPIDS MI 49502

Customer #: 555123456

Patterson Plus Level: Gold

SOLD BY PATTERSON DENTAL SUPPLY INC.
MINNESOTA BRANCH
2930 WATERS RD. SUITE 100
EAGAN, MN 55121-1557

Telephone: (651) 555-0000
Representative: 100-70
Order #: 100/1234567
Submitted: 05/11/__ 11:00 AM

Printed: 05/11/__ 11:00 AM

CUSTOMER P.O.: 222-333
Account: REGULAR

Item#	Ordered	Shipped	Pkg	Mfr	MFR Catalog #	Item Description	Unit Price	Amount
07 111-2233	1	1	DZ	ACME	112233A	TOOTHBRUSH CROSS ACTION, 35 SOFT	(18.00)	(18.00)
07 111-4455	1	1	CA	ACME	445566B	TOOTHPASTE CAVT PROTECT .85 OZ	(45.00)	(45.00)

CREDIT MEMO

Sample only- Not Valid.

Total	2	2			Subtotal		(63.00)
					State Tax	6.5%	(4.10)

Payment Terms:
Payment due upon receipt of statement. Overdue balance is subject to service charge not to exceed 1.5% per month. To pay by invoice, send a copy of invoice(s) with remittance to: PATTERSON DENTAL SUPPLY INC., 23254 NETWORK PLACE, CHICAGO, IL 60673-1232

Page 1 of 1

Buy $200 worth of Patterson Private Label bleaching products.
Contact your Patterson representative for details.

| Total | (67.10) |

Figure 13-11 Sample credit memo. (Courtesy Patterson Dental, St. Paul, MN.)

BOX 13-1

Questions to Consider in Inventory Evaluation

- Does the system distinguish between expendable, nonexpendable, and capital items?
- Is it simple to use?
- Does everyone understand the system?
- Is the line of responsibility well defined?
- Can you identify different supply sources for various materials?
- Can you determine when an item has been ordered, back-ordered, and received?
- Is stock always current?
- Are supplies stored safely?
- Is the system cost effective?

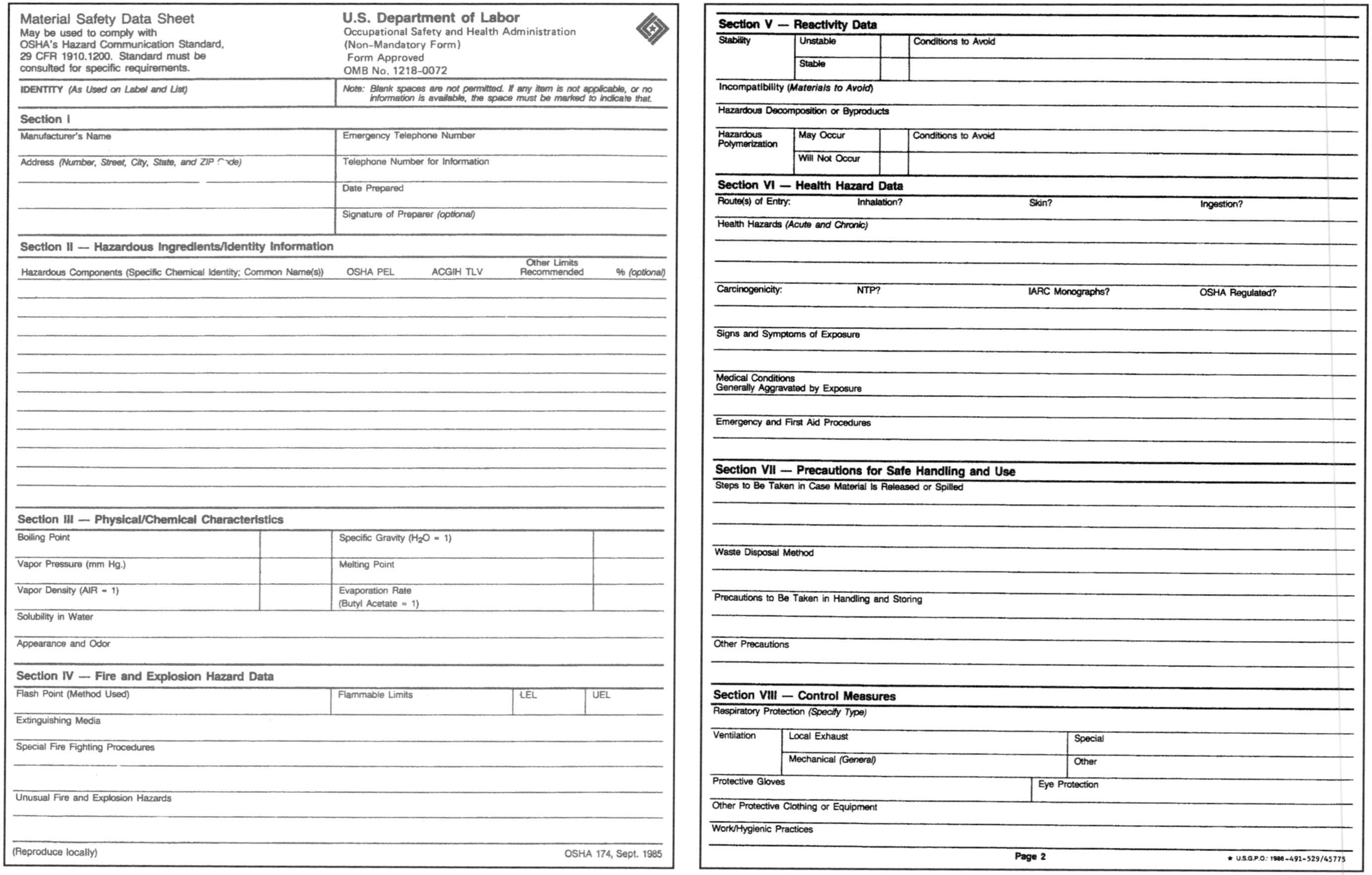

Material Safety Data Sheet
May be used to comply with
OSHA's Hazard Communication Standard,
29 CFR 1910.1200. Standard must be
consulted for specific requirements.

U.S. Department of Labor
Occupational Safety and Health Administration
(Non-Mandatory Form)
Form Approved
OMB No. 1218-0072

IDENTITY *(As Used on Label and List)*

Note: Blank spaces are not permitted. If any item is not applicable, or no information is available, the space must be marked to indicate that.

Section I

Manufacturer's Name | Emergency Telephone Number
Address *(Number, Street, City, State, and ZIP Code)* | Telephone Number for Information
Date Prepared
Signature of Preparer *(optional)*

Section II — Hazardous Ingredients/Identity Information

Hazardous Components (Specific Chemical Identity; Common Name(s))	OSHA PEL	ACGIH TLV	Other Limits Recommended	% *(optional)*

Section III — Physical/Chemical Characteristics

Boiling Point		Specific Gravity (H_2O = 1)	
Vapor Pressure (mm Hg.)		Melting Point	
Vapor Density (AIR = 1)		Evaporation Rate (Butyl Acetate = 1)	

Solubility in Water

Appearance and Odor

Section IV — Fire and Explosion Hazard Data

Flash Point (Method Used) | Flammable Limits | LEL | UEL

Extinguishing Media

Special Fire Fighting Procedures

Unusual Fire and Explosion Hazards

(Reproduce locally) OSHA 174, Sept. 1985

Section V — Reactivity Data

Stability	Unstable		Conditions to Avoid
	Stable		

Incompatibility *(Materials to Avoid)*

Hazardous Decomposition or Byproducts

Hazardous Polymerization	May Occur		Conditions to Avoid
	Will Not Occur		

Section VI — Health Hazard Data

Route(s) of Entry: Inhalation? Skin? Ingestion?

Health Hazards *(Acute and Chronic)*

Carcinogenicity: NTP? IARC Monographs? OSHA Regulated?

Signs and Symptoms of Exposure

Medical Conditions
Generally Aggravated by Exposure

Emergency and First Aid Procedures

Section VII — Precautions for Safe Handling and Use

Steps to Be Taken in Case Material Is Released or Spilled

Waste Disposal Method

Precautions to Be Taken in Handling and Storing

Other Precautions

Section VIII — Control Measures

Respiratory Protection *(Specify Type)*

Ventilation	Local Exhaust	Special
	Mechanical *(General)*	Other

Protective Gloves | Eye Protection

Other Protective Clothing or Equipment

Work/Hygienic Practices

Page 2 ★ U.S.G.P.O.: 1986-491-529/45775

Figure 13-12 Occupational Safety and Health Administration (OSHA) Material Safety Data Sheet (MSDS). (From Occupational Safety and Health Administration, U.S. Department of Labor, Washington, DC.)

KEY TERMS

Back-order memo—A form accompanying an order that notifies the purchaser that an item ordered is not currently in stock at the supply house and will be sent at a later date.

Capital supplies—Large, costly items that are seldom replaced; they include equipment such as the computer, sterilizer, and dental unit.

Credit memo—A form that indicates that the dentist's account has been credited for the cost of a returned item; the amount appears as a credit on the statement at the end of the month.

Expendable supplies—Single-use items, such as dental cements, stationery, local anesthetics, and gypsum products.

Invoice—A list of the contents of a package, the price of each item enclosed, and the total charge.

Material Safety Data Sheet (MSDS)—A form supplied by the manufacturer that provides information about a hazardous material; these forms are required by the U.S. government.

Nonexpendable supplies—Reusable items that do not constitute a major expense; this category generally includes most dental instruments.

Packing slip—An enumeration of the items included in an order; it does not include the cost per item.

Purchase order—A standardized form for ordering supplies.

Statement—A request for payment submitted by the dental supplier.

LEARNING ACTIVITIES

1. Explain the following terms: expendable, nonexpendable, capital items, invoice, statement, credit slip, and back-order inventory.
2. Explain the processing of an item from the time it is ordered until it is received in the office and the statement is paid.
3. Describe the management of chemicals and hazardous materials in the dental office. What are OSHA guidelines and how do they affect the dental office?

Please refer to the student workbook for additional learning activities.

BIBLIOGRAPHY

Govoni M: Don't agonize – organize!, *Dental Equipment and Materials* 3(7):18, 2005.

Snider CC: Smart shopping, *RDH*, 24(5):46, 2004.

DENTAL SUPPLIERS

Patterson Office Supplies
P.O. Box 9009
Champaign, IL 61826
1-800-637-1140
www.pattersonofficesupplies.com

Henry Schein, Inc.
10920 West Lincoln
West Allis, WI 53227
1-800-372-4346
www.henryschein.com

Smart Practice
(a division of Smart Health, Inc.)
3400 E. McDowell Rd.
Phoenix, AZ 85008-7899
1-800-522-0800
www.SmartPractice.com

vSupply
1475 N. Scottsdale Road
Suite 200
Scottsdale, AZ 85257
480-268-7955
www.vsupply.com

Deluxe for Business
3680 Victoria Street North
Shoreview MN55126
1-800-865-1913
www.deluxe.com

Medical Arts Press Corporation
P.O. Box 43200
Minneapolis, MN 55443-0200
1-800-328-2119
www.medicalartspress.com

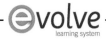

Please visit http://evolve.elsevier.com/Finkibeiner/practice for additional practice activities.

14 Dental Insurance

CHAPTER OUTLINE

LEARNING OUTCOMES

- Define key terms.
- Identify the four parties affected by dental benefit plans.
- Differentiate among the different dental plan models.
- Use the current American Dental Association (ADA) *Code on Dental Procedures and Nomenclature* and the *Code of Dental Terminology* (CDT) manual.
- Complete an ADA form.
- Submit Medicaid dental benefit claims.
- Apply the rules for coordination of benefits.
- Explain common dental benefit and claims terminology.

OVERVIEW OF DENTAL INSURANCE

Evolution

In the early twentieth century, **dental insurance** and dental benefits programs did not exist. Their emergence and growth provided access to care for people who had never considered routine dental treatment. Patient education changed the general perception of dentistry, transforming the dental office from a place best avoided to a familiar and necessary partner in personal health care.

As more companies and organizations added dental benefits to their group health coverage, the percentage of people seeking regular preventive services and restorative treatment increased. As oral health improved, patients and healthcare professionals began to notice a trend toward better overall health. By the end of the century, the connection between oral health and overall general health was clearly established. With the identification of linkages between certain oral health conditions and serious physical illnesses, dentists can use those oral indicators to help in the detection and early diagnosis of diseases such as diabetes, high blood pressure, oral cancer, anemia, and deficient immune system (HIV positive).

Group dental benefits have high value for the workforce, and more than half of the nation's population has some type of dental plan. Dental benefits continue to be a factor in treatment; statistics show that 60% of the **insured** people go to the dentist, whereas only approximately 27% of the uninsured seek any dental treatment. Although the percentage of insured patients may vary (by region, specialty, policy, etc.), nearly every dental office offers insurance billing as a service to their patients.

Prompt and efficient insurance billing of dental services can have a direct effect on the profitability of the practice. The majority of dental offices accept assignment of benefits, allowing the benefit payment to be paid to the dentist or dental office business. Correct billing procedures ensure that the payment reaches the dental office as quickly as possible and keeps the accounts receivable in a positive cash flow position. This job requires organization, perseverance, and strict attention to detail.

Parties Involved

The system of dental insurance involves four parties: the patient, the dentist, the **dental benefits carrier**, and the group or program sponsor (e.g., employer, union, or business association). The dental office administrative assistant works closely with the patient, dentist, and benefits carrier to produce the successful adjudication of dental benefit claims.

Patient

The patient is the primary resource for the following information needed to submit a claim:

- Name and address of the **benefit carrier**
- Subscriber's name, address, identification number (Social Security number [SSN] or other assigned number), and date of birth
- Subscriber's group/employer, address, and group number

Most patients aren't aware of the details of their benefit coverage, and they don't understand most of the dental terminology associated with their treatment and coverage. The administrative assistant is in the position to interpret and explain dental terms, codes, and benefit details in lay terms. This interaction gives the patient the opportunity to be an active partner in his or her dental care and promotes a good relationship between the patient and the practice. *Note:* It is important to inform patients that even though they are covered by a dental benefits program, they ultimately are liable for all treatment fees.

Dentist

The administrative assistant consults the dentist to verify the services rendered, determine the correct procedure codes, and confirm the fees. Most dental offices work closely with carriers to help their patients make the best use of their benefits; however, the dentist and his or her patient make the final decision as to the best course of treatment for that individual. The dentist's primary commitment is to discuss and render necessary treatment, establish and maintain the patient's oral health, and adhere to the standards of care that prevail in the professional community.

Dental Benefits Carrier

This may be an **insurer**, a **third-party administrator (TPA)**, or a **dental service corporation**. The administrative assistant can contact the carrier to verify the patient's eligibility and benefits, claims address, and any other details pertinent to filing claims. The benefit carrier administers the plan according to the group contract, which includes maintaining **member** eligibility, processing claims, and remitting benefit payments to the appropriate party.

Group or Program Sponsor

The **group**—for example, an employer, union, or business association—(or a broker who represents the group) contracts with the benefit carrier and selects the benefits levels, program type, maximums, limitations, and exclusions for their dental plan. Communication with the group is generally the responsibility of the patient (also called the **group member** or **subscriber**); however, occasionally the administrative assistant may contact the group on behalf of the patient.

DENTAL BENEFITS PROGRAMS

The dental carrier's method of **reimbursement** depends on the dental plan design. The two basic models of benefits programs are indemnity and capitation, although many variations of each model exist.

Many dental benefits carriers recruit dentists to participate in their programs. Generally when a dentist signs a participation contract with a benefits carrier, he or she agrees to certain terms and conditions of payment for services rendered to enrollees. Each carrier has a unique set of terms of participation, which may include: accepting the carrier's fee table (no **balance billing** or **unbundling of procedures** or fees), receiving **assignment of benefits**, and filing claims for enrollees. Although the dentist may be required to discount fees to enrollees, participation is a proven method of practice building, accelerating cash flow, and increasing patient acceptance of treatment.

Indemnity

According to Webster's *New College Dictionary,* the term *indemnity* means "compensation for damage, loss, or injury," and dental indemnity plans make reimbursement to insured persons (or the dentist through assignment of benefits) for costs incurred through covered dental treatment (**approved services**). Indemnity programs are most often referred to as **fee-for-service plans** because the reimbursement is based on each dental service rendered or received. The following list presents types of fee-for-service programs:

- **Usual, customary, and reasonable (UCR) plan:** Payment for covered benefits is based on a combination of usual (the fee most often charged for a service by a dentist), customary (the fee most often charged for a service in a geographic area or in a specialty), and reasonable (the fee that meets the other two criteria or that is adjusted according to the nature or criteria of individual circumstances) fee criteria.
- **Reasonable and customary (R&C) plan:** Payment for covered benefits is based on **reasonable fee** (the fee most often charged by the dentist or that is adjusted according to the nature or criteria of individual circumstances) and **customary fee** (the fee most often charged for a service in a geographic area or in a specialty) criteria.
- **Preferred provider organization (PPO) plan:** Payment is based on a discounted **fee schedule**. Dentists who sign an agreement with a carrier agree to accept the discounted fees and do not charge enrollees any difference between their **usual fee** and the discounted fee.
- **Exclusive provider organization (EPO) plan:** The benefits are payable only when services are rendered by participating providers. Enrollees have no benefit coverage for services received from out-of-network providers; however, some exceptions may be allowed for emergency and out-of-area services.
- **Point-of-service plan:** Fee schedules and benefit levels vary based on participation status of the dentist rendering treatment.

- **Table of allowances plan**: Also called a *schedule of allowances plan,* payment is based on a list of covered services, and each service has a fixed dollar amount for reimbursement of treatment.
- **Open panel system**: Payment can be made to the patient or the billing dentist, depending on assignment of benefits guidelines. Panels of participating dentists may be available, and enrollees may choose to receive dental treatment from any licensed dentist. Dentists may accept or refuse any enrollee in accordance with professional rules of conduct.
- **Closed panel system**: Payment can only be made for services rendered by a participating dentist.

Capitation

Capitation is a benefits delivery system in which a contracting provider receives a fixed monthly payment for providing covered dental services to enrollees who select or are assigned to his or her location. The provider receives the payment regardless of whether services were actually performed. This program type is also called a **dental health maintenance organization (DHMO)**, and it is typically a closed panel system. To be covered, enrollees must go to their primary care provider for all their dental treatment. Most plans allow the primary care dentist to refer enrollees to a participating specialist for qualified services, and exceptions may be allowed for emergency and out-of-area dental care. Enrollees may not have out-of-pocket costs for routine services, although they may have a **copayment** for more extensive, expensive services, such as fixed bridges.

Alternative Benefit Plans

Employers or associations that do not include dental coverage in their benefit package may elect to offer an **alternative benefit plan**. A variety of options are available, and following are some examples:

- *Group discounts:* Large employers or associations may contract with dentists or dental clinics to deliver dental services to their enrollees at a discounted rate. The enrollee usually pays an annual or monthly membership fee and pays the dentist directly for services rendered. The dentist does not file claims, and the plan has no **exclusions**, **limitations**, or maximums.
- *Discount card:* For an annual fee, purchasers have access to a network of participating dentists who have agreed to charge reduced fees to cardholders. The cardholder pays the dentist directly, and the dentist does not file any claims.
- *Health savings account (I):* The federal government allows eligible employers to offer their employees a pretax salary savings account for payment assistance with healthcare-related expenses. Contributions to the account are made by payroll deduction, and employees save money because no federal or state taxes are deducted. Patients with an I pay the dentist, submit a receipt to their employer, and receive reimbursement up to the limit they have selected for the I.

- *Direct reimbursement:* With **direct reimbursement**, an employer or organization can set up a self-funded program for reimbursing covered individuals based on a percentage of the amount spent for dental care.
- *Voluntary plans:* These individual dental benefit plans offer many of the same advantages of employer-sponsored plans, including lower rates and comprehensive benefit designs. **Eligible persons** who elect the coverage pay the full **premium**, so there is no cost to the employer or organization. Program administration can be assigned or shared among the employer, an insurance broker, and the benefit carrier.

PREPARING DENTAL CLAIM FORMS

Dental claims can be submitted on paper forms or in electronic format. Both modes require specific and detailed information about the patient/subscriber, treating dentist, and services rendered. One small error or omission can cause a claim to reject. Rejected claims create more work for the administrative staff and unnecessary delays in payment. Because the requirements of benefit carriers may vary, administrative assistant can further increase efficiency by becoming familiar with or keeping records on the techniques that work best with individual carriers.

Paper Claim Form

The **American Dental Association (ADA) claim form** (also known as the **attending dentist's statement**) is universal, and it is designed to meet or exceed the informational needs of nearly all dental benefit carriers. The form includes comprehensive completion instructions (Figure 14-1), and it may be purchased from the ADA or through most dental supply vendors. Some dental benefits carriers have a proprietary paper claim form, which may be brought in by the patient or available to download from their web sites.

The administrative assistant can legibly print or type the required information on the claim form or, if the office is computerized, forms can be generated and printed using the practice management software. The assistant then reviews the claims, attaches x-rays, and adds documentation where needed. Claims are batched according to carrier and mailed out.

Note: Some carriers require radiographs or documentation for a limited number of services, such as fixed bridges or miscellaneous procedures. However, sending unnecessary films or documentation may slow down processing and payment. The assistant can contact the benefit carrier for a list of procedure codes that require special handling or support documents.

Electronic Claim Form

According to a survey of dentists and dental staff members conducted in 2006 by Delta Dental of Michigan, Ohio, and Indiana, more than half of dental offices submit all or part of their dental claims electronically—through a clearinghouse, via practice management services, or on web sites.

Offices that file e-claims must comply with federal laws governing electronic transactions that include personal health

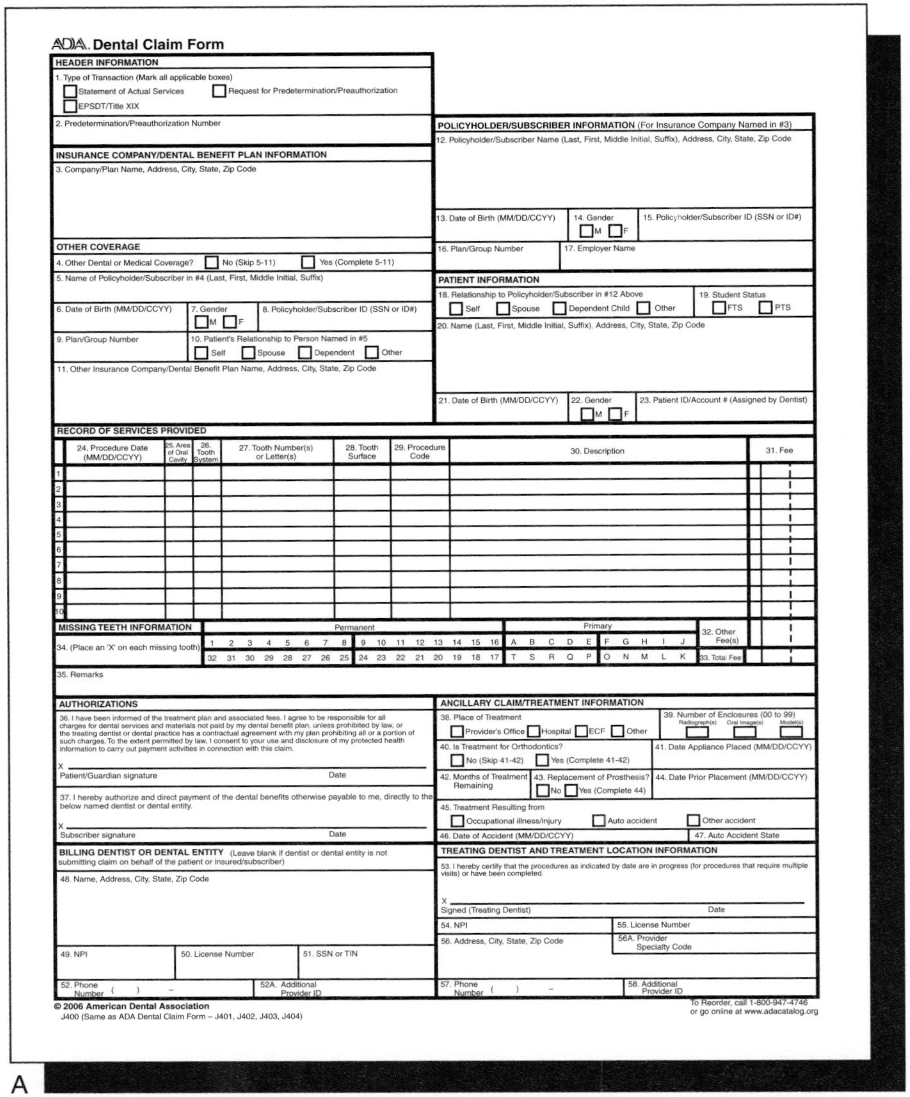
ADA Dental Claim Form

HEADER INFORMATION
1. Type of Transaction (Mark all applicable boxes)
☐ Statement of Actual Services ☐ Request for Predetermination/Preauthorization
☐ EPSDT/Title XIX
2. Predetermination/Preauthorization Number

INSURANCE COMPANY/DENTAL BENEFIT PLAN INFORMATION
3. Company/Plan Name, Address, City, State, Zip Code

OTHER COVERAGE
4. Other Dental or Medical Coverage? ☐ No (Skip 5-11) ☐ Yes (Complete 5-11)
5. Name of Policyholder/Subscriber in #4 (Last, First, Middle Initial, Suffix)
6. Date of Birth (MM/DD/CCYY) | 7. Gender ☐M ☐F | 8. Policyholder/Subscriber ID (SSN or ID#)
9. Plan/Group Number | 10. Patient's Relationship to Person Named in #5 ☐ Self ☐ Spouse ☐ Dependent ☐ Other
11. Other Insurance Company/Dental Benefit Plan Name, Address, City, State, Zip Code

POLICYHOLDER/SUBSCRIBER INFORMATION (For Insurance Company Named in #3)
12. Policyholder/Subscriber Name (Last, First, Middle Initial, Suffix), Address, City, State, Zip Code
13. Date of Birth (MM/DD/CCYY) | 14. Gender ☐M ☐F | 15. Policyholder/Subscriber ID (SSN or ID#)
16. Plan/Group Number | 17. Employer Name

PATIENT INFORMATION
18. Relationship to Policyholder/Subscriber in #12 Above ☐ Self ☐ Spouse ☐ Dependent Child ☐ Other | 19. Student Status ☐ FTS ☐ PTS
20. Name (Last, First, Middle Initial, Suffix), Address, City, State, Zip Code
21. Date of Birth (MM/DD/CCYY) | 22. Gender ☐M ☐F | 23. Patient ID/Account # (Assigned by Dentist)

RECORD OF SERVICES PROVIDED

	24. Procedure Date (MM/DD/CCYY)	25. Area of Oral Cavity	26. Tooth System	27. Tooth Number(s) or Letter(s)	28. Tooth Surface	29. Procedure Code	30. Description	31. Fee
1								
2								
3								
4								
5								
6								
7								
8								
9								
10								

MISSING TEETH INFORMATION
34. (Place an 'X' on each missing tooth)
Permanent: 1 2 3 4 5 6 7 8 9 10 11 12 13 14 15 16 / 32 31 30 29 28 27 26 25 24 23 22 21 20 19 18 17
Primary: A B C D E F G H I J / T S R Q P O N M L K
32. Other Fee(s)
33. Total Fee
35. Remarks

AUTHORIZATIONS
36. I have been informed of the treatment plan and associated fees. I agree to be responsible for all charges for dental services and materials not paid by my dental benefit plan, unless prohibited by law, or the treating dentist or dental practice has a contractual agreement with my plan prohibiting all or a portion of such charges. To the extent permitted by law, I consent to your use and disclosure of my protected health information to carry out payment activities in connection with this claim.
X
Patient/Guardian signature Date
37. I hereby authorize and direct payment of the dental benefits otherwise payable to me, directly to the below named dentist or dental entity.
X
Subscriber signature Date

ANCILLARY CLAIM/TREATMENT INFORMATION
38. Place of Treatment ☐ Provider's Office ☐ Hospital ☐ ECF ☐ Other
39. Number of Enclosures (00 to 99) Radiograph(s) Oral Image(s) Model(s)
40. Is Treatment for Orthodontics? ☐ No (Skip 41-42) ☐ Yes (Complete 41-42)
41. Date Appliance Placed (MM/DD/CCYY)
42. Months of Treatment Remaining
43. Replacement of Prosthesis? ☐ No ☐ Yes (Complete 44)
44. Date Prior Placement (MM/DD/CCYY)
45. Treatment Resulting from ☐ Occupational illness/injury ☐ Auto accident ☐ Other accident
46. Date of Accident (MM/DD/CCYY) | 47. Auto Accident State

BILLING DENTIST OR DENTAL ENTITY (Leave blank if dentist or dental entity is not submitting claim on behalf of the patient or insured/subscriber)
48. Name, Address, City, State, Zip Code
49. NPI | 50. License Number | 51. SSN or TIN
52. Phone Number ( ) - | 52A. Additional Provider ID

TREATING DENTIST AND TREATMENT LOCATION INFORMATION
53. I hereby certify that the procedures as indicated by date are in progress (for procedures that require multiple visits) or have been completed.
X
Signed (Treating Dentist) Date
54. NPI | 55. License Number
56. Address, City, State, Zip Code | 56A. Provider Specialty Code
57. Phone Number ( ) - | 58. Additional Provider ID

© 2006 American Dental Association
J400 (Same as ADA Dental Claim Form – J401, J402, J403, J404)
To Reorder, call 1-800-947-4746 or go online at www.adacatalog.org

A

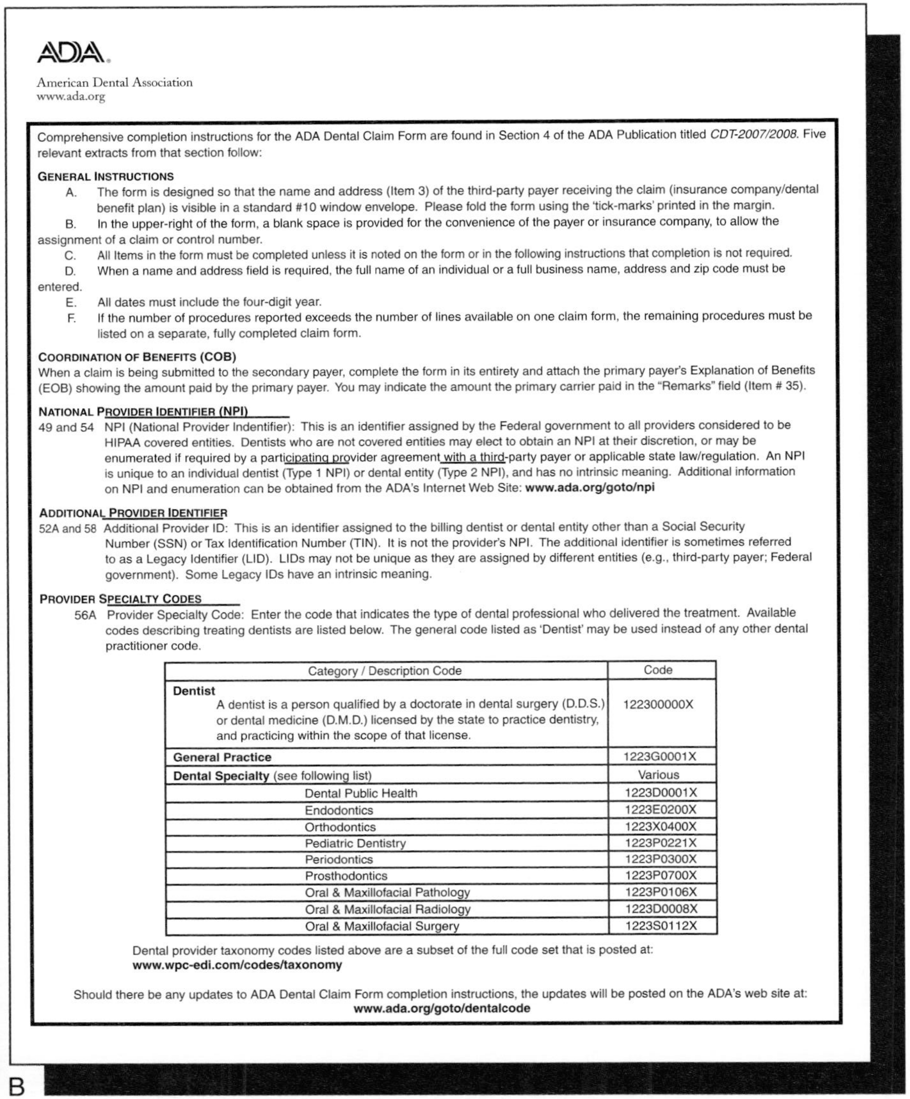
ADA.
American Dental Association
www.ada.org

Comprehensive completion instructions for the ADA Dental Claim Form are found in Section 4 of the ADA Publication titled *CDT-2007/2008*. Five relevant extracts from that section follow:

General Instructions

A. The form is designed so that the name and address (Item 3) of the third-party payer receiving the claim (insurance company/dental benefit plan) is visible in a standard #10 window envelope. Please fold the form using the 'tick-marks' printed in the margin.

B. In the upper-right of the form, a blank space is provided for the convenience of the payer or insurance company, to allow the assignment of a claim or control number.

C. All Items in the form must be completed unless it is noted on the form or in the following instructions that completion is not required.

D. When a name and address field is required, the full name of an individual or a full business name, address and zip code must be entered.

E. All dates must include the four-digit year.

F. If the number of procedures reported exceeds the number of lines available on one claim form, the remaining procedures must be listed on a separate, fully completed claim form.

Coordination of Benefits (COB)

When a claim is being submitted to the secondary payer, complete the form in its entirety and attach the primary payer's Explanation of Benefits (EOB) showing the amount paid by the primary payer. You may indicate the amount the primary carrier paid in the "Remarks" field (Item # 35).

National Provider Identifier (NPI)

49 and 54 NPI (National Provider Indentifier): This is an identifier assigned by the Federal government to all providers considered to be HIPAA covered entities. Dentists who are not covered entities may elect to obtain an NPI at their discretion, or may be enumerated if required by a participating provider agreement with a third-party payer or applicable state law/regulation. An NPI is unique to an individual dentist (Type 1 NPI) or dental entity (Type 2 NPI), and has no intrinsic meaning. Additional information on NPI and enumeration can be obtained from the ADA's Internet Web Site: **www.ada.org/goto/npi**

Additional Provider Identifier

52A and 58 Additional Provider ID: This is an identifier assigned to the billing dentist or dental entity other than a Social Security Number (SSN) or Tax Identification Number (TIN). It is not the provider's NPI. The additional identifier is sometimes referred to as a Legacy Identifier (LID). LIDs may not be unique as they are assigned by different entities (e.g., third-party payer; Federal government). Some Legacy IDs have an intrinsic meaning.

Provider Specialty Codes

56A Provider Specialty Code: Enter the code that indicates the type of dental professional who delivered the treatment. Available codes describing treating dentists are listed below. The general code listed as 'Dentist' may be used instead of any other dental practitioner code.

Category / Description Code	Code
Dentist A dentist is a person qualified by a doctorate in dental surgery (D.D.S.) or dental medicine (D.M.D.) licensed by the state to practice dentistry, and practicing within the scope of that license.	122300000X
General Practice	1223G0001X
Dental Specialty (see following list)	Various
Dental Public Health	1223D0001X
Endodontics	1223E0200X
Orthodontics	1223X0400X
Pediatric Dentistry	1223P0221X
Periodontics	1223P0300X
Prosthodontics	1223P0700X
Oral & Maxillofacial Pathology	1223P0106X
Oral & Maxillofacial Radiology	1223D0008X
Oral & Maxillofacial Surgery	1223S0112X

Dental provider taxonomy codes listed above are a subset of the full code set that is posted at:
www.wpc-edi.com/codes/taxonomy

Should there be any updates to ADA Dental Claim Form completion instructions, the updates will be posted on the ADA's web site at:
www.ada.org/goto/dentalcode

B

Figure 14-1 Front **(A)** and back **(B)** of an American Dental Association dental claim form. (Courtesy American Dental Association, Chicago.)

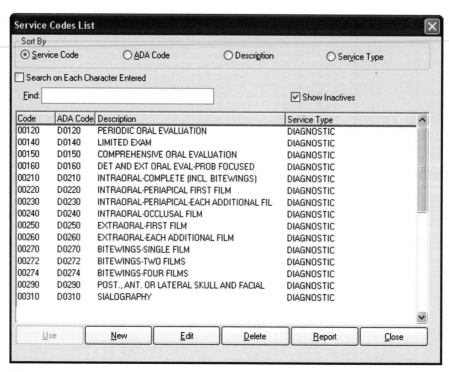

Figure 14-2 Pull-down screen of American Dental Association service codes. (Courtesy Patterson Dental, St. Paul, MN.)

information (PHI). Under the **Health Insurance Portability and Accountability Act of 1996 (HIPAA)** all healthcare providers, health plans, and healthcare clearinghouses that transmit PHI electronically must use a universal language, a standard format, and a government-assigned, unique identification number. HIPAA also mandates security and privacy standards for electronic transactions as discussed in Chapter 7.

- *The Code:* The universal language used for electronic transmission of dental data is the ADA *Code on Dental Procedures and Nomenclature (the Code)*, which is updated every 2 years (Figure 14-2). *Current Dental Terminology (CDT)* manuals, the only official source for these codes, can be purchased from the ADA, and they list the procedure codes with nomenclature and descriptors, changes from the previous code, and other helpful information (Figure 14-3).*

- *Electronic data formats:* Practice management programs, clearinghouses, and benefit carriers are required to use the same standard software formats for electronic transactions of health information. The standard formats are used for claims, remittance advice (explanation of benefits), eligibility inquiry and response, prior authorization and referral, and claims status inquiry and response. Attachments to the claim form (such as x-rays) can also be submitted electronically, although special software and scanning equipment might be needed.

- *Unique identifiers:* Dental offices that submit claims or claims attachments electronically or use the Internet to look up eligibility, benefits, or claims status are required to have and use a **National Provider Identifier (NPI)**. The NPI is provided through a designated agency, and it is a permanent 10-digit number that replaces any other identifiers used in electronic transactions. It does not replace the tax identification number (TIN) or the treating dentist's state license number as these are used for purposes other than identification.

Most dental offices have replaced the pegboard and appointment book with computers and sophisticated practice management software, and the percentage of dental offices submitting all or part of their claims electronically has grown steadily over the past 20 years. Compared with the time and expense of preparing and mailing paper claims, electronic claims submission can be faster, less expensive, and more accurate. E-claims are usually submitted through a clearinghouse or directly to the carrier, and most carriers offer payment via electronic funds transmission (EFT).

Via Clearinghouse

A clearinghouse is a company that accepts the transmission of raw data, scans for errors or missing information, and transforms it into the appropriate data format for submission to the benefit carrier. The clearinghouse charges for this service, usually either a set amount per claim or a monthly fee.

Using practice management software, the dental office administrative assistant collects the patient and treatment

---

*Council on Dental Benefit Programs: Current dental terminology: CDT-2009-2010, Chicago, 2008, American Dental Association.

information that's ready to be billed to a benefit carrier. The batch of claims information is transmitted to the clearinghouse. After reformatting the data, any claims with missing or incomplete information are transmitted back to the dental office. The finished claims are sorted by benefit carrier or insurance company, and mass transmitted to the carrier for processing. The clearinghouse can also print and mail a paper claim forms to the few carriers unable to accept electronic claims.

Direct to Carrier

The dental office has to be computerized and connected to the Internet to transmit claims directly to benefit carriers. Not all benefit carriers offer this service; however, most major carriers provide it free of charge. The dental office administrative assistant goes online to the carrier's web site or portal and enters claim information into an electronic claim form, which can begin processing immediately. Entering claims via the carrier's portal eliminates the sorting, scanning, and data entry required with paper claims, so processing time is reduced by an average of 2 to 4 days. The dental practice's transaction history, including payments, rejections, and **predeterminations**, is maintained in a highly secure system, and can be accessed or downloaded only through the dentist's unique password.

Electronic Funds Transfer

Most carriers can deposit claim payments directly into the billing dentist's designated checking account. Offices that combine e-claims and EFT can receive payment in their bank account within 24 to 48 hours of transmission of the claim. If the dentist or practice wants to use electronic funds transfer (also called *direct deposit*), enrollment forms and authorization must be filed with each carrier. Once enrolled, most carriers will pay all claims, electronic and paper, by EFT.

Note: Benefits carriers may not send out check copies or explanations of benefit (EOBs) for EFT deposits, so Internet service may be required to access payment information online from the carrier.

COORDINATION OF BENEFITS

Coordination of benefits (COB) is the procedure used to pay health care expenses when a person is covered by more than one plan. Dental benefits carriers follow rules established by state law in deciding which plan pays first (**primary carrier**) and how much the other plan (secondary carrier) or plans (tertiary carrier, etc.) must pay. The objective is to provide the **maximum allowable benefit (MAB)** without exceeding the actual fee charged.

Determining the Order of Liability

To identify the primary plan, the administrative assistant needs to know whether the patient is the subscriber or a dependent

Code on Dental Procedures and Nomenclature

The ADA *Code on Dental Procedures and Nomenclature* (commonly known as *the Code*) is used to report dental services and procedures to dental benefits plans. Per HIPAA, the ADA updates *the Code* every other year (in odd-numbered years) and publishes the Code in a reference manual called the *CDT (Current Dental Terminology)*. These procedure codes identify and describe each specific dental treatment. The codes and the dentist's fees are used to report and bill treatment to the benefits carrier. Each procedure code starts with a *D* followed by four numerals. The codes are categorized according to types of treatment:

Diagnostic	D0100-D0999
Preventive	D1000-D1999
Restorative	D2000-D2999
Endodontics	D3000-D3999
Periodontics	D4000-D4999
Prosthetics, removable	D5000-D5899
Maxillofacial prosthetics	D5900-D5999
Implant services	D6000-D6199
Prosthodontics, fixed	D6200-D6999
Oral and maxillofacial surgery	D7000-D7999
Orthodontics	D8000-D8999
Adjunctive general services	D9000-D9999

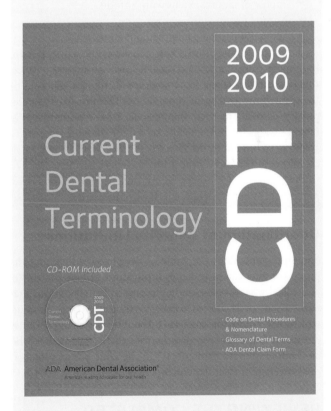

Figure 14-3 *Current Dental Terminology* (CDT), the only official source for dental service codes, is published by the American Dental Association and updated every 2 years. (Courtesy American Dental Association, Chicago.)

and any special COB rules for either plan. The primary carrier must meet *at least one* of the following criteria:

- *The plan has a no-COB clause.* If the other plan does not coordinate benefits, it is primary.
- *The patient is the employee (subscriber).* The plan covering the patient as an employee (subscriber) is always primary over a plan covering the person as a retiree, spouse, dependent, or **COBRA**-qualified beneficiary. If the patient is the subscriber for both plans, the plan covering the person as an active enrollee is primary. If the subscriber is an active **enrollee** under both plans, the plan that has covered the individual the longest is primary.
- *The patient is a dependent child.* Most carriers follow the **birthday rule**—the plan of the parent with the first birthday in a calendar year is primary for the children. For example, if the mother's birthday is in January and the father's birthday is in March, the mother's plan is primary for all their children. Some carriers may have a different coordination rule, such as the **gender rule**—the father's plan is always primary.
- *The patient is a dependent child of divorced or legally separated parents.* If a court decree makes one parent responsible for healthcare expenses, that parent's plan is primary. If a court decree does not mention health care, default rules for determining the order of liability are:
  - Natural parent with custody
  - Spouse of natural parent with custody
  - Natural parent without custody
  - Spouse of natural parent without custody

The claim for the primary carrier is always filed first. If reimbursement from the primary carrier leaves an unpaid balance, then a claim listing the same services and the amount paid by the primary carrier can be submitted to the next liable, or secondary, carrier. The total amount paid by the primary carrier must be indicated in the field reserved for the primary carrier's payment (if any) or in the *Remarks* section. Some benefit carriers may require a copy of the primary carrier's payment attached to the claim, but for others, an attachment may actually delay processing. When in doubt, check with the carrier.

Coordination of Benefits Limitations

Some programs limit the scope of benefits coordination. The group contract can have a **nonduplication of benefits** clause, also called a *carve-out*. Nonduplication of benefits means that reimbursement is limited to the maximum payable amount, which may not be the same as 100% of the fee charged. Other groups do not allow coordination of benefits for spouses who are both employees (subscribers) in the same group, although dual coverage of their **dependents** may be allowed.

REVIEWING THE COMPLETED CLAIM FORM

Figure 14-4 is an example of a paper claim form for treatment rendered by Ashley Lake, D.D.S. to a patient covered by a fictitious dental plan in Michigan. Entering the description is not necessary. This treatment plan includes the following information:

Tooth Number	Treatment	Procedure Number
3	Full cast high noble	D2790
4	Porcelain fused to high noble	D2750
13MO	Amalgam-two surfaces	D2150
14MOD	Amalgam-three surfaces	D2160

The administrative assistant must be thoroughly familiar with the Code and able to use it accurately. A close look at these entries illustrates the importance of understanding the Code and applying it correctly. For example, the number of surfaces and restorative material used on these fillings determine the procedure code number.

PAYMENT VOUCHER AND CHECK

Most carriers provide a voucher explaining the claim payment in a line-by-line breakdown, commonly called an **explanation of benefits (EOB)**. When benefits are paid to the dentist (Figure 14-5, *A*)—called the **assignment of benefits**—the voucher may have a detachable check or the check and voucher may be separate items. The administrative assistant should review each voucher to make sure all services were paid correctly. The patient also receives an EOB (Figure 14-5, *B*) to advise them that the claim is paid and the amount they are responsible for paying the dentist.

When benefits go to the patient, many carriers do not send a copy of the voucher to the dentist. Offices with Internet service can check with carriers to see if they have an online portal available for dental offices. Many carriers offer this service, and dental offices can use it to access eligibility, benefits, and claims information. The administrative assistant can also request this information from the patient.

MEDICAID CLAIM FORMS

Medicaid is a federal assistance program established as Title XIX under the Social Security Act of 1965. It provides payment for health care for certain low-income individuals and families. The program is funded jointly by the federal and state governments and is administered by each state. Medicaid should not be confused with Medicare, which only subsidizes medical expenses for citizens 65 years of age or older.

Medicaid provides comprehensive dental benefits to low-income children and young adults under age 21 as required by federal law. Dental coverage for adults enrolled in Medicaid may be limited by the state. Eligibility for Medicaid programs is determined by the state and is generally limited to individuals receiving public financial assistance.

Because each state administers its own Medicaid program, rules and regulations governing covered dental services vary. Most programs have the following general conditions:

- Reimbursement is made only to dentists participating in the Medicaid program.
- The dentist agrees to accept the amount paid by the state (or any carrier designated by the state) as payment in full; there is no patient copayment (*Note:* In states with adult Medicaid

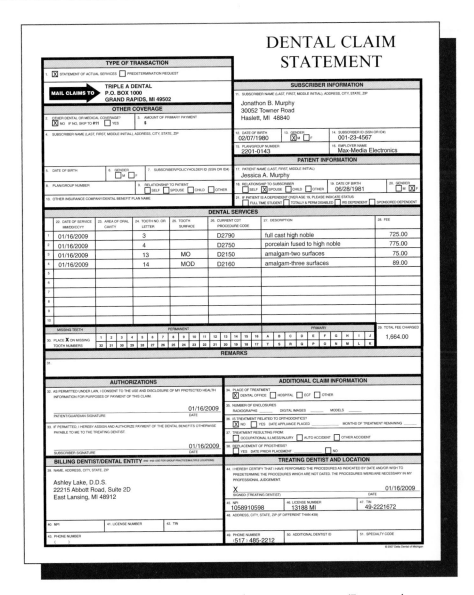

Figure 14-4 Sample completed claim form for restorative services. (Form template courtesy Delta Dental of Michigan, Ohio, and Indiana, Lansing, MI.)

dental coverage, adults over age 21 may have a minimal copayment per visit).

- Any other third-party payer is primary.
- Reimbursement to the state is required if the patient or dentist receives payment from another third-party source.
- Records must be retained for a specified length of time and may be reviewed by an authorized state or federal official.
- Patients with Medicaid coverage may not be discriminated against for reasons of race, gender, color, creed, or financial status.
- All claims must be submitted within 12 months of the date of treatment.
- Prior authorization is required for certain treatments as outlined by the state.
- All patient records remain confidential.
- Handwritten forms are not accepted; forms must be typewritten, computer generated, or submitted electronically.

Medicaid offices of the federal government accept the standard ADA paper claim form and require HIPAA compliance for all electronic submissions. In some states the Medical Services Administration (MSA) has contracted with commercial benefit carriers to partially administer alternative dental programs for children and young adults covered by Medicaid. A national model for expanding access to dental services for low-income individuals under age 21, Healthy Kids Dental (HKD), was established in Michigan and replaces Medicaid in 61 Michigan counties. Enrollee information is maintained by the state, and claims, inquiries, eligibility requests, and payments are processed by Delta Dental. Some other states, such as Tennessee, Alabama, Connecticut, and Vermont, have public-private partnerships set up to improve access to care. The ADA has a report outlining how other states are working to improve access to oral health care for children enrolled in Medicaid and the State Children's Health Insurance Program. Called *ADA State*

A

Explanation of Benefits
(THIS IS NOT A BILL)

Patient Name: CYNTHIA MARTINEZ-JONES	Business/Dentist: ASHLEY LAKE, D.D.S.
Date of Birth: 10/19/1963	License No.: 99188 / MI (NPI: 1058910598)
Relationship: SUBSCRIBER	Check No.: 80274460
Subscriber: CYNTHIA MARTINEZ-JONES	Issue Date: 01/23/2009
Subscriber ID: XXX-XX-2065	Receipt Date: 01/23/2009
Patient Acct: 0048330OR66889-2727	Claim No.: 1807411228090

Pay To: C = Custodial Parent / S = Subscriber / P = Provider

Tooth Code/ Area/Surface	Date of Service	Procedure Code	Submitted Amount	Maximum Approved Fee	Par Dentist Adjustment	Allowed Amount	Deductible / Patient Co-Pay / Office Visit	Co-Pay %	Payment	Patient Payment	Pay To
					PLAN: TRIPLE A DENTAL OF MICHIGAN						
				PRODUCT: TRIPLE A DENTAL PPO (POINT-OF-SERVICE)							
CLIENT/ID: 7743		ACME MANUFACTURING									
SUBCLIENT: 0012		INTERSTATE DIVISION									
	01/21/09	D0120	40.00	40.00	0.00	40.00		100%	40.00	0.00	P
	01/21/09	D0210	108.00	106.00	2.00	106.00		100%	106.00	0.00	P
	01/21/09	D1110	65.00	61.00	4.00	61.00		100%	61.00	0.00	P
		Total	213.00	207.00	6.00	207.00	0.00		207.00	0.00	

GENERAL MAXIMUM USED TO DATE 751.60

FOR INQUIRIES: 1-800-555-5555

CLAIMS PROCESSED BY:
TRIPLE A DENTAL
P.O. BOX 10001
LANSING, MI 48909

Payment for these services is determined in accordance with the specific terms of the member's dental plan and/or Triple A Dental's agreements with its participating dentists.

ASHLEY LAKE, D.D.S.
22215 ABBOTT ROAD, SUITE 2D
EAST LANSING, MI 48912

B

Explanation of Benefits
(THIS IS NOT A BILL)

Patient Name: CYNTHIA MARTINEZ-JONES	Business/Dentist: ASHLEY LAKE, D.D.S.
Date of Birth: 10/19/1963	License No.: 99188 / MI (NPI: 1058910598)
Relationship: SUBSCRIBER	Check No.: 80274460
Subscriber: CYNTHIA MARTINEZ-JONES	Issue Date: 01/23/2009
Patient Acct: 0048330OR66889-2727	Receipt Date: 01/23/2009
	Claim No.: 1807411228090

Pay To: C = Custodial Parent / S = Subscriber / P = Provider

Tooth Code/ Area/Surface	Date of Service	Procedure Description	Submitted Amount	Maximum Approved Fee	Par Dentist Savings	Allowed Amount	Deductible / Patient Co-Pay / Office Visit	Co-Pay %	Payment	Patient Payment	Pay To
					PLAN: TRIPLE A DENTAL OF MICHIGAN						
				PRODUCT: TRIPLE A DENTAL PPO (POINT-OF-SERVICE)							
CLIENT/ID: 7743		ACME MANUFACTURING									
SUBCLIENT: 0012		INTERSTATE DIVISION									
	01/21/09	ORAL EXAM	40.00	40.00	0.00	40.00		100%	40.00	0.00	P
	01/21/09	XRAYS	108.00	106.00	2.00	106.00		100%	106.00	0.00	P
	01/21/09	CLEANING	65.00	61.00	4.00	61.00		100%	61.00	0.00	P
		Total	213.00	207.00	6.00	207.00	0.00		207.00	0.00	

GENERAL MAXIMUM USED TO DATE 751.60

FOR INQUIRIES: 1-800-555-5555

CLAIMS PROCESSED BY:
TRIPLE A DENTAL
P.O. BOX 10001
LANSING, MI 48909

Payment for these services is determined in accordance with the specific terms of your dental plan and/or Triple A Dental's agreements with its participating dentists. For inquiries regarding participating dentists, please call the number listed. Triple A Dental's payment decisions do not qualify as dental or medical advice. You must make all decisions about the desirability or necessity of dental procedures and services with your dentist.

If your claim was denied in whole or in part so that you must pay some amount of the claim, upon a written request and free of charge, we will provide you with a copy of any internal rule, guideline or protocol or, if applicable, an explanation of the scientific or clinical judgment relied upon in deciding your claim. If you still believe your claim should have been paid in full, you may ask to have the claim reviewed. Your written request for a formal review must be sent within 180 days of your receipt of this EOB to the address listed. You may submit any additional materials you believe support your claim. A decision will be made no later than 60 days from the date we receive your request. If your claim is denied in whole or in part after the review, you have the right to seek to have your claim paid by filing a civil action in court within one year from the final denial.

CYNTHIA MARTINEZ-JONES
8404 FOXWOOD LANE
GRAND LEDGE, MI 48917

Figure 14-5 Explanation of benefit (EOB) statements are provided to both the provider **(A)** and the patient **(B)**. (Form template courtesy Delta Dental of Michigan, Ohio, and Indiana, Lansing, MI.)

Innovations Compendium Update, revised edition, the report is posted online at www.ada.org/prof/resources/topics/medicaid_reports.asp.

VETERANS ADMINISTRATION CLAIM FORM

Veterans of the U.S. armed forces may be eligible for limited dental benefits. Patients with this coverage receive a claim form from the Veterans Administration to give to the attending dentist, and the form includes all information necessary to assess benefits. Prior approval of treatment usually is required.

GUIDELINES FOR SUCCESSFUL CLAIMS ADMINISTRATION

Every team member is vital to the success of the dental office. The administrative assistant takes care of the business end of dentistry, and proper handling of the insurance accounts receivable ensures that the practice meets its financial goals. Claims must be submitted promptly and correctly, and accurate records maintained to track claims status and payments. Following are some guidelines and suggestions for controlling claims input and output:

- Keep a record of the subscriber's benefit carrier and scope of coverage. Most practice management software programs have a module that stores information by employer or organization. For offices that keeping paper records, make a standardized detail sheet for each plan, and keep them in a central file, notebook, or in the patient's personal record.
- Note any special information or procedures the carrier requires.
- Require new patients and patients of record who have a change in coverage to provide his or her benefit carrier's complete mailing address, and the telephone number for claims and inquiries.
- Ask the patient if there are any changes in coverage at each appointment. If the subscriber has been terminated, laid off, on sick leave, or changed jobs, dental benefits may not be in effect. A call to the benefits carrier can help determine eligibility/**effective dates** and **termination/expiration dates**.
- Inform each patient about his or her benefits and copayment amounts.
- Establish a routine for preparing claim forms, such as once or twice a day with daily mail-out or electronic transmission.
- Keep a current file or computer record of outstanding claims and review it frequently. Follow up with the benefit carrier on claims that are outstanding for more than 30 days.
- Submit preauthorization for treatment (**predetermination**) when required by the subscriber's plan or benefit carrier and when requested by the dentist or patient.
- Regularly verify and update patients' general information.
- If using paper claims, maintain an adequate supply of forms.
- Focus on accuracy, and complete all required fields on the claim form. If a field does not apply, leave it blank.

- Add comments only for codes that require documentation, such as miscellaneous codes (D2999, D6199).
- Use the current CDT codes, and whenever possible, use the active CDT handbook as a reference tool.
- Attend seminars presented by benefits carriers to stay current on billing practices and learn new techniques. Many seminars offer CDE credits for licensed or registered dental assistants.

INSURANCE FRAUD

Misrepresenting treatment or inaccurately reporting fees and dates of service to benefits carriers is illegal—accuracy and honesty are not negotiable. Administrative assistants who participate in any way with actions that defraud benefits carriers may be liable to legal prosecution.

The following actions, whether deliberate or unintentional, constitute fraud:

- Billing the benefits carrier for higher fees than the patient is charged
- Billing before completion of service
- Predating or postdating services on claim forms
- Improperly reporting treatment (e.g., listing a bony extraction instead of a simple extraction)
- Billing for services not rendered

KEY TERMS

Alternative benefit plan—A benefit plan other than conventional group dental coverage.

American Dental Association (ADA)—A professional association for dentists that promotes the integrity and ethics of the profession; provides services in education, research, and advocacy; and develops dental standards.

Approved services—Services covered by a benefit plan. Payment for these services may be subject to plan maximums, limitations, and deductibles.

Assignment of benefits—Authorization by the enrollee/patient for the dental benefits carrier to make payment for covered services directly to the treating dentist.

Attending dentist's statement—See *claim form.*

Balance billing—Requiring the patient to pay any difference between the dentist's actual fee and the amount reimbursed by the benefits carrier, in addition to any copayment, deductible, or maximum.

Benefit carrier—The insurance company, administrator, or other entity that manages eligibility, benefits, claims, and reimbursement for enrollees of a dental benefit contract. See *dental service corporations, insurer, third party administrator (TPA).*

Birthday rule—A method of determining the primary carrier for dependent children who are covered by more than one dental plan. With this method, the primary payer is the parent with the earlier date of birth by month and day, without regard to the year of birth.

Capitation—A benefits delivery system in which a dentist contracts with the program's sponsor or administrator to provide all or most of the dental services covered under the program in return for a fixed monthly payment per covered person. Also called a dental health maintenance organization (DHMO).

Claim form—The paper form used to request payment or predetermination for patients covered by a dental benefits program. The ADA maintains a standardized form that nearly all dental benefit carriers accept, the *ADA Dental Claim Form*. Also called an *attending dentist's statement*.

Closed panel system—A dental benefits program in which enrollees can receive benefits only when services are provided by dentists who have signed an agreement with the benefit plan to provide treatment to eligible patients.

COBRA—Consolidated Omnibus Budget Reconciliation Act, which allows a person to temporarily maintain insurance coverage even if he or she loses the job.

Code on Dental Procedures and Nomenclature—The dental procedure codes, nomenclature, and descriptors used to report dental services and procedures; also called simply *the Code*. Under HIPAA, the Code is maintained and regularly updated by the American Dental Association (ADA).

Copayment—The amount or percentage of the dentist's fee that the patient is obligated to pay.

Current Dental Terminology (CDT)—A reference manual developed by the ADA that includes the Code on Dental Procedures and Nomenclature and other instructional tools for reporting dental services to dental benefits plans and administrators.

Customary fee—The fee for a service/services determined to be representative of the fees charged by dentists in a specific region or geographic area; may be used by a benefits carrier to establish the maximum payable amount for dental procedures (also see *usual fee* and *reasonable fee*).

Dental benefits carrier—A service corporation, insurance company, or other business that contracts with employers or groups of consumers to administer dental benefits coverage.

Dental health maintenance organization (DHMO)—A dental capitation plan in which comprehensive care is provided to enrollees through participating providers. The dental provider receives a monthly payment for each enrollee accepted, and enrollees generally are required to remain in the program for a specific period. Also see Capitation.

Dental insurance—An indemnity or risk policy provided by a licensed insurance company to underwrite group or individual costs for dental treatment.

Dental service corporation—A legally constituted, non-profit organization that contracts with groups, employers, and organizations to administer dental coverage for enrolled individuals.

Dependents—Individuals, such as a spouse and children, who are legally and contractually eligible for benefits under a subscriber's dental benefits contract.

Direct reimbursement—An employer's or organization's self-funded program for reimbursing covered individuals based on a percentage of the amount spent for dental care.

Effective date—The date an individual and/or dependents become eligible for benefits under a dental benefits contract; also called the eligibility date.

Eligible person—See *enrollee*.

Enrollee—A person who is eligible for benefits under a dental benefits contract; also called *covered* or *insured individual, member, enrollee, participant, or beneficiary*.

Exclusions—Dental services that are not covered under a dental benefits program.

Exclusive provider organization (EPO) plan—A dental benefits program in which benefits are provided only if care is rendered by institutional and professional providers with whom the plan contracts. Some exceptions may be allowed for emergency and out-of-area services.

Expiration date—The date on which the dental benefits contract expires or the date an individual ceases to be eligible for benefits. Also called the *termination date*.

Explanation of Benefits (EOB)—A detailed statement of a processed claim showing the patient, provider, procedure codes, dates of service, the carrier's payment, and the patient's copayment. It may also include maximums used to date and limitations or exclusions applied to the listed services.

Fee-for-service plan—A dental benefits program in which dentists are paid for each covered service rendered to an eligible enrollee.

Fee schedule—A list of charges established by or agreed to by a dentist for specific dental services, usually listed by ADA procedure code.

Gender rule—A method of determining the primary carrier for dependent children who are covered by more than one dental plan. With this method, the primary payer is the plan that covers the father.

Group—The company or organization that contracts with a benefits carrier to administer their dental program. The group determines program type, benefit levels, maximums, and member eligibility.

Group member—See *subscriber*.

Health Insurance Portability and Accountability Act of 1996 (HIPAA)—A federal law intended to improve access to health insurance, limit fraud and abuse, and control administrative costs. Under the *Administration Simplification* section of this law, any covered entity that transmits protected health information (PHI) electronically (including dental benefit carriers, clearinghouses, and dental practices) must use a standard format, the ADA procedure codes, and use the National Provider Identifier (NPI) for all electronic transactions. Additionally, covered entities must comply with security and privacy mandates. Paper transactions are not subject to this legislation.

Insured—See *enrollee*.

Insurer—An organization that bears the financial risk for the cost of defined categories or services for a defined group of policy holders or beneficiaries.

Limitations—Restrictions stated in a dental benefits contract that limit the scope of coverage; such restrictions may include age limits for certain procedures, waiting periods before benefits are available, and payment frequency for certain services.

Maximum allowable benefit (MAB)—The highest total dollar amount a dental benefits program pays toward the cost of dental care incurred by an individual or family in a specified period, such as a calendar year, a contract year, or a lifetime.

Medicaid—A federal assistance program, established as Title XIX under the Social Security Act of 1965, that provides payment for medical care for certain low-income individuals and families. The program is funded jointly by state and federal governments and is administered by the states.

Member—See *enrollee*.

National Provider Identifier (NPI)—A unique identification number used by any healthcare entity in the electronic transmission of protected personal health information (PHI). The NPI is part of the *HIPAA* Administrative Simplification provisions.

Nonduplication of benefits—A benefit contract provision that limits coordination of benefits payments. Total reimbursement is limited to the highest amount payable by either contract, not the actual fee charged or the maximum allowable amount. Also called a *carve-out*.

Open panel system—A dental benefits program that allows (1) enrollees to receive dental treatment from any licensed dentist; (2) licensed dentists to participate; and (3) payment of benefits to either the enrollee or the dentist. The dentist may accept or refuse any enrollee.

Point-of-service plan—A dental benefits program in which the level of payment is based on the participation status of the dentist rendering treatment. In general, benefit levels are higher and patient copayments lower for services rendered by providers who participate with the enrollee's dental program. Covered services provided by out-of-network providers may be reimbursed on a lower fee scale with higher out-of-pocket costs for the enrollee.

Predetermination—A treatment plan submitted to the benefit carrier for review and estimation of payment before services are rendered. An approved predetermination is not a guarantee of payment, and payment is subject to eligibility, deductibles, and maximum used-to-date when services are rendered. Some programs require predetermination of services expected to exceed a specific amount, such as $200. Also called *precertification, preauthorization, pretreatment estimate*, and *prior authorization*.

Preferred provider organization (PPO) plan—A dental benefits program in which participating dentists agree to a discounted fee schedule for services rendered to patients enrolled in the program.

Premium—The amount charged by a dental benefits carrier for coverage or administration of benefits for a specified time.

Primary carrier—The benefit carrier that has initial responsibility for benefit payment when a patient is covered by two or more carriers.

Reasonable and customary (R&C) plan—A fee-for-service dental benefits program in which payment of benefits is based on reasonable and customary fee criteria (also see *customary fee* and *reasonable fee*).

Reasonable fee—The fee most often charged by the dentist or that is adjusted in consideration of the nature and severity of the condition treated and any medical or dental complications or unusual circumstances that may affect treatment.

Reimbursement—Payment made by a benefit carrier or other third-party payer to an enrollee or to a dentist on behalf of the enrollee as repayment of fees charged for a covered service.

Subscriber—The employee or participant who is certified by the company or organization (group) providing the dental program as eligible to receive benefit coverage. If family coverage is offered, the additional people listed on the contract will be designated as spouse or dependent(s). See *group member*.

Table of allowances plan—A dental benefits program that lists an assigned amount payable for each covered service. The payable amount is generally below the average fee charged by dentists. Also called a *schedule of allowances*.

Termination date—The date on which the dental benefits contract ends or the date when the enrollee is no longer eligible for benefits. Also called the expiration date.

Third-party administrator (TPA)—An entity that administers a health benefit plan without assuming any financial risk.

Unbundling of procedures—The division of a dental procedure into component parts and assignment of a separate charge for each; the total of these charges is higher than the single fee for the complete procedure.

Usual, customary, and reasonable (UCR) plan—A dental benefits program in which payment for covered benefits is based on a combination of usual, customary, and reasonable fee criteria (see *usual fee, customary fee,* and *reasonable fee*).

Usual fee—The fee a dentist most frequently charges for a given dental service.

DENTAL INSURANCE TERMINOLOGY

Allowed amount—The maximum dollar amount the benefit carrier allows for each dental procedure. It is not always the same as the approved amount.

Approved amount—The amount used by the benefit carrier as the basis of payment for a submitted fee.

Benefit administrator—The person or company who manages or directs a dental benefits program on behalf of the program's sponsor.

Benefit plan summary—A description or synopsis of employee benefits, which employers are legally required to distribute to employees. Also called the *summary plan description (SPD)*.

Benefit year—The 12-month period of the dental contract (not always a calendar year). Most patients have a *maximum allowable benefit* that renews at the beginning of each benefit year.

Cafeteria plan—A health coverage system under which employers offer eligible employees a list of options for health care benefits, which may include several carriers and levels of coverage. Participants may receive additional, taxable cash compensation if they select less expensive benefits.

Claim audit—An administrative or a professional review of the services reported on a claim to verify information, determine the appropriateness of treatment, or propose acceptable alternative treatment.

Claimant—A person who files a claim for reimbursement of covered costs.

Covered charges—Charges for services rendered or supplies furnished by a dentist that qualify as covered services and are paid for in whole or in part by the dental benefits program. These charges may be subject to deductibles, copayments, coinsurance, and annual or lifetime maximums as specified by the terms of the contract.

Covered services—A dental service that is payable under the terms of the benefit program.

Deductible—The amount of dental expenses a covered person must pay before the dental plan benefits begin. A deductible may be an annual or a one-time charge and can vary in amount. Individual deductibles are applied to one person; family deductibles are satisfied by combining the expenses of all covered family members.

Direct billing—Requiring payment in full from the patient/responsible party for all services rendered.

Extension of benefits—An extension of eligibility that covers treatment started before the expiration date. The duration is limited and generally expressed in days.

Individual practice association (IPA)—A legal entity representing independent dentists that contracts as a dental group with a carrier, business, or organization to provide services to enrolled populations. Dentists may practice in their own offices and provide care to patients not covered by the contract as well as to IPA patients.

Maximum allowable amount—The highest dollar amount payable by a third-party payer for a covered dental treatment. Also called *maximum allowable payment*.

Nonparticipating dentist—A dentist who does not have a contractual agreement with a dental benefits carrier.

Open enrollment—The period during which employees or group members can enroll in health care programs.

Overcoding—Reporting a more complex and/or more expensive procedure than was actually performed.

Participating dentist—A dentist who has a contractual agreement with a dental benefits carrier.

Peer review—A process for reviewing issues arising from dental treatment. A panel of licensed dentists reviews cases submitted by carriers, patients, and dentists involving quality of care, appropriateness of treatment, fee disputes, and professionalism. The review panel typically is organized by the state dental association.

Preexisting condition—An oral health condition that existed before a person enrolled in a dental program.

Schedule of benefits—A list of dental services covered by a dental benefits program.

Waiting period—The period between employment or enrollment in a dental program and the date the enrollee becomes eligible for benefits. Also a specific time frame between the date of eligibility and activation of coverage for some services.

LEARNING ACTIVITIES

1. Identify the four parties affected by dental benefits and the roles of each.
2. Describe the two main types of dental benefits programs.
3. What patient information needed to complete a standard ADA claim form?
4. Describe the *Code on Dental Procedures and Nomenclature* and explain how it is used.
5. Differentiate between filing claims on paper and electronically.
6. What is the purpose of the claim payment voucher?
7. Identify five actions that constitute dental benefits fraud.

Please refer to the student workbook for additional learning activities.

RECOMMENDED WEB SITES

www.deltadental.com
www.ada.org/prof/resources/topics/medicaid_reports.asp

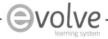

Please visit http://evolve.elsevier.com/Finkibeiner/practice for additional practice activities.

15

Financial Systems: Accounts Receivable

LEARNING OUTCOMES

- Define key terms.
- Define *bookkeeping*.
- Define *accounting*.
- Explain basic mathematical procedures.
- Describe common bookkeeping systems in dentistry.
- Explain the function of a computerized accounts receivable program.
- Explain the production of patient statements.
- Identify common payment and credit policies.
- Describe the various laws affecting credit policies and collection procedures
- Describe the "red flags" rule.
- Identify common problems in maintaining a credit policy.
- Identify the functions of a credit bureau.
- Explain the function of a collection agency.
- Compose collection letters.

As discussed in various areas of this textbook, dentistry is a business as well as a health profession. In this chapter the reader will understand that sound business practices must be integrated into the management of the dental office, to maintain a steady cash flow to maintain a solvent practice. Consequently the administrative assistant who maintains the business portion of the dental practice with a high degree of efficiency becomes a valuable asset.

The two financial systems used in a dental business office are accounts receivable and accounts payable. The administrative assistant is responsible for both. The **accounts receivable** system includes all production; data are entered for treatment rendered, payments received, and account adjustments made, and new balances are calculated. After all computations have been made, the current accounts receivable amount, or the

amount of money owed to the dentist (incoming money), is determined. **Accounts payable** refers to all the dentist's financial obligations, or money the dentist owes (outgoing money). This chapter discusses accounts receivable; Chapter 16 details accounts payable and other financial systems.

PRACTICE NOTE
The administrative assistant who maintains the business portion of the dental practice with a high degree of efficiency becomes a valuable asset.

As mentioned, records management is a primary responsibility of the administrative assistant. Financial records are as important as clinical records but should be maintained separately. They provide (1) protection for both the dentist and the patient, (2) information for tax purposes, and (3) data for a business analysis. Inaccurate records result in poor public relations and may create unnecessary litigation with the state or federal government. **Bookkeeping**, or the recording of financial transactions, is the responsibility of the administrative assistant. **Accounting**, which is the recording, classifying, and summarizing of financial and business records, generally is the job of the accountant. Most dentists have an accountant who audits the books and computes a variety of tax reports and financial statements.

UNDERSTANDING BASIC MATHEMATICAL COMPUTATIONS

Before becoming proficient at computing financial activity on various records, review some basic mathematical rules. Because computers are used to produce so many documents, it often is easy to forget how to perform basic calculations or compute percentages on insurance claim forms.

Although a computer can make the necessary calculations, the administrative assistant is responsible for entering the data in the appropriate fields to ensure that the final figures are accurate. The administrative assistant often needs to add and subtract figures with decimals and perform other business-related computations. Most people use manual or electronic calculators for these tasks; however, relying solely on technological devices without having an understanding of basic computation can result in embarrassment, patient dissatisfaction, and possibly loss of cash flow when errors are detected. Understand the computations and also be prepared for the day when the electronic functions may fail, and it becomes necessary to do the computations manually. The following descriptions cover basic mathematical procedures used for routine bookkeeping entries.

DECIMALS

Adding and Subtracting Decimals

Place the numbers to be added or subtracted in a vertical column, aligning the decimal points, before performing the addition or subtraction. To add columns of figures with decimals, add the numbers in each column, beginning with the column farthest to the right and working to the left:

$$
\begin{array}{r}
0.5 \\
2.8 \\
30.50 \\
67.945 \\
+750.000 \\
\hline
851.745
\end{array}
$$

To subtract, follow the same procedure. Place the numbers to be subtracted in a vertical column, aligning the decimal points. Each amount must have the same number of decimals;

therefore, it may be necessary to add zeros before performing this procedure. For example, to subtract 1.75 from 3.876, add one zero at the end of the 1.75:

$$
\begin{array}{r}
3.876 \\
-1.750 \\
\hline
2.126
\end{array}
$$

Multiplying Decimals

To multiply decimals, perform the procedure as for all whole numbers, except the decimal point must be placed correctly in the answer. Count the number of digits to the right of the decimal point in the multiplicand and in the multiplier; then count the same number of places from right to left in the product and insert the decimal point:

600.75	2 decimals (multiplicand)
× 0.20	2 decimals (multiplier)
120.1500	2 + 2 = 4 decimals

or

$800.50	2 decimals
× 0.75	2 decimals
$600.3750	2 + 2 = 4 decimals

or

$800	0 decimals
× 0.75	2 decimals
$600.00	0 + 2 = 2 decimals

Percentages

Working with percentages is a common function of routine posting of accounts receivable. For example, if processing insurance claim forms manually, determine the subscriber and carrier percentages and any deductible amounts. In an automated system these figures are calculated, but again, the administrative assistant must understand this process to ensure accuracy. The following are examples of some very basic procedures.

To change a percent to a fraction, drop the percent sign, place the number over 100, and reduce the fraction to the lowest terms. If the numerator is a decimal, multiply both the numerator and denominator by an appropriate power of 10 to clear the decimal. For instance,

$$5\% = \frac{5}{100} = \frac{1}{20}$$

or

$$7.5\% = \frac{7.5}{100} = \frac{75}{1000} = \frac{3}{40}$$

To change a percent to a decimal, move the decimal point two places to the left and drop the percent sign.

$$15\% = 0.15$$
$$2\% = 0.02$$
$$110\% = 1.1$$

To find a certain percent of a number, convert the percent to a decimal and multiply by the number. For instance, the following computation shows how to calculate 80% of $670:

$$\begin{array}{r} \$670 \\ \times\, 0.80 \\ \hline \$536 \end{array}$$

TYPES OF BOOKKEEPING SYSTEMS

Overview

In the past, dentistry used a variety of bookkeeping systems, including the pegboard, or "write it once," system, which until the 1990s was the system most often used in dental offices. With the pegboard system, one notation provided an entry on the daily journal sheet, the ledger card, the receipt, and in some cases a statement. The system of choice now is a computer software program, which goes beyond the basic transactions of the pegboard system to provide all financial records, insurance claim forms, future appointments and recall management, and documents for practice analysis.

A computerized bookkeeping system can be integrated into total records management. In other words, the administrative assistant can make a clinical entry on a patient record that can then be transferred to a financial record. Using designated codes, he or she can transfer this information to a patient statement, and an insurance claim form can be generated from the original data entry. This type of system is more than just a mechanism for bookkeeping.

Components of a Computerized Bookkeeping System

Chapter 5 described the use of dental office management software. One component of most of these systems is the accounts receivable program. By entering data for a patient account, one can generate a myriad of reports, forms, or other types of information.

When a dentist purchases a software management program, some type of tutorial generally is provided, and the administrative assistant probably will be given live or web-based instruction in the use of the software. Once the software has been installed in the computer and the training is completed, the administrative assistant can begin entering basic patient clinical and financial data. To generate accounts receivable data, one generally follows specific steps outlined in the software package. The following description is an overview of some of the common steps in basic data entry. Although each software package has its own distinct features, most include these steps. Table 15-1 presents some common commands used in a variety of accounts receivable programs.

Opening the Program

When the administrative assistant opens the program, he or she is commonly required to enter his or her name or user name and a password. Generally, when a password is entered, the characters are not displayed on the screen as they are keyed in. Most systems allow for reentry of the password in case an error is made, but after a specified number of entries, the program may lock the person out.

TABLE 15-1	Common Commands in Accounts Receivable Software
Command	**Meaning**
ADD	Enter additional data; create a new record
APPOINTMENT/ SCHEDULER	Enter data for a patient appointment
DEL	Delete; to eliminate part or all of the data entry
EDIT	Alter or change data
ENTER	Insert data
ESC	Leave the screen
FILE	Open, close, print, or take action on files
INSURANCE	Make a data entry or obtain a hard copy of a claim form
LIST	Provides a screen view or hard copy of lists of patients, accounts, or other data
LOCATE	Find a patient, an account, or other data
N	No
PATIENT	Enter a field of patient records
POST	Enter data, financial or other
PRINT	Produce a hard copy of a document
RECALL	Enter data about a patient for recall
REPORTS	Obtain some form of report programmed into the system
SYSTEM	Change the system setting, log in, or password
TRANSACTION	Reference to financial activity
VIEW	Changes the format of the screen view
WINDOW	Allows a different configuration of the screen
WORD PROCESSOR	Program that allows letter writing
Y	Yes

Locating Account Information

When the administrative assistant makes a selection, such as *Accounts*, a screen opens in which the account can be selected with which that person would like to work (Figure 15-1). If no account appears, a new patient can be added by clicking on the *Add* icon and creating a new patient record (Figure 15-2). Certain basic account information is common to most systems, such as an ID number, patient name and address, personal data (e.g., telephone number or numbers, Social Security number, date of birth, gender, and age), person responsible for the patient's charges, dentist of choice (the primary provider for the patient if the office has several dentists) and insurance policy holder, and insurance numbers and employment. Special notes, such as the patient's preferred pharmacy, who referred the patient to the office, school the patient may be attending, etc. may be included.

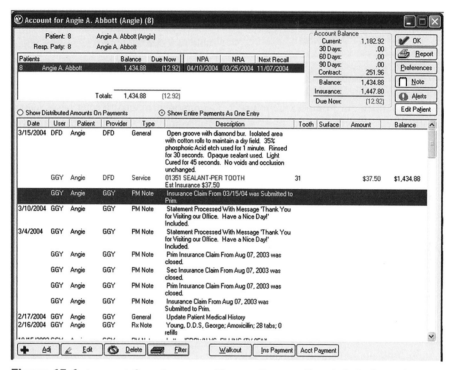

Figure 15-1 Account information screen. (Courtesy Patterson Dental, St. Paul, MN.)

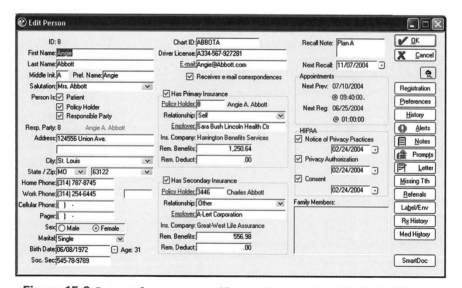

Figure 15-2 Patient information screen. (Courtesy Patterson Dental, St. Paul, MN.)

Editing Account Information

At times one will need to edit account information, such as when a patient's name or address changes. To do this, enter the *Account* window and select *Edit*. (*Edit* refers to the task of changing existing data.)

Adding, Inactivating, or Transferring a Patient

Patients may be added to an account in the system shown by selecting ADD. This is commonly done to add a spouse or dependent to an account. Inactivating a patient may be necessary because of divorce or death. Children may be transferred to their own accounts as they grow older.

Posting Transactions

Perhaps one of the most common daily activities in bookkeeping is entering transaction data. From the transaction screen (Figure 15-3), most systems are designed to allow the person to enter clinical data about treatment, for which he or she may insert appropriate codes. When the data are entered, the program computes the financial activity and produces an account **balance**. The data are then saved. There may also be a prompt to complete an insurance claim form or other activity (e.g., recall or appointment scheduling) as part of the walkout process (Figure 15-4).

Backing Up Data

As mentioned in Chapter 8, maintaining all the practice data on a computer's hard drive without a backup is dangerous. Valuable information can be lost as the result of a power surge, computer crash, or misdirected ERASE or DEL command. For

this reason, the hard drive must be backed up regularly. This can be done using a CD-ROM, DVD, external hard drive, or some other type of storage device.

The office procedures manual must describe the backup procedure step by step, and a backup log must be maintained (Figure 15-5).

Today many offices are contracting with an offsite backup service using an existing Internet connection to access the offsite backup provider. The initial step is the installation of the online backup client software. Next, a backup set is created and important files and/or records are identified. Finally, a backup schedule is selected. From that point forward, backups generally occur automatically, on schedule, without end-user intervention.

The service transfers encrypted copies of the most critical computer data to a secure remote storage vault. In the event of data loss, this process is reversed and missing data are retrieved (restored) from the storage vault and returned to the computer.

Before contracting with such a service, the company must be researched to ensure that they adhere to HIPAA standards, and such a company can be relied on exclusively to provide daily backups. Some offices may use the service as a complement to their local tape or CD/DVD backups. In these cases, only the most critical data files (financial records, patient clinical charts, etc.) are identified and backed up offsite. This better protects the dentist against physical threats such as fire, flood, and theft. An example of a provider for offsite backup service can be viewed at www.drbackup.net.

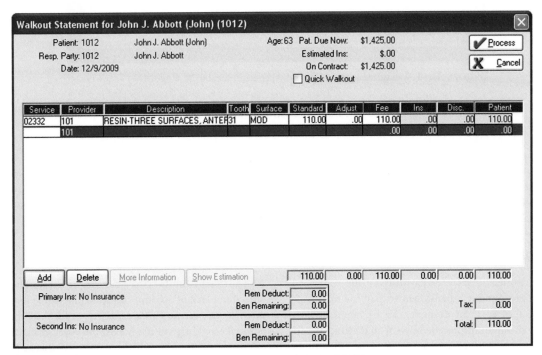

Figure 15-3 Transaction screen. (Courtesy Patterson Dental, St. Paul, MN.)

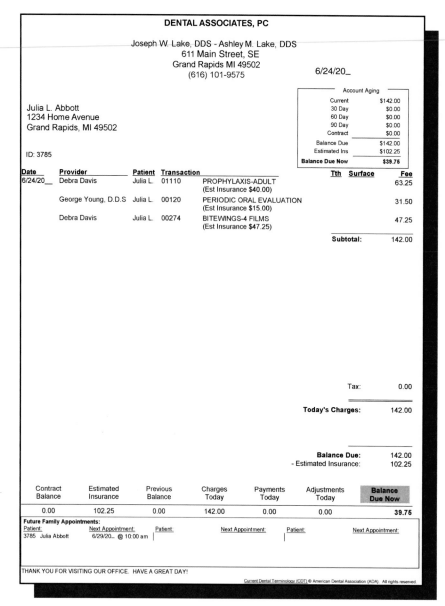

Figure 15-4 Walkout statement. (Courtesy Patterson Dental, St. Paul, MN.)

SPECIAL SITUATIONS

A day would not be complete without some unusual activity that cannot be recorded using the procedure exactly as listed previously. Several such situations and their solutions are presented in the following discussions.

Credit Balance

A credit balance often occurs when payment is made in advance, as when a patient obtains a bank loan to pay for treatment. A credit balance of $50, for example, can be noted in three ways: (1) with the amount preceded by *CR* (CR$50); (2) with the amount preceded by a minus sign (–$50); and (3) with the amount, in color, enclosed in parentheses ($50) (Figure 15-6).

Each time treatment is rendered, charges are made against the credit balance, reducing it. Remember, the credit balance represents what is owed to the patient in services. Note that the credit transaction is also shown when a patient pays on the account (Figure 15-7).

Nonsufficient Funds

Nonsufficient funds (NSF) checks, or checks returned to the office for a lack of account funds, require some form of adjustment to the account. A person may redeposit the check and not make an entry on the books. However, it may be necessary to charge the account with this returned check. Note that for the returned check in Figure 15-8, an NSF notation has been

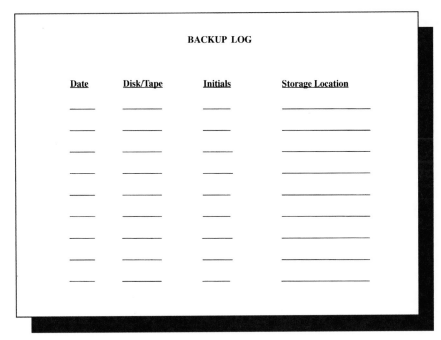

Figure 15-5 Manual backup log.

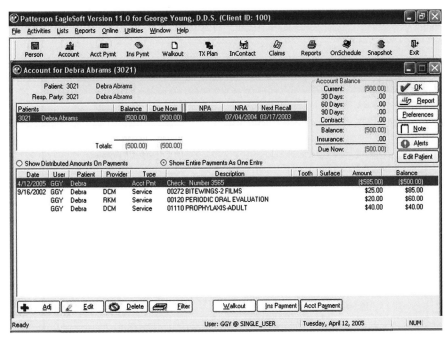

Figure 15-6 The current credit balance on the account is indicated in red and parentheses. (Courtesy Patterson Dental, St. Paul, MN.)

made and a service charge of $25 has been assessed against the account. Collection fees are paid to an agency for collecting a delinquent account, and these fees generally are deducted from the payment before it is sent to the dentist.

A courtesy discount is given when the dentist extends a professional courtesy to a patient. The courtesy discount is entered in a separate **adjustment** row (Figure 15-9).

Debit and Credit Cards

When a patient uses a debit or credit card to pay for services the *Account* window is opened and the payment is selected as a debit or credit card. A terminal to provide the debit/credit card transaction is provided either by the software company for the computer system or from the dentist's bank. If the patient pays with a debit card, a field on this same screen will be visible for the patient to

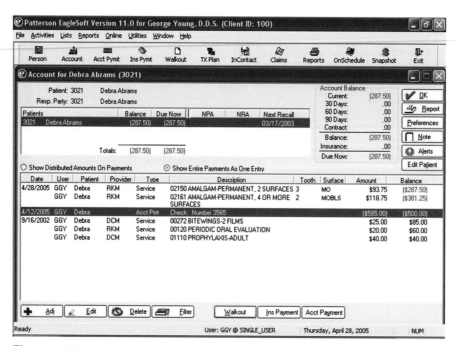

Figure 15-7 Credit is adjusted when activity occurs on the account. (Courtesy Patterson Dental, St. Paul, MN.)

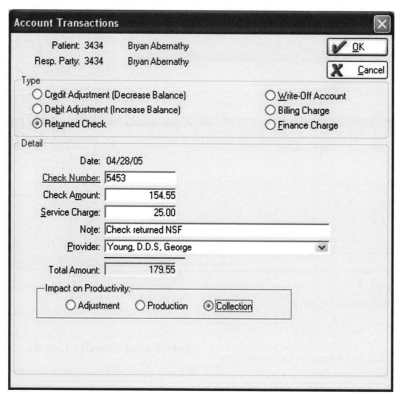

Figure 15-8 Account transaction screen indicates a nonsufficient funds (NSF) check with a service charge attached. (Courtesy Patterson Dental, St. Paul, MN.)

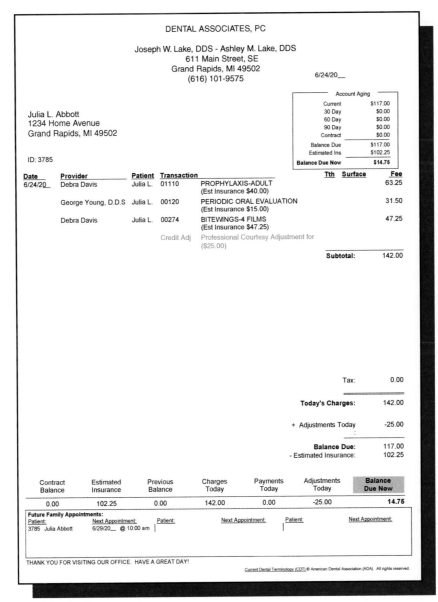

DENTAL ASSOCIATES, PC

Joseph W. Lake, DDS - Ashley M. Lake, DDS
611 Main Street, SE
Grand Rapids, MI 49502
(616) 101-9575

6/24/20___

Account Aging	
Current	$117.00
30 Day	$0.00
60 Day	$0.00
90 Day	$0.00
Contract	$0.00
Balance Due	$117.00
Estimated Ins	$102.25
Balance Due Now	**$14.75**

Julia L. Abbott
1234 Home Avenue
Grand Rapids, MI 49502

ID: 3785

Date	Provider	Patient	Transaction		Tth	Surface	Fee
6/24/20	Debra Davis	Julia L.	01110	PROPHYLAXIS-ADULT (Est Insurance $40.00)			63.25
	George Young, D.D.S	Julia L.	00120	PERIODIC ORAL EVALUATION (Est Insurance $15.00)			31.50
	Debra Davis	Julia L.	00274	BITEWINGS-4 FILMS (Est Insurance $47.25)			47.25
			Credit Adj	Professional Courtesy Adjustment for ($25.00)			
						Subtotal:	142.00

Tax: 0.00

Today's Charges: 142.00

+ Adjustments Today −25.00

Balance Due: 117.00
- Estimated Insurance: 102.25

Contract Balance	Estimated Insurance	Previous Balance	Charges Today	Payments Today	Adjustments Today	**Balance Due Now**
0.00	102.25	0.00	142.00	0.00	−25.00	**14.75**

Future Family Appointments:

Patient:	Next Appointment:	Patient:	Next Appointment:	Patient:	Next Appointment:
3785 Julia Abbott	6/29/20___ @ 10:00 am				

THANK YOU FOR VISITING OUR OFFICE. HAVE A GREAT DAY!

Current Dental Terminology (CDT) © American Dental Association (ADA). All rights reserved.

Figure 15-9 A courtesy discount is entered as credit to the account. (Courtesy Patterson Dental, St. Paul, MN.)

enter a pin number. The patient then enters his or her debit card pin number when prompted on the pin pad (Figure 15-10).

STATEMENTS

A statement informs patients of their financial status with the dentist and indicates the charges, payments, and balances of their accounts for the month just concluded. The statement is also a request for payment. Statements may be sent on the first, fifteenth, or thirtieth day of the month or on a staggered basis according to the alphabet or date of services. The important factor is consistency; that is, statements should be sent at the same time each month.

A statement can be generated on the computer with an automated bookkeeping system (Figure 15-11). The itemized statement shows the dates of payments and the treatments for each member of the family during the month. With a computerized system, a person can add special messages or aging columns to statements to enhance the collection process.

IDENTITY THEFT

Identity theft occurs in contemporary society when the thief uses a person's personal identifying information to open new accounts or misuse existing accounts. Try as one may, no small business is immune from identity theft, including the dental

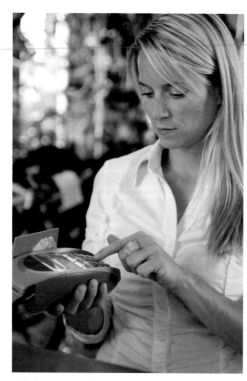

Figure 15-10 Patient entering pin number on a pin pad for a debit transaction. (Copyright 2007 Neil Speers, Canada. Image from www. BigStockPhoto.com).

office. It is likely that a dental practice may encounter such a situation only once or twice and maybe never, but in a dental practice such situations can occur. The administrative assistant should be mindful of potential unknown persons in the practice using stolen credit cards or false information. The American Dental Association provides for its members information on federal regulations that may impact the practice of dentistry. To obtain the latest in identity theft as it relates to the dental practice, visit www.ada.org and do a search for the latest in identity theft.

ESTABLISHING FINANCIAL ARRANGEMENTS

Well-Defined Policies

The adage, "Inform before you perform," still applies to the management of accounts in the dental office. A well-defined credit policy should be an integral part of the accounts receivable system. This policy must: (1) conform to community standards, (2) reflect the attitude of the dentist toward the patient's welfare, (3) represent sound business concepts, (4) be presented in written form to the patient, (5) provide options for the patient, and (6) be adhered to at all times. Many payment policies exist; therefore, including this policy as part of the office policy is a wise move.

Because financial arrangements generally are made by the administrative assistant, be well acquainted with the office

credit policy. Furthermore, be firm yet polite in adhering to the policy and avoid becoming a victim of any of the following common situations.

- The patient says he will take care of the bill in full when treatment has been completed. A patient having extensive restorative treatment should not be offended when it is explained that office expenses and laboratory fees require some form of payment before completion of the treatment.
- The patient becomes defensive or angry when asked about payment arrangements. Find out why she is irritated; patients with good intentions seldom become defensive when asked about payment.
- The patient says he will pay the bill when his income tax refund or other windfall is received. There is no way of knowing whether he will actually receive the expected money or use it to pay his dental bills.
- The patient makes promises and does not fulfill them. A consistent follow-up system must be initiated to eliminate such problems. Patients often become lax in their responsibility because the dental staff is not consistent.

Types of Payment Policies

Many payment policies are used in dentistry today, but a few are common to all practices.

Cash-Only System

The cash-only system obviously eliminates much paperwork in the business office, but it may place limitations on the dental practice.

Payment of Statement in Full

Unless other arrangements have been made with the office, the patient is expected to pay in full within 10 days of receipt of the statement. Some form of notice, such as appropriate signage or a written policy statement, must be presented to the patient.

Extended Payment

Regulation 2 of the Truth in Lending Act requires that an agreement exist between the dentist and the patient if payment for services is to be made in more than four installments. Even if no finance charge is involved, the truth in lending form (Figure 15-12) must be completed to verify that such a payment agreement has been reached. In some areas this form has been modified to include an entry for insurance coverage. A payment booklet may be used to help the patient keep track of payments and to identify the payment when the slip is mailed with the check. This system is common in practices such as orthodontics.

USING A CREDIT BUREAU

Perhaps the best way to define a credit bureau, or *consumer reporting agency (CRA)*, is to explain what it does not do: it does not lend money; it does not deny credit; and it is not a collection agency. A credit bureau reports specific information about a person's previous payment habits on deferred payment plans.

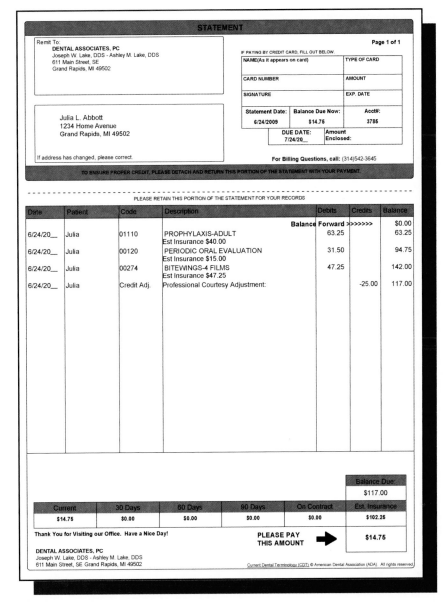

Figure 15-11 Computer-generated statement using American Dental Association (ADA) codes. (Courtesy Patterson Dental, St. Paul, MN.)

It reports on accounts placed for collection and provides information of public interest, such as that regarding bankruptcies, judgments, and lawsuits.

The Fair Credit Reporting Act (FCRA) was passed in 1992 to promote accuracy, fairness, and privacy of information in the files of all Credit Reporting Agencies (CRAs). Most CRAs are credit bureaus that gather and sell information about a person (e.g., whether a person pays bills on time or has filed bankruptcy) to **creditors**, employers, landlords, and other businesses. The full text of this legislation is available on the FTC's web site. Consumers may have additional rights under state law, and a state or local consumer protection agency or a state attorney general can provide that information.

CRAs charge a nominal fee for supplying information. When seeking information from a credit bureau, complete data should be given about the prospective creditor. This information should include the following information about the individual:

- Full name, including first and middle names. Accurate spelling is essential. The spouse's name should be used as a cross-reference for identification purposes only.
- Address or addresses for the past 3 years
- Place of employment for the past 3 years
- Names of stores and firms where credit has been established
- Name of bank or banks
- Social Security number

After this information has been given to the credit bureau, a credit report will be issued on the applicant. Care must be taken to record the information accurately. The Associated Credit Bureaus of America have designed a common language,

FINANCIAL AGREEMENT

DATE ____________

PATIENT NAME ____________________________

RESPONSIBLE PARTY ____________________________

ADDRESS ____________________________

____

HOME PHONE ____________ WORK PHONE ____________

CELL PHONE ____________ E-MAIL ____________

COST OF TOTAL TREATMENT	$______
INITIAL PAYMENT	–______
APPROXIMATE INSURANCE PAYMENTS	–______
BALANCE DUE	=______
INTEREST RATE PERCENTAGE	______
TOTAL AMOUNT OF FINANCE CHARGE	+______
AMOUNT REMAINING TO BE PAID BY PATIENT	=______

AMOUNT DUE TO BE PAID IN ____________ MONTHLY PAYMENTS OF $ ____________ STARTING ____________. BALANCE TO BE PAID IN FULL BY ____________.

I understand the financial arrangements above and agree to comply with them. I agree that parents are responsible for all fees and services rendered for treatment of a child. I understand that I am responsible for ALL fees regardless of insurance coverage. I also understand that as treatment progresses the above fees may have to be adjusted, but that I will be informed of these adjustments and how they will affect my payment plan. In the event that my payments are not received within 30 days of their due date, I agree to pay all costs of collections, including, but not limited to, reasonable attorney's fees.

____________________________ ____________

Responsible Party Signature Date

FINANCIAL AGREEMENT

ITEM 07-0513739/9054

Figure 15-12 Truth in lending form. (Redrawn from a form courtesy Patterson Office Supplies, Champaign, IL.)

which incorporates symbols, for reporting this information (Table 15-2). The symbols should mean the same things throughout the consumer credit industry, such as *O* for open, *R* for revolving, and *I* for installment.

The dentist decides whether to extend credit to a patient. If the patient is denied credit, FCRA requires that the patient be informed of the reason for denial of credit and the name of the bureau from which a credit report was obtained. The dental office is not required to report the specific data obtained from the bureau; a patient who wants this information should contact the bureau personally.

COLLECTION PROCEDURES

Collecting fees in the dental office is a critical responsibility of the administrative assistant, although sometimes it can be a difficult task. Experience has shown that patients pay medical and dental bills last. People pay their rent for fear of eviction, their car payments for fear of repossession, and their utility bills for fear of losing service. They even pay off loans before the dental bill because banks generally adhere to a stricter enforcement of collection procedures than the dentist does. Fortunately, only about 5% of patients become "uncollectable," but this 5% can be exasperating.

TABLE 15-2	Language Used in Consumer Credit Reports	
Usual Manner of Payment		**Symbol**
Open Account, 30-Day Account, 90-Day Account		**0**
Too new to rate; approved but not used		0–0
Pays (or paid) within 30 days of billing; pays 90-day accounts as agreed		0–1
Pays (or paid) in more than 30 days but not more than 60 days		0–2
Pays (or paid) in more than 60 days but not more than 90 days		0–3
Pays (or paid) in more than 90 days but not more than 120 days		0–4
Pays (or paid) in 120 days or more		0–5
Bad debt; placed for collection; suit; judgment; bankrupt; skip		0–9
Revolving or Option Account R or R $ _____ *		*****
Too new to rate; approved but not used		R-0
Pays (or paid) according to the terms agreed		R-1
Not paying (or paid) as agreed but not more than one payment past due		R-2
Not paying (or paid) as agreed and two payments past due		R-3
Not paying (or paid) as agreed and three payments past due		R-4
Bad debt; placed for collection; suit; judgment; bankrupt; skip		R-9
Installment Account I or I $ _____ *		*****
Too new to rate; approved but not used		I-0
Pays (or paid) according to terms agreed		I-1
Not paying (or paid) as agreed but not more than one payment past due		I-2
Not paying (or paid) as agreed and two payments past due		I-3
Not paying (or paid) as agreed and three payments or more past due		I-4
Repossession		I-8
Bad debt; placed for collection; suit; judgment; bankrupt; skip		I-9

*When the monthly payment is known, it should be shown (e.g., R $20 or I $78).

Aging Accounts

Each month the administrative assistant should age the accounts receivable. With a computer, this can be programmed into the system and an aging report of the accounts is automatically produced when desired. The dentist must determine a policy about aging accounts, and the administrative assistant must follow through with this policy routinely so that delinquent accounts do not become a drain on the practice.

Fair Debt Collection Practices Act

Collection procedures are regulated by the Fair Debt Collection Practices Act of 1996. This act was passed to protect the public from unethical collection procedures. The activities outlined specifically in the law are listed in Box 15-1.

BOX 15-1 Provisions of the Fair Debt Collection Practices Act

- Debtors may not be subjected to harassment, oppressive tactics, or abusive treatment. The law prohibits the collector from making any false statements to a debtor, such as claiming to be an attorney or a government agency.
- Debtors may not be called at work if the employer or debtor objects and requests no calls.
- Debtors may not be called at inconvenient places or times, such as before 9 AM or after 9 PM.
- No one except the debtors themselves may be told they are behind on their bills.

Because these regulations generally apply to collection agencies, it is important that an agency verify its stringent adherence to them. These same regulations should be considered by the administrative assistant when performing collection procedures in the office.

Collection Letters

Letters may be sent at the discretion of the dentist. In offices that use a computer, a reminder notice can be included on the statement, and the first collection letter (Figure 15-13) is automatically generated when an account becomes past due. The administrative assistant may use a series of computer-generated reminder notices automatically sent at specified intervals (e.g., 30, 60, and 90 days past due) before assigning an account to a collector. Be responsible, however, in reviewing the list of delinquent accounts. One of these accounts might be a patient of long standing who, because of extenuating circumstances, was unable to pay the account. It is not wise to risk the loss of a well-established patient relationship by adding a message or sending an account to a collector without first checking to see if a reason exists for the oversight.

Generally the collection process should have four stages: reminder, inquiry/discussion, urgency, and ultimatum. The previous discussion concerned the first stage, reminder, which is accomplished through a notice on the statement. In the second stage (inquiry), the patient is personally contacted to determine the problem. The final two stages can be completed with letters. The letter of urgency must be more persuasive and urgent (Figure 15-14). An urgent phone call may be used as a follow-up as long as it does not result in harassment. In either situation be courteous, considerate, and helpful, yet firm.

The final stage, the ultimatum, arrives when a patient has failed to respond to all messages sent thus far. Confront the patient with the ultimatum. Refrain from referring directly to lawsuits, attorneys, or collection agencies unless the intention is to follow through. Send only one ultimatum letter with a deadline date (Figure 15-15). Send this letter by certified mail with a return receipt requested to prove that the debtor has received the letter. If payment is not received by the designated date, the account must be turned over immediately to an attorney or a collection agency.

Dental Associates, PC
Joseph W. Lake, DDS – Ashley M. Lake, DDS

November 5, 20—

Mr. Marvin Beattie
1407 Colorado Street N.W.
Grand Rapids, MI 49505

Dear Mr. Beattie:

Your account of $565.00 is over 90 days past due. If you are unable to pay this account in full, perhaps we can help you in making arrangements to take care of this account.

Please contact us before November 15, 20—at 5:00 p.m.

Sincerely,

Jennifer Ellis, RDA
Administrative Assistant

611 Main Street, SE – Grand Rapids, MI 49502 Phone: *616.101.9575* Fax: *616.101.9999*
E-mail: office@dapc.com or Visit us at: www.Lakedental.com

Figure 15-13 Sample first collection letter.

The following rules can guide the composition of collection letters:

1. Keep the letter brief.
2. Make sure that data about the account are complete and accurate.
3. Use simple words and uncomplicated sentences.
4. Use phrases that will motivate the patient, such as "cooperation" or "maintenance of a good credit rating."
5. Don't make statements there is no intention to carry out. If the patient is told that the account will be sent to a collection agency in 10 days, give a specific date and then follow through if necessary.
6. Set a specific date by which payment is expected, rather than saying "by the end of the month," or "in 10 days."
7. Be firm and polite.
8. Include a "thank you" in the letter closing because this, too, can be an important part of the collection procedure, and it is a valuable aid to public relations.

Telephone as a Collection Instrument

Many assistants find it difficult to use the telephone in collecting delinquent accounts. Experience should instill confidence in the assistant, but if not, another method of collection should be pursued. The telephone allows a more personal contact with a patient. When a patient who normally pays the account on time becomes delinquent, a phone call seems less formal than a letter and helps maintain a friendly relationship.

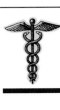

Dental Associates, PC

Joseph W. Lake, DDS - Ashley M. Lake, DDS

November 26, 20—

REGISTERED

Mr. Marvin Beattie
1407 Colorado Street N.W.
Grand Rapids, MI 49505

Dear Mr. Beattie:

Since we have not heard from you regarding your account of $565.00 from June 1, 20—, please be informed that it will be necessary to transfer this account to a collection agency.

This account must be paid in full by Friday, December 1, 20—to avoid such legal action.

Sincerely,

Jennifer Ellis, RDA
Administrative Assistant

611 Main Street, SE – Grand Rapids, MI 49502 Phone: 616.101.9575 Fax: 616.101.9999
E-mail: office@dapc.com or Visit us at: www.Lakedental.com

Figure 15-14 Sample urgent collection letter.

Specific rules should be followed when using the telephone for collections:

1. Do not call before 9 AM or after 9 PM.
2. Verify that you are speaking to the person whose account is overdue. Ask, "Is this Mr. Johnson?"
3. Identify yourself: "This is Miss Ellis, from Dr. Lake's office."
4. Ask whether it is a convenient time to talk. If not, ask when you may call back or find out when the patient will be able to call you. Do not give details to a third party or leave detailed messages on an answering machine or voicemail.
5. State the purpose of your call. Be friendly and display a helping attitude.
6. Be positive. Don't say, "I'm sorry to call you." Act as though you know the patient intends to pay and you are simply determining the arrangements for such a payment.
7. Have all of the information about the account in front of you.
8. Attempt to obtain a definite commitment; that is, the date and the amount of the payment. Follow up with written confirmation of the telephone discussion.
9. Make calls in a private area out of the hearing range of anyone in the reception room.
10. Don't threaten the patient.
11. Follow up on the promises the patient makes.
12. Don't ever discuss the account with anyone else. If you call the patient at work and the person cannot talk with you, leave a message to "Call Miss Ellis at 101-9575." Don't leave the dentist's name; the patient may not return the call.
13. Don't leave a message on the answering machine that includes the reason for the call; simply leave a message to "Call Miss Ellis at 101-9575."

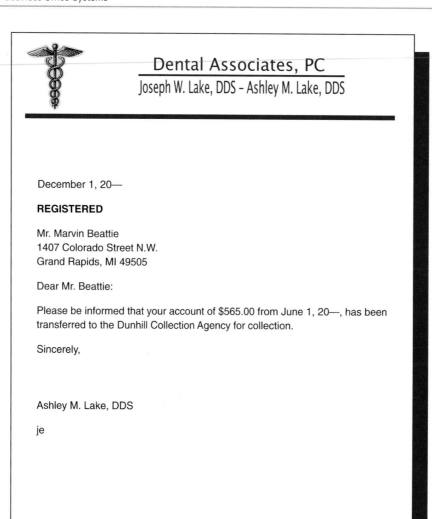

Figure 15-15 Sample final collection letter.

Collection Agency

After every attempt has been made to collect an account, it may be necessary to engage the services of a collection agency. These services are required when the patient fails to respond to a final collection letter or can no longer be located and becomes a "skip."

Delay in sending the account to a collection agency results in less chance of recovering a portion of the fee. Although the agency's fee reduces the portion recovered, continued unsuccessful attempts by the office are even less rewarding.

A collection agency should be selected that maintains high standards of professionalism. Investigate the agency thoroughly to determine its ethics and reliability.

1. Check the ownership of the agency through a banker, the local Chamber of Commerce, or the Better Business Bureau.

2. Contact the local dental society, National Retail Credit Association, or the Associated Credit Bureaus of America for information about the agency.
3. Find out whether the agency has contacts out of town to aid in collection of accounts.
4. Make sure the agency will not start legal action without the dentist's consent.
5. Make sure the agency understands a patient's needs and that a report is wanted on its activities.

Once the dentist has sought the services of an agency, the office should use these services routinely. To allow action to be taken promptly, complete data about each case should be given to the agency, including the following:

• Debtor's full name
• Last known address and phone number
• Total amount of account

- Date of last entry on account (credit or debit)
- Debtor's occupation
- Business address and phone number
- Any other pertinent information

When an account is turned over to a collection agency, the administrative assistant no longer pursues collection procedures on it. However, the dental office staff must cooperate with the agency. The staff should:

- Send no more statements.
- Indicate the transfer to the collection agency on the patient's financial record, giving the date of transfer
- Refer the patient to the agency if the person contacts the office.
- Report the amount to the agency when payment is received in the office.
- Rely on the agency staff members to do the job (i.e., don't pester them with calls of inquiry about the account).

From the time the patient enters the office until final collection of the fee, the administrative assistant has many important duties in managing the accounts receivable. The importance of accuracy in each aspect cannot be overemphasized. If the administrative assistant can carry out this responsibility, his or her value to the office becomes immeasurable.

KEY TERMS

Accounting—The recording, classifying, and summarizing of financial and business records; this generally is the task of the accountant.

Accounts payable—All the dentist's financial obligations, or money that the dentist owes (outgoing money).

Accounts receivable—A category that includes all production; data are entered for treatment rendered and payments received, and new balances are calculated.

Adjustment—Alteration of an account balance as a result of a courtesy discount, the return of a nonsufficient funds (NSF) check, or a payment.

Balance—The credit or debit amount on an account.

Bookkeeping—The process of recording of financial transactions.

Credit balance—An amount owed to the patient for services for which the dentist has been paid in advance but that have not yet been performed.

Credit bureau—An organization that reports specific information about a person's previous payment habits on deferred payment plans.

Creditor—An institution or business that sends a bill to a person, agrees to an installment payment plan, accepts insurance payments, or arranges for a loan for payment.

Nonsufficient funds (NSF) check—A check returned unpaid to the payee because insufficient funds were available in the payer's account.

Receipt—A form given to the payer (patient) that acknowledges payment on an account.

Statement—A document that informs patients of their financial status with the dentist; it indicates the charges, payments, and balances on an account for the month just concluded.

LEARNING ACTIVITIES

1. Explain the differences between accounting and bookkeeping.
2. List common types of bookkeeping systems used in dentistry.
3. List and explain the function of the components of a pegboard system.
4. List and explain the function of the components of a computer bookkeeping system.

Please refer to the student workbook for additional learning activities.

REFERENCES

American Dental Association: *Guide for compliance with the new "Red Flags" Rule*, Chicago, 2009, ADA.

McDonough D: *Dental Administrator Alert: "New Red Flags" requirements for financial in situations and creditors to help fight identity theft*, ADAA Business Beat Spring.

RECOMMENDED WEB SITES

www.ada.org
www.dentalassistant.org

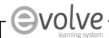

v http://evolve.elsevier.com/Finkibeiner/practice for additional practice activities.

16

Other Financial Systems

LEARNING OUTCOMES

- Define key terms
- Explain the function of a budget.
- Explain the use of electronic banking.
- Describe the steps in accessing an online bank account.
- Identify the parts of a check.
- Explain the use of financial management software.
- Prepare a check and determine the correct balance on a checkbook register.
- Identify various types of checks.
- Prepare checks for deposit with correct endorsements and complete a deposit slip.
- Reconcile a bank statement.
- Explain the purpose of a monthly expense sheet.
- Explain the purpose of a yearly summary.
- Identify the purpose of payroll records.
- Explain the purpose of the employee's earnings record.
- Calculate gross and net wages.
- Explain how withheld income tax and Social Security taxes are deposited.
- Explain how federal unemployment taxes are deposited.
- Describe how to complete a Form W-2.
- Explain the importance of retaining payroll records.
- Explain the use of an automated payroll system.
- Use the Internet as a resource for financial forms and instructions.

All dental practices, regardless of size, have financial matters that need to be addressed by either internal or external accounting staff. The administrative assistant can expect to perform many tasks in addition to the accounts receivable activities highlighted in the previous chapter. These tasks might include receiving and organizing statements, paying for materials and supplies, processing payroll or tax forms, recording and analyzing expenses, and other responsibilities. In a group practice or a larger organization, the administrative assistant may collect the data for these activities and support accounting personnel in the preparation of financial documents or be responsible for entering data in a software package such as QuickBooks® (Figure 16-1). Although some offices may still perform these tasks manually, the use of computer software will provide the practice with the benefits shown in Box 16-1. The administrative assistant must have a basic understanding of the software system involved.

In the processing of financial documents, accuracy is essential. Verification of data and attention to detail are necessary to ensure that the processed information is accurate. Incorrect data can mean improper cash flow analysis, inaccurate accounts receivable, erroneous claim form preparation, or inaccurate budget and expense figures. All of these can have very serious repercussions for the entire business.

> **PRACTICE NOTE**
>
> In the processing of financial documents, accuracy is essential. Verification of data and attention to detail are necessary to ensure that the processed information is accurate.

As the administrative assistant becomes more skilled in the business office, his or her responsibilities probably will include completing many monthly and annual forms vital to the dental practice. This chapter presents the major types of

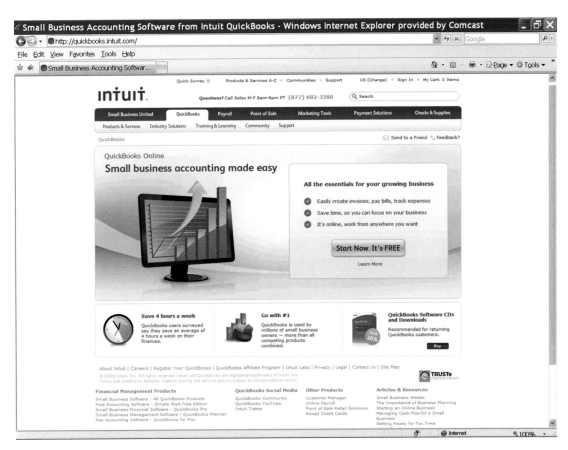

Figure 16-1 QuickBooks® software web page. (Screenshot © Intuit, Inc. All rights reserved.)

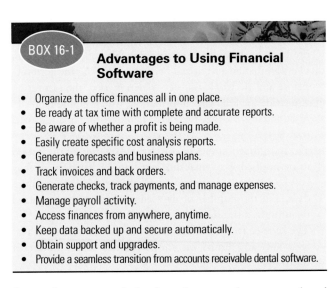

BOX 16-1 Advantages to Using Financial Software

- Organize the office finances all in one place.
- Be ready at tax time with complete and accurate reports.
- Be aware of whether a profit is being made.
- Easily create specific cost analysis reports.
- Generate forecasts and business plans.
- Track invoices and back orders.
- Generate checks, track payments, and manage expenses.
- Manage payroll activity.
- Access finances from anywhere, anytime.
- Keep data backed up and secure automatically.
- Obtain support and upgrades.
- Provide a seamless transition from accounts receivable dental software.

financial systems and the data that must be processed and managed in a modern dental practice. The chapter shows how technology is applied to the financial operations of a practice to make it more productive. In addition, it talks about the resources available through the Internet that can act as guides in procuring and filling out many of the financial forms needed by the practice.

DETERMINING A BUDGET

A budget is a dental practice's financial plan of operation for a given period, usually 1 year. The purpose of the budget is to establish the practice's financial goals. To achieve an acceptable level of profit, expenditures, the amount of money spent to operate the practice, must be kept in balance with revenue, the amount of income received by the practice. Dentists can use spreadsheet software to develop a budget so that they can plan more thoroughly and in less time than with paper and pencil methods. Spreadsheets allow planners to see how a change in one calculation affects all the related calculations. A template of a business budget created in QuickBooks® software for a dental practice is shown in Figure 16-2.

BANK ACCOUNTS

One of the daily routine functions of the dental office administrative assistant is control of the *cash flow*, or the amounts of money received and the amounts disbursed. Therefore a good understanding of banking technology and procedures is necessary. Some of the administrative assistant's banking responsibilities are check writing, accepting checks from patients for payment of services, endorsing and depositing checks, keeping an accurate bank balance, and reconciling the bank statement.

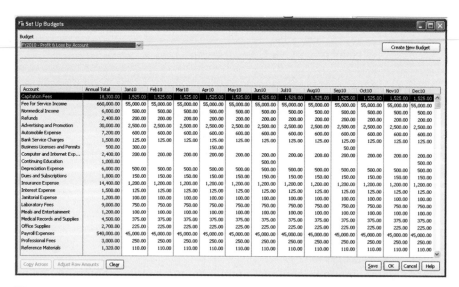

Figure 16-2 Business budget modified for a dental practice using QuickBooks®. (Screenshot © Intuit, Inc. All rights reserved.)

 PRACTICE NOTE

One of the daily routine functions of the dental office administrative assistant is control of the *cash flow*, or the amounts of money received and the amounts disbursed.

ONLINE BANKING

For many dental offices, electronic or online banking means 24-hour access to cash through an automated teller machine or direct deposit of paychecks and accounts receivable into a checking or savings account. Electronic banking now involves many different types of transactions. For instance, the federal government is even moving toward direct deposit or transfer of funds for employment taxes.

Online banking uses a computer and electronic technology as a substitute for checks and other paper transactions. Electronic fund transfers (EFTs) are initiated through devices such as cards or codes that let the dentist or those authorized by the dentist access an account. Many financial institutions use **automatic teller machines (ATMs)** or debit cards and personal identification numbers (PINs) for this purpose. Other institutions use devices such as debit cards or a signature or scan to access to an account. The federal Electronic Fund Transfer Act (EFT Act) covers some electronic consumer transactions.

ATMs, or 24-hour tellers, are electronic terminals that allow banking at almost any time. To withdraw money, make deposits, or transfer funds between accounts, an ATM card is inserted and a PIN number is entered. Generally ATMs must indicate if a fee is charged and give the amount on or at the terminal screen before the transaction is completed.

Direct deposit enables a person to make a deposit to the account on a regular basis. In this system the dentist may preauthorize recurring bills to be paid automatically, such as insurance premiums, mortgages, and utility bills.

Online banking allows the account to be accessed from a remote location, such as the office or personal computer. The account holder can view the account balance, request transfers between accounts, and pay bills electronically.

The use of electronic transfers should be monitored carefully. The dentist and any other person responsible for electronic banking must read the documents that are received from the financial institution that issued the access device. No one should know the PIN except the responsible person or persons. The steps common to accessing the account are illustrated in Figure 16-3. Each bank will set up some form of security system that verifies that an authorized person is accessing the account.

Before any electronic transfer system is used, the institution must provide the following information, which should be filed:
- A summary of the practice's liability for unauthorized transfers
- The telephone number or contact information of the person to be notified if an unauthorized transfer has been or may have been made, a statement of the institution's business days, and the number of days allowed to report suspected unauthorized transfers
- The type of transfers that can be made, the fees for transfers, and any limits on the frequency and amount of transfers
- A summary of the right to receive documentation of transfers and to stop payment on a preauthorized transfer, as well as the procedures for stopping payment
- A summary of the institution's liability
- Privacy assurance

If problems arise in the use of online banking, a complaint can be filed through the web site for the state member banks of the Federal Reserve System at www.federalreserve.gov.

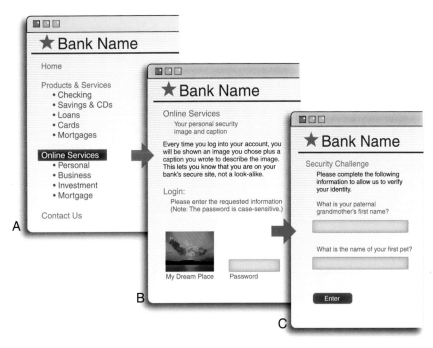

Figure 16-3 Basic security steps built into online banking account access. **A,** Home page with menu. **B,** Login screen. **C,** Security check.

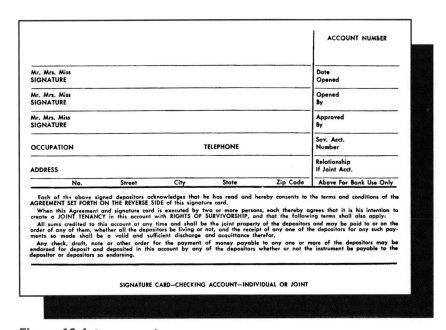

Figure 16-4 Signature card.

ESTABLISHING A CHECKING ACCOUNT

As a rule, the checking account for the dental practice will have been opened before the administrative assistant begins working for the practice. However, in opening the account, the dentist had to decide what type of an account would be used. The dentist also signed a signature card (Figure 16-4)

that permitted him or her to write checks against the account. If another person is permitted to write checks against the account, that person's signature must also appear on a signature card for the account or on the same signature card that the dentist signed. However, if the administrative assistant is allowed to sign the checks, the bank may require that the assistant be given power of attorney (Figure 16-5).

Form 2848 (Rev. 6-2008)   Page **2**

7 Notices and communications. Original notices and other written communications will be sent to you and a copy to the first representative listed on line 2.

a If you also want the second representative listed to receive a copy of notices and communications, check this box . . . ▶ ☐

b If you do not want any notices or communications sent to your representative(s), check this box . . . . ▶ ☐

8 Retention/revocation of prior power(s) of attorney. The filing of this power of attorney automatically revokes all earlier power(s) of attorney on file with the Internal Revenue Service for the same tax matters and years or periods covered by this document. If you **do not** want to revoke a prior power of attorney, check here . . . . ▶ ☐
YOU MUST ATTACH A COPY OF ANY POWER OF ATTORNEY YOU WANT TO REMAIN IN EFFECT.

9 Signature of taxpayer(s). If a tax matter concerns a joint return, **both** husband and wife must sign if joint representation is requested, otherwise, see the instructions. If signed by a corporate officer, partner, guardian, tax matters partner, executor, receiver, administrator, or trustee on behalf of the taxpayer, I certify that I have the authority to execute this form on behalf of the taxpayer.
▶ **IF NOT SIGNED AND DATED, THIS POWER OF ATTORNEY WILL BE RETURNED.**

_____	_____	_____
Signature	Date	Title (if applicable)
_____		_____
Print Name	PIN Number	Print name of taxpayer from line 1 if other than individual
_____	_____	_____
Signature	Date	Title (if applicable)
_____		
Print Name	PIN Number	

Part II   Declaration of Representative

Caution: *Students with a special order to represent taxpayers in qualified Low Income Taxpayer Clinics or the Student Tax Clinic Program (levels k and l), see the instructions for Part II.*

Under penalties of perjury, I declare that:
• I am not currently under suspension or disbarment from practice before the Internal Revenue Service;
• I am aware of regulations contained in Circular 230 (31 CFR, Part 10), as amended, concerning the practice of attorneys, certified public accountants, enrolled agents, enrolled actuaries, and others;
• I am authorized to represent the taxpayer(s) identified in Part I for the tax matter(s) specified there; and
• I am one of the following:

a   Attorney—a member in good standing of the bar of the highest court of the jurisdiction shown below.
b   Certified Public Accountant—duly qualified to practice as a certified public accountant in the jurisdiction shown below.
c   Enrolled Agent—enrolled as an agent under the requirements of Circular 230.
d   Officer—a bona fide officer of the taxpayer's organization.
e   Full-Time Employee—a full-time employee of the taxpayer.
f   Family Member—a member of the taxpayer's immediate family (for example, spouse, parent, child, brother, or sister).
g   Enrolled Actuary—enrolled as an actuary by the Joint Board for the Enrollment of Actuaries under 29 U.S.C. 1242 (the authority to practice before the Internal Revenue Service is limited by section 10.3(d) of Circular 230).
h   Unenrolled Return Preparer—the authority to practice before the Internal Revenue Service is limited by Circular 230, section 10.7(c)(1)(viii). You must have prepared the return in question and the return must be under examination by the IRS. See **Unenrolled Return Preparer** on page 1 of the instructions.
k   Student Attorney—student who receives permission to practice before the IRS by virtue of his/her status as a law student under section 10.7(d) of Circular 230.
l   Student CPA—student who receives permission to practice before the IRS by virtue of his/her status as a CPA student under section 10.7(d) of Circular 230.
r   Enrolled Retirement Plan Agent—enrolled as a retirement plan agent under the requirements of Circular 230 (the authority to practice before the Internal Revenue Service is limited by section 10.3(e)).

▶ **IF THIS DECLARATION OF REPRESENTATIVE IS NOT SIGNED AND DATED, THE POWER OF ATTORNEY WILL BE RETURNED.** See the Part II instructions.

Designation—Insert above letter (a–r)	Jurisdiction (state) or identification	Signature	Date

Form **2848** (Rev. 6-2008)

Form **2848**
(Rev. June 2008)
Department of the Treasury
Internal Revenue Service

**Power of Attorney
and Declaration of Representative**
▶ **Type or print.** ▶ **See the separate instructions.**

OMB No. 1545-0150

For IRS Use Only	
Received by:	
Name	
Telephone	
Function	
Date	/ /

Part I   Power of Attorney

Caution: *Form 2848 will not be honored for any purpose other than representation before the IRS.*

1   Taxpayer information. Taxpayer(s) must sign and date this form on page 2, line 9.

Taxpayer name(s) and address	Social security number(s)	Employer identification number
	_ _ _ _	
	Daytime telephone number	Plan number (if applicable)
	( )	

hereby appoint(s) the following representative(s) as attorney(s)-in-fact:

2   Representative(s) must sign and date this form on page 2, Part II.

Name and address	
	CAF No. _ _ _ _ _ _ _ _ _ _ _
	Telephone No. _ _ _ _ _ _ _ _ _
	Fax No. _ _ _ _ _ _ _ _ _
	Check if new: Address ☐ Telephone No. ☐ Fax No. ☐
Name and address	
	CAF No. _ _ _ _ _ _ _ _ _ _ _
	Telephone No. _ _ _ _ _ _ _ _ _
	Fax No. _ _ _ _ _ _ _ _ _
	Check if new: Address ☐ Telephone No. ☐ Fax No. ☐
Name and address	
	CAF No. _ _ _ _ _ _ _ _ _ _ _
	Telephone No. _ _ _ _ _ _ _ _ _
	Fax No. _ _ _ _ _ _ _ _ _
	Check if new: Address ☐ Telephone No. ☐ Fax No. ☐

to represent the taxpayer(s) before the Internal Revenue Service for the following tax matters:

3   Tax matters

Type of Tax (Income, Employment, Excise, etc.) or Civil Penalty (see the instructions for line 3)	Tax Form Number (1040, 941, 720, etc.)	Year(s) or Period(s) (see the instructions for line 3)

4   Specific use not recorded on Centralized Authorization File (CAF). If the power of attorney is for a specific use not recorded on CAF, check this box. See the instructions for **Line 4. Specific Uses Not Recorded on CAF** . . . . ▶ ☐

5   Acts authorized. The representatives are authorized to receive and inspect confidential tax information and to perform any and all acts that I (we) can perform with respect to the tax matters described on line 3, for example, the authority to sign any agreements, consents, or other documents. The authority does not include the power to receive refund checks (see line 6 below), the power to substitute another representative or add additional representatives, the power to sign certain returns, or the power to execute a request for disclosure of tax returns or return information to a third party. See the line 5 instructions for more information.

Exceptions. An unenrolled return preparer cannot sign any document for a taxpayer and may only represent taxpayers in limited situations. See **Unenrolled Return Preparer** on page 1 of the instructions. An enrolled actuary may only represent taxpayers to the extent provided in section 10.3(d) of Treasury Department Circular No. 230 (Circular 230). An enrolled retirement plan administrator may only represent taxpayers to the extent provided in section 10.3(e) of Circular 230. See the line 5 instructions for restrictions on tax matters partners. In most cases, the student practitioner's (levels k and l) authority is limited (for example, they may only practice under the supervision of another practitioner).

List any specific additions or deletions to the acts otherwise authorized in this power of attorney: _ _ _ _ _ _ _ _ _ _ _ _ _ _ _ _ _ _

6   Receipt of refund checks. If you want to authorize a representative named on line 2 to receive, **BUT NOT TO ENDORSE OR CASH**, refund checks, initial here _____ and list the name of that representative below.

Name of representative to receive refund check(s) ▶ _

For Privacy Act and Paperwork Reduction Act Notice, see page 4 of the instructions.   Cat. No. 11980J   Form **2848** (Rev. 6-2008)

Figure 16-5 Power of attorney (Form 2848). (From Internal Revenue Service, Department of the Treasury, Washington, DC.)

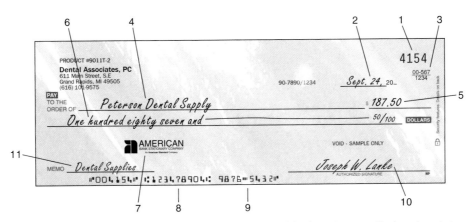

Figure 16-6 Parts of a check. *1*, Check number. *2*, Date of check. *3*, American Bankers Association (ABA) bank identification number. *4*, Payee, the person or company to be paid. *5*, Amount of check (in figures). *6*, Amount of check (in words). *7*, Drawee, the bank on which the check is drawn. *8*, Bank identification number magnetically printed for electronic processing. *9*, Customer account number magnetically printed for electronic processing. *10*, Signature of drawer. *11*, Reason the check was written.

Checks

Checks are a means of ordering the bank to pay cash from the bank customer's account. In the past, checks accounted for a majority of all financial transactions in the United States. However, the use of online banking and debit cards has risen dramatically. Patients increasingly will use debit and credit cards, rather than cash or checks, to pay their bills. However, checks still constitute a significant portion of the receipts for the dental practice.

> 📄 **PRACTICE NOTE**
> More than 90% of all financial transactions in this country are done by check.

Many parts of a check are self-explanatory; however, some parts need additional explanation. In Figure 16-6, part 3 is the **American Bankers Association (ABA)** bank identification number. Under this coding system, every bank is given its own number, which constitutes a numerical name for the bank. This number aids the sorting of checks for distribution to their proper destination. The ABA number is a fraction and usually is printed in the upper right corner of the check or slightly to the left of the check number. Part 4 of the check is the *payee*, the individual or company that will receive the money. Part 7, the *drawee*, is the bank that pays the check. Parts 8 and 9 are magnetic ink character recognition (MICR) numbers. These are encoded on all checks to facilitate high-speed handling by machine. The first number is the bank identification number (also found in the ABA identification number). The second number is the check writer's checking account number. These numbers can easily be read by people or by machine. Part 10 of the check is the signature of the *drawer* or check writer, the person who orders the bank to pay cash from the account.

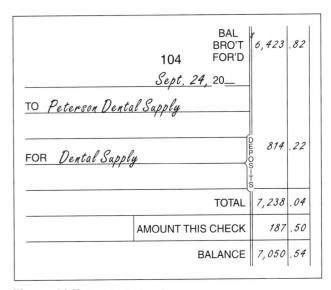

Figure 16-7 Sample check stub.

Preparing Checks

In the past the administrative assistant manually prepared checks. Today with the use of financial management software, the assistant can set aside some time during the working day, as the schedule permits, to prepare the checks using the selected software. If a manual system is used, the following steps are taken in writing the check. The check stub or checkbook register should be completed before the check is written or printed. The stub or register provides a record of the (1) check number, (2) date, (3) payee, (4) amount of the check, (5) purpose of the check, and (6) new balance brought forward after the amount of the check has been subtracted; or it provides the new balance if a deposit is to be added to the previous balance, as shown in the manual system (Figure 16-7).

Figure 16-8 presents a step-by-step procedure for manually writing a check. A check produced by a software system such as

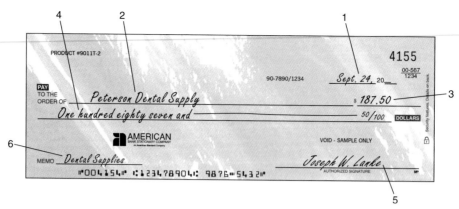

Figure 16-8 How to write a check. *1*, Date the check. *2*, Key or write the name of the person or firm to whom the check will be payable. *3*, Enter the amount of the check (in figures) opposite the dollar sign. *4*, Write the amount of the check (in words) under the "Pay to the order of" line. Start as far to the left margin as possible. *5*, The name on the signature line should be signed as it appears on the bank signature card. *6*, On the memo line, record the purpose of the payment.

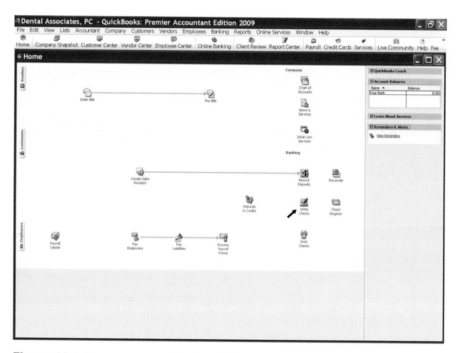

Figure 16-9 The main screen of QuickBooks® contains icons representing various accounting options, including one for check writing. (Screenshot © Intuit, Inc. All rights reserved.)

QuickBooks® requires that the user select the icon for check writing from the main screen (Figure 16-9) and then follow through with the data entry as requested on each screen. A check written to a dental supplier includes information important about the check and the account (Figure 16-10).

Types of Checks

The following list describes a few of the types of checks the administrative assistant may receive:

- *Certified check:* A **certified check** is a guarantee that funds have been set aside to cover the amount of the check. The person goes to the bank and writes a personal check for the

proper amount; the bank sets aside that amount from the customer's account, placing it in a special account, and then stamps *Certified* across the face of the check. Usually a nominal fee is charged for certifying a check.

- *Cashier's check:* A **cashier's check** is the bank's own order to make payment out of the bank's funds. When a cashier's check is purchased, the person specifies to whom the bank makes the check payable and receives a carbon or stub of the check as a record. A fee is usually charged for this type of check.

- *Money order:* A **money order** is a means of transferring money without using cash or a personal check. People who do not maintain a personal checking account often use money orders

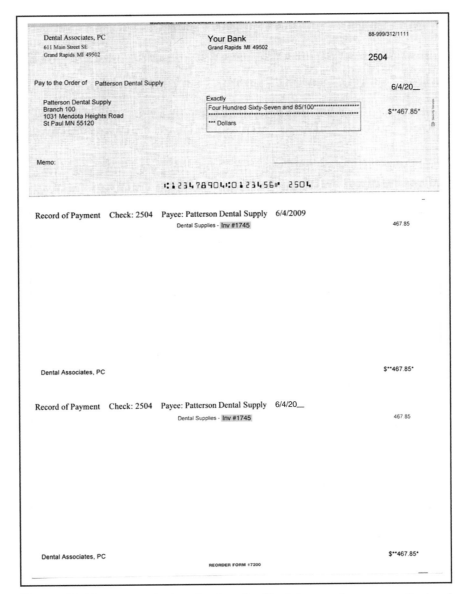

Figure 16-10 A sample check produced on QuickBooks® system for a payment for dental supplies. (Software © Intuit, Inc. All rights reserved.)

to pay their creditors. The money order may be purchased in the form of a bank money order, a postal money order, or an express money order. The money order shows the name of the purchaser and the person who is to receive the payment (the payee). A fee is charged for this service.

- *Traveler's check:* Even though the traveler's check is designed as a payment device for a person who is away from home, it is not uncommon to receive a traveler's check in payment for dental services. Traveler's checks are purchased through a bank, American Express Company, or Railway Express Agency. The checks are preprinted in various denominations, usually $10, $20, $50, and $100. A small fee, determined by the amount purchased, is charged. When the checks are purchased, the individual signs his or her name in a designated place on each check. When the checks are used for payment or are cashed, they are *countersigned*; that is, the

purchaser signs them again in the presence of the individual who cashes the check or accepts it for payment.
- *Bank draft:* A bank draft is a check drawn by the cashier of one bank on another bank where the first bank has available funds on deposit or credit. A bank draft is used if a person or company wants to send a sum of money and a personal check is not acceptable.
- *Voucher check:* A voucher check provides a detachable stub, which serves as an excellent accounting record for itemizing payment of invoices or any other type of itemization the payer would like as a reference.

Accepting and Cashing Checks

Many different types of checks may be used as payment for services. When a check is accepted, make sure that it is: (1) legibly written in ink or typewritten, (2) currently dated, (3) signed by the check writer, (4) drawn on a US bank, (5) made payable in a certain sum of money (the amount in figures and the amount in words should agree), and (6) made payable to a payee or bearer.

At times the administrative assistant may be asked to accept a check for more than the charges. This may present a problem. For example, if the individual owes $100 and wants to pay $50 but writes a check for $100 and asks for $50 to be returned, a question may arise at a later date if the patient tries to use the canceled check as a receipt for full payment of the account. Another problem that may be encountered is the acceptance of payment for more than the balance and the return of the difference in cash to the patient. If the bank returns the patient's check for insufficient funds, cash has been paid out from the business, and the patient has the cash. To avoid problems of this nature, it is better to establish a firm policy of not accepting checks for more than the amount owed. This policy should be established by the dentist and enforced at all times.

Other Forms of Payment

As mentioned, credit or debit cards (e.g., MasterCard, VISA, Discover, and American Express) increasingly are being used to pay professional fees. The dentist makes arrangements through a bank, usually the one in which the business account has been established, to use this banking service. The bank charges a fee for this service, generally 1 to 5 percent of the transactions handled. A merchant's service company provides the terminal with a scanner and pin pad.

 PRACTICE NOTE
Credit cards such as MasterCard and VISA increasingly are being used to pay professional fees.

The debit card (also known as a *bank card* or *check card*) is a plastic card which provides an alternative payment method to cash when making payments. In reality it is an electronic check, as the funds are withdrawn directly from either the bank account (often referred to as a *check card*), or from the remaining balance on a prepaid debit card.

When a patient presents a debit card, it is entered as payment and a request is made to have a PIN entered by the patient. The administrative assistant has the patient enter the PIN on the pin pad (Figure 16-11), and the transaction is then completed. A debit card for the office may be used by the dentist or authorized person to make purchases for the office. The debit card also allows for instant withdrawal of cash, acting as the ATM card for withdrawing cash and as a check guarantee card. Although not common to the dental office, merchant users can also offer "cashback" or "cashout" facilities to customers, where customers can withdraw cash along with their payment or purchase.

At the end of the day when the administrative assistant prints out a Collection Reconciliation Sheet of the day's financial activities from the dental software program, the sheet will indicate which payments were made in cash, debit, or credit card (Figure 16-12).

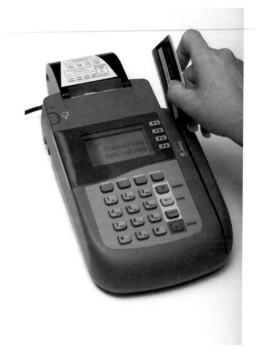

Figure 16-11 A credit or debit machine contains a card reader to allow the office to swipe the card and a PIN pad for the patient to enter the PIN number for payment. (Copyright 2008, Andre Blais, Andre Blais Photography. Image from www.BigStockPhoto.com.)

A few precautions are necessary when patients use credit or debit cards for payment. Be sure to check the card's expiration date and the signature on the back to ensure it matches the signature of the patient. Sometimes a card may be rejected for payment; the administrative assistant then must ask for an alternate form of payment. Do not discuss the card rejection, as this is the patient's private business.

Because some patients pay their accounts with cash, some cash must be kept in the office. However, large amounts of cash should not be routinely kept in the office, because it may end up being counted as part of the total cash receipts for the day. A separate cash balance can be maintained for petty cash (discussed later in the chapter).

DEPOSITS

The checks that need to be deposited should have been endorsed as soon as they were received to ensure safe keeping in the office. A stamp can be obtained from most office supply stores with the vital information about the office and the account. Figure 16-13 illustrates and describes the various types of **endorsements**. Depositing money into the practice's checking account is usually a daily routine but may vary according to the office schedule. A **bank deposit** represents the accumulation of money received for a single day or possibly a longer period. The bank provides checking account deposit slips for a nominal fee, which have the dental practice's name and account number imprinted on them. Follow the step-by-step procedure presented in Figure 16-14 when completing the deposit form.

TIME 4:24 PM   George Young, D.D.S.   DATE 7/28/2009

PAYMENT RECONCILIATION
Today
All Providers

Patient Name	Date	User	Payment	Amount
Check Payments				
3446 - Abbott, Charles K	7/28/2009	BAB	Acct Pymt Check Number: 123456	$4,756.00
1120 - Allen, Cathy	7/28/2009	BAB	Acct Pymt Check Number: 4562	$80.00
2815 - Campbell, Chris	7/28/2009	BAB	Acct Pymt Check Number: 1232123	$30.25
2815 - Campbell, Chris	7/28/2009	BAB	Acct Pymt Check Number: 1232123	$33.00
			Total Check	$4,899.25
Visa Payments				
868 - Lange, Jack	7/28/2009	BAB	Acct Pymt Visa Number: Credit card payment	$78.00
			Total Visa	$78.00
Discover Payments				
463 - Farkas, Paul	7/28/2009	BAB	Acct Pymt Discover Number: Credit card payment	$397.50
			Total Discover	$397.50
Insurance Ck Payments				
8 - Abbott, Angie A	7/28/2009	BAB		$16.28
3446 - Abbott, Charles K	7/28/2009	BAB		$807.60
3432 - Abbott, Mark	7/28/2009	BAB		$20.00
2517 - Macphee, Christy	7/28/2009	BAB		$48.50
2517 - Macphee, Christy	7/28/2009	BAB		$21.50
			Total Insurance Ck	$913.88
			TOTAL PAYMENTS:	**$6,288.63**

Figure 16-12 Payment Reconciliation Screen indicating debit and credit card use for the day. (Courtesy Patterson Dental, St. Paul, MN.)

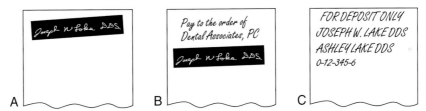

Figure 16-13 Check endorsements. **A,** *Blank endorsement,* which is an endorsement that consists of the signature of the payee. A blank endorsement makes the check payable to any holder. **B,** *Endorsement in full,* which is an endorsement that states to whom the check is to be paid and the signature of the payee. This endorsement specifies that the check can be cashed or transferred only on the order of the person, bank, or company named in the endorsement. **C,** *Restrictive endorsement,* which is an endorsement that includes special conditions or that limits the receiver of the check in the uses that can be made of it; this type of endorsement commonly is used when checks are prepared for deposit.

A duplicate copy of the deposit form may be retained for office use to verify with the check register and bank statement at the end of the month.

Another type of bank deposit slip that may be generated easily is produced from the accounts receivable software system (Figure 16-15).

Night Depository

Sometimes the practice receives large amounts of money after banking hours. The night depository is a means of depositing money in the bank vault when the bank is closed. Usually the deposit is completed the next business day by a bank teller; the depositor must go to the bank to pick up the deposit bag and receipt. However, if the depositor prefers, the deposit bag can remain locked until the person arrives at the bank to make the deposit personally.

Automatic Teller Machine

As mentioned, in conjunction with the checking account, financial institutions offer special access cards that can be used

DEPOSIT TICKET
PRODUCT 419

CHECKS AND OTHER ITEMS ARE RECEIVED FOR DEPOSIT SUBJECT TO
THE TERMS AND CONDITIONS OF THIS BANK'S COLLECTION DEPARTMENT.
PLEASE LIST EACH CHECK SEPARATELY.

PRODUCT #419-4

Dental Associates, PC
611 Main Street S.E
Grand Rapids, MI 49505
(616) 101-9575

YOUR BANK NAME HERE
321 MAIN STREET
CITY, STATE AND ZIP

Date _____

	DOLLARS	CENTS
CURRENCY		
COIN		
1 *11-82*	225	00
2 *12-416*	75	00
3 *2-412*	80	00
4 *16-308*	55	00
5 *10-012*	135	00
6 *MONEY ORDER*	40	00
7 *MASTER CHG.*	140	00
8 *AM.EXP.TRAV.CH.*	50	00
9		
10		
11		
12		
13		
14		
15		
16		
17		
18		
19		
20		
21		
22		
23		
24		
LESS CASH RETURNED		
TOTAL ITEMS *8* **TOTAL DEPOSIT**	800	00

Figure 16-14 Deposit slip. *1,* Write or type the date on the front side. *2,* List currency and coins to be deposited. *3,* Identify checks to be deposited individually; if there are more than three, use the back side of the deposit slip. Checks should be listed on the deposit slip by the ABA numbers. However, the administrative assistant may prefer to list checks with the patient's name and number. If it is a money order, traveler's check, or MasterCard or VISA charge receipt, the total amount of money and the name of the item are listed. *4,* Enter the total from the back on the front side of the deposit slip. *5,* Total the entire deposit (net deposit). *6,* Optional: some deposit slips provide a line in case the depositor wants part of the deposit back in cash. The amount desired is entered on this line and subtracted from the total line above; the net deposit then is entered as in *5.*

to perform banking transactions virtually 24 hours a day, 7 days a week. The cards can be used at ATMs, which are computer workstations that electronically prompt the user through most routine banking activities. Deposits or withdrawals can be made, or funds can be transferred between accounts. However, some precautions must be taken when using an ATM (Box 16-2).

RECONCILING THE BANK STATEMENT

Basic Steps

Although procedures may differ, most banks send a **bank statement** (Figure 16-16) to the depositor each month. The bank statement shows the balance of the account at the beginning of the month, deposits made during the month, checks drawn against the account, corrections or charges against the account (e.g., the service charge or stop payment charges), and the bank balance at the end of the month. To maintain an accurate record of the checking account, reconcile the bank statement as soon as the records are received from the bank. An online bank statement is available after the close of business on the last day of each month. This can be printed or reconciled online, thus aiding in creating a paperless office.

Use the following procedure to reconcile the bank statement.

1. Verify the amount of the canceled checks with the amounts on the bank statement. (The canceled checks are usually returned in the order listed on the statement.)
2. Arrange the canceled checks numerically.
3. Compare the amounts on the canceled checks and the deposits with the amounts written in the checkbook register. Check off all canceled checks and deposits in the checkbook register.
4. List the *outstanding checks* (checks not yet returned to the bank), including the check number and the amount.
5. Total the outstanding checks. If a deposit has been made but does not appear on the bank statement, the deposit must be added to the bank statement balance before the outstanding checks are subtracted.
6. Look for charges other than checks that have been deducted from the account; for example, service charges (SC), debit memos (DM), and overdrafts (OD). These charges must be subtracted from the checkbook register.

In Figure 16-17, a reconciliation of the bank statement has been prepared for the practice of Dental Associates, PC.

Petty Cash

Although the cash receipts are deposited in the bank and invoices and miscellaneous items are paid by check, a small amount of cash should be kept on hand in the office. This should be established as a **petty cash** fund and controlled with the same accuracy as the checking account.

October 24, 20___ at 3:05p   Page 1

DEPOSIT SLIP
PRACTICE
Dates Included: 10/24/___ to 10/24/___

Dental Associates, PC
611 Main Street S.E
Grand Rapids, MI 49505
(616) 101-9575

Account Number:

Code	Bank No.	Check No.	Amount	Reference (ID, Name)
3	87/44323	634	206.00	(7301) Gable, Catherine M
3	55/980	978	380.00	(12202) Page, Michael W
3	90/4532	709	326.00	(26901) Glass, Steven
3	77/345-0	4793	148.00	(48201) Nair, Ernest
3	445/0983	345	513.00	(50101) O'brien, Armando
3	12-9855	746	121.00	(234101) Jackewitz, Jerry

TOTAL

6 Checks Total	1694.00
Total Cash	211.00
Total Deposit	1905.00

Figure 16-15 Sample computer-generated deposit slip.

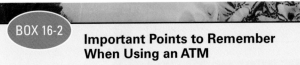

 PRACTICE NOTE

Although the cash receipts are deposited in the bank and invoices and miscellaneous items are paid by check, a small amount of cash should be kept on hand in the office.

When it has been determined how much cash will be placed in the petty cash account, a check is written against the business account and cashed, and the cash is returned to the office and kept in a separate fund. To help eliminate errors in disbursements from the fund, one person in the office should have control over the petty cash. A voucher is completed each time money is taken from the fund. The voucher shows the date, voucher number, amount of payment, what the payment was for, to whom the payment was made, and the name of the person approving the payment (Figure 16-18).

After the voucher is completed, it is placed in the drawer as a reminder of the amount of cash taken from the fund. The vouchers and cash together should equal the original balance of petty cash.

A formal record of petty cash disbursements may also be used. This record shows all the disbursements in chronological order, the voucher number, and special columns for each expense item disbursed from the fund. It also provides a complete summary of how the money was disbursed. At the end of the month, the fund must be replenished. This involves writing another check for cash purposes and charging the various expense accounts for the amount used from the petty cash.

Previous Statement Transactions on CHECKING ACCOUNT 0-12-345-6 - $35019.27 as of June 01, 20__

Date	Check Number	Description	Debit	Credit	Balance
5/4		MERCHANT SERVICE MERCH DEP 731668000667		870.50	40,698.57
5/5		MERCHANT SERVICE MERCH DEP 731668000667		684.00	41,382.57
5/6	1789	CHK	104.18		41,278.39
5/6	1794	CHK	600.00		40,678.39
5/6	1793	CHK	89.60		40,588.79
5/6	1792	CHK	175.19		40,413.60
5/6	1790	CHK	165.00		40,248.60
5/6	1791	CHK	15.00		40,233.60
5/6	1788	CHK	95.00		40,138.60
5/6	1787	CHK	706.13		39,432.47
5/6	1786	CHK	52.83		39,379.64
5/6	1785	CHK	49.51		39,330.13
5/6	1784	CHK	161.96		39,168.17
5/7		DEPOSIT		438.00	39,606.17
5/11	1795	CHK	36.10		39,570.07
5/11		MERCHANT SERVICE MERCH DEP 731668000667		787.75	40,357.82
5/12		MERCHANT SERVICE MERCH DEP 731668000667		543.50	40,901.32
5/14		MERCHANT SERVICE MERCH DEP 731668000667		658.00	41,559.32
5/14	1796	CHK	52.50		41,506.82
5/14		DEPOSIT		579.51	42,086.33
5/14	1797	CHK	10,336.00		31,750.33
5/14	1799	CHK	451.00		31,299.33
5/18		MERCHANT SERVICE MERCH DEP 731668000667		594.00	31,893.33
5/19		MERCHANT SERVICE MERCH DEP 731668000667		471.75	32,365.08
5/21		MERCHANT SERVICE MERCH DEP 731668000667		511.00	32,876.08
5/21		DEPOSIT		870.00	33,746.08
5/21		PROOF CORRECTION CREDIT		9.00	33,755.08
5/21	1801	CHK	110.00		33,645.08
5/21	1802	CHK	37.50		33,607.58
5/21	1800	CHK	11.76		33,595.82
5/25		MERCHANT SERVICE MERCH DEP 731668000667		658.75	34,254.57
5/27		MERCHANT SERVICE MERCH DEP 731668000667		261.00	34,515.57
5/28		MERCHANT SERVICE MERCH DEP 731668000667		465.00	34,980.57
5/28		DEPOSIT		369.00	35,349.57
5/31		MERCHANT SERVICE MERCH FEE 731668000667	333.16		35,016.41
5/31		INTEREST		2.86	35,019.27

Figure 16-16 Sample bank statement.

Dental Associates, PC
Bank Reconciliation

April 30, 20__

Balance per Bank statement	$41,195.10	Balance per checkbook		$41,052.13
+ Deposit of 04-01-20__ not on statement	330.24	Subtract		
		Debit Memo	$ 5.00	
		Merchant Service Fee	348.56	$ 353.56

Less Outstanding Checks

NO.	1778	$ 25.00
NO.	1779	$ 325.56
NO.	1780	$ 425.98
NO.	1782	$ 35.00
NO.	1783	$ 15.23

Total Outstanding checks $ 826.77

Adjusted Bank Balance	$40,698.57	Adjusted Checkbook Balance	$40,698.57

Figure 16-17 Sample bank reconciliation.

Petty Cash Voucher

No.________ Date________

Paid to________________________________ Amount

For________________________________ ________

Charge to________________________________

________________ ________________

Approved by Payment received

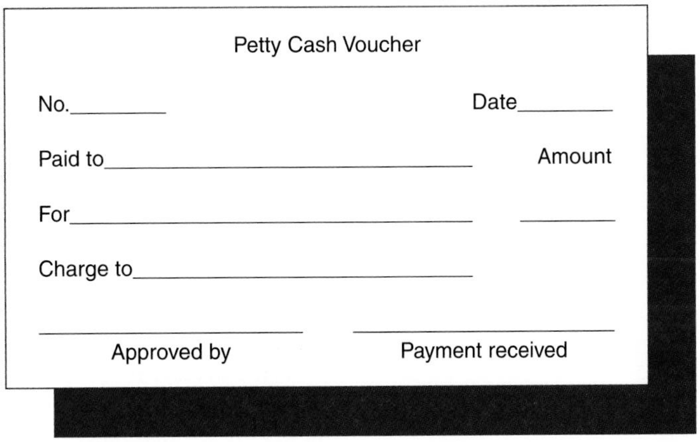

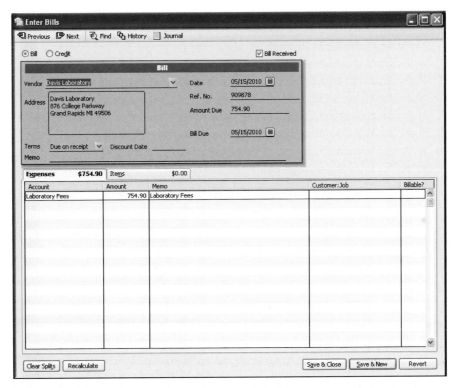

Figure 16-18 Petty cash voucher.

Figure 16-19 Sample of a bill entered into QuickBooks®. The *Enter Bills* function allows a user to keep a record of expenditures and also to pay those bills electronically if the office is set up for that functionality. (Screenshot © Intuit, Inc. All rights reserved.)

RECORDING BUSINESS EXPENSES

As invoices are processed, the expenditures represented on them need to be analyzed and verified for payment. If using a financial management software system, this information is listed in the accounts payable file. A check is then made out to each supplier for payment of these statements. The payments are automatically entered in an expense category. A monthly income and expense register provides a list of all the expenditures for the month, including the date of payment, the company to which the payment was made, the category of deduction, and the amount of payment. These totals are transferred to the annual summary. When using a system like QuickBooks®, the entries are made and the categories of expenses are updated automatically (Figure 16-19), and checks can then be produced as illustrated in Figure 16-10. QuickBooks® also allows users the option to convert the entered bills into paid bills via electronic funds transfer.

MAINTAINING PAYROLL RECORDS

Various federal and state laws require that most businesses keep records to provide information about wages paid and to help in the preparation of required tax reports. Therefore the administrative assistant must have a good working knowledge of payroll and tax records.

 PRACTICE NOTE

Various federal and state laws require that most businesses keep records to provide information about wages paid and to help in the preparation of required tax reports.

INITIAL PAYROLL RECORDS

The dentist, as an employer, must apply for an **employer identification number**, a nine-digit number assigned to sole proprietors or corporations for filing and reporting payroll information. The application, **Form SS-4**, is available from the Internal Revenue Service (IRS; Figure 16-20). Some states also require a state employer identification number.

The employer is required to have every employee complete an **Employee's Withholding Allowance Certificate (Form W-4)** (Figure 16-21). This form is needed to determine the status of each employee for income tax deductions from wages. Employees are required to complete a new Form W-4 when they change the number of withholding exemptions claimed.

Figure 16-20 Application for employer identification number (Form SS-4). (From Internal Revenue Service, Department of the Treasury, Washington, DC.)

Cut here and give Form W-4 to your employer. Keep the top part for your records.

Form **W-4** | Department of the Treasury, Internal Revenue Service

Employee's Withholding Allowance Certificate

▶ **Whether you are entitled to claim a certain number of allowances or exemption from withholding is subject to review by the IRS. Your employer may be required to send a copy of this form to the IRS.**

OMB No. 1545-0074 | **2009**

1 Type or print your first name and middle initial.	Last name	2 **Your social security number**
Home address (number and street or rural route)	3 ☐ Single ☐ Married ☐ Married, but withhold at higher Single rate. **Note.** If married, but legally separated, or spouse is a nonresident alien, check the "Single" box.	
City or town, state, and ZIP code	4 **If your last name differs from that shown on your social security card, check here. You must call 1-800-772-1213 for a replacement card.** ▶ ☐	

5 Total number of allowances you are claiming (from line **H** above **or** from the applicable worksheet on page 2) . . . 5

6 Additional amount, if any, you want withheld from each paycheck . . . . 6 $

7 I claim exemption from withholding for 2009, and I certify that I meet **both** of the following conditions for exemption.
- Last year I had a right to a refund of **all** federal income tax withheld because I had **no** tax liability **and**
- This year I expect a refund of **all** federal income tax withheld because I expect to have **no** tax liability.

If you meet both conditions, write "Exempt" here . . . . ▶ 7

Under penalties of perjury, I declare that I have examined this certificate and to the best of my knowledge and belief, it is true, correct, and complete.

Employee's signature
(Form is not valid unless you sign it.) ▶ **Date** ▶

8 Employer's name and address (Employer: Complete lines 8 and 10 only if sending to the IRS.)	9 Office code (optional)	10 Employer identification number (EIN)

For Privacy Act and Paperwork Reduction Act Notice, see page 2. Cat. No. 10220Q Form **W-4** (2009)

Form W-4 (2009) Page **2**

Deductions and Adjustments Worksheet

Note. Use this worksheet *only* if you plan to itemize deductions, claim certain credits, adjustments to income, or an additional standard deduction.

1 Enter an estimate of your 2009 itemized deductions. These include qualifying home mortgage interest, charitable contributions, state and local taxes, medical expenses in excess of 7.5% of your income, and miscellaneous deductions. (For 2009, you may have to reduce your itemized deductions if your income is over $166,800 ($83,400 if married filing separately). See *Worksheet 2* in Pub. 919 for details.) . . . 1 $

2 Enter: { $11,400 if married filing jointly or qualifying widow(er); $ 8,350 if head of household; $ 5,700 if single or married filing separately } . . . . 2 $

3 **Subtract** line 2 from line 1. If zero or less, enter "-0-" . . . . 3 $

4 Enter an estimate of your 2009 adjustments to income and any additional standard deduction. (Pub. 919) . . . 4 $

5 **Add** lines 3 and 4 and enter the total. (Include any amount for credits from *Worksheet 8* in Pub. 919.) . 5 $

6 Enter an estimate of your 2009 nonwage income (such as dividends or interest) . . . . 6 $

7 **Subtract** line 6 from line 5. If zero or less, enter "-0-" . . . . 7 $

8 **Divide** the amount on line 7 by $3,500 and enter the result here. Drop any fraction 8

9 Enter the number from the **Personal Allowances Worksheet,** line H, page 1 9

10 **Add** lines 8 and 9 and enter the total here. If you plan to use the **Two-Earners/Multiple Jobs Worksheet,** also enter this total on line 1 below. Otherwise, **stop here** and enter this total on Form W-4, line 5, page 1 10

Two-Earners/Multiple Jobs Worksheet (See *Two earners or multiple jobs* on page 1.)

Note. Use this worksheet *only* if the instructions under line H on page 1 direct you here.

1 Enter the number from line H, page 1 (or from line 10 above if you used the **Deductions and Adjustments Worksheet**) 1

2 Find the number in **Table 1** below that applies to the **LOWEST** paying job and enter it here. **However,** if you are married filing jointly and wages from the highest paying job are $50,000 or less, do not enter more than "3." 2

3 If line 1 is **more than or equal to** line 2, subtract line 2 from line 1. Enter the result here (if zero, enter "-0-") and on Form W-4, line 5, page 1. **Do not** use the rest of this worksheet 3

Note. If line 1 is *less than* line 2, enter "-0-" on Form W-4, line 5, page 1. Complete lines 4–9 below to calculate the additional withholding amount necessary to avoid a year-end tax bill.

4 Enter the number from line 2 of this worksheet 4

5 Enter the number from line 1 of this worksheet 5

6 **Subtract** line 5 from line 4 6

7 Find the amount in **Table 2** below that applies to the **HIGHEST** paying job and enter it here . . 7 $

8 **Multiply** line 7 by line 6 and enter the result here. This is the additional annual withholding needed . 8 $

9 Divide line 8 by the number of pay periods remaining in 2009. For example, divide by 26 if you are paid every two weeks and you complete this form in December 2008. Enter the result here and on Form W-4, line 6, page 1. This is the additional amount to be withheld from each paycheck . . . . 9 $

Table 1				Table 2			
Married Filing Jointly		All Others		Married Filing Jointly		All Others	
If wages from **LOWEST** paying job are—	Enter on line 2 above	If wages from **LOWEST** paying job are—	Enter on line 2 above	If wages from **HIGHEST** paying job are—	Enter on line 7 above	If wages from **HIGHEST** paying job are—	Enter on line 7 above
$0 - $4,500	0	$0 - $6,000	0	$0 - $65,000	$550	$0 - $35,000	$550
4,501 - 9,000	1	6,001 - 12,000	1	65,001 - 120,000	910	35,001 - 90,000	910
9,001 - 18,000	2	12,001 - 19,000	2	120,001 - 185,000	1,020	90,001 - 165,000	1,020
18,001 - 22,000	3	19,001 - 26,000	3	185,001 - 330,000	1,200	165,001 - 370,000	1,200
22,001 - 26,000	4	26,001 - 35,000	4	330,001 and over	1,280	370,001 and over	1,280
26,001 - 32,000	5	35,001 - 50,000	5				
32,001 - 38,000	6	50,001 - 65,000	6				
38,001 - 46,000	7	65,001 - 80,000	7				
46,001 - 55,000	8	80,001 - 90,000	8				
55,001 - 60,000	9	90,001 - 120,000	9				
60,001 - 65,000	10	120,001 and over	10				
65,001 - 75,000	11						
75,001 - 95,000	12						
95,001 - 105,000	13						
105,001 - 120,000	14						
120,001 and over	15						

Privacy Act and Paperwork Reduction Act Notice. We ask for the information on this form to carry out the Internal Revenue laws of the United States. The Internal Revenue Code requires this information under sections 3402(f)(2)(A) and 6109 and their regulations. Failure to provide a properly completed form will result in your being treated as a single person who claims no withholding allowances; providing fraudulent information may also subject you to penalties. Routine uses of this information include giving it to the Department of Justice for civil and criminal litigation, to cities, states, the District of Columbia, and U.S. commonwealths and possessions for use in administering their tax laws, and using it in the National Directory of New Hires. We may also disclose this information to other countries under a tax treaty, to federal and state agencies to enforce federal nontax criminal laws, or to federal law enforcement and intelligence agencies to combat terrorism.

You are not required to provide the information requested on a form that is subject to the Paperwork Reduction Act unless the form displays a valid OMB control number. Books or records relating to a form or its instructions must be retained as long as their contents may become material in the administration of any Internal Revenue law. Generally, tax returns and return information are confidential, as required by Code section 6103.

The average time and expenses required to complete and file this form will vary depending on individual circumstances. For estimated averages, see the instructions for your income tax return.

If you have suggestions for making this form simpler, we would be happy to hear from you. See the instructions for your income tax return.

Figure 16-21 Employee's Withholding Allowance Certificate (Form W-4). (From Internal Revenue Service, Department of the Treasury, Washington, DC.)

EMPLOYEE EARNINGS RECORDS

The employer must maintain employees' earnings records, including a summary of information for each employee (Figure 16-22). If the record has been properly designed, it provides the information needed for quarterly and annual reports. The employee's earnings record should contain the following information, which is used for various state and federal reports:

- Name, address, Social Security number, rate of pay, withholding exemptions claimed, marital status, and special deductions (e.g., credit union account, bonds, United Fund)
- The number of pay periods in a quarter and the date on which each pay period ends
- Columns for regular earnings, overtime earnings, and total earnings. (Earnings records are available that provide columns for rate of pay and hours or days worked in a pay period.)
- A column for each deduction and for total deductions
- A column for entering the net amount (net pay) received. (*Net pay* is the difference between total earnings and deductions.)
- A column for recording accumulated taxable earnings. This column provides the employer with information for taxable earnings, **Federal Insurance Contributions Act (FICA)** deductions (see the next section), and taxable wages for unemployment taxes.
- Columns for quarterly and annual totals

Determining Employee Wages

The dentist and employees must reach an agreement on an acceptable wage. This may be determined as an hourly rate, a weekly rate, or a monthly amount. After this rate has been established, the procedure must be decided for determining **net pay**.

EMPLOYEE'S EARNINGS RECORD

Exemptions ______ Name ______
Date of Birth ______ Address ______
Date Employed ______
Phone ______ Soc. Sec. No. ______
In Emergency Notify ______

REMARKS	DATE	CHECK NO.	GROSS SALARY	FEDERAL W.H. TAX	F.I.C.A.	STATE W.H. TAX	OTHER	OTHER	NET CHECK
THIRD QUARTER									
FOURTH QUARTER									
YEAR'S TOTALS									

Figure 16-22 Employee's earnings record.

The administrative assistant often is responsible for figuring the payroll and preparing the checks for the dentist's signature, as follows:

 PRACTICE NOTE
The dentist and employees must reach an agreement on an acceptable wage.

1. The administrative assistant's hourly wage is $24 per hour.
2. If the workweek is based on 36 hours per week, the **gross wages** (amount earned before deductions) are $864 (36 hours × $24 per hour = $864).
3. Deductions are made from wages as follows:
   a. *FICA deduction (Social Security and Medicare taxes)*: The amount to be withheld is determined by calculating at the combined 2009 rate (7.65 percent [or 0.0765] × $864 = $66.10). This tax rate is divided into two parts: (1) the Social Security part, which is 6.2 percent on the first $106,800 earned in 2009, and (2) the second part, for Medicare, which is 1.45 percent on all earnings, no ceiling. These tax rates are subject to change by Congress. The employer must keep track of such changes and make deductions according to the current rate. The *Employer's Tax Guide-Circular E*, available from the IRS, can be used to check the current tax rates.
   b. **Withholding** *(income tax deductions)*: The amount withheld depends on the number of exemptions indicated on Form W-4. The tax amount withheld is determined from a table in the *Employer's Tax Guide-Circular E*. According to the table in Figure 16-23, the withholding tax on $864 for a single person claiming one exemption is $105.
   c. *Local income tax*: Some cities and states have personal income taxes that must be deducted. Again, the employer must be familiar with the state and local laws regarding these taxes.
   d. *Other deductions*: In addition to the standard deductions, the administrative assistant may have a weekly deduction of $60 for the credit union (noted on the earnings record).
4. The net pay (take-home pay), and the amount for which the paycheck is written, is $632.90. The check is generated on the financial software, such as QuickBooks®, shown in Figure 16-24.

Gross Wages	Minus Deductions	Deductions Total	Net Pay
$864	FICA: $53.57 Medicare: $12.53 Withholding tax: $105 Credit union: $60	$171.10	$632.90

SINGLE Persons—WEEKLY Payroll Period
(For Wages Paid Through December 2009)

| If the wages are— | | And the number of withholding allowances claimed is— | | | | | | | | | | |
At least	But less than	0	1	2	3	4	5	6	7	8	9	10
		The amount of income tax to be withheld is—										
$780	$790	$103	$85	$73	$62	$52	$41	$31	$20	$10	$2	$0
790	800	105	88	74	64	53	43	32	22	11	3	0
800	810	108	90	76	65	55	44	34	23	13	4	0
810	820	110	93	77	67	56	46	35	25	14	5	0
820	830	113	95	79	68	58	47	37	26	16	6	0
830	840	115	98	80	70	59	49	38	28	17	7	0
840	850	118	100	83	71	61	50	40	29	19	8	1
850	860	120	103	85	73	62	52	41	31	20	10	2
860	870	123	105	88	74	64	53	43	32	22	11	3
870	880	125	108	90	76	65	55	44	34	23	13	4
880	890	128	110	93	77	67	56	46	35	25	14	5
890	900	130	113	95	79	68	58	47	37	26	16	6
900	910	133	115	98	80	70	59	49	38	28	17	7
910	920	135	118	100	83	71	61	50	40	29	19	8
920	930	138	120	103	85	73	62	52	41	31	20	10
930	940	140	123	105	88	74	64	53	43	32	22	11
940	950	143	125	108	90	76	65	55	44	34	23	13
950	960	145	128	110	93	77	67	56	46	35	25	14
960	970	148	130	113	95	79	68	58	47	37	26	16
970	980	150	133	115	98	80	70	59	49	38	28	17
980	990	153	135	118	100	83	71	61	50	40	29	19
990	1,000	155	138	120	103	85	73	62	52	41	31	20
1,000	1,010	158	140	123	105	88	74	64	53	43	32	22
1,010	1,020	160	143	125	108	90	76	65	55	44	34	23
1,020	1,030	163	145	128	110	93	77	67	56	46	35	25
1,030	1,040	165	148	130	113	95	79	68	58	47	37	26
1,040	1,050	168	150	133	115	98	80	70	59	49	38	28
1,050	1,060	170	153	135	118	100	83	71	61	50	40	29
1,060	1,070	173	155	138	120	103	85	73	62	52	41	31
1,070	1,080	175	158	140	123	105	88	74	64	53	43	32
1,080	1,090	178	160	143	125	108	90	76	65	55	44	34
1,090	1,100	180	163	145	128	110	93	77	67	56	46	35
1,100	1,110	183	165	148	130	113	95	79	68	58	47	37
1,110	1,120	185	168	150	133	115	98	80	70	59	49	38
1,120	1,130	188	170	153	135	118	100	83	71	61	50	40
1,130	1,140	190	173	155	138	120	103	85	73	62	52	41
1,140	1,150	193	175	158	140	123	105	88	74	64	53	43
1,150	1,160	195	178	160	143	125	108	90	76	65	55	44
1,160	1,170	198	180	163	145	128	110	93	77	67	56	46
1,170	1,180	200	183	165	148	130	113	95	79	68	58	47
1,180	1,190	203	185	168	150	133	115	98	80	70	59	49
1,190	1,200	205	188	170	153	135	118	100	82	71	61	50
1,200	1,210	208	190	173	155	138	120	103	85	73	62	52
1,210	1,220	210	193	175	158	140	123	105	87	74	64	53
1,220	1,230	213	195	178	160	143	125	108	90	76	65	55
1,230	1,240	215	198	180	163	145	128	110	92	77	67	56
1,240	1,250	218	200	183	165	148	130	113	95	79	68	58

$1,250 and over — Use Table 1(a) for a **SINGLE person** on page 5. Also see the instructions on page 3.

Figure 16-23 Tax withholding table. (From Internal Revenue Service, Department of the Treasury, Washington, DC.)

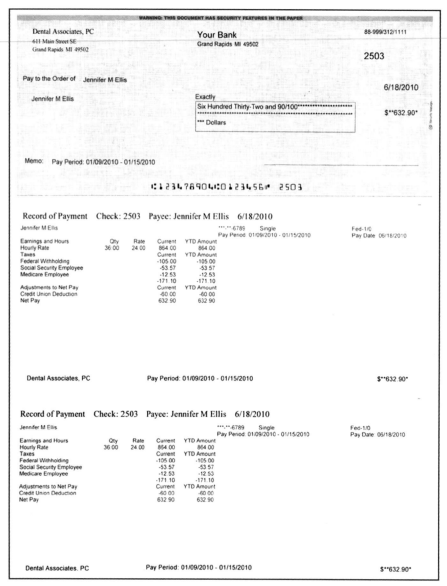

Figure 16-24 QuickBooks®-generated payroll check for single person claiming one withholding allowance. (Software © Intuit, Inc. All rights reserved.)

The net pay for each member of the office staff must be calculated. After the amounts have been determined, the paychecks are written, the information is entered on each employee's earnings record, and a record is made on the expense sheet.

Depositing Withheld Income Tax and Social Security Taxes

Generally the employer must deposit withheld income tax, Social Security, and Medicare taxes in an authorized commercial bank or a Federal Reserve bank. Coupon forms are used for depositing taxes. The IRS sends the employer a Federal Tax Deposit (FTD) coupon book (Form 8109) containing 15 coupons for depositing all types of taxes. FTD forms are no longer mailed out periodically. If additional forms are needed, the FTD Reorder Form (Form 8109A) provided in the coupon book is used. If the administrative assistant does not have a coupon book, one may be requested from the IRS district office.

The amount of taxes determines the frequency of deposits. These taxes are owed when the employer pays the wages (or makes the payments from which the taxes are withheld), not when the payroll period ends. To determine when the taxes are due and the amount on which they are based, the administrative assistant should check the instructions on the reverse side of the Employer's Quarterly Federal Tax Return (Form 941; Figure 16-25).

Although the employer probably will make monthly deposits for the withholding taxes and FICA deductions, he or she

▼ Detach Here and Mail With Your Payment and Form 941. ▼

Form **941-V**
Department of the Treasury
Internal Revenue Service

Payment Voucher

▶ Do not staple this voucher or your payment to Form 941.

OMB No. 1545-0029
2009

1 Enter your employer identification number (EIN).

2 **Enter the amount of your payment.** ▶ Dollars | Cents

3 Tax period

1st Quarter	3rd Quarter
2nd Quarter	4th Quarter

4 Enter your business name (individual name if sole proprietor).

Enter your address.

Enter your city, state, and ZIP code.

Form **941 for 2009: Employer's QUARTERLY Federal Tax Return** 950109
(Rev. April 2009) Department of the Treasury — Internal Revenue Service OMB No. 1545-0029

(EIN) Employer identification number ☐☐ – ☐☐☐☐☐☐☐

Name *(not your trade name)*

Trade name *(if any)*

Address Number Street Suite or room number

City State ZIP code

Report for this Quarter of 2009
(Check one.)

☐ **1:** January, February, March
☐ **2:** April, May, June
☐ **3:** July, August, September
☐ **4:** October, November, December

Read the separate instructions before you complete Form 941. Type or print within the boxes.

Part 1: Answer these questions for this quarter.

1 **Number of employees who received wages, tips, or other compensation for the pay period including:** ***Mar. 12*** **(Quarter 1),** ***June 12*** **(Quarter 2),** ***Sept. 12*** **(Quarter 3),** ***Dec. 12*** **(Quarter 4)** 1

2 **Wages, tips, and other compensation** 2

3 **Income tax withheld from wages, tips, and other compensation** 3

4 **If no wages, tips, and other compensation are subject to social security or Medicare tax** ☐ Check and go to line 6.

5 **Taxable social security and Medicare wages and tips:**

	Column 1		Column 2
5a **Taxable social security wages**	.	× .124 =	.
5b **Taxable social security tips**	.	× .124 =	.
5c **Taxable Medicare wages & tips**	.	× .029 =	.

5d **Total social security and Medicare taxes** (*Column 2*, lines 5a + 5b + 5c = line 5d) . 5d

6 **Total taxes before adjustments** (lines 3 + 5d = line 6) 6

7 **CURRENT QUARTER'S ADJUSTMENTS,** for example, a fractions of cents adjustment. See the instructions.

7a **Current quarter's fractions of cents** . . . . . .

7b **Current quarter's sick pay** . . . .

7c **Current quarter's adjustments for tips and group-term life insurance**

7d **TOTAL ADJUSTMENTS.** Combine all amounts on lines 7a through 7c 7d

8 **Total taxes after adjustments.** Combine lines 6 and 7d 8

9 **Advance earned income credit (EIC) payments made to employees** 9

10 **Total taxes after adjustment for advance EIC** (line 8 – line 9 = line 10) 10

11 **Total deposits for this quarter, including overpayment applied from a prior quarter and overpayment applied from Form 941-X or Form 944-X** . . . .

12a **COBRA premium assistance payments** (see instructions) . . .

12b **Number of individuals provided COBRA premium assistance reported on line 12a** . . . .

13 **Add lines 11 and 12a** 13

14 **Balance due.** If line 13 is more than line 13, write the difference here 14
For information on how to pay, see the instructions.

15 **Overpayment.** If line 13 is more than line 10, write the difference here . Check one ☐ Apply to next return. ☐ Send a refund.

▶ You **MUST** complete both pages of Form 941 and **SIGN** it. Next ➔

For Privacy Act and Paperwork Reduction Act Notice, see the back of the Payment Voucher. Cat. No. 17001Z Form **941** (Rev. 4-2009)

Figure 16-25 Employer's Quarterly Federal Tax Return (Form 941). (From Internal Revenue Service, Department of the Treasury, Washington, DC.)

(Continued)

Figure 16-25, cont'd Employer's Quarterly Federal Tax Return (Form 941). (From Internal Revenue Service, Department of the Treasury, Washington, DC.)

must file a quarterly return on Form 941. The returns and tax payments are due on the following dates:

Quarter	Quarter Ending	Due Date
January to March	March 31	April 30
April to June	June 30	July 31
July to September	September 30	October 31
October to December	December 31	January 31

The employer completes Form 941 by entering the summarized payroll data for the quarter. Information about total wages and taxable FICA wages is obtained from the employee's earnings record. Further instructions are available in the IRS pamphlet instructions for Form 941.

Federal Unemployment Tax

The employer is subject to a federal unemployment tax under the provisions of the Federal Unemployment Tax Act (FUTA). This tax is 8 percent of wages paid and applies to the first $7000 of wages paid during the calendar year. Generally a credit may be taken against the federal unemployment tax for contributions to be paid into state unemployment funds. The federal unemployment tax is imposed on employers and must not be deducted from employees' wages. On or before January 31, the employer must file an unemployment tax return (i.e., Employers' Annual Federal Unemployment [FUTA] Tax Return [Form 940]) (Figure 16-26) and deposit or pay the balance of the tax in full. For deposit purposes, the employer must compute the federal

Detach Here and Mail With Your Payment and Form 940.

Form **940-V**
Department of the Treasury
Internal Revenue Service

Payment Voucher

► Do not staple or attach this voucher to your payment.

OMB No. 1545-0028

2008

1 Enter your employer identification number (EIN).

2 **Enter the amount of your payment.** ►

Dollars   Cents

3 Enter your business name (individual name if sole proprietor).

Enter your address.

Enter your city, state, and ZIP code.

Form **940 for 2008:**   Employer's Annual Federal Unemployment (FUTA) Tax Return   850108
Department of the Treasury — Internal Revenue Service

OMB No. 1545-0028

(EIN)
Employer identification number

☐☐ – ☐☐☐☐☐☐☐

Name (not your trade name)

Trade name (if any)

Address
Number   Street   Suite or room number
City   State   ZIP code

Type of Return
(Check all that apply.)

☐ a. Amended
☐ b. Successor employer
☐ c. No payments to employees in 2008
☐ d. Final: Business closed or stopped paying wages

Read the separate instructions before you fill out this form. Please type or print within the boxes.

Part 1: Tell us about your return. If any line does NOT apply, leave it blank.

1 If you were required to pay your state unemployment tax in ...

　1a **One state only**, write the state abbreviation . . **1a** ☐☐

　- OR -

　1b **More than one state** (You are a multi-state employer) . . . . . . **1b** ☐ Check here. Fill out Schedule A.
　　Skip line 2 for 2008 and go to line 3.

2 If you paid wages in a state that is subject to CREDIT REDUCTION . . . . **2** ☐ Check here. Fill out Schedule A (Form 940), Part 2.

Part 2: Determine your FUTA tax before adjustments for 2008. If any line does NOT apply, leave it blank.

3 Total payments to all employees . . . . **3** ☐

4 Payments exempt from FUTA tax . . . . **4** ☐

　Check all that apply: **4a** ☐ Fringe benefits **4c** ☐ Retirement/Pension **4e** ☐ Other
　　　　　　　　　　4b ☐ Group-term life insurance **4d** ☐ Dependent care

5 Total of payments made to each employee in excess of $7,000 . . . . **5** ☐

6 **Subtotal** (line 4 + line 5 = line 6) . . . . . . **6** ☐

7 Total taxable FUTA wages (line 3 – line 6 = line 7) . . . . . . **7** ☐

8 FUTA tax before adjustments (line 7 × .008 = line 8) . . . . **8** ☐

Part 3: Determine your adjustments. If any line does NOT apply, leave it blank.

9 If ALL of the taxable FUTA wages you paid were excluded from state unemployment tax, multiply line 7 by .054 (line 7 × .054 = line 9). Then go to line 12 . . . . . **9** ☐

10 If SOME of the taxable FUTA wages you paid were excluded from state unemployment tax, OR you paid ANY state unemployment tax late (after the due date for filing Form 940), fill out the worksheet in the instructions. Enter the amount from line 7 of the worksheet onto line 10 . **10** ☐

　　Skip line 11 for 2008 and go to line 12.

11 If credit reduction applies, enter the amount from line 3 of Schedule A (Form 940) . . . **11** ☐

Part 4: Determine your FUTA tax and balance due or overpayment for 2008. If any line does NOT apply, leave it blank.

12 Total FUTA tax after adjustments (lines 8 + 9 + 10 + 11 = line 12) . . . . . **12** ☐

13 FUTA tax deposited for the year, including any payment applied from a prior year . . **13** ☐

14 **Balance due** (If line 12 is more than line 13, enter the difference on line 14.)
　• If line 14 is more than $500, you must deposit your tax.
　• If line 14 is $500 or less, you may pay with this return. For more information on how to pay, see the separate instructions . . . . **14** ☐

15 **Overpayment** (If line 13 is more than line 12, enter the difference on line 15 and check a box below.) . . . . **15** ☐

Check one: ☐ Apply to next return.　☐ Send a refund.

► You **MUST** fill out both pages of this form and **SIGN** it.

Next ►

For Privacy Act and Paperwork Reduction Act Notice, see the back of Form 940-V, Payment Voucher.   Cat. No. 11234O   Form **940** (2008)

Figure 16-26 Employer's Annual Federal Unemployment (FUTA) Tax Return (Form 940). (From Internal Revenue Service, Department of the Treasury, Washington, DC.)

(Continued)

850208

Name (not your trade name)

Employer identification number (EIN)

Part 5: Report your FUTA tax liability by quarter only if line 12 is more than $500. If not, go to Part 6.

16   Report the amount of your FUTA tax liability for each quarter; do NOT enter the amount you deposited. If you had no liability for a quarter, leave the line blank.

16a   **1st quarter** (January 1 – March 31) 16a

16b   **2nd quarter** (April 1 – June 30) 16b

16c   **3rd quarter** (July 1 – September 30) 16c

16d   **4th quarter** (October 1 – December 31) 16d

17   **Total tax liability for the year** (lines 16a + 16b + 16c + 16d = line 17) **17**   Total must equal line 12.

Part 6: May we speak with your third-party designee?

Do you want to allow an employee, a paid tax preparer, or another person to discuss this return with the IRS? See the instructions for details.

☐   **Yes.**   Designee's name and phone number   (   )   –

Select a 5-digit Personal Identification Number (PIN) to use when talking to IRS

☐   **No.**

Part 7: Sign here. You MUST fill out both pages of this form and SIGN it.

Under penalties of perjury, I declare that I have examined this return, including accompanying schedules and statements, and to the best of my knowledge and belief, it is true, correct, and complete, and that no part of any payment made to a state unemployment fund claimed as a credit was, or is to be, deducted from the payments made to employees. Declaration of preparer (other than taxpayer) is based on all information of which preparer has any knowledge.

X **Sign your name here**

Print your name here

Print your title here

Date   /   /

Best daytime phone   (   )   –

Paid preparer's use only   Check if you are self-employed   .   .☐

Preparer's name

Preparer's SSN/PTIN

Preparer's signature

Date   /   /

Firm's name (or yours if self-employed)

EIN

Address

Phone   (   )   –

City   State   ZIP code

Page **2**   Form **940** (2008)

Figure 16-26, cont'd Employer's Annual Federal Unemployment (FUTA) Tax Return (Form 940). (From Internal Revenue Service, Department of the Treasury, Washington, DC.)

unemployment tax on a quarterly basis. The deposit must be made on or before the last day of the first month after the close of the quarter.

To determine whether the employer must make a deposit for any of the first three quarters in a year, compute the total tax as follows:

1. Multiply the first $7000 of each employee's annual wages paid during the quarter by 0.008.
2. If the amount subject to deposit (plus the amount subject to deposit but not deposited for any prior quarter) is more than $100, a deposit should be made during the first month after the quarter.

Wage and Tax Statement (Form W-2)

A federal Wage and Tax Statement (Form W-2) for a calendar year must be provided for each employee no later than January 31 of the following year (Figure 16-27). The Form W-2 is prepared in six parts and distributed in the following

manner: one copy for IRS use; one copy to state, city, or local tax departments; three copies to the employee (one for filing federal tax returns, one for state or local tax purposes, and one for the employee's files); and one copy retained by the employer.

Form W-2 includes the following information:
- Employer's identification number, name, and address
- Employee's Social Security number, name, and address
- Federal income tax withheld
- Total sum of wages paid to the employee
- Total FICA employee tax withheld (Social Security and Medicare)
- Total wages paid that are subject to FICA
- State and local taxes withheld when applicable

To correct a Form W-2 after one has been issued to an employee, a corrected statement must be issued. The corrected statement must completely replace the original statement and be clearly marked as "CORRECTED RETURN" in capital letters directly above the title, Wage and Tax Statement. If a

22222 | a Employee's social security number | OMB No. 1545-0008

b Employer identification number (EIN)
1 Wages, tips, other compensation
2 Federal income tax withheld
c Employer's name, address, and ZIP code
3 Social security wages
4 Social security tax withheld
5 Medicare wages and tips
6 Medicare tax withheld
7 Social security tips
8 Allocated tips
d Control number
9 Advance EIC payment
10 Dependent care benefits
e Employee's first name and initial | Last name | Suff.
11 Nonqualified plans
12a
13 Statutory employee | Retirement plan | Third-party sick pay
12b
14 Other
12c
12d
f Employee's address and ZIP code
15 State | Employer's state ID number
16 State wages, tips, etc.
17 State income tax
18 Local wages, tips, etc.
19 Local income tax
20 Locality name

Form **W-2** Wage and Tax Statement 2009 Department of the Treasury—Internal Revenue Service
Copy 1—For State, City, or Local Tax Department

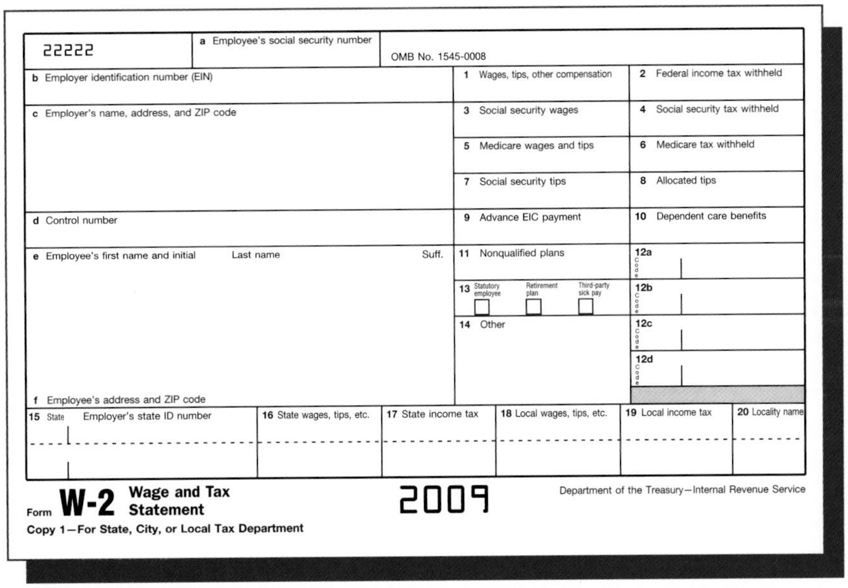

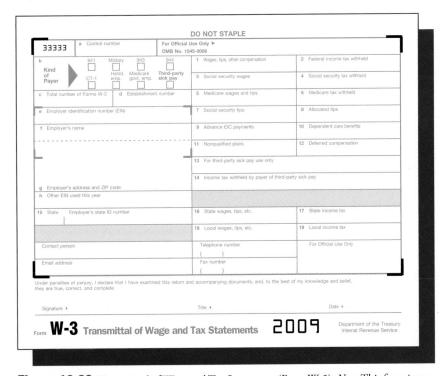

Figure 16-27 Wage and Tax Statement (Form W-2). (From Internal Revenue Service, Department of the Treasury, Washington, DC.)

DO NOT STAPLE

33333 | a Control number | For Official Use Only ▶ OMB No. 1545-0008

b Kind of Payer: 941 | Military | 943 | 944 | CT-1 | Hshld. emp. | Medicare govt. emp. | Third-party sick pay
1 Wages, tips, other compensation
2 Federal income tax withheld
3 Social security wages
4 Social security tax withheld
c Total number of Forms W-2 | d Establishment number
5 Medicare wages and tips
6 Medicare tax withheld
e Employer identification number (EIN)
7 Social security tips
8 Allocated tips
f Employer's name
9 Advance EIC payments
10 Dependent care benefits
11 Nonqualified plans
12 Deferred compensation
13 For third-party sick pay use only
14 Income tax withheld by payer of third-party sick pay
g Employer's address and ZIP code
h Other EIN used this year
15 State | Employer's state ID number
16 State wages, tips, etc.
17 State income tax
18 Local wages, tips, etc.
19 Local income tax
Contact person
Telephone number ( )
For Official Use Only
Email address
Fax number ( )

Under penalties of perjury, I declare that I have examined this return and accompanying documents, and, to the best of my knowledge and belief, they are true, correct, and complete.

Signature ▸ Title ▸ Date ▸

Form **W-3** Transmittal of Wage and Tax Statements 2009 Department of the Treasury Internal Revenue Service

Figure 16-28 Transmittal of Wage and Tax Statements (Form W-3). *Note:* This form is provided for informational purposes. Employers should **not** file this red copy downloaded from www.irs.gov but should instead call and order an official form: 1-800-TAX-FORM (1-800-829-3676). (From Internal Revenue Service, Department of the Treasury, Washington, DC.)

Form W-2 is lost or destroyed, the substitute copy issued to the employee is marked as "Reissued Return."

Report of Withheld Income Tax (Form W-3)

On or before February 28, copy A of all Form W-2s issued for the year and Form W-3, Transmittal of Wage and Tax Statements (Figure 16-28), must be sent to the IRS.

Retention of Payroll and Tax Records

The employer must keep all records pertaining to employment taxes available for inspection by the IRS. Although no form has been devised for such records, the employer must be able to supply the following information:

- Amounts and dates of all wages paid
- Names, addresses, and occupations of employees

- Periods of employees' employment
- Periods for which employees were paid while absent because of sickness
- Employees' Social Security numbers
- Employees' income tax withholding allowance certificates
- Employer's identification number
- Duplicate copies of returns filed and the dates and amounts of deposits made

 PRACTICE NOTE

The employer must keep all records pertaining to employment taxes available for inspection by the Internal Revenue Service.

These tax records should be kept for at least 4 years after the date the taxes to which they apply become due.

Employer's Responsibility for Tax Information

The *Employer's Tax Guide-Circular E*, mentioned previously, summarizes the employer's responsibilities for withholding, depositing, paying, and reporting federal income tax, Social Security taxes, and federal unemployment tax. The circular is available to all employers and may be obtained from a local IRS office. Because tax rates increase so often, the administrative assistant would be wise to check with the IRS to make sure the most up-to-date forms and percentages are used for tax calculations. A Quick and Easy Access to Tax Help and Forms is shown in Figure 16-29. Additional information and help are available at the American Payroll Association web site, www.american-payroll.org.

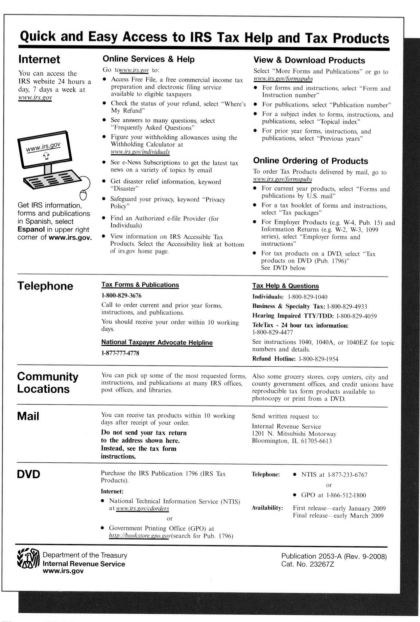

Figure 16-29 A Quick and Easy Access to Tax Help and Forms. (From Internal Revenue Service, Department of the Treasury, Washington, DC.)

KEY TERMS

American Bankers Association (ABA)—A national organization of banks and holding companies of all sizes that deals with issues of importance to national institutions.

Automatic teller machine (ATM)—A computer workstation that electronically prompts the user through most routine banking activities.

Bank deposit—Represents the accumulation of money received for a single day or possibly a longer period.

Bank draft—A check drawn by the cashier of one bank on another bank in which the first bank has available funds on deposit or credit.

Bank statement—A printed statement from the bank showing the balance of the account at the beginning of the month, deposits made during the month, checks drawn against the account, corrections or charges against the account (e.g., service charge or stop payment charges), and the bank balance at the end of the month.

Budget—A financial plan of operation for a given period, usually 1 year.

Cashier's check—The bank's own order to make payment out of the bank's funds.

Certified check—A check for which a guarantee exists that funds have been set aside to cover the amount of the check.

Check—A means of ordering the bank to pay cash from a bank customer's account.

Employee's Withholding Allowance Certificate (Form W-4)—The federal form used to determine the status of each employee for income tax deductions from wages.

Employer identification number—A nine-digit number assigned to sole proprietors or corporations for filing and reporting payroll information.

Endorsement—The signature or stamp of the payee.

Expenditures—The amount of money spent to operate a business or practice.

Federal Insurance Contributions Act (FICA)—A law that requires deductions for Social Security and Medicare taxes.

Form SS-4—The application form used to obtain an employer identification number.

Gross wages—The total amount of earnings before deductions.

Money order—A means of transferring money without using cash or a personal check.

Net pay—The total amount of earnings after deductions.

Petty cash—A small amount of cash kept on hand in the office to pay for small expenses.

Revenue—The amount of income received by a business or practice.

Traveler's check—A payment device purchased through a bank or other agency that serves as cash for a person who is away from home.

Voucher check—A check that provides a detachable stub, which can be used as an accounting record for itemizing payment of invoices or any type of itemization the payer would like as a reference.

Wage and Tax Statement (Form W-2)—A wage and tax statement for a calendar year must be provided for each employee no later than January 31 of the following year.

Withholding—The amount of money withheld for federal and/or state taxes.

LEARNING ACTIVITIES

1. Name and define the parts of a check.
2. List the necessary steps in writing a check.
3. Explain how a certified check and a cashier's check are different.
4. Describe the procedure for making a bank deposit.
5. Define the following:
   a. Blank endorsement
   b. Endorsement in full

Please refer to the student workbook for additional learning activities.

BIBLIOGRAPHY

Fulton-Calkins PJ: *The administrative professional*, ed 13, Mason, OH, 2007, Thomson South-Western.

Internal Revenue Service: *Employer's tax guide, pub no 15, circular E (revised)*, Washington, DC, 2009, U.S. Department of the Treasury.

RECOMMENDED WEB SITES

www.ftc.gov
http://americanbankassociation.com
www.federalreserve.gov

www.fdic.gov
www.irs.gov/publications
www.quickbooks.com/support (Additional terms and conditions may apply.)
www.intuit.com

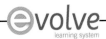

Please visit http://evolve.elsevier.com/Finkibeiner/practice for additional practice activities.

17

Infection Control Systems

CHAPTER OUTLINE

LEARNING OUTCOMES

- Define key terms.
- Identify the importance to the administrative assistant of an understanding of disease transmission.
- Identify the routes of disease transmission.
- Describe basic infection control procedures.
- Identify the various regulatory agencies that impact the dental office.
- Identify the various records required by the Occupational Safety and Health Administration that must be maintained in the business office.
- Explain routine procedures that the administrative assistant might perform to maintain quality assurance in the office.

The administrative assistant generally has no direct patient contact. Nevertheless, he or she must understand both the risks and management of occupational exposures to **blood-borne pathogens**. Although his or her primary duties are in the business office, the administrative assistant may be called upon to perform some clinical task that could cause exposure to such a risk. The assigned job, therefore, does not make it impossible to contract a **communicable disease**. The role of the administrative assistant in infection control is vital, because it involves the following responsibilities:

- Acquiring a thorough understanding of the routes of disease transmission
- Maintaining an adequate inventory of acceptable **disinfectants**, sterilants, **personal protective equipment (PPE)**, and barrier covers
- Maintaining records verifying compliance with the requirements of the **Occupational Safety and Health Administration (OSHA)**
- Transmitting spore samples to the appropriate monitoring agencies for determination of sterilization effectiveness
- Attending training sessions
- Verifying employee compliance with OSHA
- Maintaining employee records
- Scheduling continuing education courses for the staff

- Verifying quality assurance
- Maintaining all Material Safety Data Sheets (MSDSs)
- Arranging for the disposal of **hazardous waste**
- Providing infection control training for new employees as designated by the employer
- Interacting with outside agencies

A variety of diseases can be transmitted by means of routine dental care. Fortunately the dental profession, through the American Dental Association (ADA), the Organization for Safety and Asepsis Procedures (OSAP) and the **Centers for Disease Control and Prevention (CDC)**, has worked vigorously to establish infection control and safety procedures for the **dental healthcare worker (DHCW)** to prevent the transmission of disease.

The CDC report, *Guidelines for Infection Control in Dental Health Care Settings*, was revised in 2003. Every dental office should have direct access to these guidelines through a link on the ADA's web site (www.ada.org) or the CDC's web site (www. cdc.gov). This report consolidates previous recommendations and adds new ones for infection control in dental settings. It provides recommendations on: (1) educating and protecting dental healthcare personnel; (2) preventing the transmission of blood-borne pathogens; (3) hand hygiene; (4) PPE; (5) contact dermatitis and latex hypersensitivity; (6) **sterilization** and disinfection of patient care items; (7) environmental infection control; (8) dental unit water lines, biofilm, and water quality; and (9) special considerations (e.g., dental handpieces and other devices, radiology, parenteral medications, oral surgical procedures, and dental laboratories). These recommendations were developed in collaboration with and after review by authorities on infection control from the CDC and other public agencies, academia, and private and professional organizations.

DISEASE TRANSMISSION

Dental treatment involves several sources by which infectious diseases can be transmitted, including blood, saliva, nasal discharge, dust, hands, clothing, and hair. Any of these media can transmit a microbial or viral **infection**. Table 17-1 presents a list of several communicable diseases and their routes of transfer.

 PRACTICE NOTE
Infectious diseases can be transmitted by several media during dental treatment, including blood, saliva, nasal discharge, dust, hands, clothing, and hair.

Types of Infections

Infections common to dental treatment generally can be divided into two categories, autogenous infections and cross infections. **Autogenous infections** are infections for which the patient is the source. For example, a patient who undergoes dental treatment, such as an extensive scaling procedure, may subsequently develop endocarditis; this condition can result from the introduction of virulent organisms (e.g., staphylococci or pneumococci) that live in the mouth and can be introduced into the bloodstream during the scaling procedure.

 PRACTICE NOTE
With autogenous infections, the patient is the source of the infection.

Cross infections are transferred from one patient or person to another. For example, when a child has an infection and coughs or sneezes, the caregiver may contract the infection through airborne or droplet transmission.

 PRACTICE NOTE
Cross infections are transferred from one patient or person to another.

Routes of Infection Transmission

Microbial transmission through dental-related secretions and exudates occurs by three general routes: (1) direct contact with a lesion, organisms, or debris during intraoral procedures; (2) indirect contact through contaminated dental instruments, equipment, or records; and (3) inhalation of microorganisms aerosolized from a patient's blood or saliva during the use of high-speed or ultrasonic equipment, such as a high-speed handpiece or an ultrasonic scaler.

In many dental practices, treatment providers may not realize the dissemination potential of saliva and blood by these routes. Potential dangers often are missed, because much of the spatter

TABLE 17-1	Common Communicable Diseases and Routes of Transmission	
Disease	**Medium of Transmission**	**Route of Transmission**
Acquired immunodeficiency syndrome (AIDS)	Blood, semen, or other body fluids, including breast milk	Inoculation by use of contaminated needles or by direct contact so that infected body fluids can enter the body
Gonococcal disease	Lesions, discharge from infected mucous membranes	Direct contact, as in sexual intercourse; towels, bathtubs, toilets; hands of infected individuals soiled with their own discharges; through breaks in hands of attendant
Hepatitis B, viral	Blood and serum-derived fluids, including semen and vaginal fluids	Contact with blood and body fluids
Herpes	Cold sore; genital sores	Direct skin-to-skin contact as through kissing or sexual intercourse
Measles (rubella)	Discharges from nose and throat	Direct contact, hands of healthcare worker, articles used by and about patient
Mumps	Discharges from infected glands and throat	Direct contact with affected person
Pneumonia	Sputum and discharges from nose and throat	Direct contact, hands of health care worker, articles used by and about the patient
Rubeola	Secretions from nose and throat	Through mouth and nose
Streptococcal sore throat	Discharges from nose and throat, skin lesions	Through mouth and nose
Syphilis	Infected tissues, lesions, blood, transfer though placenta to fetus	Direct contact, kissing or sexual intercourse, contaminated needles and syringes
Tuberculosis	Saliva, lesions, feces	Direct contact, droplet infection from a person coughing with mouth uncovered, saliva transferred from mouth to fingers and then to food and other articles

from the patient's mouth is not readily noticeable. For example, **bioburden** (blood, saliva, exudate) may be transparent and may dry as a clear film on contaminated surfaces. Consequently the administrative assistant must understand the potential risk of handling contaminated surfaces.

INFECTION CONTROL IN THE DENTAL OFFICE

Because patient care actually begins in the business office, it is important to identify the role of the administrative assistant as it relates to infection control in the clinical area. Every dental healthcare worker is responsible for breaking the cycle of **disease transmission** (Figure 17-1). Safe practice is based on the following principles:

- A complete and accurate patient history must be obtained and screening must be done.
- Aseptic techniques must be observed using personal protective equipment.
- Healthcare workers must strictly adhere to acceptable sterilization procedures.
- Acceptable disinfection procedures must be practiced.
- Equipment asepsis and dental laboratory asepsis must be practiced.

The administrative assistant is responsible for the first step in safe practice, obtaining complete and detailed information about the patient. The records discussed in Chapter 7 must be completed, dated, signed, and reviewed thoroughly by the dentist. During treatment procedures, the administrative assistant

  PRACTICE NOTE
Every dental healthcare worker is responsible for breaking the cycle of disease transmission.

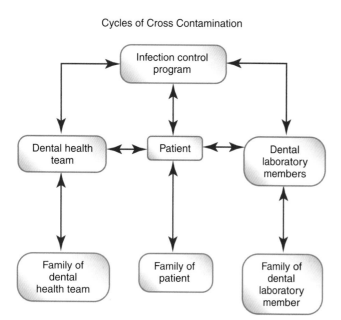

Figure 17-1 Cycle of disease transmission.

must make sure that protocols are followed and the necessary barrier materials are available for use. Finally the administrative assistant ensures that the records used during the treatment procedure are transferred safely from the clinical site to the business office without **cross contamination**.

Table 17-2 presents several situations that the administrative assistant may encounter in attempting to maintain safe practice in the office. The administrative assistant must be able to distinguish between right actions and wrong actions and must understand the consequences of a wrong action in infection control. Box 17-1 presents a self-assessing list of points the administrative assistant should live by when working in the dental office to make sure that disease transmission is not being promoted.

Health Protection Program for the Dental Staff

The administrative assistant plays a role in maintaining the health and safety of the patients and healthcare workers in the office. Although not usually assigned the task of infection control coordinator, he or she should be familiar with the aspects of this process. After all, the administrative assistant is responsible for managing the office, and must be able to access all records.

The office's personnel policy must include a health service program for the staff that covers the following:

- Education and training
- Immunizations
- Exposure prevention and postexposure management
- Medical conditions, work-related illness, and work restrictions
- Allergies or sensitivities to work-related materials, such as latex
- Records maintenance, data management, and confidentiality issue
- A referral arrangement with a medical physician who is available to treat staff members for emergencies and perform medical evaluation and treatment quickly and appropriately
- Confidential, up-to-date medical records for all workers, including documentation of immunizations and tests

The administrative assistant and the dentist must work together to maintain the safety of all staff members and patients. Attention to records maintenance and continual education and training can ensure safe practice.

Government Regulations

All dental professionals are expected to comply with current guidelines and regulations governing infection control, hazard communication, and medical waste disposal. Several agencies are responsible for providing the dental professional with the current regulations affecting each of these areas. The employer is primarily responsible for maintaining current copies of all state

TABLE 17-2 **Recognizing Wrong from Right in Infection Control**

Wrong	Effect	Right
Shaking hands while wearing contaminated gloves	Disease transmission may occur during cross-contamination.	Remove gloves and wash hands prior to leaving examination gloves treatment room; nod and speak greetings to the individual.
Pulling mask on and off	Contact with the face with contaminated gloves can expose unprotected tissues to disease. If mask is contaminated, contact with gloved or ungloved hands will also allow disease transmission.	Always leave mask in place; if movement for repositioning is necessary, either do it with clean gloves or slight readjustment may be made by using the upper arm or shoulder.
Wearing the same mask for more than one patient	Masks become moist field, allowing penetration of particles through the mask.	Always change masks between patients and use more than one mask if treatment procedure is lengthy.
Reusing same gloves	Most gloves have microscopic openings allowing penetration of microbes. Washing gloves increases the potential for disease transmission.	Gloves are always changed between patients; gloves may need to be changed during a treatment procedure that is lengthy.
Placing patient records in treatment room	Records may become exposed to aerosols or through handling; these records are transferred to the business office after treatment, thus exposing the business personnel to the potential for disease.	Records other than radiographs should be kept outside the treatment room to avoid contamination. If the records must be in the treatment room, they should be kept out of reach of aerosols and handled with clean hands or with overgloves rather than examination gloves.
Storing instruments in trays or drawers instead of sealed bags in treatment rooms	Instruments not individually bagged (if not part of a tray set-up) may be exposed to aerosols or other contact during treatment and may become contaminated.	All instruments processed through sterilization should be bagged to ensure their sterility when used. Instruments, even in closed drawers, may not remain sterile.
Eating in the laboratory or other contaminated site	Surfaces can become contaminated from instruments or materials exposed to patient aerosols or handling.	A staff lounge or eating area must be available in a site away from potentially contaminated materials.
Wearing a V-neck laboratory coat	Garments under lab coat can become contaminated. If wearing a V-neck shirt underneath, skin will be exposed.	Always wear high neck lab coat when working with patients or in the laboratory. These coats should be removed before leaving the workplace.
Wearing dangling earrings, piercings, necklaces, bracelets and/or ties	Items can become contaminated. They may hang in the patient's face or catch on something.	Minimize jewelry to only wearing wedding bands and small post earrings.

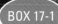

BOX 17-1 **Self-Assessment for the Administrative Assistant**

If the administrative assistant can agree with each of the following statements, he or she probably can perform the duties safely and free of potential risks. If the administrative assistant cannot agree with one of these statements, the person may jeopardize his or her own health and the safety of others with whom he or she has had contact.

1. I completely understand the Occupational Safety and Health Administration (OSHA) concepts and the need to perform my duties safely.
2. I understand the need for immunizations.
3. I am sure that the pencils, pens, and records with which I come in contact regularly are free of contamination.
4. I am never in contact with exposed surfaces, body fluids, or contaminated areas or involved with sterilization processes.
5. I never receive materials from the hands of a dental healthcare worker (DHCW) who is wearing contaminated examination gloves.
6. I never retrieve dental floss or toothbrushes that were used in a patient education treatment room.

7. I never subject myself to the potential for disease transmission by performing simple tasks such as removing armamentaria from a treatment room.
8. I will never be required to provide emergency care to patients or others without protective personal barriers.
9. I never come in contact with infectious waste or patient laboratory cases.
10. I have never encountered my colleagues wearing their clinical attire into a public area.
11. I never assume that because the patient is a family member or personal friend, he or she is not potentially contagious.

If the administrative assistant answers "no" to any of the preceding points, he or she must do so only if he or she strictly adheres to the appropriate barriers and protocols provided by the Centers for Disease Control and Prevention (CDC), OSHA, or the American Dental Association (ADA).

and federal regulations that relate to the dental office. These guidelines must be reviewed, and their implementation in the office must be documented.

OSHA established guidelines to protect workers from occupational exposure to blood-borne diseases. Regulations now require that employees in direct contact with blood or infectious materials and substances are required to use **standard precautions**; that is, all patients must be treated as if they are potentially infectious with the **human immunodeficiency virus (HIV)**, the **hepatitis B virus (HBV)**, or other infectious diseases. An overview of the latest required OSHA standards is presented in Box 17-2.

> ## PRACTICE NOTE
> All dental professionals are expected to comply with current guidelines and regulations governing infection control, hazard communications, and medical waste disposal.

When standard precautions are used, additional procedures are not necessary for treating a patient known to have an infectious disease. Under standard precautions, each workplace must meet the following goals:
- Be hazard free
- Provide personal protective clothing and equipment
- Maintain employee training and health records

> ## PRACTICE NOTE
> If standard precautions are used, additional procedures are not necessary for treating a patient known to have an infectious disease.

The **Environmental Protection Agency (EPA)**, a federal regulatory agency, developed a program for overseeing the handling, tracking, transportation, and disposal of medical waste once it has left the dental office.

The CDC, a division of the US Public Health Service, also provides recommendations for healthcare workers. It is responsible for investigating and controlling various diseases, such as dental caries, hepatitis, and tuberculosis, which currently is on the rise.

BOX 17-2 **Overview of Standards Established by the Occupational Safety and Health Administration (OSHA)**

- Employers must identify and train workers "reasonably anticipated" to be at risk of exposure. They also must reduce or eliminate exposure and offer medical care and counseling if exposure occurs.
- Employers must have written exposure control plans, identifying workers with occupational exposure to blood and other infectious materials and specifying ways to protect and train those workers.
- Employers must have a plan that includes protocols for **barrier techniques**, sterilization, disinfection, hepatitis B vaccination, and the handling of office accidents, including exposure to infectious materials. They must also have plans to protect and train employees; these plans must be reviewed and updated annually and must be available to employees at all times.
- The use of puncture-resistant containers, hand washing as gloves are changed, and proper personal protective equipment are required.
- Employers must provide laundering of protective clothing. Laundering of protective clothing at home is prohibited.
- Sharps must be recapped with a one-handed technique or a mechanical recapping device.
- Employees must wear gowns and gloves when a risk exists of exposure to or skin contact with blood, body fluids, or saliva.
- General work clothes are not considered protection against exposure to blood, body fluids, or saliva.

- Employees must wear masks, eyewear, or a face shield during exposure to splashes, spray, spatter, droplets of blood, body tissue, or saliva.
- Eyewear must have fixed side shields.
- Employers must provide personal protective equipment to be worn by all employees (i.e., gowns, gloves, masks, and eyewear) at no expense to employees.
- **Sharps containers** must be labeled and easily accessible to areas where sharps are used.
- Hepatitis B vaccinations must be offered to employees at no cost after training is completed but within 10 days of placement in a position that involves occupational exposure.
- If a worker declines the hepatitis B vaccination, access is still required if the employee has a change of mind.
- Employers must provide a training program during working hours for all employees in occupational exposure positions by June 4, 1992, and annually in subsequent years.
- Training records must be kept for 3 years after the training sessions.
- The following must be handled as infectious waste (i.e., placed in special, labeled containers): pathological waste sharps; blood and body fluid items that release blood, body fluid, or saliva when compressed; and items caked with dried blood, body fluid, or saliva if such contaminants can be released from the materials during handling.

From Occupational Safety and Health Administration: *CP2–2.69: Exposure procedures for occupational exposure to bloodborne pathogens,* Washington, DC, 2001, U.S. Department of Labor.

Maintaining Regulatory Records

The dentist may assign the administrative assistant the job of maintaining the myriad records required to meet the various standards and regulations. To aid this process, many companies and organizations have provided brochures and manuals, such as the ADA's *Regulatory Compliance Manual* (Figure 17-2). An implementation control form (Figure 17-3) can help ensure that all records are kept as required. Examples of all records should be included in the office procedures manual or the *Regulatory Compliance Manual*.

These records should be kept confidential and should include the following:

- Exposure determination forms (see Figure 17-4 on p. 309), which describe the office infection control program and procedures
- Employee training records (see Figure 17-5 on p. 310), which describe HBV vaccination availability, requirements, and implementation
- Employee medical records (see Figure 17-6 on p. 312)
- Informed refusal for hepatitis B vaccination (see Figure 17-7 on p. 313)
- Postexposure evaluation and follow-up training
- Employee informed refusal of postexposure medical evaluation (see Figure 17-8 on p. 314)
- Incident report of exposure to occupational illness (see Figure 17-9 on p. 315)

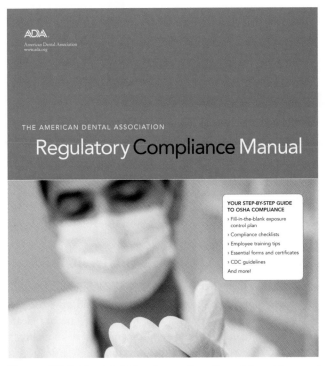

Figure 17-2 The ADA's Regulatory Compliance Manual is a good resource to help the administrative assistant ensure that the dental office is complying with the necessary standards and regulations related to infection control. (Courtesy of American Dental Association, Chicago.)

Hazard Communication Program

OSHA's hazard communication standards require all dental professionals to develop and implement a program involving employee training, compilation of a list of hazardous chemicals, maintenance of MSDSs, and proper labeling of all chemicals in the office. This program must apply to all activities in which an individual may be exposed to hazardous chemicals under normal working conditions or during an emergency.

One individual (often the administrative assistant) is designated the hazard communication program coordinator. This person is responsible for the following:

- Disseminating information about the program
- Recognizing the hazardous properties of chemicals found in the workplace
- Keeping up-to-date on procedures for safe handling of chemicals
- Implementing measures for protecting the office staff from hazardous chemicals

Material Safety Data Sheet

If assigned the job of hazard communication program coordinator, the administrative assistant should make and maintain a list of all products in the office that contain hazardous chemicals (see Figure 17-10 on p. 316). MSDSs, which are a government-approved or equivalent forms that provide specific information about chemicals purchased for use in a workplace, are an important part of the records. MSDSs for all products with hazardous potential are compiled and kept updated in a master list available to all individuals. An MSDS should include the manufacturer's name and address, the product name, the generic name (if applicable), potential routes of entry, the organs affected by the chemical, and means of protecting against or reducing the effects of chemical exposure (e.g., **eyewash**).

Labeling of Hazardous Materials

The hazard communication program coordinator also is responsible for properly labeling hazardous chemicals and substances. Many products purchased from dental supply companies arrive with permanently affixed information about hazardous chemicals. When items are purchased in bulk and then transferred to smaller containers, hazard communication labels must be put on these containers. The label must show that the MSDS was obtained and must designate the chemical's hazard class, the routes of entry into the body, and the organs affected. Labeling kits (see Figure 17-11 on p. 317) and informational materials are available from a variety of companies.

Equipment for Hazardous Situations

The administrative assistant may be responsible for ordering equipment and training office staff members in the use of a variety of materials during a hazardous situation. Spills of chemicals, gypsum products, and flammable materials may produce

Implementation Records of OSHA Requirements

SECTION	DATE
Exposure determination	_____
Infection control program	_____
HBV vaccination	_____
Postexposure evaluation and follow-up	_____
Training	_____
Recordkeeping	_____

Figure 17-3 An implementation control form can help ensure that the necessary infection control records are kept in order.

different reactions, depending on the hazardous chemical. Again, even though the administrative assistant may not work directly with hazardous materials, it becomes his or her responsibility to ensure that safe practice is implemented, understand how to prevent accidents, and know how to react in the event of an accident.

The following equipment should be kept readily available for use in preventing or dealing with a hazardous spill:
- Fire extinguisher
- Eyewash stations
- Amalgam spill kit
- Masks approved by the National Institute for Occupational Safety and Health (NIOSH)
- Protective clothing (long sleeves, high neck, fluid-impervious fabric)
- Kitty litter and broom and dustpan
- Protective mitral gloves and glasses

- Bags in which to seal spilled materials and contaminated objects
- Well-ventilated areas for work (which allow the ventilation to be turned off if an accident occurs)
- Scavenging system (for use with nitrous oxide)

INFECTION CONTROL TECHNIQUES

In the course of dental treatment, some bioburden contamination of equipment, surfaces, instruments, and other devices occurs; sometimes these items and areas simply are not clean. The goal of any infection control program must be to maintain aseptic techniques to prevent cross infection.

Aseptic Technique

The term *aseptic technique*, or *asepsis*, refers to procedures that break the circle of infection (**sepsis** indicates the presence of

Exposure determination form

All employees holding the following positions in my office have occupational exposure.

Position   Names
1._____   1._____
2._____   2._____
3._____   3._____

Some employees holding the following positions in my office have occupational exposure. That is, they are occasionally called upon to perform tasks that may result in occupational exposure.

Position   Names
1._____   1._____
2._____   2._____
3._____   3._____

This table contains tasks and procedures that might result in occupational exposure to employees in job classifications in which only some employees have occupational exposure.

Position   Name   Tasks that may
                                result in exposure

1._____   1._____   1._____
                                _____
                                _____
                                _____

2._____   2._____   2._____
                                _____
                                _____
                                _____

Positions listed below have no occupational exposure

Position   Names
1._____   1._____
2._____   2._____

The office of   _____
located at   _____
                 _____

Figure 17-4 Sample exposure determination form.

pathogens) and, ideally, eliminate **cross contamination**. With cross contamination, a previously sterile environment is exposed to harmful agents. In some situations such as hand scrubbing an **antiseptic**, an antimicrobial agent that can be applied to a body surface, usually skin or raw mucosa, to try to prevent or minimize infection in the area of application, is used.

Procedures commonly used to maintain asepsis and prevent cross contamination include the following:
- Barrier coverings are used on surfaces that cannot be sterilized.
- Exposed surfaces are cleaned and disinfected.
- Sterile disposable items are used whenever possible.
- All contaminated reusable items are cleaned and sterilized.
- Contaminated gloved hands are not allowed to touch protective eyewear, masks, or the hair.

- Patients are asked to use a pretreatment antimicrobial mouth rinse.
- The hands are washed regularly throughout the day with an antimicrobial cleanser, such as before and after lunch and just before and immediately after the treatment of each patient. This is the single most important way to prevent cross contamination.
- Alcohol hand rubs may be used in appropriate situations.
- A complete and comprehensive health history is obtained for every patient.

Under OSHA standards, employees are allowed access to a patient's health history information. This is especially important if an employee is exposed to blood-borne pathogens in the dental office. Such information is maintained as part of a confidential medical record for employees. OSHA requires that these records be kept for all employees at risk of blood-borne pathogen transmission in an occupational setting such as the dental office.

All patients should be treated in the same manner, as potentially infectious for HBV, HIV, or other blood-borne pathogens or infectious diseases. Consistent adherence to these standard precautions is a primary professional standard of care and reduces the guesswork of determining a patient's infection status.

The following sections describe techniques that can be used to minimize contamination during treatment procedures (Box 17-3).

Personal Protection

Personal protection involves two basic considerations, immunologic protection (immunization) and barrier protection.

Immunization

Immunization is the process by which resistance to an infectious disease is induced or augmented. The human body can produce immunity to particular diseases or conditions. When no natural immunity exists for a disease, immunization may be provided through certain vaccinations.

Immunization to prevent and control cross infection is an important aspect of healthcare for dental professionals. The HBV vaccine, for example, is effective and widely available. However, several other diseases may also pose a threat to the health and well-being of dental personnel and potentially to patients.

Dental healthcare workers should receive the appropriate vaccines, which prevent the onset of clinical or subclinical infection, when symptoms of the disease are not apparent. The occupational risks for hepatitis B, measles, rubella, influenza,

Hazard Communication Training Record

This office facility has conducted a training session for individuals incorporating OSHA Hazard Communication Standard.

Name of Employer ______________________

Office Address ______________________

Date ______________________

Conducted by ______________________

Signature ______________________

Attended by ______________________

Signatures ______________________

A

Figure 17-5 **A,** Sample employee training record.

Employee Comment Form

Please provide your view of the training program to the program coordinator.

Name of Employer _____

Office Address _____

Date of training session _____

What items did you find useful? _____

_____

_____

_____

What items would you like to be covered in more detail? _____

_____

_____

_____

_____

_____

What suggestions can you offer for improvement in the training program? _____

_____

_____

B

Figure 17-5, cont'd **B,** Sample employee evaluation form for training session.

and certain other microbial infections can be minimized considerably by stimulation of artificial active immunity. Approved vaccines are available for each of these, and individuals who provide patient care should have them.

Common childhood immunizations may be given for several diseases, including diphtheria, tetanus, pertussis, polio, and rubella. Other vaccinations help prevent rubeola, mumps, and influenza. The tuberculin Mantoux test, which is not a vaccine, can determine whether an individual has been exposed to or has tuberculosis. This test is extremely important, because tuberculosis, once thought to be almost nonexistent in North America, is on the rise. Dental healthcare workers should have this test done annually.

Barrier Protection

Although vaccines are effective at minimizing the transmission of certain infections, they are not sufficient protection against the wide variety of potential pathogens encountered during patient treatment. Physical barriers are a fundamental component of an infection control program. Disposable examination gloves, overgloves, and utility gloves should be used, and during treatment, face masks and protective clinic attire and eyewear should be worn. The administrative assistant should maintain an adequate inventory of all necessary barrier equipment. A variety of barrier covers can be used during treatment (Box 17-4).

Instrument Sterilization

Sterilization is the process of rendering an item free of germs; dental sterilization commonly is achieved by steam under pressure, dry heat, or chemical vapor. The processing of dental instruments and armamentarium is the primary responsibility of the clinical assistant and requires the use of utility gloves. To maintain

Confidential employee medical record

Employee medical record
Employee name———————————————————————————
Employee address—————————————————————————————

Employee social security number ————————————————————
Employee starting date———————————————————————————
Employee termination date (if any) ——————————————————
History of HBV vaccination (date received, or, if not received, a brief explanation of
why not) ———————————————————————————————

History of other immunizations ————————————————————

History of exposure incident(s) (dates, brief explanation, attachments)——————————

Results of medical exams and follow-up procedures regarding exposure incident or
hepatitis B immunity, including written opinion of healthcare professional
(dates, brief explanation, attachments)

Information provided to the health care professional regarding hepatitis B vaccination
and/or exposure incident(s)
(dates, brief explanation, attachments)

Attach pre-employment health records to this document.
Note: maintain the record for duration of employment plus 30 years

Figure 17-6 Sample employee medical record.

sterility, many dental professionals bag instruments before the sterilization process. Color-coded indicators signify whether an instrument bag has reached sterilizing temperatures. Instruments are also bagged as tray setups to aid the efficiency of the clinical dental assistant.

The administrative assistant may assume a major role in monitoring the efficiency of the sterilization systems. Several factors may diminish the effectiveness of the various sterilizers used in the office. Frequent problems include improper wrapping of instruments; prevention of adequate penetration to the instrument surface; human error in timing the cycle; defective control gauges that do not reflect actual conditions inside the sterilizer; and sterilizer malfunction.

Although chemically treated tapes are available to determine color changes or biological controls as a means of checking for proper sterilizer function, the use of calibrated biological controls remains the gold standard of sterilization. A test strip with harmless active spores is placed in the sterilization chamber with a normal load of instruments. The test strip is returned to the manufacturer or a monitoring agency for verification that sterilization has occurred. The office receives written documentation that is maintained as a record.

Disposables

Disposable items are manufactured and identified for single use only. These items, which may include needles, saliva ejectors, prophylaxis cups, sealant, and composite brushes, should not be reused. Disposables are becoming even more widely available as manufacturers, distributors, and office personnel recognize their usefulness. Examples of recently marketed items include disposable prophylaxis angles, rag wheels, evacuation line traps, and HVE tips. These products pose less of

Informed Refusal for Hepatitis B Vaccination

I, _____ am employed as a dentist/dental assistant/
dental hygienist/laboratory technician in the office of _____ . I have been provided training
regarding the hepatitis B vaccine. I understand the effectiveness of the vaccine, the risks of contracting
hepatitis B in the dental office, and the importance of taking active steps to reduce the risk.

However, I, of my own free will and volition, and despite the urging of Dr. _____,
have elected not to be vaccinated against hepatitis B. I have personal reasons for making the decision
not to be vaccinated.

_____
Signature

Witness   _____
                                                                   Name

                                                                   _____
                                                                   Address

                                                                   _____
                                                                   City   State   Zip Code

                                                                   _____
                                                                   Date

Figure 17-7 Sample form for informed refusal of hepatitis B vaccination.

a risk of cross contamination because they do not undergo recleaning and recycling; however, they must be disposed of properly.

Laboratory Asepsis

Special handling is required when impressions, prosthetic devices, and other materials are transferred from the dental office to a commercial dental laboratory. These items, which are contaminated with the patient's saliva, blood, or other substances, can be a source of disease transmission. The ADA's councils on Dental Therapeutics and Prosthetic Services and Dental Laboratory Relations updated guidelines for infection control in dental laboratories in 1988. The ADA and the CDC recommend that impressions, appliances, and other items removed from a patient's mouth be cleaned and disinfected before they are sent to the laboratory. Items received from the laboratory for delivery to a patient should be cleaned and disinfected before placement. All items must be disinfected according to product directions. Because the administrative assistant often prepares cases for and receives them from the dental laboratory, this person should have a clear understanding of the recommended guidelines.

Disinfection of dental impressions and prostheses must be done carefully to avoid distortion of impressions or damage to metal, porcelain, or acrylic surfaces of prostheses. The administrative assistant should always consult the dentist or the dental laboratory before disinfecting any material.

Employee Informed Refusal of Postexposure Medical Evaluation

I, _____ , am employed by _____ as a dentist, dental assistant, dental hygienist, or laboratory technician. Dr. _____ has provided training for me regarding infection control and the risk of disease transmission in this dental facility.

On _____ ,20___ , I was involved in an exposure incident when I

_____

_____

_____

(describe details of needlestick, etc.) I have been offered follow-up medical evaluation in order to ensure that I have full knowledge of whether I have been exposed to or contracted an infectious disease from this incident.

However, I, of my own free will and volition, and despite Dr. _____ 's offer, have elected not to have a medical evaluation. I have personal reasons for making this decision.

_____
Signature

_____
Witness   Name

_____
Address

_____
City   State   Zip Code

_____
Date

Figure 17-8 Sample employee form for informed refusal of postexposure medical evaluation.

EDUCATING PATIENTS ABOUT INFECTION CONTROL PROGRAMS

Effective infection control must become a routine component of professional activity. The use of standard precautions in the treatment of all patients greatly minimizes occupational exposure to microbial pathogens, because it addresses the reality that most potentially infectious individuals are asymptomatic and therefore undiagnosed.

PRACTICE NOTE
Effective infection control must become a routine component of professional activity.

Procedures aimed at preventing the spread of infectious disease during dental treatment are constantly evaluated by the profession as well as by consumer agencies. Therefore the best course of action is to educate the staff and patients about the importance of safe practice and the use of standard precautions for all patients. The dental professional should be willing to freely discuss infection control with patients, using valid data. Remember, the two best ways to avoid potential litigation and OSHA inspections are prevention and good documentation.

The dental profession has done much in the past 40 years in the clinical application of infection control techniques and procedures. The implementation of appropriate recommendations by many dental professionals and government organizations continues to have a major impact on the way dental

Bureau of Statistics
Supplementary Record of
Occupational Injuries and Illnesses

U.S. Department of Labor

This form is required by Public Law 91-596 and must be kept in the establishment for 5 years. Failure to maintain can result in the issuance of citations and assessment of penalties. | Case or File No. | Form approved O.M.B. No. 1220-0029

Employer

1. Name

2. Mail address *(No. and street, city or town, State, and zip code)*

3. Location, if different from mail address

Injured or Ill Employee

4. Name *(First, middle, and last)* | Social Security No.

5. Home address *(No. and street, city or town, State, and zip code)*

6. Age | 7. Sex: *(Check one)* Male ☐ Female ☐

8. Occupation *(Enter regular job title, not the specific activity he was performing at the time of injury.)*

9. Department *(Enter name of department or division in which the injured person is regularly employed, even though he may have been temporarily working in another department at the time of injury.)*

The Accident or Exposure to Occupational Illness

If accident or exposure occurred on employer's premises, give address of plant or establishment in which it occurred. Do not indicate department or division within the plant or establishment. If accident occurred outside employer's premises at an identifiable address, give that address. If it occurred on a public highway or at any other place which cannot be identified by number and street, please provide place references locating the place of injury as accurately as possible.

10. Place of accident or exposure *(No. and street, city or town, State, and zip code)*

11. Was place of accident or exposure on employer's premises? Yes ☐ No ☐

12. What was the employee doing when injured? *(Be specific. If he was using tools or equipment or handling material, name them and tell what he was doing with them.)*

13. How did the accident occur? *(Describe fully the events which resulted in the injury or occupational illness. Tell what happened and how it happened. Name any objects or substances involved and tell how they were involved. Give full details on all factors which led or contributed to the accident. Use separate sheet for additional space.)*

Occupational Injury or Occupational Illness

14. Describe the injury or illness in detail and indicate the part of body affected. *(E.g., amputation of right index finger at second joint; fracture of ribs; lead poisoning; dermatitis of left hand, etc.)*

15. Name the object or substance which directly injured the employee. *(For example, the machine or thing he struck against or which struck him; the vapor or poison he inhaled or swallowed; the chemical or radiation which irritated his skin; or in cases of strains, hernias, etc., the thing he was lifting, pulling, etc.)*

16. Date of injury or initial diagnosis of occupational illness | 17. Did employee die? *(Check one)* Yes ☐ No ☐

Other

18. Name and address of physician

19. If hospitalized, name and address of hospital

Date of report | Prepared by | Official position

OSHA No. 101 (Feb. 1981)

Figure 17-9 Sample incident report of exposure to occupational illness. (From Bureau of Statistics, Department of Labor, Washington DC.)

treatment is practiced in the twenty-first century. It is important for dental professionals to keep up with developments and incorporate new technology into their practices as it becomes available. Membership in the Organization for Safety and Asepsis Procedures (OSAP) is most beneficial for the practice. This organization is dedicated to promoting infection control and safety policies and practices supported by science and research to the global dental community. OSAP is a method of remaining on the cutting edge. To obtain information about this organization visit the web site at www.OSAP.org.

WASTE DISPOSAL IN THE DENTAL OFFICE

Two basic types of waste are found in the dental office—regulated and nonregulated waste. Nonregulated waste refers to the total discarded solid waste that is generated from patient diagnosis, treatment, or other management areas. This includes items such as gloves, face masks, et al., but not sharps or other infectious or hazardous waste. According to OSHA, "Infectious or regulated waste means blood and blood products, contaminated sharps, pathological wastes, and microbiological wastes." In the past years, differences among federal agencies concerning the definition of infectious medical waste have narrowed. Some states and local jurisdictions may supersede these definitions, but no state or local agency can mandate a regulation that does not first encompass all federal rules.

In general all **infectious waste** destined for disposal should be placed in closable, leak-proof containers or bags that are color coded or labeled appropriately. Miller and Palenik in the book *Infection Control and Management of Hazardous Materials for the Dental Team*, 4th edition, state that "the prevailing view is that no epidemiologic evidence suggests that most medical waste is any more infective than residential waste. Also, no

Hazardous Chemicals and the Dental Products in Which They Are Found

CHEMICAL NAME	MAY BE FOUND IN:	CHEMICAL NAME	MAY BE FOUND IN:
acetic acid	photographic solutions	nickel (metal and soluble compounds)	nickel-based casting alloys, stainless steel orthodontic appliances
acetone	solvents		
aluminum oxide	polishing disks		
aluminum soluble salts	astringent agents	nitric acid	pickling solutions, some bleaching solutions
asbestos	some cast ring liners		
benzoyl peroxide	resin systems, denture resins	nitrous oxide	nitrous oxide
beryllium	nickle based casting alloys	oil mist, mineral	handpiece lubricants
calcium carbonate	polishing agents	petroleum distillates	solvents, waxes, jellies
carbon tetrachloride	solvents	phenol	disinfectants
chloroform	solvents	phosphoric acid	etching agents, phosphate cements
chromium	casting alloys		
cobalt	casting alloys	phthalic anhydride	resins
copper	amalgam, casting alloys	picric acid	pickling agents
cresol, all isomers	endodontic materials	platinum soluble salts	impression materials (addition silicones)
cyanide as CN	plating solutions		
dibutylphthalate	impression materials	platinum	casting alloys
ethyl acetate	solvents	propane	burners
ethyl acrylate	resins	rouge	polishing agents
ethyl alcohol	solvents, sterilizing agents	silica, amorphous including natural distomaceous earth	composite resins, materials
ethyl chloride	solvents, topical refrigerants		
ethyl silicate	silicate investments, impression materials (condensation silicones)	silica, crystalline (quartz)	composite resins, porcelain, investments
ethylene oxide	sterilizing agents	silicon carbide	polishing disks, cutting wheels
fluoride dust	fluoride-containing composites	silver (metal and soluble compounds)	amalgam, endodontic points, casting alloys, photographic solutions
formaldehyde	sterilizing agents		
glutaraldehyde	sterilizing agents		
hydrochloric acid	pickling solutions, bleaching agents	sulfuric acid	etchant for alloys, copper plating solutions
hydrogen fluoride	etching agents for porcelain	talc, nonasbestos form	gloves
hydroquinone	methacrylate and denture base resins, photographic solutions	tantalum	nickel-chromium-cobalt alloys
		tin, inorganic compounds	amalgam, polishing pastes
		tin, organic compounds	impression material (condensation silicones)
iodine	iodophor disinfectants and antimicrobial hand cleansers	titanium dioxide	porcelain, impression materials
isopropyl alcohol	solvents, wiping agents	toluene	solvents
lead/inorganic lead compounds	impression materials (some polysulfides)	trichloroethane	solvents
		uranium, insoluble compounds	porcelain
LPG (liquid petroleum gas)	burners	vinyl chloride	maxillofacial plastics, mouth guard trays
mercury	amalgam		
mercury/organic	topical antiseptics		
methyl acetate	solvents	xylene	solvents
methyl alcohol	denatured alcohol	zirconium compounds	porcelain, polishing pastes
methyl methacrylate	denture base resins		
methylene chloride	solvents		
molybdenum, insoluble compounds	casting alloys (chromium-cobalt alloys, stainless steel)		

Figure 17-10 List of common chemicals found in a dental office. (From Finkbeiner BL, Johnson CS: *Mosby's comprehensive dental assisting*, St Louis, 1995, Mosby.)

epidemiologic evidence indicates that current medical/dental waste handling and disposal procedures have caused disease in the community. Therefore identifying wastes for which special precautions are necessary is largely a matter of judgment concerning the relative risk of disease transmission."

The primary factor in defining regulated medical waste is determined by the presence of blood or other potentially infectious material (OPIM). In dentistry OPIM is mainly saliva. Most of the regulated waste in dental offices consists of contaminated sharps and extracted teeth. Some offices involved with surgeries may also generate a small amount of nonsharp solid medical waste such as 2 × 2s or cotton rolls saturated/caked with blood or saliva.

Warning labels should be affixed to containers of infectious waste, refrigerators and freezers containing blood, other

containers used to store or transport blood or other potentially infectious materials, and any potentially infectious materials. The labels required by OSHA should be used in the office. These labels should be fluorescent orange or orange-red or predominantly so and should have lettering or symbols in a contrasting color (see Figure 17-11, *B* and *C*).

Although the administrative assistant is not directly responsible for preparation of the waste, this person should be aware that all infectious material is disposed of in accordance with federal, state, and local regulations and that appropriate forms are maintained. A medical waste tracking form (see Figure 17-12 on p. 319) is completed for medical waste disposal, and a shipment log (see Figure 17-13 on p. 319) is used to verify the mode of transport and other vital information.

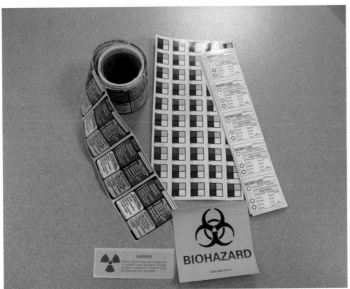

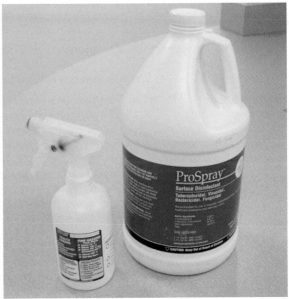

A

B

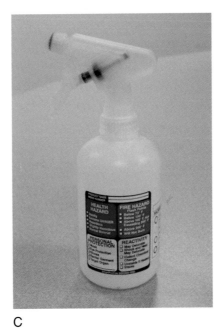

C

Figure 17-11 A, Supply kit for hazardous materials labeling. **B** and **C,** Hazardous labels affixed to containers.

BOX 17-3 **Flowchart for Management of Occupational Exposures to Blood-Borne Pathogens**

Before an Exposure Occurs . . .

Dental Worker
- Receives training in risks of occupational exposures, immediate reporting of injuries/ exposures, and reporting procedures within the practice setting

Employer /Infection Control Coordinator
- Establishes referral arrangements and protocol for employees to follow in the event of exposures to blood or saliva via puncture injury, mucous membrane, or non-intact skin
- Trains occupationally exposed employees in postexposure protocols
- Makes available and pays for hepatitis B vaccine for workers at occupational risk

Qualified Healthcare Provider
- Contracts with dentist-employer to provide medical evaluation, counseling, and follow-up care to dental office employees exposed to blood or other potentially infectious materials.
- Keeps current on public health guidelines for managing occupational exposure incidents and is aware of evaluating healthcare provider's responsibilities ethically and by law.

(Continued)

BOX 17-3

Flowchart for Management of Occupational Exposures to Blood-Borne Pathogens—cont'd

When an Exposure Incident Occurs...

Dental Worker

1. Performs first aid
2. Reports injury to employer
3. Reports to the designated healthcare professional for medical evaluation and follow-up care, as indicated

Employer/Infection Control Coordinator

1. Documents events in the practice setting
2. Immediately directs employee to evaluating healthcare professional
3. Sends to evaluating healthcare professional:
   - copy of standard job description of employee
   - exposure report
   - source patient's identity and bloodborne infection status (if known)
   - employee's HBV status and other relevant medical information
   - copy of the Occupational Safety and Health Administration (OSHA) Bloodborne Pathogen Standard
4. Arranges for source patient testing, if the source patient is known and has consented
5. Pays for postexposure evaluation and, if indicated, prophylaxis

Qualified Healthcare Provider

1. Evaluates exposure incident, worker, and source patient for HBV, HCV, and HIV, maintaining confidentiality
   - Arranges for collection and testing (with consent) of exposed worker and source patient as soon as feasible (if serostatus is not already known)
   - In the event that consent is not obtained for HIV testing arranges for blood sample to be preserved for up to 90 days (to allow time for the exposed worker to consent to HIV testing)
   - Arranges for additional collection and testing as recommended by the U.S. Public Health Service/CDC
   - Notifies worker of results of all testing and of the need for strict confidentiality with regard to source patient results
   - Provides counseling
   - Provides postexposure prophylaxis, if medically indicated
2. Assesses reported illnesses/side effects.
3. Within 15 days of evaluation sends to ← the employer a Written Opinion, which contains (only)*
   - documentation that the employee was informed of evaluation results and the need for any further follow-up
   - whether HBV vaccine was indicated and if it was received

6. Receives Written Opinion from evaluating healthcare professional
   - Files copy of Written Opinion in employee's confidential medical record (if maintained by the dentist employer)
4. Receives copy of Written ← • Provides copy of Written Opinion to exposed employee
   Opinion

* All other findings or diagnoses remain confidential and are not included in the written report.
Courtesy Organization for Safety & Asepsis Procedures (OSAP): *CDC guidelines: from policy to practice*, Annapolis, MD, 2007, Author.

BOX 17-4

Commonly Used Barrier Covers

Barriers coverings may be used on a variety of surfaces to lessen the need for surface disinfection

Treatment Room

- Light handle covers
- On/off switch on operating light
- Plastic bag over dental chair and adjustment buttons
- Paper towel folded to cover working end of thumb forceps used to retrieve instruments from the mobile cabinetry
- Plastic tubing over hoses of unit (when accessible)
- Plastic bag attached to mobile cabinetry for debris
- Overgloves to retrieve armamentaria and charts

Radiography Treatment Room

- Plastic bag over radiographic head and PID
- Plastic covering over on/off switch
- Plastic covering over touch/control panel
- Plastic bag over dental chair
- Barrier-type film packets
- Covering over area from which each dental film is retrieved. (If the film is laid out on a surface before exposure, a covering placed under the film before use eliminates disinfection of the surface.)

MEDICAL WASTE TRACKING FORM

GENERATOR

1. Generator's Name and Mailing Address

2. Tracking Form Number

4. State Permit or ID No.

3. Telephone Number ( )

5. Transporter's Name and Mailing Address

6. Telephone Number ( )

7. State Transporter Permit or ID No.

EPA Med. Waste ID No.

8. Destination Facility Name and Address

9. Telephone Number ( )

10. State Permit or ID No.

11. US EPA Waste Description	12. Total No. Containers	13. Total Weight or Volume
a. Regulated Medical Waste (Untreated)		
b. Regulated Medical Waste (Treated)		
c. State Regulated Medical Waste		

14. Special Handling Instructions and Additional Information

15. **Generator's Certification:**
Under penalty of criminal and civil prosecution for the making or submission of false statements, representations, or omissions, I declare, on behalf of the generator _____ that the contents of this consignment are fully and accurately described above and are classified, packaged, marked, and labeled in accordance with all applicable State and Federal regulations, and that I have been authorized, in writing, to make such declarations by the person in charge of the generator's operation.

Printed/Typed name   Signature   Date

INSTRUCTIONS FOR COMPLETING MEDICAL WASTE TRACKING FORM

Copy 1 — GENERATOR COPY: Mailed by Destination Facility to Generator
Copy 2 — DESTINATION FACILITY COPY: Retained by Destination Facility
Copy 3 — TRANSPORTER COPY: Retained by Transporter
Copy 4 — GENERATOR COPY: Retained by Generator
As required under 40 CFR Part 259:
1. This multicopy (4-page) shipping document must accompany each shipment of regulated medical waste generated in a Covered State.
2. Items numbered 1-14 must be completing before the generator can sign the certification. Items 4, 7, 10, 11c, & 19 are optional unless required by the State. Item 22 must be completed by the destination facility.

For assistance in completing this form, contact your nearest State office or Regional EPA office, or call (800) 424-9346.

TRANSPORTER

16. **Transporter 1** (Certification of Receipt of Medical Waste as described in items 11, 12, & 13)

Printed/Typed name   Signature   Date

17. **Transporter 2 or Intermediate Handler** (name and address)

18. **Telephone Number** ( )

19. **State Transporter Permit or ID No.**

EPA Med. Waste ID No.

20. **Transporter 2 or Intermediate Handler** (Certification of Receipt of Medical Waste as described in items 11, 12, &13)

Printed/Typed name   Signature   Date

21. **New Tracking Form Number** (for consolidated or remanifested waste)

DESTINATION

22. **Destination facility** (Certification of Receipt of Medical Waste as described in items 11, 12, & 13)
☐ Received in accordance with items 11, 12, &13

Printed/Typed name   Signature   Date
(If other than destination facility, indicate address, phone, and permit or ID no. in box 14.)

23. **Discrepancy Box** (Any discrepancies should be noted by item number and initials)

Figure 17-12 Sample medical waste tracking form.

Transporter Name and Address	Transporter State Permit or ID Number	Quantity and Category of Waste Transported		Date of Shipment	Signature of Representative Accepting Waste for Transport
		Containers	Pounds		
		Untreated		__/__/__	
		Treated			
		Untreated		__/__/__	
		Treated			
		Untreated		__/__/__	
		Treated			
		Untreated		__/__/__	
		Treated			
		Untreated		__/__/__	
		Treated			
		Untreated		__/__/__	
		Treated			
		Untreated		__/__/__	
		Treated			

Figure 17-13 Sample generator shipment log.

KEY TERMS

Acquired immunodeficiency syndrome (AIDS)—A disease caused by a retrovirus known as the human immunodeficiency virus type 1 (HIV-1). A related but distinct retrovirus (HIV-2) has recently appeared in a limited number of patients in the United States.

Antiseptic—An antimicrobial agent that can be applied to a body surface, usually skin or raw mucosa, to try to prevent or minimize infection in the area of application.

Autogenous infection—Self-produced infection; originating within the body.

Barrier techniques—Protocols used in infection control to prevent cross contamination between healthcare worker and patient or between patients.

Bioburden—Any substance that interferes with the sterilization process.

Blood-borne pathogens—Organisms transmitted through blood or blood products that can cause infectious diseases, such as human immunodeficiency virus (HIV) infection, AIDS, and hepatitis B virus (HBV) infection.

Centers for Disease Control and Prevention (CDC)—A federal agency responsible for investigating the incidence of disease, monitoring diseases throughout the world, and conducting research directed toward controlling and preventing disease.

Communicable disease—A disease that may be transmitted directly or indirectly from one individual to another.

Cross contamination—The transfer of impurities, infection, or disease from one source to another.

Dental healthcare worker (DHCW)—A dental professional who provides care to patients or has some contact with dental patients in the office.

Disease transmission—The spread of disease-causing organisms from one person to another.

Disinfectants—Chemicals used to destroy some forms of pathogenic microorganisms.

Disinfection—The process of destroying some pathogenic microorganisms.

Environmental Protection Agency (EPA)—A federal agency that regulates the use and disposal of hazardous materials. Workplace management of hazardous materials falls under the jurisdiction of OSHA.

Eyewash—An OSHA-required device used to flush the eyes with water when exposure to unnatural contaminants has occurred.

Hazardous waste—Materials identified as hazardous to human health; local, state, and federal regulations require special handling of such materials.

Hepatitis B virus (HBV)—Virus that causes a form of hepatitis B that is transmitted in contaminated serum in blood transfusions, the passing of contaminated fluids, or by use of contaminated needles and instruments. *Caution*: Any DHCW who comes in contact with blood, body fluids, or body tissues has an increased risk of developing this type of hepatitis. A DHCW who does not have the protection of the HBV antigen should be immunized with a hepatitis B vaccine.

Human immunodeficiency virus (HIV)—See *Acquired immunodeficiency virus (AIDS)*.

Infection—Invasion of body tissues by disease-producing microorganisms and the reaction of the tissues to these microorganisms or their toxins (or both).

Infectious waste—Blood and blood products, contaminated sharps, pathologic wastes, and microbiological wastes.

Occupational Safety and Health Administration (OSHA)—A federal agency that establishes guidelines and regulations for worker safety. These guidelines include the storage and disposal of toxic chemicals and hazardous materials and the safe and proper use of clinical and office equipment.

Personal protective equipment (PPE)—Materials used to protect the employee when occupational exposure is possible. Such equipment includes but is not limited to disposable gloves, disposable surgical masks and gowns, laboratory coats and scrubs, and face shields or eye protection with side shields.

Sanitization—The act of making something sanitary, or clean and free of dirt.

Sepsis—A pathologic state characterized by the presence of pathogens.

Sharp containers—Enclosed containers from which an article cannot be retrieved. They are used for the disposal of sharp items that may cause punctures or cuts when handled, such as broken medical glassware, needles, scalpel blades, and suture needles.

Sterilization—The process of rendering an item free of germs; dental sterilization commonly is achieved by steam under pressure, dry heat, or chemical vapor.

Standard precautions—Protocols used to maintain an aseptic field and to prevent cross contamination and cross infection between healthcare providers, between healthcare providers and patients, and between patients. Such measures, formerly called *universal precautions*, include but are not limited to sterilization of instruments and other equipment; isolation and disinfection of the immediate clinical environment; use of sterile disposables; scrubbing; use of personal protective equipment (e.g., mask, gown, protective eyewear, and gloves); and proper disposal of contaminated wastes.

LEARNING ACTIVITIES

1. Explain why it is important that each member of the dental team understand the concepts of infection control and the need for immunization.
2. Identify common barrier materials and explain their use.
3. Explain the term standard (formerly universal) precautions.
4. Describe the role the administrative assistant plays in infection control.
5. Review various office situations and identify incidents that might require special attention to prevent the transmission of disease-causing organisms from the treatment room or dental laboratory to the business office.

Please refer to the student workbook for additional learning activities.

BIBLIOGRAPHY

American Dental Association: *ADA regulatory compliance manual. Chicago*, The Association.

Centers for Disease Control and Prevention: Guidelines for infection control in dental health-care settings, *MMWR* 52(RR-17):2003.

Centers for Disease Control and Prevention: *Guidelines for preventing M. Tuberculois in health care settings 2005*, Washington, DC, 2005, Author.

Miller CH, Palenik CJ: *Infection control and management of hazardous materials for the dental team*, ed 4, St Louis, 2010, Mosby.

Molinari JA: Infection control: its evolution to the current standard (formerly universal) precautions, *JADA* 134(5):569, 2003.

Molinari JA, et al: *Cottone's practical infection control in dentistry*, Philadelphia, 2009, Lippincott Williams & Wilkins.

RECOMMENDED WEB SITES

www.cdc.gov/Handhygiene/ (CDC hand hygiene fact sheet.)
ww.ada.org (General guidelines for dentistry.)
www.needlestick.com (Managing needle sticks.)
www.cdcresources.org (Links to CDC resources.)
www.osha.gov/fso/osp/index.html (State OSHA plans.)
www.osap.org (Membership in the organization and updates on aseptic procedures.)
www.hepfi.org/Hepinfo/Fact5201-99.htm

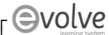

evolve
learning system

Please visit http://evolve.elsevier.com/Finkibeiner/practice for additional practice activities.

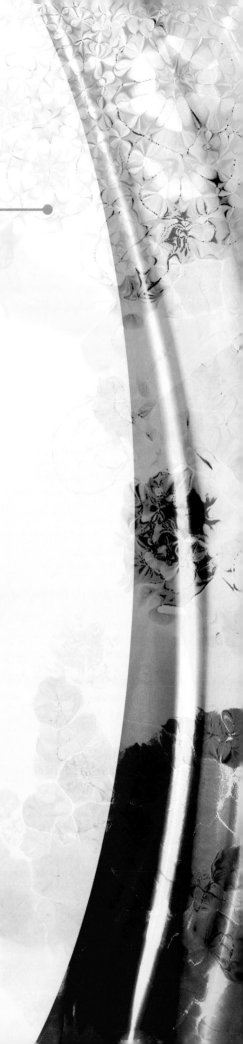

PART IV

THE DENTAL ASSISTANT IN THE WORKPLACE

18

Planning and Managing Your Career Path

CHAPTER OUTLINE

Preparing for the Job Search
Planning and Organizing
Five Important Questions

Self-Assessment
Critical Analysis
Identifying Personal Assets and Liabilities

Marketing Your Skills

Job Priorities
Determining Your Career Philosophy
Determining Your Worth to a Practice

Potential Areas of Employment
Private Practice
Institutional Dentistry
Insurance Offices
Research
Dental Manufacturers
Management Consulting Firms
Teaching

Where Do You Begin to Find Employment Opportunities?
School Placement
Newspaper Advertisements
Employment Agencies
Professional Organizations and Journals
Internet and World Wide Web
Personal Networks

Preparing Employment Data
Preparing a Letter of Application
Contacting an Office by Telephone
Creating a Résumé
Optional Areas

Completing the Job Application Form

Preparing for an Interview
The Personal Interview
Other Formats for Interviewing
Concluding the Interview
Following Up the Interview
Regular Self-Evaluation on the Job

Hints for Success as Part of the Dental Team
Learn the Names of Staff Members
Listen Attentively
Establish Meaningful Social Friendships
Use a Notebook and Calendar to Record Important Activities and
    Procedures
Observe Office Hours

Use Judgment in Working Overtime and Taking Breaks
Do Not Flaunt Your Education and Abilities
Seek Honest Performance Evaluations
Maintain Office Policies
Be Yourself

Asking for a Raise
Job Termination
Attitudes for Continued Success

LEARNING OUTCOMES

- Define key terms.
- Determine your career goals.
- Identify your personal assets and liabilities for a job.
- Identify legal considerations in hiring.
- Explain the use of preemployment testing.
- Describe new employee orientation.
- Determine desirable characteristics for a job you might seek.
- Determine methods of marketing your skills.
- Identify personal priorities for a potential job.
- Develop a career/life philosophy.
- Identify factors to consider in salary negotiations.
- Identify potential areas of employment.
- Prepare data for job applications and interviews.
- Identify potential interview questions.
- List suggestions for a successful interview.
- Prepare an interview follow-up letter.
- Explain how to advance on the job.
- List hints for success in a job on the dental team.
- Describe how to terminate a job.

PREPARING FOR THE JOB SEARCH

Planning and Organizing

At this juncture in reading this textbook you have mastered a variety of skills. It is now time to begin a job search. You may have completed a formal educational program or course of study as a clinical or administrative assistant, and you may already have passed a certification examination or other credentialing examination. Now you are ready to begin the job search. A successful job search requires organization and effort. You cannot simply walk out the door and wander around asking about jobs. Nor can you look for work only when you feel like it or when it's convenient. Planning and organizing are critical to job search success. This chapter will aid you in planning and organizing yourself to begin the most important career task of your working life.

When you apply for various jobs, your prospective employers will assume that you have completed your studies and obtained your credentials as a Certified Dental Assistant, a Registered Dental Assistant, a state credential, or have some form of business specialty credentials. This chapter emphasizes the tasks necessary to market your skills as a highly educated dental assistant with special training in business office management.

You sometimes may feel nervous about the prospect of taking a credentialing examination or finding a job. Even after attending formal classes or studying for a specific job, your self-confidence may falter. However, cultivating positive attitudes and taking time to reflect on career goals often help a person get on track in seeking a job. This is the time in your career when you must reflect on all the skills you have acquired. The top eight *hard skills* listed by dentist employers are:

1. Interpersonal skills
2. Teamwork skills
3. Verbal communication skills
4. Critical thinking skills
5. Technical skills
6. Computer skills
7. Written communications skills
8. Leadership skills

 PRACTICE NOTE
Cultivating positive attitudes and taking time to reflect on career goals often help a person get on track in seeking a job.

In addition to hard skills, you have gained *soft skills*, such as value clarification, self-discipline, ethical behavior, positive attitudes, creativity, and anger and stress management. As you reflect on your skills, both hard and soft, you should analyze what they mean to your career path.

Five Important Questions

Before you venture into the job market as an administrative assistant, you must identify your career goals. Obviously you are interested in the business office, because you have spent considerable time studying in this field. Therefore at this juncture, you should explore ways your career can develop in that field in the future. A career path is based on careful planning and preparation, but it can be altered by unexpected opportunities and luck. To begin preparation, you should ask yourself the series of questions shown in the job preparation ladder (Figure 18-1). Prospective employers will put your résumé on the top of the job application pile if you spend some time reflecting on each of these questions: Where have I been? Where am I now? Where am I going? How am I going to get there? How will I know when I have arrived?

Before going to any job interviews, you should share your thoughts about these questions with peers or spend some time alone reflecting on them. This sharing and introspection can help you build confidence in your plans and goals for a career.

Where Have I Been?

This question helps you to review your past and identify some of the reasons you arrived where you are. It is your origin and thus forms the foundation of your preparation ladder. Some individuals may find looking at the past depressing, whereas others may yearn for the comfort of the past. Regardless of the impact of your past, reflection is worthwhile. Some personal information is confidential, and certain types of questions may not be asked during a job interview; however, it is wise to be prepared for questions about your past employment. For instance, if you have worked at several jobs in the past, you may be asked about your reasons for having changed jobs frequently. You should explain your job history honestly.

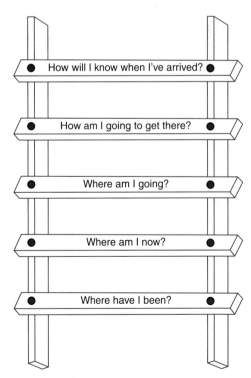

Figure 18-1 Job preparation ladder. Questions to ask yourself when preparing for a job search.

Where Am I Now?

This question seems obvious, yet you need to reassure yourself about where you are in your career path. You have just completed a course of study, you are secure or insecure in a personal or family relationship, and you are looking forward to finding a job soon or sometime in the future. Knowing where you are at the present time enables you to continue on the career path.

Where Am I Going?

This is a goal-oriented question that requires you to identify what you want to do. As you progress up the preparation ladder, you must stop to think about what you want in both the near and the distant future. For some individuals, getting a job and gaining independence are their primary goals. For others, the job may be the means to a future goal. Obtaining a job now, gaining experience, and continuing with one's education may be several short-range goals that are needed to reach the ultimate goal of teaching, obtaining a business degree, or even going to dental school. Regardless of your goals, you must realize that they may change; remaining flexible in your goals enables you to accept challenges along the way.

How Am I Going to Get There?

This question identifies the route or steps that must be taken to achieve your goals. For some, a job means independence or a sense of security and self-worth. For others, who are pursuing additional education, a short-term job supports a return to school for another degree.

How Will I Know When I Have Arrived?

This is the top rung of the ladder. To answer this question, you must define what success means to you. For some people, the definition of success is always changing. Money, material goods, or a feeling of security and satisfaction can represent success. No one answer is correct for this question. It is an individual response that only you can give.

Taking time to prepare yourself for your future career can influence a job interview. When a dentist or office manager asks you to describe yourself, your background, and your career goals, you will be prepared. Simply saying, "Oh, I don't know, there isn't much to tell," indicates that you have not given your career much thought, and a potential employer might think you feel the same about employment.

SELF-ASSESSMENT

Critical Analysis

As you begin the job search, ask yourself, "What skills and characteristics can I bring to a job and a prospective employer?" Take the time to write down your skills, strengths, and weaknesses with a prospective job in mind.

> **PRACTICE NOTE**
> Take time to write down your skills, strengths, and weaknesses with a prospective job in mind.

As you begin this exercise, you may find that you seem to concentrate on your weaknesses. This is not uncommon. Parents, teachers, and associates share criticism willingly, thinking it improves a person, but sincere praise might not be given as freely. Criticism may be so common that when praise is offered, it might be difficult to accept. Learn to accept praise, identify your positive characteristics, and develop your assets.

Identifying Personal Assets and Liabilities

How do you begin? First identify your positive characteristics and your skills. Then identify your liabilities, but analyze how these weaknesses can be overcome. For instance if you are prompt and seldom absent and you pay attention to details, you have characteristics that employers seek in a new employee (Box 18-1). You may find it difficult to use a specific type of software, or you may have a problem remembering all the American Dental Association (ADA) insurance codes; however, these skill deficiencies can be improved with experience. If a prospective employer asks about any weaknesses, you could explain that, although you have had difficulty using a specific type of software, you would like to improve this skill and are willing to spend some extra time on your own to do so. This is a positive attitude that shows an interest in improving yourself, rather than an attitude of not caring.

MARKETING YOUR SKILLS

A well-educated, experienced administrative assistant with the appropriate credentials has valuable bargaining power for obtaining a job that requires these skills and provides adequate compensation. Stating that you are a graduate of a dental assistant or business program is a credible assertion; however, supporting

---

BOX 18-1 Desirable Characteristics of an Administrative Assistant

- Promptness
- Initiative
- Dependability
- Creativity
- Flexibility
- Self-motivation
- Enthusiasm
- Honesty
- Sense of humor
- Good general health
- Willingness to accept change
- Good listener
- Willingness to work with a team
- Effective organizational skills
- Knowledge of automated equipment
- Use of proper language skills in verbal and written communications
- Attention to detail

this claim with valid data that demonstrate the positive effect you can have on the practice is likely to win you the job.

If a dentist were to state that he or she couldn't afford a well-educated administrative assistant, your response might be, "I don't believe you can afford not to have a well-educated administrative assistant." Consider the following rebuttals to the dentist's reluctance:

- Credentialed administrative assistants have proved by some form of study and perhaps by a test given by a valid national dental or business board that they have a basic understanding of dental knowledge and business procedures. Delegating business functions to an inexperienced person with no formal knowledge of business principles or the standards required by the Occupational Safety and Health Administration (OSHA) is opening the door to potential penalties and litigation.
- Losses caused by errors in records management, claim form management, appointment scheduling, payroll, accounts receivable, banking, accounts payable, or patient communication can be significantly reduced if a qualified, educated administrative assistant is put in charge of those elements of the practice. Although an initial orientation period is necessary in any office, an educated administrative assistant is already aware of the procedures and terminology used in business and dentistry.
- Mature students who return to school from other careers, such as homemaking, teaching, and nursing, can bring with them many life experiences that are valuable assets to an administrative assistant position.
- An educated person remains in the profession longer than an inexperienced person because the former has made a commitment to the profession through the educational process.

You must develop a caring, positive attitude about your ability to become an asset to the dental office. It is your responsibility, however, to live up to the claims you make. Your skills, knowledge of dentistry, investment in your education, and credentials are all tools that can be used to achieve compensation commensurate with that of other allied health or business professionals with similar backgrounds and responsibilities.

 PRACTICE NOTE
You must develop a caring, positive attitude about your ability to become an asset to the dental office.

JOB PRIORITIES

Everyone dreams of the ideal job. Yet many people are so excited to be given an interview that they take the first job offer without considering their goals, needs, and priorities. Before applying for a job or preparing for a job interview, decide what you need and want in a job and what your basic philosophy is about your career.

Determining Your Career Philosophy

As mentioned, before seeking employment, you should determine your needs and clarify your life goals and a philosophy that is consistent with them. Unfortunately, a dental assistant may accept the first job offer with little consideration given to how his or her philosophy coincides with the philosophy of the prospective employer. Carefully evaluate yourself and establish some realistic goals. Then ask yourself the following questions: Are my professional, moral, and social values compatible with those of my prospective employer? With what type of work environment do I want to be associated, a solo practice or a large group practice? Which of my skills in dental assisting or business do I want to use to the greatest extent? What are my strengths? What are my weaknesses? How can I compensate for my weaknesses? What do I want to be doing in 5 years, in 10 years? How important are salary, hours, and location?

Once you have written down your philosophy of life and enumerated your goals, remind yourself that these goals will be ever changing, and you undoubtedly will reevaluate your philosophy as you gain confidence from your new experiences.

After you have reviewed the various factors involved in job selection, decide your top five priorities for a job and then rate each job offer. A decision-making grid such as the one shown in Table 18-1 may be helpful for this purpose. The job offers are listed in the left vertical column, and the priorities are listed across the top. Starting on the left, the priorities are given a point value based on your personal needs. Each job is evaluated, and the points totaled. If a tie occurs, other characteristics might be added.

Remember, you may need to do more than one or two interviews to find the job that satisfies your goals, needs, and priorities, but remain steadfast in your job search.

Determining Your Worth to a Practice

Although many elements may be considered important in deciding whether to accept a job offer, for most people salary and benefits are the primary factors in job selection. The difficulty

---

TABLE 18-1 Job Decision-Making Grid

	Practice Environment	Salary	Benefits	Location	Challenge	Hours	Total
Point Value	6	5	4	3	2	1	
Job Offer #1		√	√	√	√	√	15
Job Offer #2	√		√	√			13
Job Offer #3	√	√		√			14

often arises when a dentist asks you during an interview what salary you expect. You need to prepare yourself for this question and not say simply, "Oh, I don't know; what have you paid your other assistants?" You need to have a firm understanding of the cost of living in your area, the comparable salaries for similar responsibilities and educational attainment, the local and national salary data available for reference, and what you are really worth in terms of your skills and knowledge. The following discussion provides ideas for formulating a benefits and salary package that could reasonably be suggested to a prospective employer. Box 18-2 lists several benefits that are commonly offered to employees.

Salary is often a difficult subject to bring up, yet it must be discussed openly before you accept a job. You need to know the beginning salary, how salary increases are obtained, and when salary increases are awarded. An employer must expect to pay a fair salary that is based on education, experience, credentials, and merit performance. The salary should be competitive with other allied health professionals who have equal responsibilities, yet it should be cost-effective.

PRACTICE NOTE
An employer must expect to pay a fair salary that is based on education + experience + credentials + merit performance.

The economics of dental assisting vary widely across the country, depending on the specific position and its responsibilities and the geographical location of the practice. According to the DANB, the average median salary of a dental assistant in 2008 was $18 per hour.[1] Data broken down by geographic location and type of practice as well as benefits can be found online at www.danb.org. A survey done by the *Dental Assisting Digest* e-Newsletter in 2008 indicated only 2.3% of the assistants who responded made more than $30 an hour, but 19% made more than $22 an hour.[2] Salary data also may be obtained from the ADA web site (www.ada.org) for various areas of the country. Dental assistants who have a formal education, management skills, and appropriate credentials are likely to receive significantly higher salaries. Realize that this is a median national hourly salary with no benefits included. It is sometimes stated that some dental professionals make higher hourly salaries than others. When salaries are discussed, care must be

taken to determine that all factors related to the salaries compared are the same. Some dollar value must be given to each of the benefits to determine the total salary and benefits package. Determine whether the job responsibilities are equitable. Education, experience, credentials, and performance evaluations are factored into the salary. Some value must be placed on job environment. Remember, no skilled administrative or clinical assistant in today's market should be making a salary that does not reflect an honest respect for the individual's productivity. It is wise to ask for a contract or an employment agreement that verifies in writing the conditions of employment. These conditions might include the salary scale, an explanation of the merit performance evaluation, the required probationary period, and how the benefits package is to be administered.

POTENTIAL AREAS OF EMPLOYMENT

An administrative assistant can choose from myriad opportunities for potential employment. These can range from a small solo practice to a large clinic. They also can include the public or the private sector, practice management consulting firms, dental manufacturers, job placement, and teaching.

Private Practice

The dental assistant may seek employment in a private practitioner's office, a group practice, or a clinic with several dentists. The practice may be a general dental practice, which means that all phases of dental treatment are rendered for a patient, or it may be limited to one of the dental specialties recognized by the ADA (i.e., endodontics, orthodontics and dentofacial orthopedics, oral and maxillofacial surgery, oral and maxillofacial pathology, pediatric dentistry, periodontics, prosthodontics, oral and maxillofacial radiology, and dental public health). In private practice, the dental assistant may find a position that is limited specifically to clinical assisting, office management, or laboratory duties or that is a combination of all these responsibilities. Private practice affords many opportunities to work closely with the dentist and patients, as well as diversification of duties, individuality, and considerable personal responsibility. As the value of a highly skilled dental assistant continues to increase, compensation and benefits in this area will continue to rise.

Institutional Dentistry

As the federal, state, and local governments demonstrate increased interest in the delivery of dental care, more facilities are being established to provide more dental services for the public. One institution that should be considered as a source of employment is a dental school. Schools offer many areas of potential employment, such as working with undergraduate or graduate dental students at chairside, supervising clinical activities, or managing business functions. Other institutions are a part of the civil service programs and offer employment in prisons, public clinics, and Veterans Administration hospitals. Additionally, hospitals, some of which are associated closely

BOX 18-2 **Potential Job Benefits**

- Dress/uniform allowance
- Retirement plan
- Health insurance
- Vision insurance
- Dental care/insurance (for self and family)
- Profit sharing
- Child care
- Membership in professional organizations
- Travel and expenses for professional meetings
- Special bonuses for holidays or production achievement

with dental schools, offer employment in various departments. The dental assistant working in an institution has the opportunity to work with a larger staff than is possible in private dental practice. Diversification of duties, participation in newly developed techniques, potential advancement to several levels of supervision, and possibly more liberal vacations (in learning institutions, vacations are often coordinated with school calendars) may be available in this setting.

Insurance Offices

Work in insurance offices is especially appealing to the dental assistant who aspires to perform various business tasks and become involved in management. With the increase in dental insurance coverage, more companies are seeking highly qualified dental assistants to work in management positions, because a broad knowledge of dentistry is an asset to their business. A position in insurance may also involve public speaking activities and travel.

Research

Hospitals and dental schools hire many dental assistants to work in research laboratories. Individuals who enjoy working with data, mathematical computations, and details and who enjoy being independent often seek positions in research.

Dental Manufacturers

An area of potential employment that should not be overlooked is the dental manufacturers, which employ dental assistants for sales and teaching. Such employment would limit contact with dentistry to a specific type or line of products, but it also offers a great opportunity to travel throughout the country and meet people.

Management Consulting Firms

Experienced dental assistants with a broad knowledge of clinical and business concepts are turning their interest into profitable businesses. Many highly qualified administrative assistants have joined management consulting firms or created their own

companies to assist dental practices in increasing their productivity through more efficient practices and marketing.

Teaching

Numerous colleges and universities have developed occupational education programs that include dental assisting. A graduate of a dental assistant program who is a Certified Dental Assistant (CDA) or Registered Dental Assistant (RDA) may transfer into a baccalaureate degree program. Anyone who has broad experience in dental assisting, is highly motivated to teach, and is patient and objective, should perhaps contact a college or university about entering their program. Another source of information is the American Dental Assistants Association (www.dentalassistant.org).

WHERE DO YOU BEGIN TO FIND EMPLOYMENT OPPORTUNITIES?

After surveying some of these potential areas of employment, where do you begin looking for the right job? Many prospects are available, and several different avenues may be used.

School Placement

The school placement office or faculty members often are notified of job opportunities in the area. Instructors frequently know employers who are interested in hiring new graduates, and they also know their students' qualifications and abilities. Most schools spend considerable time and effort obtaining information about potential job opportunities, and they take a great deal of pride in placing their graduates.

Newspaper Advertisements

Both local and out-of-area newspapers have classified sections of jobs available. Advertisements in the classified section state the qualifications required and other details about the job, including whether it is for an administrative or clinical assistant (Figure 18-2). However, in some cases the employer does not give the name of the practice or the telephone number,

---

A

> Clinical Dental Assistant needed to join a large team-oriented practice. Must have credentials for advanced functions in this state and experience in periodontics. Challenging opportunity for a skilled, ambitious professional assistant. Many benefits included. Salary commensurate to education and credentials. Send résumé to: Joseph W. Lake, 611 Main St., SE, Grand Rapids, MI 49502

B

> Dental Administrative Assistant needed for a busy orthodontic office. This position requires an energetic, ambitious person who has a broad knowledge of dentistry and business applications. For a person who enjoys a fast pace, this office provides a challenging career opportunity in practice management utilizing modern electronic business systems. Current practice management education preferred. Write to: Ashley M. Lake, DDS, 611 Main St., SE, Grand Rapids, MI 49502

Figure 18-2 A, Job advertisement for a clinical chairside assistant. **B,** Job advertisement for an administrative assistant.

Dental Administrative Assistant: Interested in an exciting position in a small, professional office? A group dental practice is expanding its clinical facilities. Position demands strong supervisory skills; ability to work effectively under pressure, use good judgment, and accept responsibility; and a working knowledge of OSHA standards. Forward your résumé to: Box #2589, Grand Rapids News, Grand Rapids, MI 49502

Figure 18-3 A sample blind ad.

but instead places a **blind ad** asking the applicant to submit a résumé (Figure 18-3). This type of ad should not be overlooked, because it becomes the employer's first means of screening applicants.

In composing a letter of application and a résumé, always remember that although first impressions are not necessarily the most accurate, they often are the most influential. A little more initiative is required of the applicant to construct a résumé than to pick up the telephone and call for an interview. The letter of application and the résumé give the prospective employer an opportunity to evaluate the applicant's keyboarding skills, communication skills, and neatness.

Employment Agencies

Both free and private employment agencies are available. Most states provide an employment service, and applicants may register with this service without charge.

Private employment agencies, which are service enterprises, provide many good job opportunities but charge a fee. Before registering with an employment agency, always check its reputation. This can be done locally or through the National Employment Association in Washington, DC. In fact, in many states dental professionals have begun their own employment agencies, and this type of firm is more likely to provide applicants with a dental background, determined by the agency's screening processes. After selecting a reputable agency, the applicant should find out about testing and placement procedures.

Professional Organizations and Journals

Local dental societies and dental assistant organizations frequently maintain employment placement services. By checking your local telephone directory or the Internet, you can quickly establish contact with one of these organizations. State and national professional journals generally have a classified section devoted to job offerings for dental assistants. Many of these jobs offer unique opportunities, possibly even relocation. State and local dental associations often allow new graduates to post their contact information in the association's newsletters or journals free of charge.

Internet and World Wide Web

The Internet is a group of computers connected all over the world, which allows people to communicate with each other. For instance, on the Internet you can obtain information about companies or dental offices worldwide.

If you are interested in working with a large dental manufacturing company or a dental school, you can use the Internet and the computer files of the World Wide Web (www) to find information about them. Many major companies and dental schools post company profiles and employment opportunities on the Internet. Smaller dental practices may not use this system, but several "temp" agencies and employment agencies seek prospective employees this way. Many web sites are available (e.g., www.jobweb.com, www.monster.com, www.yourmissinglink.com, www.careerbuilder.com) that can provide information for your job search or allow you to post your résumé.

Personal Networks

Networking is "the process of identifying and establishing a group of acquaintances, friends, and relatives who can assist you in the job search process." This approach is one of the best strategies for finding a job. In fact some studies have shown that as many as 80% of jobs are obtained through some form of networking. Friends, relatives, business associates, local dental assistant societies, dental associations, dental supply houses, and dental schools all offer myriad contacts, which can provide potential contacts in the profession, which may lead to a job opportunity. If a friend is leaving a job and knows you are interested in the same area of dentistry and are available for work, a good recommendation from your friend is always welcome.

How do you go about networking? If you have a part-time job or have had a clinical rotation in an office while you are a student, let the dentist or other staff members know that you are ready for a full-time position. If these individuals know you are interested in a full-time job, they can talk with friends in the community about your skills and often can serve as an excellent reference for you. You may want to consider a social networking website such as Facebook, My Space, Twitter, or others that provide an opportunity to interact with a network of friends, personal profiles, groups, and other professional worldwide.

PREPARING EMPLOYMENT DATA

Several steps must be taken between the determination of your goals and choice of employment and the time you actually begin work. The steps, in addition to career preparation planning, include searching for job information, writing the letter of application, creating a personal résumé, preparing for the interview, completing a job application, participating in the interview, touring the facility and meeting the staff, and following up on the interview (Figure 18-4).

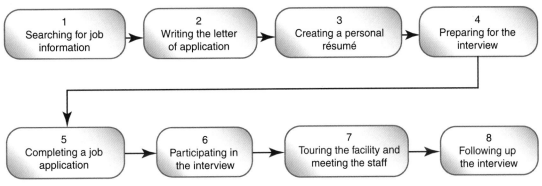

Figure 18-4 The career planning process.

Preparing a Letter of Application

The **letter of application**, or *cover letter*, has three basic goals: to arouse interest, describe your abilities, and request an interview. The letter of application should be kept to a single page, including the date and the closing signature. Every effort must be made to customize this letter and to express your philosophy, motivations, and character in a less formal format than the résumé. In fact, this letter may very well be the most important business letter you ever write.

Arouse Interest

In the opening, introduce yourself to the prospective employer and include a brief description of your personal qualifications. This opening essentially gives you the opportunity to promote yourself. The letter should make the reader interested enough in your skills and abilities and to grant you an interview.

> *Example 1*: The position you have advertised in the *Grand Rapids News* sounds challenging. My certificate in Dental Assisting and my credential as a Certified Dental Practice Management Assistant have provided me the skills necessary to perform the job well. You will find that I have the necessary tasks to become an asset to your practice.

> *Example 2*: Your employment announcement posted on my school bulletin board calls for a clinical chairside assistant who is interested in applying the latest concepts of four-handed dentistry. My education at Grand Rapids Community College has provided me with the skills necessary to be an asset to your office while increasing your productivity.

> *Example 3*: Your employment announcement calls for an administrative assistant who is interested in learning the latest technology and has good computer skills. My education at Grand Rapids Community College for the past 2 years has provided me with these skills and I am ready to become a valuable member of your dental team.

In each of these cases, the applicant lets the prospective employer know that she or he is interested in the position and believes that she or he has the skills needed for the job. Note that each paragraph is "you" or, reader, oriented.

Describe Your Skills and Abilities

The second paragraph of the letter should describe your skills in more detail. It should also call attention to your enclosed résumé, curriculum vitae, or data sheet (explained in the next section).

> *Example*: In August of this year I will graduate from Grand Rapids Community College. I will have completed courses in business office procedures, clinical procedures, laboratory and radiographic procedures, and dental specialties, as well as 300 hours of clinical practice in the local community. I had taken courses in accounting, management, business communications, and computers before entering the Dental Assisting Program. While in school I have worked part time as a clinical dental assistant in a local dental office.

This brief description includes an overview of basic skills. Further details about the skills and the dates of education and work experience are included in the attached résumé.

Request an Interview

Because the purpose of a cover letter is to obtain an interview, you should ask for the interview directly.

> *Example*: Please give me an opportunity to discuss my qualifications with you. My telephone number is 616-999-2041" Or "I look forward to an appointment with you so we can discuss how I can become an asset to your dental team.

Box 18-3 presents a list of action verbs that can be used to describe your activities. General guidelines for creating a cover letter are provided in Box 18-4.

Figures 18-5 to 18-7 show letters of application submitted by three applicants with varying backgrounds.

Contacting an Office by Telephone

If you have been informed of a job opening by an instructor or a friend, time may not allow you to write a letter of application; in such cases a telephone call is required. This situation requires a different approach. First place a call to the office and indicate to the individual receiving your call who you are and why you

---

BOX 18-3   **Action Verbs for Use in Résumés and Cover Letters**

- Accomplished
- Achieved
- Active in
- Assisted
- Attained
- Attended
- Brought about
- Communicated
- Completed
- Conducted
- Contributed
- Cooperated
- Coordinated
- Counseled
- Created
- Demonstrated
- Designed
- Formed
- Founded
- Generated
- Graduated
- Headed
- Implemented
- Improved
- Increased
- Initiated
- Installed
- Instructed
- Interviewed
- Kept
- Lectured
- Led
- Maintained
- Managed
- Mediated
- Motivated
- Observed
- Obtained
- Operated
- Ordered
- Organized
- Originated

- Overcame
- Participated
- Perfected
- Performed
- Persuaded
- Placed
- Planned
- Prepared
- Presented
- Printed
- Processed
- Produced
- Programmed
- Proposed
- Proved
- Provided
- Publicized
- Realized
- Received
- Recognized
- Recommended
- Recruited
- Reevaluated
- Refined
- Regulated
- Represented
- Restored
- Reviewed
- Scheduled
- Secured
- Served
- Set up
- Simplified
- Sold
- Spearheaded
- Staffed
- Streamlined
- Substituted
- Trained
- Transformed
- Updated
- Validated

BOX 18-4   **Guidelines for Writing a Letter of Application**

1. Create a professional letterhead that includes vital data; that is, your full name, address, telephone number (home, cell, and fax) and your e-mail address.
2. Use standard business letter format.
3. Use personal stationery made of quality bond paper; do not use your current employer's stationery.
4. Make sure your spelling, grammar, punctuation, and capitalization are correct. If you are composing your letter on a computer, always use the spell checker, but remember to have someone else look over the letter as spell checker is not always correct.
5. Avoid opening with "My name is…" Your name is on the letterhead and in the closing signature line.
6. Keep the letter short, three to four paragraphs. Put details in the résumé.
7. Limit the letter to one page.
8. Address the letter to a specific person. Never address an application letter "To Whom It May Concern." Take time to find out the name of the employer. If it is not available, use "Dear Doctor" or, if the letter is going to a larger organization, "Dear Human Resources Manager."
9. Put the employer's needs first by making the letter "you" oriented; avoid "I."
10. Send an original letter for each application. Do not send photocopies.
11. Do not copy a letter of application from a book. Make your letter representative of your personal characteristics.
12. Consider mailing your letter and résumé in a large envelope so that it will stand out from the more commonly used No. 10 envelopes on the employer's desk.

---

are calling. Second, explain how you learned about the position. Finally, if the job is available, ask for an interview.

Whether you plan to send a letter of application or decide to contact the office by telephone, you must prepare a résumé, either to enclose with the letter or take with you to the office.

Creating a Résumé

A **résumé**, personal data sheet, or personal history should be prepared to accompany the letter of application or take with you to the interview. A résumé is a marketing tool, and the product

is you. The objective is to capture the attention of the reader and maintain the person's interest. From the employer's point of view, the résumé is a time-saver, because it gives a quick account of what you have done, what you can do, and for what you are striving. A résumé needs to be a brief, well-documented account of your qualifications. A simple résumé is best suited for those who are entering the job market or who have limited work experience. Remember, your objective is to be granted an interview; therefore, you want to impress the reader with a résumé that is concise and presents a positive presentation of your abilities and qualifications. A résumé may be prepared in a functional or chronological format. (See Figure 18-5 through 18-6, *C*, to determine which format appeals to you.) Both are acceptable formats, but sometimes the person who has more extensive educational and professional skills may prefer to use the chronological résumé, as it lists these categories more succinctly.

 PRACTICE NOTE

A résumé is a marketing tool, and the product is you.

Prepare a customized résumé. Never use a one-size-fits-all document. If you are in an educational program, avoid copying

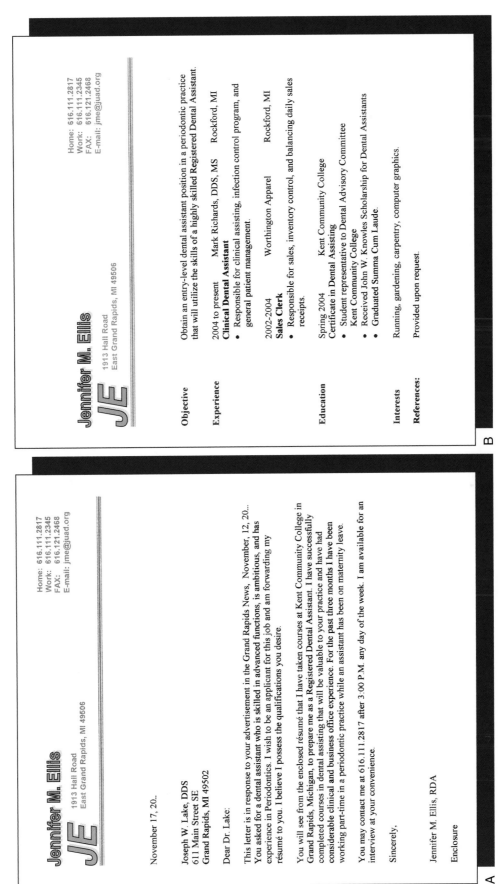

Figure 18-5 A, Letter of application for an entry-level position as a clinical assistant. **B,** Personal résumé to accompany the letter applying for an entry-level position as a clinical assistant.

A

Jennifer M. Ellis

JE 1913 Hall Road
East Grand Rapids, MI 49506

Home: 616.111.2817
Work: 616.111.2345
FAX: 616.121.2468
E-mail: jme@juad.org

November 17, 20..

Joseph W. Lake, DDS
611 Main Street SE
Grand Rapids, MI 49502

Dear Dr. Lake:

This letter is in response to your advertisement in the Grand Rapids News, November, 12, 20.. You asked for a dental assistant who is skilled in advanced functions, is ambitious, and has experience in Periodontics. I wish to be an applicant for this job and am forwarding my résumé to you. I believe I possess the qualifications you desire.

You will see from the enclosed résumé that I have taken courses at Kent Community College in Grand Rapids, Michigan, to prepare me as a Registered Dental Assistant. I have successfully completed courses in dental assisting that will be valuable to your practice and have had considerable clinical and business office experience. For the past three months I have been working part-time in a periodontic practice while an assistant has been on maternity leave.

You may contact me at 616.111.2817 after 3:00 P.M. any day of the week. I am available for an interview at your convenience.

Sincerely,

Jennifer M. Ellis, RDA

Enclosure

B

Jennifer M. Ellis

JE 1913 Hall Road
East Grand Rapids, MI 49506

Home: 616.111.2817
Work: 616.111.2345
FAX: 616.121.2468
E-mail: jme@juad.org

Objective   Obtain an entry-level dental assistant position in a periodontic practice that will utilize the skills of a highly skilled Registered Dental Assistant.

Experience   2004 to present   Mark Richards, DDS, MS   Rockford, MI
Clinical Dental Assistant
* Responsible for clinical assisting, infection control program, and general patient management.

2002-2004   Worthington Apparel   Rockford, MI
Sales Clerk
* Responsible for sales, inventory control, and balancing daily sales receipts.

Education   Spring 2004   Kent Community College
Certificate in Dental Assisting
* Student representative to Dental Advisory Committee Kent Community College
* Received John W. Knowles Scholarship for Dental Assistants
* Graduated Summa Cum Laude.

Interests   Running, gardening, carpentry, computer graphics.

References: Provided upon request.

a sample from this or any textbook as others in your class may do the same. Remember you want to make your résumé stand out and grasp the attention of the reader.

Customize the résumé to fit the position for which you are applying. It is best to create the document in word processing on the computer and then save it for future reference. Most software provides several optional templates that allow you to create a professional personal letterhead and a matching résumé. Other suggested templates are available at www.womenforhire.com/advice/resumes_examples_and_cover_letter_templates as well as a variety of other web sites geared to job searches. Remember, you want to get the attention of the prospective employer when the person reads the letter, so take time to create an attractive professional image through your stationery. After the letter has been completed, create an original copy on résumé quality stationery and remember never to send a copied résumé. If this is not possible, try to obtain the finest quality copy possible from a commercial printer. You should also keep a copy for yourself to take when going for an interview.

In general, your résumé should be designed with the following suggestions in mind:
- Put yourself in the position of your prospective employer. Try to determine the qualities the person may be seeking and emphasize these qualifications.
- Be as impressive as possible but do not deviate from the truth. This is not the time to be shy and modest. You must tell the reader what you can do; no one else will do it for you. You are in the position to sell yourself and you must be positive without being overly assertive.
- Review the material carefully to make sure you didn't forget anything. An overlooked item may be just the one the employer is seeking. Box 18-5 presents some hints for writing a résumé.

1847 Sheffield
Ann Arbor, MI 48105
Home: 734.673.1235
Work: 734.768.2800
E-Mail: amy@hotmail.com

From the Desk of Amy S. March

February 5, 20 —

Ashley M. Lake, DDS
611 Main St., SE
Grand Rapids, MI 49502

Dear Dr. Lake:

You will find enclosed a resumé I am sending in response to your advertisement in the *Grand Rapids News* for an administrative assistant in your busy orthodontic practice. I believe, after you review this resumé, you will find that I have the qualifications needed to fill this position.

Over the past two years, I have gained a great deal of experience in a large orthodontic practice in Ann Arbor, Michigan. During the second year, I was in charge of insurance management and appointment scheduling. I have attended seminars sponsored by noted insurance companies and had an opportunity recently to attend a practice management course in Chicago on automated claim forms management.

My spouse has recently accepted a position with a law firm in the Grand Rapids area. Since our families both reside in nearby communities, we are delighted to be returning to Grand Rapids. In fact, we will be in the area looking for housing during the next thirty days, so I would welcome a call for an interview.

You may reach me at 734.673.1235 after 6 p.m. or you may leave a message on our answering machine and I will return the call as soon as possible.

Sincerely,

Amy S. March, RDA

Enclosure

A

Figure 18-6 A, Letter of application for an office manager in a specialty practice.

From the Desk of Amy S. March

1847 Sheffield
Ann Arbor, MI 48105
Home: 734.673.1235
Work: 734.768.2800
E-Mail: amym@hotmail.com

PROFESSIONAL SUMMARY

I am seeking a position that needs a highly conscientious, detail-minded professional with education and clinical experience in orthodontics. Accustomed to working with a diverse patient clientele. Excellent communication and motivational skills with an interest in a challenging career in dental assisting.

EXPERIENCE

2005-Present	Orthodontic Associates Ann Arbor, MI *Business office manager*	
2002-2005	Gerald Wilson, DDS, MS Ann Arbor, MI *Clinical dental assistant*	
1998-2002	University of Michigan School of Dentistry Ann Arbor, MI	
	♦ Operative Dentistry Department	
	♦ Oral Diagnosis Department	

EDUCATION

June 2000	Delta Midwest Insurance Lansing, MI ♦ Processing claim forms seminar
June 1998	Washtenaw Community College Ann Arbor MI ♦ Certificate, Dental Assisting ♦ WCC Dental Departmental Scholarship

CREDENTIALS

December 1998	Michigan Board of Dentistry Licensure RDA
August 1998	Dental Assisting National Board CDA

REFERENCES

Provided upon request.

B

Figure 18-6, cont'd B, Personal résumé, chronological style, to accompany the letter applying for the position of office manager in a specialty office.

(Continued)

Every résumé should have certain types of information. These include a professional summary or objective, personal data, qualifications, experience, and education. Optional areas might include objectives, affiliations, and references. The arrangement of and headings for this information can vary, depending on the person's work experience, education, and general goals. It is wise to select a standard format and emphasize sections in which you have the greatest assets. Regardless of the format selected, there are do's and don'ts to creating an effective résumé; these are presented in Box 18-6.

Personal Data

Personal data include the following:
- Full name
- Address
- Telephone number (home and cell, if available)
- Fax number and e-mail address (if you have one)

Professional Summary

The **professional summary** section lets the reader know instantly in two or three sentences what you offer and what you seek. Avoid using generic or vague phrases such as "looking for a position at a well-known practice with room to grow." Instead, use this section to promote specific goals and accomplishments, and tout your desire to work in a specific field or area of a dental practice.

> *Example*: Professional summary: Administrative assistant with 5 years of exceptional dental practice management experience. Extensive knowledge in practice management software, insurance management, and staff supervision. Seeking management role that will use my technology, dental, and human relations skills.

Amy S. March
1847 Sheffield
Ann Arbor, MI 48105
Home: 734-673-1235
Cell phone: 734.768.1111
E-mail: amym@hotmail.com

CAREER OBJECTIVE

Highly conscientious, detailed minded with great ability to multitask and able to work with a diverse clientele. Excellent communication and motivational skills and am seeking an opportunity in a challenging orthodontic practice.

PROFESSIONAL SKILLS

EXCEPTIONAL PATIENT SERVICE: Strong communication skills to understand patient needs and provide exceptional results. Track record of successfully managing difficult patients.

ADAPTABLE TO TECHNOLOGY: Proficient in several types of dental software, Microsoft Office including Word, Excel, and PowerPoint and able to operate all major office equipment.

INDEPENDENT AND TEAM PLAYER: Enjoy collaborating with colleagues, patients as well as completing tasks independently. Eager to motivate and inspire others to deliver their best.

LANGUAGE SKILLS: Conversant in Spanish.

PROFESSIONAL (AND/OR VOLUNTEER) EXPERIENCE

2005-Present	Orthodontic Associates Ann Arbor, MI *Business office manager*
2002-2005	Gerald Wilson, DDS, MS Ann Arbor, MI *Clinical dental assistant*
1998-2002	University of Michigan School of Dentistry Ann Arbor. MI
	♦ Operative Denstistry Department
	♦ Oral Diagnosis Department

EDUCATION

June 2000	Delta Midwest Insurance Lansing, MI ♦ Processing claim forms seminar
June 1998	Washtenaw Community College Anna Arbor MI ♦ Certificate, Dental Assisting ♦ WCC Dental Departmental Scholarship

CREDENTIALS

December 1998 August 1998	Michigan Board of Dentistry Licensure RDA Dental Assisting National Board CDA

REFERENCES

Provided upon request.

C

Figure 18-6, cont'd C, Personal résumé, functional style, to accompany the letter applying for the position of office manager in a specialty office.

Notice that this summary did not specify what type of dental practice, but rather emphasized the person's interest in an office management position. You might also list your long-term goals. In that case, the summary might be concluded with the following statement:

Example: Professional summary: A position as an administrative assistant in a dental office, with a long-range goal of supervisory management.

Education

Be sure to include relevant information about your educational background. List all colleges and universities attended and the date you graduated. (List most recent schools first.) List diplomas or degrees, as well as awards and scholarships or special achievements. Courses that you took when completing the dental assistant program might be listed (e.g., dental science, dental laboratory procedures, clinical practice, dental radiography, and dental practice management).

Work Experience

A chronological résumé begins with your most recent job and experience dates of employment, name and address of employer, position held, and a brief description of the job. Summer and part-time jobs may be lumped in a single category; however, if work experiences have been limited, you may want to list them separately. Box 18-7 presents the advantages and disadvantages of a **chronological résumé**. If using a functional résumé you will list your skills first and then your work experience. Box 18-8 lists the advantages and disadvantages of the **functional résumé**.

Michelle M. Schaffer

1913 Hall Road
East Grand Rapids, MI 49506

Objective

To obtain a management position in a team-oriented practice that will utilize my maturity, experience, communication, and motivational skills to maximum advantage and provide a setting in which safe quality care is a primary objective.

Experience

2004-Present	Hillsdale Dental Clinic	Hillsdale, MI
Office Manager		
2001-2004	Kent Community College	Grand Rapids, MI
Admissions Office Clerk		
1997-2001	Burlington Country Club	Rockford, MI
Dining Room Hostess		

Education

July 2008	OSHA Update Seminar Presented by GRDS	Grand Rapids, MI
	Harriet Beamer, DDS, MS Lecturer	
June 2008	CDC Guidelines for Dentistry	Grand Rapids, MI
	Presented by MDA John Molinari, PhD Lecturer	
1999-2001	Aquinas College	Grand Rapids, MI
	B.A., Business Administration and Computer Science	
	Graduated Summa Cum Laude	
1997-1999	Kent Community College	Grand Rapids, MI
	Certificate in Dental Assisting	

Credentials

CDPMA	Dental Assisting National Board
CDA	Dental Assisting National Board
CPR Certificate	American Heart Association

References

Provided upon request.

Home: 231.789.0909   Pager: 616.757.1010   E-Mail: SchaM6@hotmail.com

---

Michelle M. Schaffer

5200 Blueberry Lane
Cutlerville, MI 49509
Phone: 231.765.8899

November 7, 20—

P.O. Box 2589
Grand Rapids News
Grand Rapids, MI 49502

Dear Doctor:

Please accept my résumé directed toward the position you advertised in the *Grand Rapids News*. The position interested me since you are seeking a person with strong supervisory skills, good judgment, and ability to work under pressure, and a knowledge of OSHA standards. I have successfully managed a large clinical facility for the past six years and believe I have all of the qualifications you are seeking.

As you review my résumé you will note I am a highly motivated individual who has completed course work in numerous areas of value to your office. Since I am especially interested in infection control in a dental health care environment, I have attended a variety of seminars on this subject.

I look forward to hearing from you concerning this position and hope to meet you for an interview in the near future. You may reach me by calling in the evening at 231.675.8899. Thank you very much for your consideration of this application.

Sincerely,

Michelle M. Schaffer, CDA, CDPMA

Enclosure

E-mail: Scham6@hotmail.com
Pager: 231.789.0909

A

Figure 18-7 A, Letter of application in response to a blind advertisement for an office manager. **B,** Personal résumé to accompany the letter applying for the office manager position.

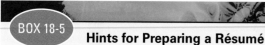

BOX 18-5   Hints for Preparing a Résumé

- Use all the layout, formatting, and finishing techniques available to you.
- Use headings that allow the reader to find information easily.
- Be succinct.
- Use a spell checker and have the résumé reviewed by a competent person.
- Make the résumé easy to read (e.g., print size, font styles, and arrangement of information).
- Put your education and experience information in chronological order unless using a functional format.
- Leave sufficient white space to avoid a cluttered look.

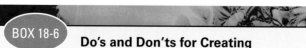

BOX 18-6   Do's and Don'ts for Creating an Effective Résumé

Do

- Emphasize your qualities and experience.
- Substantiate your educational and experience qualifications to justify the abilities you claim.
- Be clear and concise in your descriptions.
- Choose a format that is easy to read.
- Be consistent in using the format.

Don't

- Include on the résumé the date the résumé was written.
- Include a physical description of yourself (e.g., height, weight, age).
- Include race or religion.
- Mention your health status.
- Include salary information (unless specifically requested; then include it in the cover letter).
- Use abbreviations or acronyms that may not be understood.

BOX 18-7   Advantages and Disadvantages of a Chronological Résumé

Advantages

- Highlights titles and company/dental practice names, which is advantageous when the names or titles are relevant or impressive
- Highlights consistent progress from one position to another
- Highlights length of time in each organization

Disadvantages

- Readily shows gaps in the work history
- Shows frequent job changes
- Does not show the most impressive or relevant work experience first if it is not the most recent

BOX 18-8   Advantages and Disadvantages of a Functional Résumé

Advantages

- Highlights your strengths such as key skills, capabilities, and community service
- If you are looking for a career in a field that you do not have specific qualifications in, highlight some transferable and marketable skills that you do have.
- When you have had extensive experience in a variety of areas, use this opportunity to express this experience with terms such as *exceptional customer service, highly responsible and ethical,* and *adaptable to new technology—proficient in Microsoft Office.*

Disadvantages

- Not effective for inexperienced persons.
- Does not indicate chronology of job history.

In some instances, if your work experience is more recent than your education, the work experience should be listed before your education. At this point in your career, work experience is of greater value to a prospective employer than education.

Optional Areas

Affiliations and Activities

If you have participated in school or community activities or received awards or honors, this information would be valuable to the prospective employer, and it should be included. Activities and hobbies are optional, but can indicate that you are a well-rounded individual and get along well with others.

References

Generally references are provided upon request and not before the personal interview. Be prepared with the names, addresses, and telephone numbers of at least two people who are willing to verify your abilities and skills and one character reference.

If your work experience has been limited, list instructors or clinical supervisors who can evaluate your abilities. Always obtain the individual's permission to use his or her name as a reference and be sure that person is willing to give you a good recommendation.

Remember, do not give information on the résumé that might be detrimental to you. Details can be given when you are interviewed. At the interview, be prepared to discuss your weaknesses honestly, confidently, and in a way that puts your present self in the best light.

Figures 18-5, *B*, 18-6, *B*, and 18-7, *B*, show the ways résumés were designed to accompany each of the letters in Figures 18-5, *A*, 18-6, *A*, and 18-7, *A*, respectively.

COMPLETING THE JOB APPLICATION FORM

The type of dental assisting job for which you are applying determines the detail and complexity of the application form. The job application form is a series of questions requesting comprehensive data about you and your past education, work, and professional experience. It often may require you to complete a narrative statement about yourself and give the reasons you are seeking a particular job. You may have had the opportunity to complete the application form before arriving for the interview or you may be asked to complete the form when you arrive. Figure 18-8 presents an example of an application used for private practice.

Regardless of the job for which you are applying, you must keep several things in mind when completing the application form, as follows:

- If possible, try to obtain two forms, one to use as a working copy and the other to submit to the employer.
- Before entering data on the application form, read through the application very thoroughly and avoid asking unnecessary questions. The application form often is used as the first employment test. It tests your ability to follow directions.
- The directions may indicate that the form can be keyed on a computer or hand written. If you are required to complete the form in your own handwriting, this may be another test of neatness and also gives the employer a sample of how well or poorly you write.
- Answer all the questions. If the question does not relate to you, write N/A (not applicable) or draw a line through the question. The employer then realizes you have read the question and have not overlooked it.
- Be truthful when answering interview questions. Dates, names, and places must be accurate. Make a list of your former addresses, schools, family names, and references to take along when going for the interview. It is better to have the information available even if it is not needed. Be sure that no discrepancies exist between your reported date of birth and your age. If you are residing at a temporary address, be sure to give a permanent address. Be particularly careful with your spelling. A small pocket dictionary is a great item to take along as a handy reference.

 PRACTICE NOTE
Be truthful when answering interview questions.

PREPARING FOR AN INTERVIEW

The day you receive a response from a prospective employer, you will be elated to know that someone is interested in your qualifications after reviewing the résumé and now wishes to meet you in person. This elation is immediately followed by a feeling of fear—fear of the unknown. You may or may not know anything about this prospective position, but one thing is certain: You do know yourself. The following steps can be used to prepare for an interview. At a later time, you should go through each of these steps and apply them to your situation:

1. *Learn about the dental practice or clinic.* Once you have identified the dental practice or clinic to which you are interested in applying, spend time learning more about the office or clinic,

its mission, and its vision. Find out about its reputation and how it treats its employees. This can be done in several ways:
   a. Ask friends, relatives, and acquaintances what they know about this office or clinic.
   b. Check the office or clinic web site if one is available. For example, dental schools have a web site from which you could learn about staffing and the various types of jobs and clinics in the institution.
   c. Search the dental society web sites to identify professional memberships.
   d. If you are a student, consult with local professional contacts or dental faculty.
   e. Search the state Board of Dentistry to identify any possible disciplinary action.

2. *What do I wear?* Wear something that looks businesslike. You may have a new outfit that you would like to wear but cannot decide if it is the proper thing. If you question whether an outfit is right, don't wear it. Your hair should be worn up and off the shoulders, with natural looking makeup and minimal jewelry. Avoid a fragrance that is too heavy. Your well-groomed polished image shows that you value and respect your patients and the practice. You may even want to look at photos or video footage of yourself to see what the prospective employer will view with an objective eye. Do you look the part of a confident, up-to-date, healthy professional? It is prudent to follow the old adage, "First appearances are lasting ones." You may know all the answers and have a lot of skill, but you must win the approval of the dentist before you will ever have an opportunity to display these skills.

3. *What do I take with me?* The day you receive the call for the interview, write down the time, place, and name of the interviewer. Prepare the materials to take with you to the interview. These should include a ballpoint pen, a pencil, an eraser, a small spiral notebook, a pocket dictionary, and a copy of your college transcripts and your résumé. In the notebook list many of your outstanding characteristics that you may wish to bring to the attention of the dentist, a list of questions you hope to cover during the interview, and the names, addresses, and telephone numbers or e-mail addresses of your references.

 PRACTICE NOTE
You may know all the answers and have a lot of skill, but you must win the approval of the dentist before you will get the opportunity to display those skills.

Depending on the type of job for which you are applying, you may want to take a **portfolio**, which is a compilation of samples of your work. If you are applying for an administrative assistant position, a portfolio might include the following:
- Letters you have written, which show your writing style
- Spreadsheets you have prepared
- Reports, including graphics
- PowerPoint slides

EMPLOYMENT APPLICATION

All information listed on this application will be considered and handled as personal and confidential. Please write or print legibly.

AN EQUAL OPPORTUNITY EMPLOYER

This employer provides equal opportunity to all persons without regard to handicap, race, color, religion, sex, age, or national origin.

		Date of Application:
Name:		
Address:	City:	State:	Zip:
Home Phone:	Cell Phone:	Social Security Number:

GENERAL INFORMATION

Position applied for:

Available to work: ☐ Full-Time ☐ Part-Time ☐ Temporary

Date available to start work:

Are you over 18 yrs. of age? ☐ Yes ☐ No   Will transportation be a problem for you? ☐ Yes ☐ No

If you are not a U.S. Citizen, do you have the right to work in the United States?
☐ Yes ☐ No

Have you ever been convicted of a felony? ☐ Yes ☐ No

(A conviction is not an automatic bar to employment. Each case will be considered on its own merits.)

Does the sight of blood bother you? ☐ Yes ☐ No

EDUCATION

	Name and address of School	Major/Degree(s)	No. of Years Completed	Did you Graduate?
High School				
Community College				
4 Year Institution				
Vocational				
Other (specify)				

Describe Specialized Training, Apprenticeship, Skills, Seminars, Courses, Extra-Curricular Activities

SKILLS

Task	Circle One		Task	Circle One	
Keyboarding WPM _____	Yes	No	Pour Models	Yes	No
Bookkeeping	Yes	No	Cavitron	Yes	No
Computer Operations	Yes	No	Cast Onlays	Yes	No
Handling Group Insurance	Yes	No	Plaque Control Instruction	Yes	No
Expose, Process, and Mount X-rays	Yes	No	Oral Evacuator	Yes	No
Panoramic X-Rays	Yes	No	Knowledge of Dental Instruments	Yes	No
Have you used insurance software?	Yes	No	Knowledge of Dental Terms	Yes	No
Other: (Describe if yes)					

EMPLOYMENT RECORD

Beginning with your current employer, please list your work experience over the past ten years. You may include pertinent volunteer activities.

Name of Employer		Start Date	End Date
Address	Phone	Start Salary	End Salary
Job Title	Supervisor	Phone	
Duties			
Reason for Leaving			

Name of Employer		Start Date	End Date
Address	Phone	Start Salary	End Salary
Job Title	Supervisor	Phone	
Duties			
Reason for Leaving			

Name of Employer		Start Date	End Date
Address	Phone	Start Salary	End Salary
Job Title	Supervisor	Phone	
Duties			
Reason for Leaving			

Figure 18-8 A sample application for employment.

REFERENCES

Please provide the name, address, and phone number of at least two non employer/relatives as references.

NAME	ADDRESS	PHONE

EMERGENCY CONTACT

Name	Relationship	
Address	Phone	Alt. Phone

DUTY PERFORMANCE

Are you able to perform the essential duties of the position for which you are applying, either with or without reasonable accommodations? ☐ Yes ☐ No

If yes, please indicate what type(s) of reasonable accommodations are needed:

In the course of making an employment decision, this employer makes it a practice to verify with previous employers information such as dates of employment, description of job duties, attendance records, reason for leaving, etc. If there are any employers you want us to contact, please indicate their names below and reasons why:

I understand that if I am employed and any statement herein is not true, I may be released immediately, I will be paid only through the day of release and this employer may cancel any rights to accrued benefits.

_____ Date   _____ Signature

Figure 18-8, cont'd A sample application for employment.

The Personal Interview

Preparing a portfolio and presenting it during the job interview allows you to show what you can do rather than merely talk about it.

Plan to arrive a few minutes early at the office. Your first contact may be with the office manager. The office manager plays an important role in the office; therefore it is important to be friendly and courteous to this person. You may want to introduce yourself by saying, "Good morning, I am Jennifer Ellis (use your own name!), and I have a 10:30 appointment for an interview with Dr. Lake." The office manager will acknowledge you and may ask you to complete an application form similar to that shown in Figure 18-8. After the form is completed, the office manager may review your résumé and application and escort you to meet Dr. Lake. If you are not introduced, take the time to introduce yourself by saying, "Good morning, Dr. Lake, I am Jennifer Ellis." At this point you will be asked to be seated, and the interview will begin. Look directly at the interviewer and respond to the questions clearly and distinctly; don't be evasive. An evasive answer leaves doubt in the interviewer's mind.

In general the applicant should be responsive and answer in complete sentences. Box 18-9 presents helpful hints on things to avoid during an interview. Box 18-10 provides a series of commonly asked interview questions.

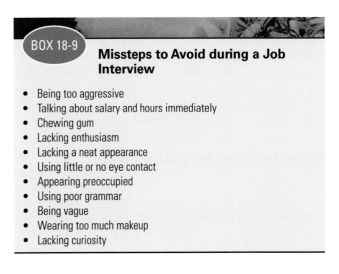

BOX 18-9 Missteps to Avoid during a Job Interview

- Being too aggressive
- Talking about salary and hours immediately
- Chewing gum
- Lacking enthusiasm
- Lacking a neat appearance
- Using little or no eye contact
- Appearing preoccupied
- Using poor grammar
- Being vague
- Wearing too much makeup
- Lacking curiosity

BOX 18-10   Commonly Asked Interview Questions

Initial Questions

- How did you learn about this position?
- What do you know about our practice?
- Why are you interested in this practice?
- Tell me about yourself.
- Why do you think you are qualified for this position?
- Describe your most significant accomplishment.
- What is your definition of "being on time"?
- What qualities are important to you in your work environment?
- If you make a decision and it is questioned, how do you react?

Interest in the Job

- Are you currently employed? If so, does your current employer know you are seeking a new position?
- What would our current employer say makes you most valuable to him or her?
- Why do you want to change jobs?
- What do you consider the ideal job for you?
- What are your long- and short-range goals?

Education

- What formal education have you had?
- Why did you choose to study dental assisting?
- What was your academic average when you were in school?
- What do you consider your greatest strength? Your greatest weakness?

Experience

- Have you ever been fired or asked to resign from a position?
- Which duties performed in the past have you liked the best? The least? Why?
- Why should I hire you?
- What salary do you expect?

Future on the Job

- What would you like to know about this practice?
- Describe how you would demonstrate compassion in this practice.
- How would you want to integrate into this practice?

After the series of questions, salary and job responsibilities generally are discussed. If the salary the dentist offers you is lower than you are willing to accept, you may reply that you had hoped to start at a higher salary but you are willing to accept an opportunity to demonstrate your ability and value to the practice. This undoubtedly will result in further discussion, whereupon you should be prepared to give firm answers on what you will accept. Also you should inquire what the benefits are that might offset the lower salary.

After an interview that included many of the questions in Box 18-10, a prospective applicant, Jennifer Ellis, was offered an acceptable salary, although it was lower than her initial request. She replied, "I feel I have the skills you need, and it is going to save you a great deal of time in not having to teach me about all the technical skills. I would be willing to start at the lower salary for a minimal amount of time if you will explain to me what the total salary scale is and how I will be evaluated for salary raises. I would like the opportunity to advance by merit or production, since I am certain you will be pleased with my ability and production in your office." Dr. Lake explained the numerous benefits and outlined the salary system to Jennifer. Remember, as discussed earlier, salary is not the primary aspect of the job, but you must be able to earn enough to adequately support yourself in a comfortable lifestyle. Also the benefits of a job often outweigh the basic salary, so don't overlook this aspect.

Other Formats for Interviewing

Some dentists like to have team interviews, in which several members of the staff who will work with you participate in the interview. Generally a team interview in a private practice setting involves three or four people. Although this type of interview may sound intimidating, it may not be. Pay attention to the individuals' names as they are introduced so that later you can refer to them by name. Listen carefully and answer questions succinctly, giving your attention to the individual who asked the question. Make eye contact with all participants if the question or statement is meant for the group.

Working Interview

Often a dentist uses the working interview format to assess a clinical assistant applicant. The dentist will invite you for a day of work at the office, for which some form of compensation is prearranged. This would serve as an opportunity to observe the office activity and give you a sense of how well the office is organized.

Virtual Interview

Virtual interviews are not common in small dental practices, but some situations may warrant them. For example, if you are applying for a job in Torrance, California, and you live in Biltmore, New Jersey, it might be feasible to conduct a virtual interview. In other words, rather than having you fly to California for the interview, the dental clinic would make arrangements for you to go to go to a facility that has a teleconferencing center. This allows the interviewer from California to see you, and you can see the interviewer. It is possible to accomplish a similar type of interview if necessary by using a web camera system or even video conferencing on your computer. This concept enables you to send pictures and sound files that say more than a résumé or telephone conversation. Two companies that provide such a format include, interview process using web cams: www.livehire.com and www.hirevue.com. Virtual interviews enable the prospective employer and employee to interact and have an opportunity to visually meet each other.

If you are going to participate in a virtual interview, careful planning must be done in advance. Many of us get a little nervous when we know we are going to be videotaped or observed on camera, but a virtual interview is a two-way system that allows you to communicate with the other person as if you were in the same room. You still greet the interviewer warmly and with a smile, just as you would in person. Sit in the chair provided and avoid nervous habits. Try to forget that the camera is present and concentrate on the interviewer and the questions. Avoid wearing black, gray, white, or distracting patterns, because they do not come across well on camera. Also avoid wearing jewelry that is distracting or that makes noise on camera.

Concluding the Interview

An interview is not a lengthy process, and it often is terminated with a tour of the office. Do not be overly flattering to the staff, but thank them for their time before you leave. You may not receive a job offer during the interview, because the dentist may have other applicants to interview. However, you may inquire as to when the dentist anticipates arriving at a decision. Remember, do not be discouraged if you do not get the job. Each interview is a learning experience, regardless of whether it produces a job offer, and it should not be treated as a disappointment.

Following Up the Interview

A good follow-up letter (Figure 18-9) should be written 1 or 2 days after the interview. This is an indication to the interviewer that you are interested in the position, and it may make you a priority applicant.

The follow-up letter does not have to be long. It simply restates your interest in the job and mentions some of the facts that interested you about the position.

Another type of follow-up may be necessary if you have not had a reply from the prospective employer. If the job is still available and you are interested, it is permissible to call the interviewer in a day or two after the interview. A telephone call lets the interviewer know of your continued interest; however, too many telephone calls can be annoying.

If you decide later that you are not interested in the position, you should send a letter explaining your decision. Not only is this thoughtful, but a time may come when you find yourself in a position to go back to this employer.

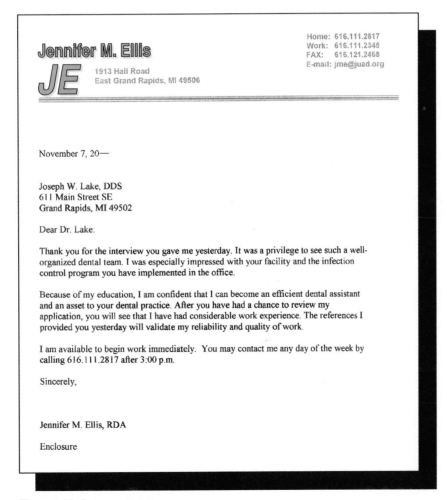

Figure 18-9 A sample follow-up letter.

Regular Self-Evaluation on the Job

Regular self-evaluation is necessary to retain your position in the dental office. People often carefully evaluate themselves before they are hired but may become careless after working in the office for a time.

Don't become negligent about evaluating yourself. As a clinical or administrative assistant, you are constantly in the public eye and must maintain a good image in your employer's office. In addition, once you have obtained the position, you must maintain your skills and acquire new ones as changes occur in dentistry through expanded use of auxiliary staff. You should promptly join your professional organizations, which offer information about educational activities in relevant techniques.

HINTS FOR SUCCESS AS PART OF THE DENTAL TEAM

When you begin your new job on the dental health team, you should gear yourself for success. The following sections can help make this experience more pleasant and result in personal success. These suggestions are summarized in Box 18-11.

Learn the Names of Staff Members

Learning and remembering the names of your immediate associates should not be difficult. If the staff is large, learning the names of those not in your immediate department may be more difficult. It is wise to learn the names as quickly as possible. It may even be wise to maintain a list of names and the position of each employee until you are able to remember them.

Listen Attentively

You will be eager to learn as much as possible about your new position as quickly as possible. Listen carefully to directions and avoid talking persistently. If you relax and listen well, often the questions you are eager to ask will be answered. If not, do not hesitate to ask for clarification of a procedure.

BOX 18-11 **Hints for Success in a New Job**

- Learn the names of staff members.
- Listen attentively.
- Establish meaningful social friendships.
- Use a notebook and calendar to record important activities and procedures.
- Use judgment in working overtime and taking breaks.
- Do not flaunt your education and abilities.
- Seek honest evaluations.
- Maintain office policies.
- Observe office hours.
- Be yourself.

Establish Meaningful Social Friendships

Most employers do not object if employees develop personal friendships with other employees. However, many traps can develop in your first days on a new job. One of these is developing a close relationship with one or two people too quickly, which can cost you friendship with others at a later time. Office cliques frequently create rivalry. Although you must have a friendly attitude toward other employees in the office, you need not feel you must participate in all the social activities or interests the others have. However, you should avoid a superior attitude that can be interpreted as snobbish.

Use a Notebook and Calendar to Record Important Activities and Procedures

When you begin your new job, many unfamiliar rules and regulations and other information will be given to you. To avoid misunderstandings or neglecting important information, develop the "notebook habit" and write down each bit of information. It is surprising how many successful people use this system.

Observe Office Hours

In most cases the office hours have been determined before your arrival. The efficiency of an office depends on your being prompt at all times. Your tardiness delays the work process for which you are responsible. You should ensure your means of transportation at all times. It is your responsibility to anticipate inclement weather and compensate for any potential delay. It is better to be 20 minutes early for work than 2 minutes late. The dentist will not be interested in your excuses.

 PRACTICE NOTE
It is better to be 20 minutes early for work than 2 minutes late.

Use Judgment in Working Overtime and Taking Breaks

Employees sometimes try to impress their employer by working extra hours or skipping lunch hours or breaks. However, you should avoid continual overtime and loss of lunch hours because it may cause friction with other employees. Your actions may be misinterpreted, and other employees may make life miserable for you. This does not mean you cannot use your discretion on days when legitimate emergencies arise and your presence is necessary to maintain office efficiency.

Do Not Flaunt Your Education and Abilities

Nothing is more irritating than a new employee who constantly informs other employees of his or her exceptional abilities. It is better to prove your ability through your work than to tell everyone about your great potential. Your coworkers may have had many years of experience, and you might learn something from them if you give them a chance to help you.

Seek Honest Performance Evaluations

Most employees want to learn about their performance. Before accepting the new job, you should have asked how and when your performance would be evaluated. As time passes, periodic reviews of your performance should be obtained from the employer, and you should have an opportunity to discuss the performance evaluation and determine ways in which you are performing satisfactorily and areas that need improvement. Figure 18-10 is an example of a performance evaluation form. Such forms are reviewed periodically with you to evaluate your day-to-day performance. It is wise to use this evaluation form first as a self-evaluation, before your employer completes it.

Maintain Office Policies

Most offices have established policies for grooming and uniform styles. You should carefully review the office policy and adhere to it. In addition, you should take home any other handbooks the office uses for its employees and read them carefully so that you will be well informed. If you do not understand a policy, ask for clarification to avoid making an embarrassing mistake.

Performance Evaluation Form

Employee Name ______________________

Job Title ______________________

Supervisor ______________________

EVALUATION

4 Excellent performance that demonstrates consistent and important contributions that meet and frequently surpass expectations of the position.

3 Performs with a very acceptable degree of skill that demonstrates the expectations of the position.

2 Performance has not met satisfactory level. Makes mistakes but usually corrects errors after further instruction. Improved performance is needed to achieve defined expectations of this position.

1 Performance indicates deficiencies that seriously interfere with attainment of the defined expectations of the position.

	Evaluation			
Attendance				
Adheres to scheduled work hours.	4	3	2	1
Uses leave appropriately.	4	3	2	1
Adjusts work schedule to office needs.	4	3	2	1
Job Knowledge				
Uses required job skills.	4	3	2	1
Updates skills periodically.	4	3	2	1
Demonstrates knowledge of procedures needed to perform the job.	4	3	2	1
Organizational Skills				
Prioritizes tasks.	4	3	2	1
Plans steps in advance to accomplish tasks.	4	3	2	1
Meets deadlines.	4	3	2	1
Work Quality				
Performs work accurately.	4	3	2	1
Demonstrates thoroughness and attention to detail.	4	3	2	1
Demonstrates neatness.	4	3	2	1
Human Relations/Communications				
Demonstrates a sense of humor.	4	3	2	1
Demonstrates good listening skills.	4	3	2	1
Maintains eye contact when speaking to another person.	4	3	2	1
Displays good manners and professional etiquette.	4	3	2	1
Conveys ideas effectively.	4	3	2	1
Responds to ideas conveyed by others.	4	3	2	1
Demonstrates sensitivity to diverse staff and patients.	4	3	2	1
Problem Solving Skills				
Remains calm in stressful situations.	4	3	2	1
Demonstrates ability to identify the problem.	4	3	2	1
Demonstrates ability to select the best solution.	4	3	2	1
Takes action to prevent future problems.	4	3	2	1
Does not require supervision to accomplish routine tasks.	4	3	2	1
Follows through on chosen solution.	4	3	2	1
Gives constructive criticism in a positive manner.	4	3	2	1
Responds to supervision in a positive manner.	4	3	2	1
Cooperation				
Respects responsibilities of others.	4	3	2	1
Provides assistance and guidance to others.	4	3	2	1
Accepts guidance from supervisor/employer.	4	3	2	1
Works as a team member.	4	3	2	1
Initiative				
Seeks work that needs to be done.	4	3	2	1
Seeks new methods and ideas to improve work.	4	3	2	1
Exhibits self-motivation to achieve team goals.	4	3	2	1
Integrity				
Respects other people and their property.	4	3	2	1
Maintains confidentiality.	4	3	2	1
Can be trusted with money that belongs to the office.	4	3	2	1
Refrains from gossip.	4	3	2	1
Is truthful regardless of potential consequences.	4	3	2	1

Supervisor/Employer Comments ______________________

Employee Comments ______________________

Employee's Signature ______________________ **Date** ______________

Supervisor/Employer Signature ______________________ **Date** ______________

Figure 18-10 Performance appraisal form.

Be Yourself

As you make your first impression in the office, it is wise to be yourself. Remember, you may admire characteristics in another person, but you cannot be that person. If you attempt to be someone else, you only destroy yourself and all of the finer parts of your character. Be yourself, and you will be a happier person.

ASKING FOR A RAISE

Pay increments should be discussed before you begin work, and you may find that raises are given after 6 months or 1 year of successful employment. To avoid any misunderstanding, determine how and when these raises can be obtained before accepting the job. Few dentists would consider performing extensive treatment on patients before informing them of the anticipated fees. Similarly you should not be working unless you are aware of your potential salary and anticipated promotions. It is wise to obtain written verification of employment conditions and responsibilities and a salary scale before beginning work. This can be accomplished in an office procedures manual (see Chapter 2). However, if pay increments have not been discussed and you have completed a year of employment, you might wonder when and how the subject can be raised.

Before approaching the dentist about a raise, you should do a self-evaluation to determine that you are justified in making such a request. The questions listed in Box 18-12 might be considered in such an evaluation. A salary conference should be a two-way discussion that allows you to identify your assets for the job and explain your performance success and allows the employer to relate the performance to a monetary amount that will reward your performance and inspire increased productivity.

If you have given serious thought to the factors mentioned previously, and you feel you deserve a raise, how do you approach the dentist? Select an opportunity when the work schedule allows enough time for a discussion of the subject. Do not wait until the end of the day, when the dentist is tired and ready to leave the office. It also is not wise to start the day by asking for a raise, especially if the schedule is rather heavy.

Let the dentist know why you believe you deserve a raise. If he or she asks why you should have one, be prepared to answer; for example, cite the rising cost of living, transportation costs, insurance, increased office production because of your efforts, or simply compensation for good performance.

Very often employees do not assert themselves enough to make the dentist aware that a raise should be given. If you become passive and content with a salary, naturally you will continue to be paid at this rate; however, if your professional skills are an asset, and because of these skills the dentist can perform the job with greater efficiency, you should be given a raise. If the employer cannot raise your salary, consider the benefits in Box 18-2 as alternatives to a salary increase.

If you are unsuccessful in getting a raise, express your appreciation for the dentist's understanding and consideration and consider your alternatives; of course, if you receive a raise, be sure to thank the responsible person.

Salary matters should be treated confidentially and are not discussed with other members of the team. Salary problems destroy positive attitudes and productivity and should be resolved as quickly as possible.

JOB TERMINATION

Terminating a job can be an obstacle for some individuals, especially when the job change is from one private practice to another in the same general locale. When you change jobs, make sure the change is to your advantage. Circumstances over which you have no control may be the reason for a change in jobs. However, an assistant who frequently changes jobs with inadequate notification or reason soon gains a poor professional reputation. Whatever the reason for terminating the job, do it ethically, remembering the following courtesies:

- Give the reason for leaving the job.
- Give sufficient notice, at least 2 weeks or longer if your job requires an extensive training period for a new assistant.
- Write a letter of resignation as a follow-up to your verbal resignation.
- Do not discuss the termination of your job with other members of the team until you are ready to inform the dentist that you will be leaving. The grapevine is a poor method of informing.
- If you terminate a job in which serious conflicts exist, it is best to leave these conflicts where they originated and not carry the feelings to another job. When beginning a new position, you should not make negative comments about a former employer. This is simply good ethics.

ATTITUDES FOR CONTINUED SUCCESS

A highly qualified and educated administrative assistant is the key to production, patient management, organization, accuracy, safe operation, and protection from potential litigation.

BOX 18-12   Questions to Consider before Asking for a Raise

1. Have I performed my duties well enough to deserve a raise?
2. Have I improved or advanced my skills since beginning the job?
3. Have I been cooperative with other members of the dental team?
4. Have I continued to maintain good patient management skills?
5. Can I verify that my attendance and punctuality have been above average?
6. Have I continually maintained professional ethics, safe practice, and quality standards?
7. Can I verify that the practice's productivity has increased because of my performance?
8. Do economic factors in the practice and the economy warrant a raise?

The right individual can significantly reduce the stress on the dental team. As you grow past your entry-level position on the job, you will discover that your future success depends more and more on your attitude and human relations skills. Completing a course in dental practice management is only the beginning.

PRACTICE NOTE

A highly qualified and educated administrative assistant is the key to production, patient management, organization, accuracy, safe operation, and protection from potential litigation.

Your willingness to be a team player and cooperate with patients and staff members as well as your good communication skills will be assets to the dental practice. Your initiative, self-motivation, creativity, and enthusiasm indicate an eagerness to accept leadership and challenges in the office. Your desire to learn, your curiosity, and your flexibility will enable you to attain new skills and advance your career.

Continue to market your skills, maintain an interest in new technologies, and accept changes no matter where you are on your career path. Good luck!

KEY TERMS

Blind ad—An advertisement that does not show the person or organization that placed the ad.

Chronological résumé—A résumé that includes education and experience information in chronological order.

Functional résumé—A résumé that will list your skills first and then your work experience.

Job application—A form with a series of questions that request comprehensive data about the applicant, including educational background and work and professional experience.

Letter of application—The letter that accompanies a personal résumé; it introduces the applicant and tries to arouse interest, prompting an interview with the prospective employer; also called a *cover letter.*

Portfolio—A compilation of samples of the applicant's work; it may include letters, spreadsheets, reports, PowerPoint slides, or other items.

Professional summary—An element of a résumé that may also be referred to as an *objective.* It is a succinct listing of personal data, qualifications, experience, education, and the goal for seeking a job.

Résumé—A listing of all the applicant's vital data, as well as information about the person's education and career experiences.

LEARNING ACTIVITIES

1. Write a philosophy in which you describe who you are, where you are going, and what you hope to accomplish. This philosophy should include your goals for life, your basic values, and your strengths and weaknesses.
2. List six areas of potential employment and explain briefly the benefits of each.
3. Choose one of the advertisements in Figure 18-2 or 18-3. Respond to the advertisement by writing a letter of application for the position. Also prepare a résumé to accompany the letter. Make a copy of the letter and the résumé for your personal files. Assume that you have been interviewed for the position mentioned in question 3 and write an appropriate follow-up letter.
4. List five assets you have to offer that you think would attract the favorable attention of a future employer.
5. Give five ways an application form might attract unfavorable attention. List 10 questions that you might be asked during an interview.

Please refer to the student workbook for additional learning activities.

REFERENCES

1. Dental Assisting National Board: *Show me the money: The 2008 DANB certificant salary survey,* Chicago, 2008, DANB. Available at www.danb.org/PDFS/2008SalarySurvey.pdf. Accessed June 5, 2009.

2. More on dental assistant salaries, *Dental Assisting Digest* [e-Newsletter], 2008. Available at http://dentalassistingdigest.com/articles/article_display.html?id=345340. Accessed June 4, 2009.

BIBLIOGRAPHY

Alexander B: 2008 salary survey: how does your income stack up? *RDH* (1), 2009. Available at www.proofs.com/display_article/350738/56/none/none/Feat/2008-Salary-Survey. Accessed June 5, 2009.

Fulton-Calkins PJ: *The administrative professional: technology & procedures*, ed 13, Mason, Ohio, 2007, South-Western Educational.

Henry K: You're worth every penny you earn and much, much more, *Dental Assisting Digest* [e-Newsletter, 2009].

Hook, line, and sinker, *Dental Office* 12(3), 2007. Available at www.proofs.com/display_article/293528/55/none/none/Feat/Hook,-Line,-&-Sinker. Accessed June 5, 2009.

Johnson T: Job hunting: tips to get your foot in the door, *Good Morning America* 2008. Available at www.abcnews.com/GMA/Parenting/Story?id=5765536&page=1 Accessed June 5, 2009.

Locker KO: *Business & administrative communication*, ed 8, New York, 2008, McGraw-Hill/Irwin.

Sabin WA: *The Gregg reference manual: a manual of style, grammar, usage, and formality*, ed 10, New York, 2005, McGraw-Hill/Irwin.

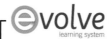

Please visit http://evolve.elsevier.com/Finkibeiner/practice for additional practice activities.

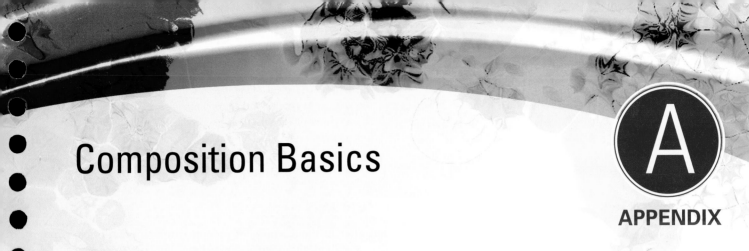

Composition Basics

GRAMMAR

Subject and Verb Agreement

1. When the subject consists of two singular nouns or pronouns connected by *or, either...or, neither...nor*, or *not only...but also*, a singular verb is required.

   Jane or *Bob has* the letter.

   Either *Ruth* or *Marge plans* to attend.

   Not only a *book* but also *paper is* needed.

2. When the subject consists of two plural nouns or pronouns connected by *or, either...or, neither...nor*, or *not only...but also*, a plural verb is required.

   Neither the *secretaries* nor the *typists have* access to that information.

3. When the subject is made up of both singular and plural nouns or pronouns connected by *or, either...or, neither...nor*, or *not only...but also*, the verb agrees with the last noun or pronoun mentioned before the verb.

   Either *Ms. Rogers* or the *assistants have* access to that information.

   Neither the *men* nor *Jo is* working.

4. Disregard intervening phrases and clauses when establishing agreement between subject and verb.

   One of the men *wants* to go to the convention.

5. The words *each, every, either, neither, one*, and *another* are singular. When they are used as subjects or as adjectives modifying subjects, a singular verb is required.

   Each person *is* deserving of the award.

   Neither boy *rides* the bicycle well.

6. The following pronouns are always singular and require a singular verb: *anybody, everybody, nobody, somebody, anyone, everyone, nothing, something, anything, everything, no one, someone*

   Everyone plans to attend the meeting.

   Anyone is welcome at the concert.

7. *Both, few, many, others*, and *several* are always plural. When these five words are used as subjects or adjectives modifying subjects, a plural verb is required.

   Several members *were* asked to make presentations.

   Both women *are* going to apply.

8. *All, none, any, some, more*, and *most* may be singular or plural, depending on the noun to which they refer.

   Some of the *supplies are* missing.

   Some of that *paper is* needed.

9. A collective noun is a word that is singular in form but represents a group of people or things. Some examples of collective nouns are: *committee, company, department, public, class*, and *board*. The following rules determine the form of the verb to be used with a collective noun.

   - When the members of a group are thought of as one unit, the verb should be singular.

     The *committee has voted* unanimously to begin the study.

   - When members of the group are thought of as separate units, the verb should be plural.

     The *board are* not in agreement on the decision that should be made.

10. *The number* has a singular meaning and requires a singular verb; *a number* has a plural meaning and requires a plural verb.

    The number of requests *is* surprising.

    A number of people *are* planning to attend.

PRONOUNS

1. A pronoun agrees with its antecedent (the word for which the pronoun stands) in number, gender, and person.

   Roger wants to know if *his* book is at your house.

2. A plural pronoun is used when the antecedent consists of two nouns joined by *and*.

   Mary and *Tommie* are bringing *their* stereo.

3. A singular pronoun is used when the antecedent consists of two singular nouns joined by *or* or *nor*. A plural pronoun is used when the antecedent consists of two plural nouns joined by *or* or *nor*.

   Neither *Elizabeth* nor *Johanna* wants to do *her* part.

   Either the *men* or the *women* will do *their* share.

4. Do not confuse certain possessive pronouns and contractions that sound alike.

   its (possessive) *it's* (it is)

   their (possessive) *they're* (they are)

   theirs (possessive) *there's* (there is)

From Fulton PJ: *General office procedures for colleges*, ed 8, Cincinnati, 1983, South-Western, a part of Cengage Learning, Inc.

your (possessive) *you're* (you are)
whose (possessive) *who's* (who is)

As a test for the use of a possessive pronoun or a contraction, try to substitute *it is, they are, it has, there has, there is,* or *you are.* Use the corresponding possessive form if the substitution does not make sense.

Your wording is correct.

You're wording that sentence incorrectly.

Whose book is it?

Who's the owner of this typewriter?

5. Use *who* and *that* when referring to people.

He is the boy *who* does well in keyboarding.

She is the type of person *that* we like to employ.

6. Use *which* and *that* when referring to places, objects, and animals.

The *card that* I sent you was mailed last week.

The *fox, which* is very sly, caught the skunk.

PLURALS

In most English words the plurals are formed by merely adding an *s* or *es*, but in Greek and Latin the plural may be designated by changing the ending.

-ae, as in fasciae (singular form, fascia)

-ia, as in crania (singular form, cranium)

-i, as in glomeruli (singular form, glomerulus; when the singular form ends in *us*, the plural form is made by adding *i* and dropping the *us*)

-ata, as in adenomata (singular form, adenoma)

SPELLING

The aforementioned rules for pronunciation and the formation of plurals are essential for spelling, but it is important that you consult a dental or medical dictionary if you are not sure. Phonetic spelling has no place in medicine or dentistry because a misspelled word may give the wrong meaning to a diagnosis. Furthermore, some terms are pronounced alike but spelled differently; for example, *ileum* is a part of the intestinal tract, but *ilium* is a pelvic bone.

From Fulton PJ: *General office procedures for colleges*, ed 8, Cincinnati, 1983, South-Western, a part of Cengage Learning, Inc.

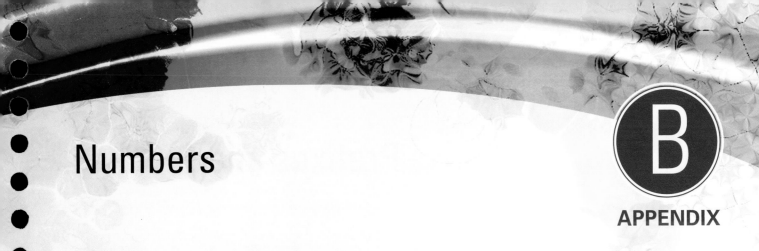

Numbers

1. Spell out numbers 1 through 10; use figures for numbers above 10.

   We ordered *ten* coats and *four* dresses.
   About *60* letters were keyed.

2. If there are numbers above and below 10 in correspondence, be consistent; either spell out all numbers or place all numbers in figures. If most of the numbers are below 10, spell them out. If most are above 10, express them all in figures.

   Please order *12* memo pads, *2* reams of paper, and *11* boxes of envelopes.

3. Numbers in the millions or higher may be expressed in the following manner to aid comprehension:

   3 billion (rather than 3,000,000,000)

4. Always spell out a number that begins a sentence.

   Five hundred books were ordered.

5. If the numbers are large, rearrange the wording of the sentence so that the number is not the first word of the sentence.

   We had a good year in *1976*.
   Not: Nineteen hundred and seventy-six was a good year.

6. Spell out indefinite numbers and amounts.

   A *few hundred* voters.

7. Spell out all ordinals (e.g., *first, second, third*) that can be expressed in words.

   The store's *twenty-fifth* anniversary was held this week.

8. When adjacent numbers are written in words or in figures, use a comma to separate them.

   On Car 33, *450* cartons are being shipped.

9. House or building numbers are written in figures. However, when the number *one* appears by itself, it is spelled out. Numbers one through ten in street names are spelled out; numbers above ten are written in figures.

   When figures are used for both the house number and the street name, use a hyphen that is preceded and followed by a space.

   101 Building
   2301 Fifth Avenue
   One Main Place
   122 - 33rd Street

10. Ages are usually spelled out except when the age is stated exactly in years, months, and days. When ages are presented in tabular form, they are written in figures.

    She is *eighteen years* old.
    He is *2 years, 10 months, and 18 days* old.
    Jones, Edward 19
    King, Ruth 21

11. Use figures to express dates written in normal month-day-year order. Do not use *th, nd,* or *rd* after the date.

    May 8, 1987
    Not: May 8th, 1987

12. Fractions should be spelled out unless they are part of mixed numbers. Use a hyphen to separate the numerator and denominator of fractions written in words when the fraction is used as an adjective.

    three-fourths inch
    5½

13. In legal documents, numbers may be written in both words and figures.

    One hundred thirty-four and 30/100 dollars
    ($134.30)

14. Amounts of money are usually expressed in figures. Indefinite money amounts are written in words.

    $100
    $3.27
    several hundred dollars

15. Express percentages in figures; spell out the word *percent*.

    10 percent

16. To form the plural of figures, add *s*.

    Technological advances will increase in the *1980s*.

17. In times of day, use figures with *A.M.* and *P.M.*; spell out numbers with the word *o'clock*. In formal usage, all times are spelled out.

    9 A.M.
    10 P.M.
    eight o'clock in the evening

From Fulton PJ: *General office procedures for colleges*, ed 8, Cincinnati, 1983, South-Western, a part of Cengage Learning, Inc.

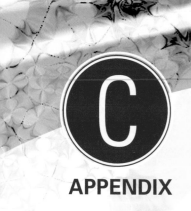

APPENDIX C

Prefixes and Suffixes

PREFIXES

Prefixes, the most frequently used elements in the formation of medical and dental words, are one or more syllables placed before words or roots to show various kinds of relationships. They are never used independently, but when added before verbs, adjectives, or nouns, they modify the meaning. Most prefixes are a part of words in ordinary speech and do not refer specifically to medical-dental or scientific terminology, but many occur frequently in medical terminology. Studying them is an important step in learning medical terms and building a medical-dental vocabulary.

Prefix	Translation	Examples
a- (an- before a vowel)	Without, lack of	Apathy (lack of feeling), anemia (lack of blood)
ab-	Away from	Abductor (leading away from), aboral (away from mouth)
ad-	To, toward, near to	Adductor (leading toward), adhesion (sticking to)
ambi-	Both	Ambidextrous (ability to use hands equally), ambilaterally (both sides)
amphi-	About, on both sides, both	Amphibious (living on both land and water)
ampho-	Both	Amphogenic (producing offspring of both sexes)
ana-	Up, back, again, excessive	Anatomy (a cutting up)
ante-	Before, forward	Antecubital (before elbow), anteflexion (forward bending)
anti-	Against, opposed to, reversed	Antisepsis (against infection)
apo-	From, away from	Aponeurosis (away from tendon), apochromatic (abnormal color)
bi-	Twice, double	Bilateral (two sides), bifurcation (two branches)
cata-	Down, according to, complete	Catabolism (breaking down), catalepsia (complete seizure)
circum-	Around, about	Circumference (surrounding), circumscribe (to draw around)
com-	With, together	Commissure (sending or coming together)
con-	With, together	Conductor (leading together), concentric (having a common center)
contra-	Against, opposite	Contraception (prevention of conception), contraindicated (not indicated)
de-	Away from	Dehydrate (remove water from), decompensation (failure of compensation)
di-	Twice, double	Diplopia (double vision), dichromatic (two colors)
dia-	Through, apart, across, completely	Diaphragm (wall across), diapedesis (ooze through), diagnosis (complete knowledge)
dis-	Reversal, apart from, separation	Disinfection (apart from infection), dissect (cut apart)
dys-	Bad, difficult, disordered	Dyspepsia (bad digestion), dyspnea (difficult breathing)
e-, ex-	Out, away from	Enucleate (remove from), exostosis (outgrowth of bone)
ec-	Out from	Ectopic (out of place), eccentric (away from center)
ecto-	On outside, situated on	Ectoderm (outer skin), ectoretina (outer layer of retina)
em-, en-	In	Empyema (pus in), encephalon (in the head)
endo-	Within	Endodont (within tooth)
epi-	Upon, on	Epidural (upon dura), epidermis (on skin)
exo-	Outside, on outer side, outer layer	Exogenous (produced outside)
extra-	Outside	Extracellular (outside cell)
hemi-	Half	Hemiplegia (partial paralysis), hemianesthesia (loss of feeling on one side of body)
hyper-	Over, above, excessive	Hyperemia (excessive blood), hypertrophy (overgrowth), hyperplasia (excessive formation)
hypo-	Under, below, deficient	Hypotension (low blood pressure)
im-, in-	In, into	Immersion (act of dipping in), injection (act of forcing liquid into)
im-, in-	Not	Immature (not mature), involuntary (not voluntary), inability (not able)
infra-	Below	Infraorbital (below eye), infraclavicular (below clavicle or collarbone)
inter-	Between	Intercostal (between ribs), intervene (come between)

From *Mosby's dental dictionary*, ed 2, St Louis, 2008, Mosby.

Prefix	Translation	Examples
intra-	Within	Intracerebral (within cerebrum), intraocular (within eyes)
intro-	Into, within	Introversion (turning inward), introduce (lead into)
meta-	Beyond, after, change	Metamorphosis (change of form), metastasis (beyond original position)
opistho-	Behind, backward	Opisthotic (behind ears), opisthognathous (behind jaws)
para-	Beside, by side	Paraplegia (paralysis of both sides), paracentesis (puncture along side of)
per-	Through, excessive	Permeate (pass through), perforate (bore through)
peri-	Around	Periosteum (around bone), periatrial (around atrium)
post-	After, behind	Postoperative (after operation), postocular (behind eye)
pre-	Before, in front of	Premolar (in front of molars), preoral (in front of mouth)
pro-	Before, in front of	Prognosis (foreknowledge), prophase (appear before)
re-	Back, again, contrary	Reflex (bend back), revert (turn again to)
retro-	Backward, located behind	Retrograde (going backward), retrolingual (behind tongue)
semi-	Half	Semicartilaginous (half cartilage), semiconscious (half conscious)
sub-	Under	Subcutaneous (under skin), subungual (under nail)
super-	Above, upper, excessive	Supercilia (upper brows), supernumerary (excessive number)
supra-	Above, upon	Suprarenal (above kidney), suprascapular (on upper part of scapula)
sym-, syn-	Together, with	Symphysis (growing together), synapsis (joining together)
trans-	Across, through	Transection (cut across), transmit (send beyond)
ultra-	Beyond, in	Ultraviolet (beyond violet end of spectrum), ultrasonic (sound waves beyond the upper frequency of hearing by human ear)

SUFFIXES

Suffixes are one or more syllables or elements added to the *root* of a word (the part that indicates the essential meaning) to alter the meaning or indicate the intended part of speech.

To make the word pronounceable, the last letter or letters of the root to which the suffix is attached may be changed. The last vowel may be changed to an *o*, or *o* may be inserted if it is not already present before a suffix beginning with a consonant, as in *cardiology*. The final vowel in the root may be dropped before a suffix beginning with a vowel, as in *neuritis*.

Most suffixes are in common use in English, but some are peculiar to medical science. The suffixes most commonly used to indicate disease are *-itis*, meaning "inflammation," *-oma*, meaning "tumor," and *-osis*, meaning "a condition," usually morbid. The following suffixes occur often in medical-dental terminology but are also used in ordinary language:

Suffix	Use	Examples
-ise, -ize, -ate	Add to nouns or adjectives to make verbs expressing to use and to act like; to subject to; make into	Visualize (able to see), hypnotize (put into state of hypnosis)
-ist, -or, -er	Add to verbs to make nouns expressing agent or person concerned or instrument	Anesthetist (one who practices the science of anesthesia), donor (giver)
-ent	Add to verbs to make adjectives or nouns of agency	Recipient (one who receives), concurrent (happening at the same time)
-sia, -y	Add to verbs to make nouns expressing action, process, or condition	Therapy (treatment), anesthesia (process or condition of feeling)
-ia, -ity	Add to adjectives or nouns to make nouns expressing quality or condition	Septicemia (poisoning of blood), disparity (inequality), acidity (condition of excess acid), neuralgia (pain in nerves)
-ma, -mata, -men, -mina, -ment, -ure	Add to verbs to make nouns expressing result of action or object of action	Trauma (injury), foramina (openings), ligament (tough, fibrous band holding bone or viscera together), fissure (groove)
-ium, -olus, -olum, -culus, -culum, -cule, -cle	Add to nouns to make diminutive nouns	Bacterium, alveolus (air sac), follicle (little bag), cerebellum (little brain), molecule (little mass), ossicle (little bone)
-ible, -ile	Add to verbs to make adjectives expressing ability or capacity	Contractile (ability to contract), edible (capable of being eaten), flexible (capable of being bent)
-al, -c, -ious, -tic	Add to nouns to make adjectives expressing relationship, concern, or pertaining	Neural (referring to nerve), neoplastic (referring to neoplasm), cardiac (referring to heart), delirious (suffering from delirium)
-id	Add to verbs or nouns to make adjectives expressing state or condition	Flaccid (state of being weak or lax), fluid (state of being fluid or liquid)

(Continued)

Suffix	Use	Examples
-tic	Add to verbs to make adjectives showing relationships	Caustic (referring to burn), acoustic (referring to sound or hearing)
-oid, -form	Add to nouns to make adjectives expressing resemblance	Polypoid (resembling polyp), plexiform (resembling a plexus), fusiform (resembling a fusion), epidermoid (resembling epidermis)
-ous	Add to nouns to make adjectives expressing material	Ferrous (composed of iron), serous (composed of serum), mucinous (composed of mucin)

The following verbs or combining forms of verbs are derived from either Greek or Latin. They may be attached to other roots to form words, or suffixes and prefixes may be added to them to form words. In the following examples, the part or root of the word to which the verb is attached is underlined, and the meaning, if not clear, is given in parentheses.

Root	Translation	Examples
-algia-	Pain	Cardialgia (heart), gastralgia (stomach), neuralgia (nerve)
-audi-, -audio-	Hear, hearing	Audiometer (measure), audiophone (voice instrument for deaf)
-bio-	Live	Biology (study of living), biogenesis (origin)
cau-, -caus-	Burn	Caustic (suffix added to make adjective), cauterization, causalgia (burning pain), electrocautery
-centesis-	Puncture, perforate	Thoracentesis (chest), pneumocentesis (lung), arthrocentesis (joint), enterocentesis (intestine)
-clas-, -claz-	Smash, break	Osteoclasis (bone), odontoclasis (tooth)
-duct-	Lead	Ductal (suffix added to make adjective), oviduct (egg uterine tube or fallopian tube), periductal (peri means "around")
-dynia-	Pain	Mastodynia (breast), esophagodynia (esophagus)
-ecta-, -ectas-	Dilate	Venectasia (dilation of vein), cardiectasis (heart), ectatic (suffix added for adjective)
-edem-	Swell	Myoedema (muscle), lymphedema (lymph), (*a* is a suffix added to make a noun)
-esthes-	Feel	Esthesia (suffix added to make noun), anesthesia (*an* is a prefix)
-flex-, -flec-	Bend	Flexion (suffix added to make noun), flexor (suffix added), anteflect (prefix added meaning "before" bending forward)
-fiss-	Split	Fissure, fission (suffixes added to make nouns)
-flu-, -flux-	Flow	Fluctuate, fluxion, affluent (abundant flowing)
-geno-, -genesis-	Produce, origin	Genotype, homogenesis (same origin), pathogenesis (disease, origin of disease), heterogenesis (prefix added meaning "other," alteration of generation)
-iatro-, -iatr-	Treat, cure	Geriatrics (old age), pediatrics (children)
-kine-, -kino-, -kineto-, -kinesio-	Move	Kinetogenic (Producing movement), kinetic (suffix added to make adjective), kinesiology (study)
-liga-	Bind	Ligament (suffix added to make noun) ligate, ligature
-logy-	Study	Parasitology (parasites), bacteriology (bacteria), histology (tissues)
-lysis-	Breaking up, dissolving	Hemolysis (blood), glycolysis (sugar), autolysis (self-destruction of cells)
-morph-, -morpho-	Form	Morphology, amorphous (not definite form), pleomorphic (more, occurring in various forms), polymorphic (many)
-olfact-	Smell	Olfactophobia (fear), olfactory (suffix added to make adjective)
-op-, -opto-	See	Amblyopia (dull, dimness of vision), presbyopia (old, impairment of vision in old age), optic myopia (*myo*, to wink, half close the eyes)
-palpit-	Flutter	Palpitation
-pep-	Digest	Dyspepsia (bad, difficult), peptic (suffix added to make adjective)
-phag-, -phago-	Eat	Phagocytosis (eating of cells), phagomania (madness, mad craving for food or to eat), dysphagia (difficulty eating or swallowing)
-phan-	Appear, visible	Phanerosis (act of becoming visible), phantasia, phantasy
-pexy-	Fix	Mastopexy (fixation of breast), nephrosplenopexy (surgical fixation of kidney and spleen)
-phas-	Speak, utter	Aphasia (unable to speak), dysphasia (difficulty in speaking)
-phobia-	Fear	Hydrophobia (fear of water), claustrophobia (fear of close places)
-phil-	Like, love	Hemophilia (blood, a hereditary disease characterized by delayed clotting of blood), acidophilia (acid stain, liking or straining with acid stains), philanthropy (love of humankind)

From *Mosby's dental dictionary*, ed 2, St Louis, 2008, Mosby.

Root	Translation	Examples
-phrax-, -phrag-	Fence off, wall off	Diaphragm (across, partition separating thorax from abdomen), phragmoplast (formed)
-plas-	Form, grow	Neoplasm (new growth), rhinoplasty (nose operation for formation of nose), otoplasty (ear)
-plegia-	Paralyze	Paraplegia (paralysis of lower limbs), ophthalmoplegia (eye), hemiplegia (partial paralysis)
-pne-, -pneo-	Breathe	Dyspnea (difficult breathing), apnea (lack of breathing), hyperpnea (overbreathing)
-poie-	Make	Hematopoiesis (blood), erythropoiesis (red blood cells), leukopoiesis (making white cells)
-rrhagia-	Burst forth, pour	Menorrhagia (abnormal bleeding during menstruation), hemorrhage (blood)
-rrhaphy-	Suture	Herniorrhaphy (suturing or repair of hernia), hepatorrhaphy (liver), nephrorrhaphy (kidney)
-rrhea-	Flow, discharge	Leukorrhea (white discharge from vagina), rhinorrhea (nasal discharge)
-rrhexis-	Rupture	Enterorrhexis (intestines), metrorrhexis (uterus)
-schiz-	Split, divide	Schizophrenia (mind, split personality), schizonychia (nails), schizotrichia (hair)
-scope-	Examine	Microscopic, cardioscope, endoscope (endo means "within," an instrument for examining the interior of a hollow internal organ)
-stasis-	Stop, stand still	Hematostasis (pertaining to stagnation of blood), epistasis (checking or stopping of any discharge)
-stazien-	Drop	Epistaxis (nosebleed)
-teg-, -tect-	Cover	Tegmen, tectum (rooflike structure), integument (skin covering)
-therap-	Treat, cure	Therapy, neurotherapy (nerves), chemotherapy (chemicals), physiotherapy
-tomy-	Cut, incise	Phlebotomy (incision of vein), arthrotomy (joint), appendectomy (ectomy, meaning "cutout," excision of appendix)
-topo-	Place	Topography, toponarcosis (numbing, hence numbing of a part or localized anesthesia)
-tropho-	Nourish	Hypertrophy (enlargement or overnourishment), atrophy (undernourishment), dystrophy (difficult or bad)

The following roots and combining forms are derived from Greek or Latin adjectives. Adjectives appear most often in compounds and are joined to either nouns or verbs. Suffixes may be added to make them into nouns. In the following examples, the part or root of the word the adjective modifies is underlined, and the meaning is given in parentheses if not clear.

Root	Translation	Examples
-auto-	Self	Autoinfection, autolysis, autopathy (disease), autopsy (view, postmortem examination)
-brachy-	Short	Brachycephalia (head), brachydactylia (fingers), brachychelia (lip), brachygnathous (jaw)
-brady-	Slow	Bradypnea (breath), bradypragia (action), bradyuria (urine), bradypepsia (digestion)
-brevis-	Short	Brevity, breviflexor (short flexor muscle)
-cavus-	Hollow	Cavity, cavernous, vena cava (vein)
-coel-	Hollow	Coelarium (lining membrane of body cavity), coelom (body cavity of embryo)
-cryo-	Cold	Cryotherapy, cryotolerant, cryometer
-crypto-	Hidden, concealed	Cryptorchid (testis), cryptogenic (origin obscure of doubtful), cryptophthalmos (eye)
-dextro-	Right	Ambidextrous (using both hands with equal ease), dextrophobia (fear of objects on right side), dextrocardia (heart)
-dys-	Difficult, bad, disordered, painful	Dysarthria (speech), dyshidrosis (sweat), dyskinesia (motion), dystocia (birth), dysphasia (speech), dyspepsia (digestion)
-eu-	Well, good	Euphoria (well-being), euphagia, eupnea (breath), euthyroid (normal thyroid), eutocia (normal birth)
-eury-	Broad, wide	Eurycephalic (head), euryopia (vision), eurysomatic (body, squat thickset body)
-glyco-	Sugar, sweet	Glycohemia (sugar in blood), glycopenia (poverty of sugar, low blood sugar level)
-gravis-	Heavy	Gravida (pregnant woman), gravidism (pregnancy)
-haplo-	Single, simple	Haploid (having a single set of chromosomes), haplodermatitis (simple inflammation of skin), haplopathy (simple uncomplicated disease)
-hetero-	Other, different	Heterogeneous (kind, dissimilar elements), heteroinoculation, heterology (abnormality of structure), heterointoxication
-homo-	Same	Homogeneous (same kind of quality throughout), homozygous (possessing identical pair of genes), homologous (corresponding in structure)

(Continued)

Root	Translation	Examples
-hydro-	Wet, water	Hydronephrosis (kidney, collection of urine in kidney, pelvis), hydrophobia (fear of water, water causes painful reaction in this disease)
-iso-	Equal	Isocellular (similar cells), isodontic (all teeth alike), isocytosis (equality of size of cells), isochromatic (having same color throughout)
-latus-	Broad	Latitude, latissimus dorsi (muscle adducting humerus)
-leio-	Smooth	Leiomyosarcoma (smooth muscle, fleshy malignant tumor), leiomyofibroma (tumor of muscle and fiber elements), leiomyoma (tumor of unstriped muscle)
-lepto-	Slender	Leptosomatic (body), leptodactylous (fingers)
-levo-	Left	Levocardia (heart), levorotation (turning to left)
-longus-	Long	Adductor longus (muscle of thigh), longitude
-macro-	Large, abnormal size	Macrocephalic (head), macrochiria (hands), macromastia (breast), macronychia (nails)
-magna-	Large, great	Magnitude, adductor magnus (thigh muscle)
-malaco-	Soft	Malacia (softening), osteomalacia (bones)
-malus-	Bad	Malady, malaise, malignant, malformation
-medius-	Middle, median, medium	Gluteus medius (femur muscle)
-mega-	Great	Megacolon (large colon), megacephaly (head)
-megalo-	Huge	Megalomania (delusion of grandeur), hepatomegaly (enlarged liver), splenomegaly (enlarged spleen)
-meso-	Middle, mid	Mesocarpal (wrist), mesoderm (skin), mesothelium (a lining membrane of cavities)
-micro-	Small	Microglossia (tongue), microblepharia (eyelids), microorganism, microphonia (voice)
-minimus-	Smallest	Gluteus minimus (smallest muscle of hip), adductor minimus (muscle of thigh)
-mio-	Less	Mioplasmia (plasma, abnormal decrease in plasma in blood), miopragia (perform, decreased activity)
-mono-	One, single, limited to one part	Monochromatic (color), monobrachia (arm)
-multi-	Many, much	Multipara (bear, woman who has borne more than one child), multilobar (numerous lobes), multicentric (many centers)
-necro-	Dead	Necrosed, necrosis, necropsy (postmortem examination), necrophobia (fear of death)
-neo-	New	Neoformation, neomorphism (form), neonatal (first 4 weeks of life), neopathy (disease)
-oligo-	Few, scanty, little	Oligophrenia (mind), oligopnea (breath), oliguria (urine), oligodipsia (thirst)
-ortho-	Straight, normal, correct	Orthodont (teeth, normal), orthogenesis (progressive evolution in a given direction), orthograde (walk, carrying body upright), orthopnea (breath, unable to breathe unless in an upright position)
-oxy-	Sharp, quick	Oxyesthesia (feel), oxyopia (vision), oxyosmia (smell)
-pachy-	Thick	Pachyderm (skin), pachysulemia (blood), pachypleuritis (inflammation of pleura), pachycholia (bile), pachyotia (ears)
-paleo-	Old	Paleogenetic (origin in the past), paleopathology (study of diseases in mummies)
-platy-	Flat	Platybasia (skull base), platycoria (pupil), platycrania (skull)
-pleo-	More	Pleomorphism (forms), pleochromocytoma (tumor composed of different colored cells)
-poikilo-	Varied	Poikiloderma (skin mottling), poikilothermal (heat, variable body temperature)
-poly-	Many, much	Polyhedral (many bases or faces), polymastia (more than two breasts), polymelia (supernumerary limbs), polymyalgia (pain in many muscles)
-pronus-	Face down	Prone, pronation
-pseudo-	False, spurious	Pseudostratified (layered), pseudocirrhosis (apparent cirrhosis of liver), pseudohypertrophy
-sclero-	Hard	Sclerosis (hardening), arteriosclerosis (artery), scleronychia (nails), sclerodermatitis (skin)
-scolio-	Twisted, crooked	Scoliodontic (teeth), scoliosis, scoliokyphosis (curvature of spine)
-sinistro-	Left	Sinistrocardia, sinistromanual (left-handed), sinistraural (hearing better in left ear)
-supinus-	Face up	Supine, supination, supinator longus (muscle in arm)
-steno-	Narrow	Stenosis, stenostomia (mouth), mitral stenosis (mitral valve in heart)
-stereo-	Solid, three dimensions	Stereoscope, stereometer
-tachy-	Fast, swift	Tachycardia (heart), tachyphrasia (speech)
-tele-	End, far away	Telepathy, telecardiogram
-telo-	Complete	Telophase
-thermo-	Heat, warm	Thermal, thermometer, thermobiosis (ability to live in high temperature)
-trachy-	Rough	Trachyphonia (voice), trachychromatic (deeply staining)
-xero-	Dry	Xerophagia (eating of dry foods), xerostomia (mouth), xerodermia (skin)

From *Mosby's dental dictionary*, ed 2, St Louis, 2008, Mosby.

PRONUNCIATION OF MEDICAL-DENTAL TERMS

Medical terms are hard to pronounce, especially if you have read them but have never heard them spoken. The following are some helpful shortcuts.

ch is sometimes pronounced like *k*. Examples: *chromatin, chronic.*

ps is pronounced like *s*. Examples: *psychiatry, psychology.*

pn is pronounced with only the *n* sound. Example: *pneumonia.*

c and *g* are given the soft sound of *s* and *j*, respectively, before *e*, *i*, and *y* in words of both Greek and Latin origin. Examples: *cycle, cytoplasm, giant, generic.*

c and *g* have a harsh sound before other letters. Examples: *gastric, gonad, cast, cardiac.*

ae and *oe* are pronounced *ee*. Examples: *coelom, fasciae.*

e and *es*, when forming the final letter or letters of a word, are often pronounced as separate syllables. Examples: *rete (reetee), nares (nayreez).*

i at the end of a word (to form a plural) is pronounced *eye*. Examples: *alveoli, glomeruli, fasciculi.*

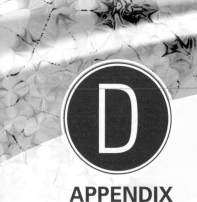

APPENDIX

Abbreviations

A amp
@ at
aa of each (F. ana)
a.c. before meals (L., *ante cibum*)
ad Latin preposition, -to, up to
a.d. alternating days (L., *alternis diebus*)
ad lib at pleasure, as needed or desired (L., *ad libitum*)
adm admission
Ag silver (L., *argentum*)
alt. dieb. every other day (L., *alternis diebus*)
alt. hor. every other hour (L., *alternis horis*)
alt. noct. every other night (L., *alternis noctibus*)
a, am, ag amalgam
AM, a.m., A.M. before noon (L., *ante meridiem*)
amp ampule
amt amount
anat anatomy, anatomical
anes anesthesia
ant anterior
AP anteroposterior
appl applicable, application, appliance
approx approximate
aq water (L., *aqua*)
av average
bact bacterium (-ia)
BF bone fragment
bib drink (L., *bibe*)
b.i.d. twice a day (L., *bis in die*)
biol biological, biology
BP blood pressure
BS blood sugar
BW bite-wing radiograph
Bx biopsy
C centigrade
C one hundred (L., *centum*)
c̄ with (L., *cum*)
CA cardiac arrest
CA chronological age
Ca calcium
Ca carcinoma
cal calorie
caps capsules
cav cavity

CBC complete blood count
CC chief complaint
cc cubic centimeter
CDA or C.D.A. Certified Dental Assistant
cent centigrade
CHD childhood disease
CHF congestive heart failure
chr chronic
cm centimeter
c.m. tomorrow morning (L., *cras mane*)
CO₂ carbon dioxide
comp compound
conc concentrated
cond condition
CP centric position
cpd compound
Cu copper (L., *cuprum*)
cu cubic
cur curettage
CV cardiovascular
CVA cerebrovascular accident
Cx convex
CY calendar year
d dose (L., *dosis*)
D, dist distal
dbl double
dc direct current
DDS or D.D.S. Doctor of Dental Surgery/Science
deg degree
dev develop, development
Dg diagnosis
diag diagnosis
dil dilute (L., *dilue*)
DO distocclusal
dis disease
disp dispensary
dist distal
DMF decayed, missing, and filled (teeth)
DOA dead on arrival
DOB date of birth
doz dozen
Dr. doctor
d.t.d. give of such a dose (L., *datur talis dosis*)

Modified from Zwemer TJ: *Boucher's clinical dental terminology*, ed 4, St Louis, 1993, Mosby.

dwt pennyweight
Dx diagnosis
EAC external auditory canal
ed effective dose
EDDA expanded duties dental assistant (auxiliary)
EENT ears, eyes, nose and throat
EFDA expanded (extended) function dental assistant (auxiliary)
e.g. for example (L., *exempli gratia*)
EKG elektrokardiogram (German)
emerg emergency
EMT emergency medical treatment
ENT ears, nose, and throat
epith epithelial
equiv equivalent
esp especially
est estimate, estimation
et and, Latin conjunction
et al. and others (L., *et alia*)
etc. and so on, and so forth, and others (L., *et cetera*)
eval evaluate, evaluation
ext extract, external
F Fahrenheit
F female
F field (of vision)
F formula
FB foreign body
FBS fasting blood sugar
FD fatal dose
ff following
FH family history
fl fluid
FLD full lower denture
fld field
fl. dr. fluid dram
fl. oz. fluid ounce
FMX full mouth x-ray examination
frac fracture
frag fragment
freq frequent, frequency
ft foot
ft let it be made (L., *fiat/fiant*)
FUD full upper denture
func function
Fx fracture
g gram
gal gallon
ging gingiva, gingivectomy
glob globulin
gm gram
GP general practitioner
gr grain
gt drop (L., *gutta*)
gtt drops (L., *guttae*)
H, h, hr hour (L., *hora*)
H₂O water
Hb, hgb hemoglobin

Hdpc handpiece
h.d. at hour of lying down at bedtime (L., *hora decubitus*)
hosp hospital
hr hour
h.s. hour of sleep (L., *hora somni*)
ht. height
Hx history
I & D incision and drainage
IA incurred accidentally
ibid. in the same place (L., *ibidem*)
id the same (L., *idem*)
i.e. that is (L., *id est*)
IH infectious hepatitis
IM intramuscular
imp impression
in inch
inc incisal, incisive incise
in d. daily (L., *in dies*)
inf infected, inferior, infusion
inj injection, injury
inop inoperable, inoperative
int internal
IQ intelligence quotient
i.q. the same as (L., *idem quod*)
IS interspace
IV intravenous
kg, kgm kilogram
kilo kilogram
kV kilovolt
L Latin
L, l liter
lab laboratory
lac laceration
LASER (laser) light amplification by stimulated emission of radiation
lat lateral
lb pound (L., *libra*)
lig ligament
ling lingual
liq liquid, liquor
LN lymph node
lt left
m murmur
m meter
m. dict. as directed (L., *modo dictu*)
m male
m, mes mesial
ma milliampere
mand mandibular
MASER (maser) microwave amplification by stimulated emission of radiation
max maximum, maxillary
MDR minimum daily requirement
med medical, medicine
mg, mgm milligram
micro microscopic

min minute, minimum
ML midline
ml milliliter
MM mucous membrane
mm millimeter
MO mesiocclusal
MOD mesiocclusodistal
mo month
MS multiple sclerosis
msec millisecond
N₂O nitrous oxide
narc narcotic, narcotism
neg negative
non. rep. do not repeat
norm normal
NPC no previous complaint
NPH no previous history
n.p.o. nothing by mouth (L., *nil per os*)
NR normal record
n.r. not to be repeated (L., *non repetatur*)
N/S normal saline
O oxygen
O₂ oxygen gas
obl oblique
occ occlusal
ODC oral disease control
o.d. every day (L., *omni die*)
o.d. right eye
OH oral hygiene
o.h. every hour (L., *omni hora*)
o.m. every morning (L., *omni mane*)
o.n. every night (L., *omni nocte*)
op operation
OPC outpatient clinic
OPD outpatient department
opp opposite, opposed
OR operating room
org organism, organic
oz ounce
P pulse
P after (L., *post*)
p- para-
PA posteroanterior
Pan panoral x-ray examination
PATH pituitary adrenotropic hormone
path pathology
p.c. after meal (L., *post cibum*)
PCN penicillin
PDR *Physicians' Desk Reference*
perf *perforating*
PLD partial lower denture
P.M. PM, p.m. after noon (L., *post meridiem*)
PM after death (L., *post mortem*)
PO postoperative

p.o. by mouth (L., *per os*)
POH personal oral hygiene
pos positive
postop postoperative
prep preparation, prepare (for surgery)
p.r.n. as required, as the occasion arises (L., *pro re nata*)
prog prognosis
pt patient
PUD partial upper denture
Px prophylaxis
q every (L., *quaque*)
q.d. every day (L., *quaque die*)
q.h. every hour (L., *quaque hora*)
q.2h every second hour (L., *quaque secunda hora*)
q.i.d. four times a day (L., *quater in die*)
q.l. as much as pleased (L., *quantum libet*)
q.n. every night (L., *quaque nocte*)
q.p. at will (L., *quantum placeat*)
q.q.h. every 4 hours (L., *quaque quarta hora*)
qt quart
q.v. as much as liked (L., *quantum vis*)
r roentgen
R respiration
RX take (thou) a recipe
rad radiograph
RC retruded contact position
RC root canal
R.D.A. Registered Dental Assistant
RDH Registered Dental Hygienist
reg regular
rem(s) roentgen-equivalent-man
req requires, required
rep(s) roentgen-equivalent-physical
resp respiration
Rh Rh factor in blood (L., *Rhesus*)
RHD rheumatic heart disease
RN Registered Nurse
rt right
Rx treatment (L., *recipe*)
s without (L., *sine*)
SBE subacute bacterial endocarditis
SD sterile dressing
sec second, secondary
Sig. write on label
sol solution
spec specimen
ss one half signs and symptoms (L., *semis*)
stat immediately (L., *statim*)
std standard
stim stimulator, stimulate
strep *Streptococcus* organisms
sup superior
surg surgeon, surgery
Sx symptom

sym symmetric
symp symptom
sys system
T temperature
tab tablet
TB, TBC tuberculosis
tbsp tablespoon
temp temperature
t.i.d. three times a day (L., *ter in die*)
tinc tincture
TLC tender loving care
TM temporomandibular
TMJ temporomandibular joint
TPR temperature, pulse, respiration
tsp teaspoon
U, u unit
ung ointment (L., *unguentum*)
unk unknown
USP United States Pharmacopoeia
ut. dict. As directed
V, v volt
VD venereal disease
vert vertebra, vertical
visc viscous
VIT vitamin
viz that is, namely (L., *videlicet*)
VO verbal order
vol volume
vs versus
WF white female
wh white
WM white male
w-n well-nourished

wnd wound
wt weight
x times, 4×, four times; ×4, times four yard
xt extract, extracted
xyl, xylo Xylocaine
yd yard
YOB year of birth
yr year

Symbols

& and
* birth
† death
↓ decrease
° Degree
= equal
' feet, minutes
♀ Female
> greater than, or indicating increase
" inches, seconds
↑ increase
< less than, or indicating decrease
♂ male
− minus, negative
number, pound
i, ii, iii one, two, or three (as in number of grams)
℥iss one and one-half drams
℥T one ounce
℥ss one-half ounce
/ per
% percent
+ plus, positive

Modified from Zwemer TJ: *Boucher's clinical dental terminology*, ed 4, St Louis, 1993, Mosby.

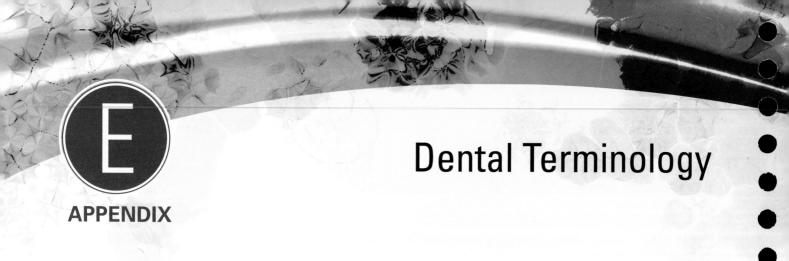

abrasion Mechanical wearing away of teeth by abnormal stressors. This could result from abnormal toothbrushing habits or other abnormal stress on the teeth.

accessional Permanent teeth that do not replace deciduous teeth but rather become an accession (addition) to the deciduous or succedaneous teeth, or both types.

accessory root canals Extra openings into the pulp; usually located on the sides of the roots or in the bifurcations.

acquired Pertaining to something obtained by oneself; not inherited.

ala Latin for "wing," referring to the sides of the nostrils of the nose; plural *alae*.

alignment Arrangement of teeth in a row.

allergenic Being hypersensitive to something.

allergic reaction Body's reaction to an allergen; an example of such a reaction is hives.

alveolar bone Bone that forms the sockets for the teeth.

alveolar crest Highest part of the alveolar bone closest to the cervical line of the tooth.

alveolar eminences Bulges on the facial surface of alveolar bone that outline the position of the roots.

alveolar mucosa Mucosa between the mucobuccal fold and gingiva.

alveolar process Part of the bone in the maxillae and mandible that forms the sockets for the teeth.

alveolus (alveoli) Cavity, or socket, in the alveolar process in which the root of the tooth is held.

anatomical crown That part of the tooth covered by enamel.

angle of the mandible Point at the lower border of the body of the mandible where it turns up onto the ramus.

Angle's classification System of dental classifications based primarily on the relationship of the permanent first molars to each other and to a lesser degree on the relationship of the permanent canines to each other.

ankyloglossia See *tongue-tie*.

ankylosis Fusion of the cementum of a tooth with alveolar bone.

anodontia The absence of teeth in the jaw.

anomaly Any noticeable difference or deviation from that which is ordinary or normal.

anterior Situated in front of; a term commonly used to denote the incisor and canine teeth or the area toward the front of the mouth.

anterior pillar Fold of tissue extending down in front of the tonsil.

antihistamine Drug that controls the body's histamine reaction, which causes congestion of tissues.

apex (apices) End point, or furthest tip, as of the tooth root.

apical foramen Aperture, or opening, at or near the apex of a tooth root through which the blood and nerve supply of the pulp enters the tooth.

arch, dental See *dental arch*.

atrophic Pertaining to the wasting away of a tissue, organ, or part from disease, defective nutrition, or lack of use.

atrophy Wasting away of a tissue, organ, or part from disease, defective nutrition, or lack of use.

attached gingiva Tightly adherent gingiva that extends from free gingiva to alveolar mucosa.

attrition Process of normal wear on the crown.

autonomic nervous system Automatic nervous system of the body that is not willfully controlled. It controls the functions of the glands and smooth and cardiac muscle.

bicuspid See *premolars*.

bifurcation Division into two parts or branches, as any two roots of a tooth.

body of the mandible Horizontal portion of the mandible, excluding the alveolar process.

bone Hard connective tissue that forms the framework of the body. The hardness is attributable to the hydroxyapatite crystal.

bruxism Abnormal grinding of the teeth.

bucca Latin word for cheek.

buccal Pertaining to the cheek; toward the cheek or next to the cheek. Also called *facial*.

buccal development groove Groove that separates the buccal cusps on a buccal surface.

buccal glands Small minor salivary glands in the cheek.

buccinator Muscle of facial expression that extends from the back buccal portion of the maxilla and mandible and pterygomandibular raphe forward in the cheek to the corner of the mouth.

From Brand RW, Isselhard DE: *Anatomy of orofacial structures*, ed 7, St Louis, 2003, Mosby.

calcification Process by which organic tissue becomes hardened by a deposit of calcium salts within its substance. The term, in a liberal sense, connotes the deposition of any mineral salts that contribute to the hardening and maturation of hard tissue.

canal Long tubular opening through a bone.

canines Third teeth from the midline, at corner of mouth; used for grasping; also called *cuspids*.

capsule Fibrous band of tissue surrounding a joint.

cell Basic functioning component of the body; capable of reproducing itself in most instances. Tissues are made up of groups of cells.

cementoenamel junction (CEJ) Junction of enamel of the crown and cementum of the root. This junction forms the cervical line around the tooth.

cementoma Cementum tumor at root tip that destroys surrounding bone.

cementum Layer of bonelike tissue covering the root of the tooth.

central developmental groove Developmental groove that crosses the occlusal surface of a tooth from the mesial to the distal side; divides the tooth into buccal and lingual parts.

centric occlusion (central occlusion) Relationship of the occlusal surfaces of one arch to those of the other when the jaws are closed and the teeth are in maximum intercuspation.

centric relation Arch-to-arch relationship of the maxilla to the mandible when the condyles are in their most upward position, the mandible is in its most posterior position, and the jaw is most braced by its musculature.

cervical Portion of a tooth near the junction of the crown and root. Pertaining to the neck region, for example, nerves of the neck.

cervical line Line formed by the junction of the enamel and cementum on a tooth.

cervical third Portion of the crown or root of a tooth at or near the cervical line.

cervicoenamel ridge Prominent ridge of enamel immediately near the cervical line on the crown of a tooth.

cervix Constricted structure; the narrow region at the junction of the crown and root of the tooth.

circumvallate papillae Large V-shaped row of papillae lying on the posterior dorsum of the tongue. Also called *vallate papillae.*

class I occlusal relationship Normal relationship between maxillary and mandibular molars.

class II occlusal relationship Relationship in which a mandibular molar is posterior to its normal position.

class III occlusal relationship Relationship in which a mandibular molar is anterior to its normal position.

cleft lip Gap in the upper lip that occurs during development.

cleft palate Lack of joining together of the hard or soft palates.

clinical crown Part of the tooth protruding from the gingiva.

clinical root Part of the tooth embedded in the gingiva and socket.

concavity Depression in a surface.

congenital Occurring at or before birth; may or may not be hereditary.

contact area Area of contact of one tooth with another in the same arch.

contact point Specific point at which a tooth from one arch occludes with another tooth from the opposing arch.

cross-bite Condition in which the cusps of a tooth in one arch exceed the cusps of a tooth in the opposing arch, buccally or lingually.

cross-section Cutting through a tooth perpendicular to the long axis.

crown Part of the tooth that is covered with enamel.

cusp Major pointed or rounded eminence on or near the occlusal surface of a tooth.

cusp of Carabelli Fifth lobe of a maxillary first molar.

cyst Sac of fluid lined by epithelium that may grow to varying sizes.

cytoplasm Fluid substance of cells.

débrided To have accomplished the removal (débridement) of nerve tissue and other debris from the pulp cavity to leave a surgically cleaned area.

deciduous That which will be shed; specifically, the first dentition of humans or animals.

deglutition The action of swallowing.

dental arch All teeth in either the maxillary or mandibular jaw that form an arch.

dentin (formerly dentine) Calcified tissue that forms the inside body of a tooth, underlying the cementum and enamel and surrounding the pulpal tissue.

dentinal tubule Space in the dentin occupied by the ontoblastic process.

dentinocemental junction Location in the root where the dentin joins the cementum.

dentinoenamel junction Line marking the junction of the dentin and the enamel.

dentinogenesis imperfecta Hereditary imperfect dentin formation.

dentition General character and arrangement of the teeth, taken as a whole, as in carnivorous, herbivorous, and omnivorous dentitions. *Primary dentition* refers to the deciduous teeth, and *secondary dentition* refers to the permanent teeth. *Mixed dentition* refers to a combination of permanent and deciduous teeth in the same dentition.

depression Lowering of the mandible or opening of the mouth.

developmental depression Noticeable concavity on the formed crown or root of a tooth; occurs at the junction of two lobes, as on the mesial surface of the maxillary first premolars, or at the furcation of roots.

developmental grooves Fine depressed lines in the enamel of a tooth that mark the union of the lobes of the crown.

diastema Any spacing between teeth in the same arch.

distal Distant; farthest from the median line of the face or from the origin of a structure.

distal proximal surface Proximal surface on the posterior side of a tooth.

distal third Viewed from the facial or lingual surface, the third of the surface farthest from the midline.

distobuccal developmental groove Developmental groove that extends on the buccal surface of a lower first or third molar between the distobuccal and distal cusps.

distocclusion See *class II occlusal relationship.*

dorsum of the tongue Top surface of the tongue.

edema Swelling of tissue.

edge, incisal See *incisal edge.*

embrasure Open space between the proximal surfaces of two teeth where they diverge buccally, labially, or lingually and occlusally from the contact area.

enamel Hard calcified tissue that covers the dentin of the crown portion of a tooth.

enamel dysplasia Abnormalities of enamel growth.

enamel hypocalcification Enamel that is not as dense as regular enamel.

enamel hypoplasia Enamel that is thin or pitted.

endocrine Gland or type of secretion that is carried away from the producing cells by blood vessels; the secretion is used in other parts of the body to control certain functions; has no duct system.

enzyme Agent capable of producing chemical changes in processes such as the digestion of foods.

epiglottis Cartilage that helps cover the laryngeal opening.

epinephrine Substance produced by the body or synthetically produced that causes many reactions; in dentistry, used to constrict blood flow in tissues.

epithelial Pertaining to epithelium.

epithelial attachment Substance produced by the reduced enamel epithelium that helps secure the attachment epithelium at the base of the gingival sulcus to the tooth.

epithelium Layer or layers of cells that cover the surface of the body or line the tubes or cavities inside the body; one of the four basic tissues.

equilibrium Sense of balance.

eruption Movement of the tooth as it emerges through surrounding tissue so that the clinical crown gradually appears longer.

eruptive stage Period of eruption from the completion of crown formation until the teeth come into occlusion.

exfoliation Shedding or loss of a primary tooth.

facial Term used to designate the outer surfaces of the teeth collectively (buccal or labial).

facial surface See *facial.*

facial third From a proximal view, the third of the surface closest to the facial side.

fauces Space between the left and right palatine tonsils.

FDI system The Federation Dentaire Internationale (International Dental Federation); system for tooth identification.

filiform papillae Small, pointed projections that heavily cover most of the dorsum of the anterior two thirds of the tongue.

fissure Deep cleft; developmental line fault usually found in the occlusal or buccal surface of a tooth; commonly the result of imperfect fusion of the enamel of the adjoining dental lobes.

flange Projecting edge; the edge of the denture.

fluorosis Discolored enamel resulting from excessive fluoride intake during crown development.

foliate papillae Poorly developed papillae that appear as small vertical folds in the posterior part of the sides of the tongue.

foramen Short circular opening through a bone.

fossa Round, wide, relatively shallow depression in the surface of a tooth as seen commonly in the lingual surfaces of the maxillary incisors or between the cusps of molars; also a shallow depression in bone.

free gingiva Gingiva that forms the gingival sulcus.

frenulum Little frenum or fold of tissue.

frontal sinus Air sinus in frontal bone above the eye that opens into the hiatus semilunaris in the middle meatus.

fungiform papillae Small circular papillae scattered throughout the anterior two thirds of the dorsum of the tongue.

fusion Two teeth that fuse at their dentin while developing.

gingiva Part of the gum tissue that immediately surrounds the teeth and alveolar bone.

gingival crest Most occlusal or incisal extent of the gingiva.

gingival crevice Subgingival space that, under normal conditions, lies between the gingival crest and the epithelial attachment.

gingival papillae Portion of the gingiva found between the teeth in the interproximal spaces gingival to the contact area; also called *interdental papillae.*

gingival sulcus Space between the free gingiva and the tooth surface.

gingivitis Inflammation involving the gingival tissues only.

hematoma Escape of blood from injured blood vessel into tissue spaces.

hemoglobin Component of red blood cells that carries oxygen.

hereditary Inherited through the genes of parents or grandparents.

immunity Body's resistance to certain organisms or diseases.

impacted Teeth that are not completely erupted and are fully or partly covered by bone or soft tissue.

incisal edge Edge formed at the labioincisal line angle of an anterior tooth after an incisal ridge has worn down.

incisal ridge Rounded ridge form of the incisal portion of an anterior tooth.

From Brand RW, Isselhard DE: *Anatomy of orofacial structures,* ed 7, St Louis, 2003, Mosby.

incisal third From a proximal, lingual, or labial view of an anterior tooth, the third of the surface closest to the incisal edge.

incisive papilla Small, rounded, oblong mound of tissue directly behind or lingual to the maxillary central incisors and lying over the incisive foramen.

incisors The four center teeth in either arch; essential for cutting.

inflammatory reaction Body's mechanism to combat harmful organisms by bringing more plasma and blood cells to the injured area.

inherited Passed on from parents or grandparents.

interdental Located between the teeth.

interdental papilla Projection of gingiva between the teeth.

interproximal Between the proximal surfaces of adjoining teeth in the same arch.

interproximal space Triangular space between adjoining teeth; the proximal surfaces of the teeth form the sides of the triangle; the alveolar bone, the base, and the contact area of the teeth form the apex.

labia Latin word for lips; singular, *labium*.

labial Of or pertaining to the lips; toward the lips.

labial frenum Fold of tissue that attaches the lip to the labial mucosa at the midline of the lips.

larynx Voice box; the trachea begins just below it.

lingual Pertaining to or affecting the tongue; next to or toward the tongue.

lingual frenum Fold of tissue that attaches the undersurface of the tongue to the floor of the mouth.

lingual glands Minor salivary glands of the tongue.

lingual groove Developmental groove on the lingual side of the tooth.

lingual surface See *lingual*.

lingual third From a proximal view, the third of the surface closest to the lingual side.

macrodontia Condition in which the teeth are too large for the jaw.

malocclusion Abnormal occlusion of the teeth.

mamelon One of the three rounded protuberances of the incisal surface of a newly erupted incisor tooth.

mandible Lower jaw.

mandibular Pertaining to the lower jaw.

mandibular arch First pharyngeal arch that forms the area of the mandible and maxilla; the lower dental arch.

mandibular condyle Rounded top of the mandible that articulates with the mandibular fossa.

mandibular foramen Opening on the medial surface of the ramus of the mandible for entrance of nerves and blood vessels to the lower teeth.

mandibular process Portion of the mandibular pharyngeal arch that forms the mandible.

mandibular tori Bony growths on the lingual cortical plate of bone opposite the mandibular canines.

marginal ridge Ridge or elevation of enamel forming the margin of the surface of a tooth; specifically, at the mesial and distal margins of the occlusal surfaces of premolars and molars, and the mesial and distal margins of the lingual surfaces of incisors and canines.

mastication Act of chewing or grinding.

maxilla Paired main bone of the upper jaw.

maxillary Pertaining to the upper arch.

maxillary arch Upper dental arch.

maxillary sinus Largest of the paired paranasal sinuses, located in the maxilla.

maxillary tuberosity Bulging posterior surface of the maxilla behind the third molar region.

median line Vertical (central) line that divides the body into right and left; the median line of the face.

mesial Toward or situated in the middle; for example, toward the midline of the dental arch.

mesial drift Phenomenon of permanent molars continuing to move mesially after eruption.

mesial third From a facial or a lingual view, the third of the surface closest to the midline.

microdontia Condition in which the teeth are too small for the jaw.

mixed dentition State of having primary and permanent teeth in the dental arches at the same time.

molars Large posterior teeth used for grinding.

mucosa Moist epithelial linings of the oral cavity and the respiratory and digestive systems.

mucous Pertaining to mucus, the thick viscous secretion of a gland.

mulberry molars Molars with multiple cusps that are caused by congenital syphilis.

multiple root Root with more than one branch.

muscle One of the four basic tissues; has the property of contraction or shortening of the fibers, which accomplishes work. The three types of muscle are skeletal, cardiac, and smooth muscle.

nasal septum Wall between the left and right sides of the nasal cavity, made up of the ethmoid and vomer bones.

nervous tissue One of the four basic tissues. Groups of cells (neurons) carry messages to and from the brain and perform many other tasks.

neuron Nerve cell.

nonsuccedaneous Permanent teeth that do not succeed or replace deciduous teeth.

occluding Contacting opposing teeth.

occlusal Articulating or biting surface.

occlusal plane Side view of the occlusal surfaces.

occlusal relationship Way in which the maxillary and mandibular teeth touch each other.

occlusal third From a proximal, lingual, or buccal view of a posterior tooth, the third of the surface closest to the occlusal surface.

occlusal trauma Injury brought about by one tooth prematurely hitting another during closure of the jaws.

occlusion Relationship of the mandibular and maxillary teeth when closed or during excursive movements of the mandible; when teeth of the mandibular arch come in contact with teeth of the maxillary arch in any functional relationship.

odontoma Tumor made up of enamel, dentin, cementum, and pulp.

opaque Not easily able to transmit light.

open bite Space left between the teeth when the jaws close.

open contact Space between adjacent teeth in the same arch; an interproximal opening instead of a contact area where the teeth touch.

overbite Relationship of teeth in which the incisal ridges of the maxillary anterior teeth extend below the incisal ridges of the mandibular anterior teeth when the teeth are in a centric occlusal relationship.

overhanging restoration Excess of filling material extending past the confines of the tooth preparation; an overextension of filling material.

overjet Relationship of teeth in which the incisal ridges or buccal cusp ridges of the maxillary teeth extend facially to the incisal ridges or buccal cusp ridges of the mandibular teeth when the teeth are in a centric occlusal relationship.

palatal Pertaining to the palate or roof of the mouth.

Palmer notation system System of coding teeth using brackets, numbers, and letters.

papillary gingiva Gingiva that forms the interdental papillae.

paramolar Small supernumerary tooth located buccally or lingually to a molar.

parasympathetic nervous system Part of the autonomic (automatic) nervous system that originates from some of the cranial nerves and some of the sacral nerves. It controls a number of functions, including stimulation of the salivary glands.

parathyroid gland Small gland embedded in the thyroid gland that helps control calcium metabolism in the body.

passive eruption Condition in which the tooth does not move but the gingival attachment moves farther apically.

peg-shaped lateral Poorly formed maxillary lateral incisor with a cone-shaped crown.

periapical Around the tip of the root of a tooth.

periodontal Surrounding a tooth.

periodontium Supporting tissues surrounding the teeth.

periosteum Fibrous and cellular layer that covers bones and contains cells that become osteoblasts.

periphery Circumferential boundary; outer border.

pharynx Throat area, from the nasal cavity to the larynx.

philtrum Small depression at the midline of the upper lip.

pillars Folds of tissue appearing in front of and behind the palatine tonsils.

pit Small pointed depression in dental enamel, usually at the junction of two or more developmental grooves; a small hole anywhere on the crown.

posterior Situated toward the back, as premolars and molars.

posterior pillars Folds of tissue behind the tonsil that contain the palatopharyngeus muscle.

posterior teeth Teeth of either jaw located to the rear of the incisors and canines.

pre-eruptive stage Period when the crown of the tooth is developing.

premature contact area Area in which an upper and a lower tooth touch and hit each other before the rest of the teeth occlude.

premaxilla Bony area of the upper jaw that includes the alveolar ridge for the incisors and the area immediately behind it.

premolars Permanent teeth that replace the primary molars.

primary dentin Dentin formed from the beginning of calcification until tooth eruption.

primary dentition First set of teeth; also called *baby teeth, milk teeth,* and *deciduous teeth.*

primary palate The early developing part of the hard palate that originates from the medial nasal process and forms a V-shaped wedge of tissue that runs from the incisive foramen forward and laterally between the lateral incisors and canines of the maxilla.

primary teeth See *deciduous.*

prosthetic appliance Any constructed appliance that replaces a missing part.

protrusion Condition of being thrust forward, as protrusion of the anterior teeth, referring to the teeth being too far labial; the forward movement of the mandible.

proximal Nearest, next, immediately adjacent to; distal or mesial.

proximal contact areas Proximal area of a tooth that touches an adjacent tooth on the mesial or distal side.

pulp canal Canal in the root of a tooth that leads from the apex to the pulp chamber. Contains dental pulp tissue under normal conditions.

pulp cavity Entire cavity within the tooth, including the pulp canal and pulp chamber.

pulp chamber Cavity or chamber in the center of the crown of a tooth that normally contains the major portion of the dental pulp. The pulp canals lead into the pulp chambers.

pulp, dental Highly vascular and innervated connective tissue contained within the pulp cavity of the tooth. It is composed of arteries, veins, nerves, connective tissues and cells, lymph tissue, and odontoblasts.

pulp horn (horn of pulp) Extension of pulp tissue into a thin point of the pulp chamber in the tooth crown.

pulp stones Small, dentinlike calcifications in pulp.

quadrants One fourth of the dentition. The four quadrants are divided into right, left, maxillary, and mandibular.

ramus of the mandible Vertical portion of the mandible.

recession Migration of the gingival crest in an apical direction, away from the crown of the tooth.

referred pain Pain that seems to originate in one area but originates in another.

reparative dentin Localized formation of dentin in response to local trauma, such as occlusal trauma or caries.

resorption Physiological removal of tissues or body products, as of the roots of deciduous teeth, or of some alveolar process after the loss of the permanent teeth.

retromolar pad Pad of tissue behind the mandibular third molars.

retromolar triangle Triangular area of bone just behind the mandibular third molars.

retrusion Act or process of retraction or moving back, as when the mandible is placed in posterior relationship to the maxilla.

ridge Long narrow elevation or crest, as on the surface of a tooth or bone.

root Portion of a tooth that is embedded in the alveolar process and covered with cementum.

root canal See *pulp canal.*

root planing Process of smoothing the cementum of the root of a tooth.

rugae Small ridges of tissue extending laterally across the anterior of the hard palate.

sebaceous glands Small oil-producing glands that are usually connected to and lubricate hairs.

secondary dentin Dentin formed throughout the pulp chamber and pulp canal from the time of eruption.

secondary dentition Permanent dentition.

single root Root with one main branch.

slough Loss of dead cells from the surface of tissue; pronounced *sluff.*

soft tissue Noncalcified tissue, such as nerves, arteries, veins, and connective tissue.

spasm Constant contraction of muscle.

submucosa Supporting layer of loose connective tissue under a mucous membrane.

succedaneous Permanent teeth that succeed, or take the place of, deciduous teeth after the latter have been shed; that is, the incisors, canines, and premolars.

sulcus Long V-shaped depression or valley in the surface of a tooth between the ridges and the cusps. A sulcus has a developmental groove at the apex of its V-shape. Sulcus also refers to the trough around the teeth formed by the gingiva.

supplemental groove Shallow linear groove in the enamel of a tooth. It differs from a developmental groove in that it does not mark the junction of lobes; it is a secondary, or smaller, groove.

supplemental tooth Supernumerary tooth that resembles a regular tooth.

supraeruption Eruption of a tooth beyond the occlusal plane.

taste buds Small structures in vallate, fungiform, and foliate papillae that detect taste.

temporomandibular ligament Thickened part of the temporomandibular joint (TMJ) capsule on the lateral side.

tongue-tie, tongue-tied Condition in which the lingual frenum is short and attached to the tip of the tongue, making normal speech difficult. Also called *ankyloglossia.*

tonsillor pillars Vertical folds of tissue that lie in front of and behind the palatine tonsils in the lateral throat wall.

tooth germ Soft tissue that develops into a tooth.

tooth migration Movement of the tooth through the bone and gum tissue.

torus palatinus Large bony growth in the hard palate.

transverse ridge Ridge formed by the union of two triangular ridges, traversing the surface of a posterior tooth from the buccal to the lingual side.

trauma Wound; bodily injury or damage.

trifurcation Division of three tooth roots at their point of junction with the root trunk.

Universal system, Universal Code System of coding teeth using the numbers 1 to 32 for permanent teeth and the letters *A* to *T* for deciduous teeth.

uvula Small, hanging fold of tissue in back of the soft palate.

vallate papillae See *circumvallate papillae.*

vascular Relating to blood supply.

vasoconstrictor Substance that constricts blood vessels.

vermillion zone Red part of the lip where the lip mucosa meets the skin.

vestibule Space between the lips or cheeks and the teeth.

From Brand RW, Isselhard DE: *Anatomy of orofacial structures,* ed 7, St Louis, 2003, Mosby.

Index

Note: Page numbers followed by *b,* indicate boxes; *f,* figures; *t,* tables.